DRUG METABOLISM AND DRUG TOXICITY

Drug Metabolism and Drug Toxicity

Editors

Jerry R. Mitchell, M.D., Ph.D.
Professor of Chemical Toxicology
and Internal Medicine
Baylor College of Medicine
Houston, Texas

Marjorie G. Horning, Ph.D.
Professor of Biochemistry
Baylor College of Medicine
Houston, Texas

Sponsored by the American Society for Pharmacology and Experimental Therapeutics

Raven Press ■ New York

Raven Press, 1140 Avenue of the Americas, New York, New York 10036

Made in the United States of America

Library of Congress Cataloging in Publication Data
Main entry under title:

Drug metabolism and drug toxicity.

Based on Workshop on Drug Metabolism and Drug Toxicity held Oct. 1980, at the Baylor College of Medicine.
Includes bibliographies and index.
1. Drugs—Metabolism—Congresses. 2. Drugs—Toxicology—Congresses. I. Mitchell, Jerry R. II. Horning, Marjorie G. III. American Society for Pharmacology and Experimental Therapeutics. [DNLM: 1. Drugs—Metabolism—Congresses. 2. Drugs—Toxicity—Congresses. QV 38 D7933 1980]

RM301. 55.D76 1984 615.9 83-24540
ISBN 0-89004-997-1

Preface

For many years the metabolism of drugs was equated with detoxification and inactivation. Indeed the first major monograph in the field by R. Tecwyn Williams in 1947 was titled *Detoxication Mechanisms—The Metabolism of Drugs and Allied Organic Chemicals.* Since the early 1960s, however, it has been increasingly recognized that drugs and environmental chemicals can be metabolized to toxic and/or pharmacologically active as well as inactive metabolites. This volume was initiated by the Drug Metabolism Division of the American Society for Pharmacology and Experimental Therapeutics in response to a perceived need for a textbook in drug metabolism and disposition that incorporated current principles and methods for studying metabolic transformations in relation to toxicology.

The book has been organized into six sections. The first section discusses metabolic pathways; that is, specific enzymes or enzyme complexes that are responsible for the metabolism of drugs and environmental chemicals. The first chapter presents a status report on the cytochrome-P_{450} complex. The oxygenation of organic nitrogen and sulfur compounds and halogenated hydrocarbons as well as the role of activated oxygen in chemical toxicity are discussed in the following chapters.

The second section is concerned with metabolism and toxicity at the cellular and organ level. Studies on the metabolic pathways involved in toxicity in isolated mammalian cells are presented in the chapter by Smith and Orrenius. In the following chapter by Bend, the role of tissues and more specifically the role of certain types of cells in these extrahepatic tissues in chemically mediated toxicity is discussed.

Although drug metabolism and drug toxicity can be directed or moderated by enzymic reaction and cellular responses, environmental and genetic factors also are important. The influence of genetic factors and the use of recombinant DNA technology to define genetic differences in drug metabolizing enzymes is discussed by Nebert.

The relationship of metabolism to toxicity and carcinogenicity is discussed in section three. The importance of DNA repair in preventing toxicity in human cells is reviewed by McCormick. Thorgeirsson discusses the importance of several metabolic pathways in converting the aromatic amides into carcinogenic or inactive metabolites.

The fourth section consists of three chapters (Benet, Wilkinson, and Gillette) that discuss quantitative approaches which help to define the relationship between drug metabolism and drug toxicity. The basic principles of pharmacokinetics are reviewed by Benet; the problems involved in applying these principles in studies of toxicity in whole animals and man are discussed by Wilkinson and Gillette.

The pathophysiological mechanisms by which reactive metabolites interact with cells and cell constituents are discussed in section five. Trump and colleagues review current concepts about the role of sodium and calcium regulation in the pathogenesis of lethal injury in cell culture studies. They categorize the major mechanisms resulting in lethal cell injury and discuss their possible extrapolation to lethal injury from chemically reactive metabolites. Mitchell and colleagues focus on the chemical nature of individual reactive metabolites; they critique the relative importance of alkylation and peroxidation reactions with tissue macromolecules, the validity of the current data base and conclusions drawn, and known pathophysiological interactions with glutathione and calcium. Lauterburg and colleagues conclude the section with a review of the dynamic regulation of glutathione homeostasis *in vivo.* They examine current opinions about glutathione compartments in the liver, about excretion of glutathione disulfide into blood, about the role of the liver in exporting glutathione, and about the extrapolation of data obtained *in vitro* to the dynamic state that exists *in vivo*.

The last section is concerned with methods for the isolation, separation, quantitation, and identification of metabolites. Perfused organs provide a simple model for studying the relationship of pharmacokinetic parameters of metabolism to drug toxicity. The methodology and applications of perfusion techniques in toxicity studies are described by Pang. Procedures for profiling drug metabolites by high pressure liquid chromatography and gas chromatography, as well as the information that can be obtained from these profiles are discussed by M. G. Horning and colleagues. The final chapter by E. C. Horning and colleagues discusses the identification of metabolites by mass spectrometric analysis. The many recent developments that have made the identification of polar, nonvolatile, and high molecular weight compounds possible are reviewed.

The intent of the editors in compiling this book was to document the role of drug metabolism in various toxic responses (mutagenicity, carcinogenicity, cytotoxicity, cell death) that may follow drug administration or chemical exposure. Considerable progress has been made in understanding the mechanisms by which metabolites can elicit a toxic response. However, information in this interdisciplinary field can only be described as fragmentary. It is hoped that the experimental approaches for investigating toxicity that are described in this book will be helpful both to graduate students and established investigators in pulling together important information and concepts from the different disciplines. For this reason the book is selective in its approach rather than comprehensive, with emphasis placed particularly on several topics either not reviewed adequately elsewhere or reviewed in the literature of disciplines not commonly followed by most pharmacologists, toxicologists, and biochemists. We also hope that the book will stimulate readers to develop new ideas and experimental approaches for solving many of the fascinating and important problems that drug toxicity presents.

Contents

Metabolic Pathways

Contributors

M. W. Anders, *Department of Pharmacology, University of Rochester, 601 Elmwood Avenue, Rochester, New York 14642*

John R. Bend, *Laboratory of Pharmacology, National Institute of Environmental Health Sciences, National Institutes of Health, P.O. Box 12233, Research Triangle Park, North Carolina 27709*

Leslie Z. Benet, *Department of Pharmacy, University of California, San Francisco, California 94143*

Irene K. Berezesky, *Department of Pathology, University of Maryland School of Medicine, 10 South Pine Street, Baltimore, Maryland 21201*

James S. Bus, *Chemical Industry Institute of Toxicology, P.O. Box 12137, Research Triangle Park, North Carolina 27709*

D. I. Carroll, *Department of Medicine and Institute for Lipid Research, Baylor College of Medicine, Houston, Texas 77030*

G. B. Corcoran, *Department of Medicine and Institute for Lipid Research, Baylor College of Medicine, Houston, Texas 77030*

Ronald W. Estabrook, *Department of Biochemistry, University of Texas Health Science Center, 5323 Harry Hines Boulevard, Dallas, Texas 75235*

James E. Gibson, *Chemical Industry Institute of Toxicology, P.O. Box 12137, Research Triangle Park, North Carolina 27709*

James R. Gillette, *Laboratory of Chemical Pharmacology, National Heart, Lung, and Blood Institute, National Institutes of Health, Bethesda, Maryland 20205*

Irene B. Glowinski, *Laboratory of Carcinogen Metabolism, Division of Cancer Cause and Prevention, National Cancer Institute, National Institutes of Health, Bethesda, Maryland 20205*

Evan C. Horning, *Institute for Lipid Research, Baylor College of Medicine, Houston, Texas 77030*

Marjorie G. Horning, *Institute for Lipid Research, Baylor College of Medicine, Houston, Texas 77030*

H. Hughes, *Department of Medicine and Institute for Lipid Research, Baylor College of Medicine, Houston, Texas 77030*

Khingkan Lertratanangkoon, *Institute for Lipid Research, Baylor College of Medicine, Houston, Texas 77030*

Bernhard M. Lauterburg, *Department of Medicine and Institute for Lipid Research, Baylor College of Medicine, Houston, Texas 77030*

Veronica M. Maher, *Department of Biochemistry, Michigan State University, East Lansing, Michigan 48824*

J. Justin McCormick, *Carcinogenesis Laboratory, Michigan State University, Fee Hall, East Lansing, Michigan 48824*

Michael E. McManus, *Laboratory of Carcinogen Metabolism, Division of Cancer Cause and Prevention, National Cancer Institute, National Institutes of Health, Bethesda, Maryland 20205*

Jerry R. Mitchell, *Department of Medicine and Institute for Lipid Research, Baylor College of Medicine, Houston, Texas 77030*

Daniel W. Nebert, *Laboratory of Developmental Pharmacology, National Institute of Child Health and Human Development, National Institutes of Health, Bethesda, Maryland 20205*

Masahiko Negishi, *Laboratory of Developmental Pharmacology, National Institute of Child Health and Human Development, National Institutes of Health, Bethesda, Maryland 20205*

J. G. Nowlin, *Department of Medicine and Institute for Lipid Research, Baylor College of Medicine, Houston, Texas 77030*

Sten Orrenius, *Department of Forensic Medicine, Karolinska Institutet, S-104 01 Stockholm, Sweden*

K. Sandy Pang, *Faculty of Pharmacy, University of Toronto, 19 Russel Street, Toronto, Ontario M5S 1A1, Canada*

Long-Sheng Sheng, *Institute for Lipid Research, Baylor College of Medicine, Houston, Texas 77030*

Cosette J. Serabjit-Singh, *Laboratory of Pharmacology, National Institute of Environmental Health Sciences, National Institutes of Health, P.O. Box 12233, Research Triangle Park, North Carolina 27709*

Charles V. Smith, *Department of Medicine and Institute for Lipid Research, Baylor College of Medicine, Houston, Texas 77030*

Martyn T. Smith, *Department of Forensic Medicine, Karolinska Institutet, S-104 01 Stockholm, Sweden*

R. N. Stillwell, *Department of Medicine and Institute for Lipid Research, Baylor College of Medicine, Houston, Texas 77030*

Snorri S. Thorgeirsson, *Laboratory of Carcinogen Metabolism, Division of Cancer Cause and Prevention, National Cancer Institute, National Institutes of Health, Bethesda, Maryland 20205*

Benjamin F. Trump, *Department of Pathology, University of Maryland School of Medicine, 10 South Pine Street, Baltimore, Maryland 21201*

Grant R. Wilkinson, *Department of Pharmacology, Vanderbilt University, Nashville, Tennessee 37232*

D. M. Ziegler, *Clayton Foundation Biochemical Institute and Department of Chemistry, The University of Texas at Austin, Austin, Texas 78712*

DRUG METABOLISM AND DRUG TOXICITY

Drug Metabolism and Drug Toxicity,
edited by J. R. Mitchell and M. G. Horning.
Raven Press, New York © 1984.

Cytochrome P-450 and Oxygenation Reactions: A Status Report

Ronald W. Estabrook

Department of Biochemistry, University of Texas Health Science Center, Dallas, Texas 75235

Oxygen is the key to the survival of life as we know it. The suitability of oxygen to play this unique role in biological and chemical reactions has been eloquently discussed by P. George (25). Molecular oxygen, a gas, is a diradical of relatively low reactivity. However, it can serve as an electron acceptor, wherein it progressively undergoes reduction to the protonated four-electron reduced product, water. During the course of this stepwise reduction (Fig. 1), there is sequential formation of the free radical, the superoxide anion (or its protonated form, the perhydroxyl radical), hydrogen peroxide, and the hydroxyl radical. In addition, oxygen at its two-electron reduced state, in the presence of a metal ion, can give rise to an electrophilic atom of oxygen containing six electrons—the so-called oxenoid species of oxygen (33).

Considerable interest has focused on the reactivity of these intermediary states of oxygen reduction, in particular, the oxenoid species and the hydroxyl radical, in regard to possible mechanisms for oxygenase reactions. Indeed, the shared characteristic of monooxygenase reactions is the "activation of oxygen"; therefore, a better understanding of the reactions of oxygen will be a necessary framework on which to construct the complex chemistry associated with these biologically important reactions.

REACTIONS OF OXYGEN IN BIOLOGICAL SYSTEMS

The diversity of reactions in which oxygen participates is extensive. Central to higher organisms is the need for the transport of oxygen from the lungs to the tissues where oxygen is utilized. An elegant series of reactions involving the reduced hemeprotein, hemoglobin, have been a topic for investigation since the beginnings of biochemistry. Today we have detailed knowledge of the chemistry of this "oxygen transferase" and its companion hemeprotein, myoglobin. Much of what we know about the chemistry of oxygen reactions with other cellular hemeproteins is based on these fundamental studies with hemoglobin.

When oxygen is presented to a cell that is active in metabolism, it can undergo a number of fates. Most prominent is the reduction of oxygen to water by the mitochondrial enzyme, cytochrome *c* oxidase. The critical role that the mitochondrial electron transport system plays in the generation of cellular energy (ATP) dictates the avidity of this enzyme system for the limited amount of oxygen available to the cell. Indeed, it has been estimated that over 90% of the oxygen utilization by life on this planet occurs as a result of the action of cytochrome oxidase (66). Despite

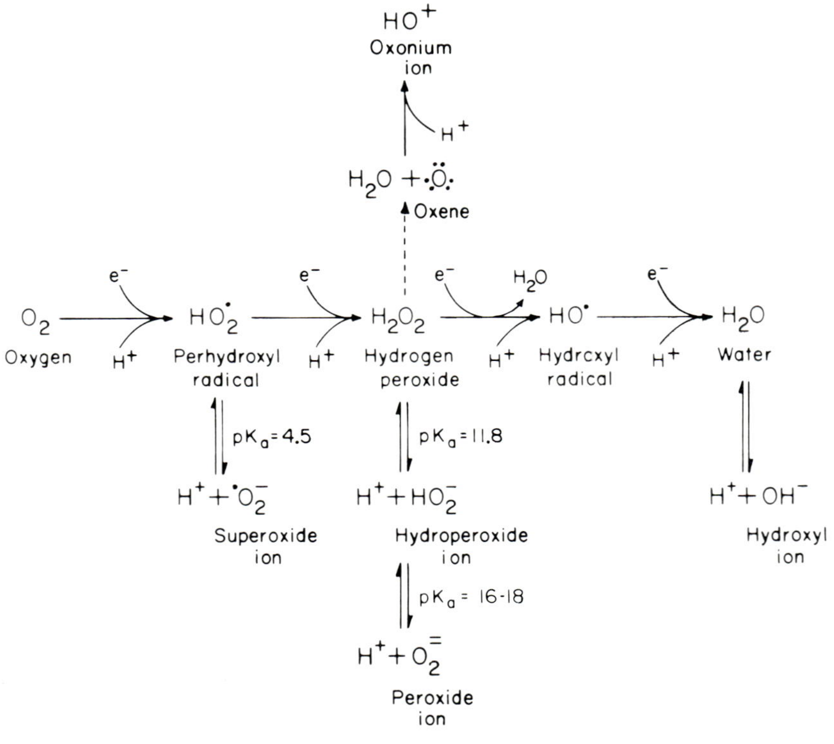

FIG. 1. Steps in the sequential reduction of oxygen.

major efforts to better understand the reactions of molecular oxygen with this hemeprotein–copper complex, our knowledge is still rudimentary, and only recently have some of the intermediates of oxygen reduction been observed during electron transport associated with the reaction of cytochrome oxidase and oxygen (8).

Other reactions of oxygen with enzymes in mammalian cells can involve special flavoproteins or metal-containing proteins. Generally, these catalyze the oxidation of specific substrates concomitant with the formation of hydrogen peroxide (many times with the superoxide anion as an intermediate), e.g., xanthine oxidase or *d*-gluconolactone oxidase. In recent years, however, considerable interest has turned to understanding the reaction of molecular oxygen with a class of enzymes that catalyze "oxygen fixation," i.e., oxygenases. In this case, molecular oxygen can be demonstrated to be incorporated into the substrate molecule that is oxidized (35,36). The requisite enzymes may contain a metal ion, such as iron or copper, or they may be hemeproteins. The reaction may be of the "dioxygenase" type, whereby both atoms of molecular oxygen are incorporated into the oxidized substrate, or they may be "monooxygenases" or mixed-function oxidases (49), where only one atom of molecular oxygen is found in the product, and the other atom is presumed to be simultaneously reduced to water.

A monooxygenase that has gained increasing attention during the last 20 years is the hemeprotein, cytochrome P-450. Although a relative newcomer to the inventory of cellular hemeproteins, cytochrome P-450 is now recognized to play a key role in the oxidative biotransformation of a diversity of "endogenous substrates," such as steroids and fatty acids, as well as "exogenous chemicals," including many drugs and other xenobiotics. For this reason, the reactions catalyzed by cytochrome P-450 may regulate the duration of effectiveness of many pharmacologically active agents or the rate of biotransformation of steroid hormones essential for cellular homeostasis. However, substrate oxidations catalyzed by cytochrome P-450 frequently have the undesired consequence of leading to highly reactive metabolites responsible for cellular toxicity, many times leading to the modification of the genomic information essential for maintenance of the characteristics of a cell. In this case, cell death can occur or there can be initiation of uncontrolled cell growth, as seen with many neoplasias. Thus, an understanding of those factors that regulate and control the action of cytochrome P-450 is of importance for determining the consequences when new agents are introduced for therapeutic purposes or when new chemicals are produced for use in the expansion of our standard of living.

The main theme of this chapter is a status report on our present knowledge of mammalian cytochrome P-450 with particular emphasis on the enzymes responsible for the metabolism of xenobiotics.

CYTOCHROME P-450

Properties of Cytochrome P-450

Cytochrome P-450 is a hemeprotein containing one molecule of iron–protoporphyrin IX as its prosthetic group (53,54). It is readily identified by a pronounced absorbance band at 450 nm in the Soret region of the visible spectrum when the carbon monoxide adduct of the reduced hemeprotein is formed—hence the name P-450. This property of cytochrome P-450 is attributed to the presence of a thiolate group as a ligand of the hemeprotein (39,59). The ability to observe a spectral absorbance band at 450 nm, displaced from the absorbance bands of comparable carbon monoxide complexes of other hemeproteins (55), has provided a simple and convenient method for readily determining the concentration of this hemeprotein in various tissue fractions (19).

The hemeprotein, P-450, as isolated from mammalian tissues, has a molecular weight ranging from about 48,000 to 56,000. Since cytochrome P-450 of mammalian tissues is associated with membrane structures, it has hydrophobic characteristics that require the use of detergents and stabilizing agents for its solubilization. This property of P-450 had rendered it refractory to isolation and purification for many years, since it is readily denatured to a protein hemochromogen called P-420 (54). In the last 10 years, great advances have been made in establishing procedures for the purification of a number of different cytochromes P-450 from mammalian tissues (10).

One can classify the cytochromes P-450 into two general categories, as shown in Fig. 2. Class A represents the types of P-450 that require an FAD-containing flavoprotein and an iron–sulfur protein for electron transport from reduced pyridine nucleotide (NADPH) to the hemeprotein (20). This class of P-450 is most frequently found associated with the mitochondria of steroid-metabolizing tissues and also is typical of the P-450s associated with bacteria (30,61). The P-450s of class A are usually involved in the metabolism of endogenous compounds such as cholesterol, deoxycorticosterone, or cholecalciferol and generally possess a high degree of substrate specificity. The class B types of cytochromes P-450 require an unusual type of flavopro-

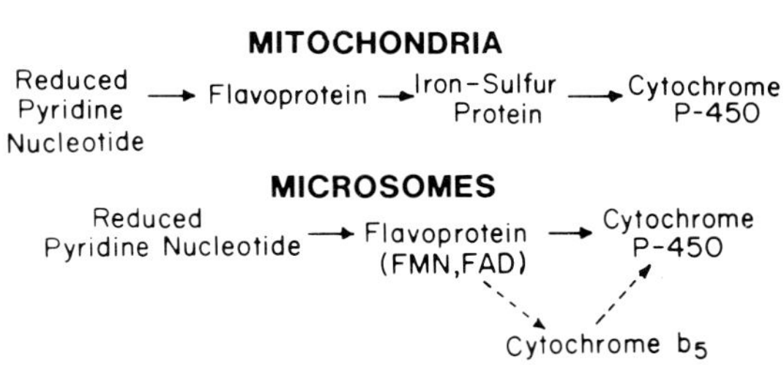

FIG. 2. Two general categories of cytochrome P-450. The specific reduced pyridine nucleotide interacting flavoproteins required for the transfer of electrons are designated, and the role of the iron–sulfur protein is indicated.

tein, which contains both FAD and FMN as prosthetic groups (43,75,77), for the transfer of reducing equivalents from reduced pyridine nucleotide to the hemeprotein. In general, this class of P-450s is found associated with the microsomal fraction of tissue homogenates in close association with another hemeprotein, termed cytochrome b_5. Recent studies have also demonstrated the presence of a similar type of P-450 associated with the nucleus of some tissues (6). Although cytochrome P-450 is widely distributed in nature, most studies for the isolation and purification of the pigment have been carried out using tissues such as the liver or adrenal, principally because of the high concentration of the hemeprotein in these tissues.

Concentration of Cytochrome P-450

In the liver of a rat or rabbit, the concentration of cytochrome P-450 is about 30 to 40 nmole per gram wet weight of tissue, i.e., the equivalent of 30 to 40 μM (17). Following treatment of animals with chemicals known to induce P-450 (see below), the concentration of cellular P-450 can increase three- to fourfold, attaining levels in excess of 0.1 mM. Thus, cytochrome P-450 is the major intracellular pigment of organs such as the liver, frequently approaching the concentration of myoglobin seen in tissues such as heart and muscle. In a tissue such as liver, the vast majority of the P-450 is associated with the endoplasmic reticulum, and it can be readily separated from other cellular organelles by differential centrifugation of the "microsomal fraction." This is in contrast to the intracellular distribution of P-450 in a tissue such as the adrenal cortex. In this case, approximately 75% of the P-450s are localized in the mitochondrion.

In the microsomal fraction of the livers of untreated rodents, the concentration of cytochrome P-450 is about 0.6 to 1.0 nmole per milligram of microsomal protein. Following treatment of the animal with a drug such as phenobarbital, this concentration can increase to as much as 5 nmole of P-450 per milligram of microsomal protein. In the latter case, it can be calculated that the hemeprotein, P-450, represents as much as 25% of the protein of the endoplasmic reticulum. Indeed, it is fair to say that P-450 is a major contributor to the structure of these membranes in liver tissue.

Induction of Cytochrome P-450

Shortly after the discovery of the role of cytochrome P-450 in the oxidative transformation of many drugs and steroids (11,16), Remmer and Merker (64) recognized that this hemeprotein may be responsible for the development of the drug tolerance seen following repeated treatment of animals with various barbiturates. Today we know that the intracellular concentration of cytochrome P-450 can easily be perturbed by a wide variety of agents, including diet, drug, or other xenobiotic treatment of the animal and events that modify the pattern of heme biosynthesis or degradation.

An example of the response of P-450 of liver to treatment of rats with phenobarbital is shown in Fig. 3. In this case, the concentration of cytochrome P-450 was determined spectrophotometrically in both a homogenate of liver and the microsomal fraction following daily treatment of animals by the intraperitoneal injection of the drug. It should be noted that the concentration of P-450 starts increasing within a short time following initiation of treatment and that repeated injections of phenobarbital continue the onset of increased synthesis of P-450 until intracellular levels four- to fivefold higher than that seen in the untreated animal are obtained (also see above). This property of enhanced enzyme synthesis has served as a convenient method for the enrichment of the tissue concentration of P-450 for subsequent studies on the isolation and purification of the various types of the hemeprotein (63).

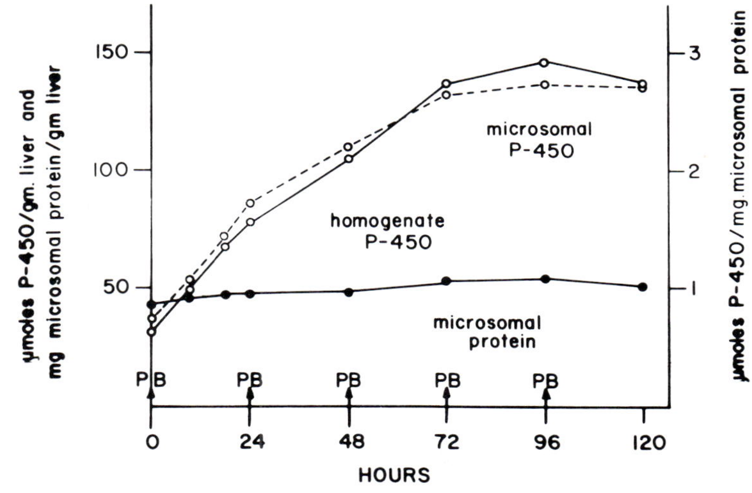

FIG. 3. Changes in the concentration of cytochrome P-450 of liver following repeated treatment of rats by the daily intraperitoneal injection of phenobarbital.

Multiplicity of P-450s

The term P-450 is the generic name for a family of hemeproteins that can be identified by differences in their physical and immunoreactive properties. The number of known isozymes of P-450 continues to grow as more refined means of recognition of unique proteins are developed.

Early studies to examine the response of animals to different "inducing agents" suggested the presence of more than one enzyme responsible for the metabolism of the many different types of compounds oxidatively transformed by cytochrome P-450 (9). That this implied different P-450s was initially confirmed by spectrophotometric studies in which differences in the reaction of carbon monoxide or ethyl isocyanide with the hemeprotein were noted (1,37,48). As shown in Fig. 4, difference spectra of the CO-reactive hemeproteins present in liver microsomes from animals pretreated with either phenobarbital or 3-methylcholanthrene show the presence of a small but measurable difference in the location of the absorbance maxima; i.e., the former is located at 450 nm, and the latter at 448 nm. For comparison,

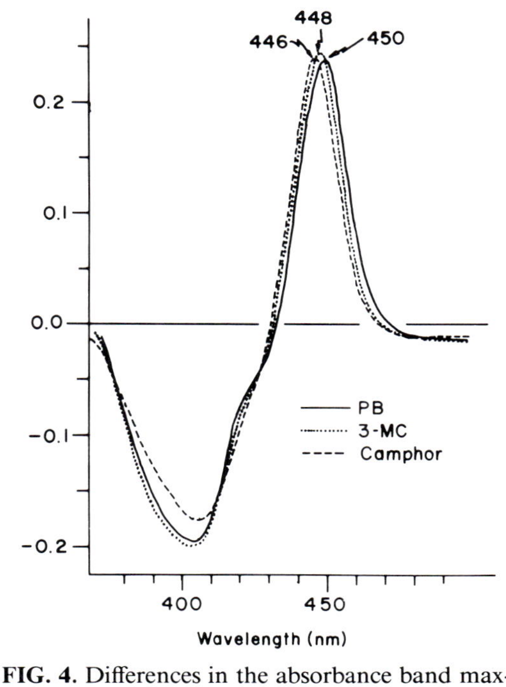

FIG. 4. Differences in the absorbance band maxima of the carbon monoxide complexes of different cytochromes P-450 as measured by difference spectrophotometry. The concentrations of cytochrome P-450 in liver microsomes from rats treated with phenobarbital or 3-methylcholanthrene have been adjusted to be equal to that of the P-450 isolated from *P. putida.*

the difference spectrum of the P-450 isolated and purified from the bacterium *Pseudomonas putida* is shown, illustrating that this P-450 has its absorbance band maximum at 446 nm.

This difference in the location of the absorbance band maxima of the CO adduct of the reduced hemeprotein, as measured by difference spectrophotometry, has been used as the basis for one type of nomenclature to distinguish different P-450s. Thus, the terminology of P-448, P-450, etc. was introduced. One must recognize, however, the imprecision of this method and the care and special instrumentation required in order to obtain meaningful results.

A second type of nomenclature, based on the inducing agent used to treat the animal, has also been used by some, e.g., $P\text{-}450_{PB}$ or $P\text{-}450_{MC}$. A third type of nomenclature has developed based on the presence of P-450s with various organs, such as $P\text{-}450_{K}$ for the pigment of kidney cortex microsomes. Further, some prefer to name P-450s based on their specific functions, such as the $P\text{-}450_{SCC}$ or $P\text{-}450_{11\beta}$, representing those hemeproteins of the adrenal cortex functional for the side chain cleavage of cholesterol or the 11-β hydroxylation of deoxycorticosterone, respectively, or $P\text{-}450_{cam}$ for the hemeprotein isolated from *P. putida* responsible for the initial step in the oxidative metabolism of camphor. At this time, no systematic method of nomenclature has yet been accepted by the workers in this area of research.

A major development in the characterization of multiple forms of P-450 occurred when the methodologies were established for the isolation and purification of the hemeproteins from their membrane environment (47,73). Application of the technique of polyacrylamide gel electrophoresis of detergent-solubilized proteins to monitor the purity of the isolated hemeproteins showed readily discernible differences in the physical properties of different P-450s (34). Following the nomenclature convention for isozymes, a more discriminating type of nomenclature for the various P-450s has developed (34). Based on their relative electrophoretic mobility on SDS gels, the P-450s are named $P\text{-}450_{LM2}$ or $P\text{-}450_{LM4}$, etc., where LM stands for the source, in this case liver microsomes, and the numeral stands for the relative position on the gel, with the lower number representing the lower-molecular-weight form. This approach has expanded our knowledge of the inventory of various P-450s from the limited few noted spectrophotometrically and permits a comparison of various P-450s isolated and purified in different laboratories.

Seen in recent years is a proliferation of studies directed to the isolation of P-450s from many different sources. This has led to the nonuniform pattern of nomenclature described above. The result has been very confusing to investigators not intimately concerned with the details of P-450 isolation and characterization. As the procedures for the purification of P-450 become more sophisticated, this problem is certain to be exacerbated; e.g., recent reports show that at least 11 distinct types of P-450 can now be isolated from the livers of untreated rabbits (2).

The ability to recognize different P-450s posed the important question of the relative concentration of each type of P-450 in a tissue and the commonality of P-450s isolated from different sources. The availability of pure proteins permitted the development of antibodies that would react preferentially with a specific type of P-450 (71). Although only a limited number of antibodies to different P-450s are now available, the power of this approach has already been demonstrated (70) for evaluating the content and composition of a tissue's inventory of different P-450s (Table 1). The exciting possibility of developing monoclonal antibodies is now being tested (58), and this method will markedly expand the usefulness of this approach for the identity of different P-450s.

The last year has seen a surge of activity applying the techniques of molecular biology to the study of P-450. The ability to prepare unique species of cDNA that will be useful

TABLE 1. *Antibody titer of P-450 content of liver microsomes*

	Total P-450 (nmole/mg protein)	Percent of total P-450[a]			
		$P\text{-}450_a$	$P\text{-}450_b$	$P\text{-}450_c$	Unknown
Adult male					
Control	1.11	3	2	1	94
Phenobarbital	2.51	1	43	1	55
3-Methylcholanthrene	1.93	3	1	68	28
Adult female					
Control	0.89	6	1	1	92
Phenobarbital	1.72	8	43	2	47
3-Methylcholanthrene	1.38	14	1	74	11

[a] Data from the paper of Thomas et al. (72). The nomenclature for designation of specific P-450s and the use of antibodies for the quantitation of the various forms of the hemeprotein is that described by Thomas et al. (72).

as probes to evaluate the genomic content of cellular information for a specific type of P-450, supported by knowledge of the nucleotide sequence coding for any P-450, offers a major step in furthering our knowledge of the extent of and basis for the multiplicity of P-450s (5,14,24,52).

Catalytic Cycle of Cytochrome P-450

Central to our understanding of the role of cytochrome P-450 in the oxidative metabolism of many drugs and other xenobiotics is the need to know the various steps in the catalytic function of this hemeprotein. A schematic representation of our present understanding of the sequence of reactions occurring during catalysis is presented in Fig. 5 together with other electron transfer reactions of liver microsomes that might be related to the function of cytochrome P-450. These reactions may be briefly summarized as follows.

Oxidized cytochrome P-450 (designated Fe^{+3}) can react reversibly with a molecule of substrate to be metabolized (designated as R) to form the equivalent of an enzyme–substrate complex. Many factors can influence the affinity of different P-450s for different substrates and the associated equilibrium constant for this reaction.

The complex of oxidized hemeprotein and substrate can accept an electron transferred from NADPH via the flavoprotein, NADPH–cytochrome P-450 reductase (designated as fp_1).

The resultant complex of the reduced (ferrous) hemeprotein, designated by Fe^{+2}, and substrate can react with oxygen to form a ternary complex called oxycytochrome P-450. A number of isoelectronic structures for this intermediate can be written, indicating the potential for distribution of electrons with any of the three components. In the absence of oxygen and presence of carbon monoxide, the complex of reduced cytochrome P-450 and substrate can react to form the ternary complex of hemeprotein, substrate, and carbon monoxide. It is this product that is characterized spectrophotometrically by the appearance of an absorbance band at about 450 nm.

The one-electron reduced ternary complex of oxygen, substrate, and hemeprotein can then be transformed in at least three ways:

1. The molecule of oxygen associated with this complex can dissociate or be displaced, regenerating the complex of substrate and reduced hemeprotein.
2. The bound molecule of oxygen can dissociate in a form equivalent to its one-electron state of reduction (the superoxide anion), thereby reforming the complex of oxidized cytochrome P-450 with substrate. The superoxide formed in this type

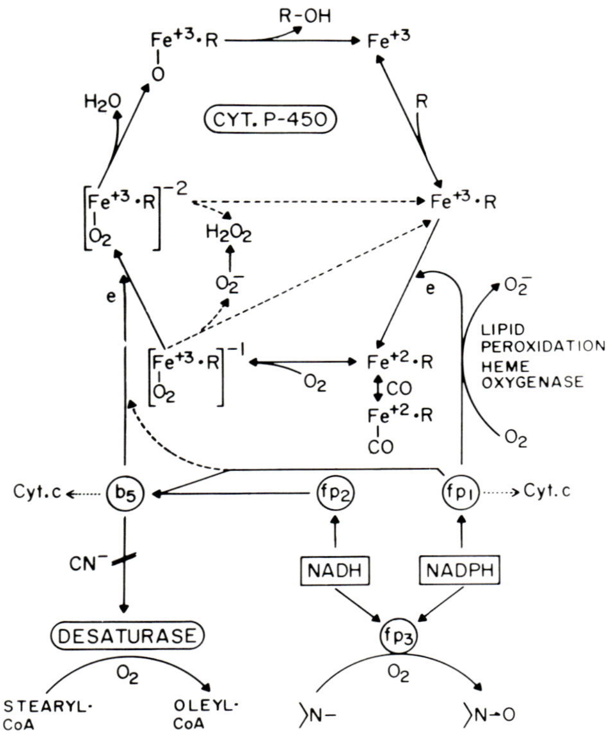

FIG. 5. The catalytic cycle of cytochrome P-450 and associated electron transfer reactions of liver microsomes.

of reaction can then dismutate (after protonation), giving rise to hydrogen peroxide. It has been suggested that this is the dominant pathway operative during the NADPH oxidase activity of liver microsomes, where hydrogen peroxide is formed concomitant with the oxidation of NADPH.

3. Oxycytochrome P-450 may accept an additional electron to form the equivalent of a two-electron reduced complex of oxygen, substrate, and hemeprotein. This intermediate has been termed peroxycytochrome P-450. The source of the electron for this reduction step is a matter of controversy. It has been proposed that reduced cytochrome b_5 can function as a suitable electron donor for this reaction. Alternatively, it has been proposed that the flavoprotein, NADPH–cytochrome P-450 reductase, because of its unique property of possessing two different flavin prosthetic groups, might better serve as the source of electrons for the reduction of oxycytochrome P-450. The possibility must also be considered that peroxycytochrome P-450 can dissociate, after protonation, to form hydrogen peroxide, although no direct experimental evidence has been reported in support of this hypothesis.

The key reactions of "oxygen activation" occur subsequent to the formation of peroxycytochrome P-450. Considerable interest now centers on these reactions. At least two possibilities can be seriously considered on the basis of present evidence:

1. It has been proposed that peroxycytochrome P-450 can be protonated, followed by removal of a molecule of water, to generate a complex of substrate and hemeprotein with an atom of oxygen that is highly electrophilic, the so-called oxenoid species of oxygen (see Fig. 1). Once

this reactive species of oxygen is formed, it is possible to envision its rapid interaction with an unsaturated bond of arenes or alkenes to form epoxides.

2. An alternate hypothesis suggests that an electron can be withdrawn from the molecule of substrate, e.g., by hydrogen abstraction, resulting in the formation of a free-radical form of the substrate and the highly reactive three-electron reduced form of oxygen, the hydroxyl radical (see Fig. 1). The process of substrate oxidation can then proceed by a radical-mediated reaction pathway.

The series of cytochrome P-450-directed reactions is concluded when the product of substrate oxidation dissociates from cytochrome P-450, thereby reforming the ferric hemeprotein. Essentially nothing is known about this reaction, although it is recognized that it may be of importance during the steady state of drug metabolism. In this way, a cycle of substrate binding, reduction, oxygenation, further reduction, rearrangement (assisted perhaps by protonation), and product dissociation accomplishes the catalytic oxidative transformation of the substrate together with the regeneration of cytochrome P-450 in a form capable of interacting with yet another molecule of substrate.

The sequence of reactions described above has most features common for all types of cytochromes P-450, regardless of source. Much of our knowledge about the chemistry of the intermediates formed has been provided by elegant studies with the soluble and purified P-450 that is readily isolated from the bacterium, *P. putida* (28,31,32). The primary differences that should be noted are that some P-450s interact with a reduced iron–sulfur protein as the donor for the needed electron whereas others require other electron transport carriers (see Fig. 2).

Associated with the function of microsomal-bound cytochrome P-450 is the operation of other oxidation–reduction reactions such as those catalyzed by the microsomal hemeprotein, cytochrome b_5, or a variety of microsomal flavoproteins. A few of these are also included in the reaction scheme presented in Fig. 5. As noted, the flavoprotein, fp_1, NADPH–cytochrome P-450 reductase, can also transfer electrons for the reduction of cytochrome b_5 or cytochrome *c*. Under special circumstances, this flavoprotein can react with molecular oxygen and a protein carrier for the degradation of heme to bile pigments (the heme oxygenase activity of microsomes). It has also been reported that this flavoprotein (in the presence of an iron chelate) can transfer electrons from NADPH to trigger the cascade of oxygen-dependent radical-mediated reactions known as lipid peroxidation (3,4,22,45).

Liver microsomes also contain a flavoprotein (fp_2) that catalyzes the transfer of reducing equivalents from NADH to cytochrome b_5 (68,69). The reduced cytochrome b_5 can then serve as an electron carrier to another protein, the fatty acid desaturase, which catalyzes the oxygen-dependent and cyanide-sensitive oxidation of various long-chain acyl coenzyme As to form unsaturated fatty acids (12,56,57). Likewise, liver microsomes frequently have an additional flavoprotein which participates in the reduced pyridine nucleotide- and oxygen-dependent transformation of some secondary and tertiary amines. This enzyme, responsible for the *N*-oxidation of a number of different compounds, has been described in detail by D. M. Ziegler (*this volume*).

SELECTED TOPICS OF CURRENT INTEREST

Substrate Binding

The hypothesis is proposed that the site of oxygen addition to a substrate molecule undergoing oxidative metabolism by the cytochrome P-450 system may be dictated by the topology of the heme-containing active site, leading to a unique spatial orientation of the substrate as it is bound to the hemeprotein. Shortly after the discovery of the function of cytochrome P-450 in the metabolism of many drugs, spectrophotometric studies revealed (40,51,65) that the addition of various substrates caused a marked change in the optical properties of the hemeprotein. Since studies at this time were restricted to an examination of optical changes occurring with the membrane-bound P-450, the method of difference spectrophotometry was applied. Although this method is very sensitive and reproducible, it can be subject to misinterpretation and the introduction of artifacts (19).

Today we recognize that oxidized cytochrome P-450 can exist in at least three interconvertible states that can be readily observed spectrophotometrically. These are illustrated in Fig. 6A. Oxidized cytochrome P-450 in the absence of a substrate is characterized by an absorbance band with a maximum at about 418 nm in the Soret re-

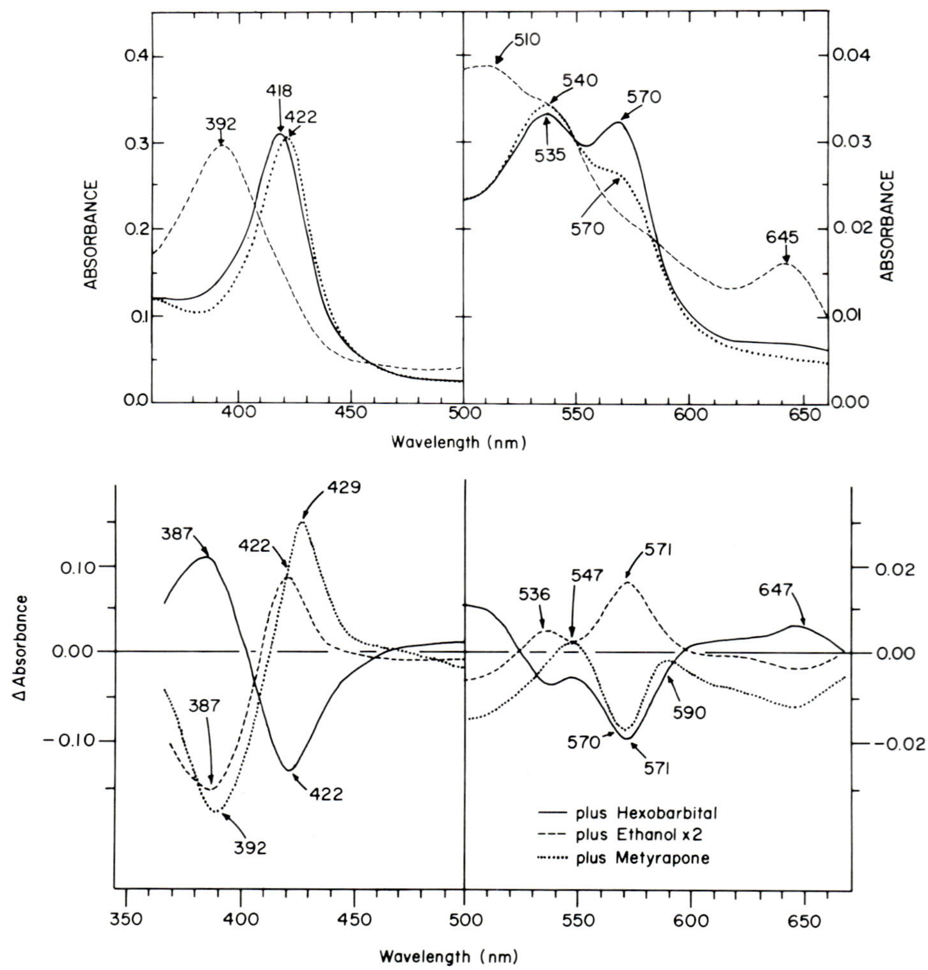

FIG. 6. Absorbance spectra of the three forms of oxidized cytochrome P-450. **A:** The absolute spectra of cytochrome P-450 isolated and purified from *P. putida.* The *dashed curve* is the spectrum obtained in the presence of excess camphor, whereas the *dotted curve* is the spectrum observed in the presence of metyrapone. **B:** Difference spectra obtained using liver microsomes from phenobarbital-treated rats. Spectral changes observed in the presence of hexobarbital, ethanol, and metyrapone are illustrated.

gion of the spectrum and two absorbance bands (535 and 570 nm) in the visible region. Addition of many substrates causes the substrate-dependent transition of this spectrum to one that has an absorbance band maximum at 392 nm together with broad absorbance at about 510 nm and a weak absorbance band at 645 nm. This spectrum is characteristic of the substrate-complexed ferric P-450 state of the hemeprotein. A third type of spectrally discernible intermediate can be formed in the presence of many nitrogen-containing aromatic compounds such as aniline, pyridine, and metyrapone. In this case, the spectrum has absorbance bands at 422, 540, and 570 nm, characteristic of a protohemochromogen. Studies have shown that either the substrate-free or the substrate-bound state of P-450 can be transformed to this hemochromogen-type intermediate (46). As mentioned above, many studies have been carried out using P-450 bound to membrane fragments, and this method necessitates the use of difference spectrophotometry. As shown in Fig. 6B, spectral differences can be measured following addition of a substrate (the so-called type 1 spectral change characterized by a loss of absorbance at about 420 nm concomitant with the appearance of an absorbance band at about 385 nm) or the addition of aromatic amines (the so-called type 2 spectral change characterized by the appearance of an absorbance band at about 430 nm and the loss of absorbance between 385 and 400 nm). In the latter case, the location of the wavelengths of absorbance change will vary depending on the relative mix of substrate-bound and substrate-free P-450 in the initial reaction system.

The fact that cytochrome P-450 exists as such a mixture is frequently overlooked by those venturing to use difference spectrophotometry to evaluate the interaction of various compounds with cytochrome P-450. An example of this is shown by the difference spectrum presented in Fig. 6B obtained following the addition of an alcohol to the liver microsomal suspension. This type of spectral change has been called the "inverse type 1" spectral change. It is undoubtedly caused by

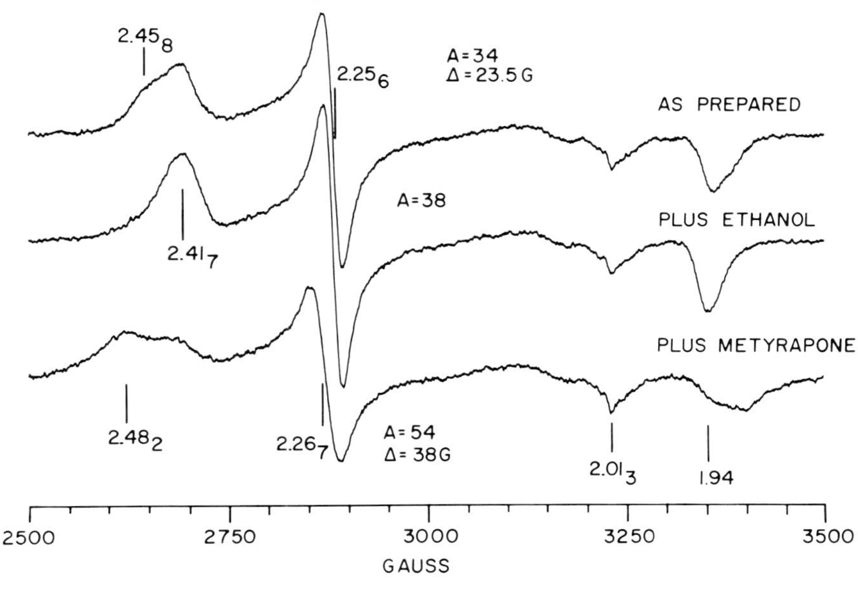

FIG. 7. The electron paramagnetic resonance spectra of liver microsomal cytochrome P-450 in the presence of ethanol and metyrapone. Spectra were recorded using a Varian E-4 EPR with the samples maintained at the temperature of liquid nitrogen.

the displacement of an "endogenous" substrate from the P-450 by the alcohol. This type of spectral change is often overlooked in difference spectrophotometry with addition of a highly lipophilic substrate that is dissolved in a solvent vehicle such as acetone or alcohol. Although many investigators add an equivalent volume of the solvent to the contents of the reference cuvette, they frequently ignore the fact that the solvent alone may cause such a spectral perturbation and thereby confuse the interpretation of the results purported to be only those of substrate interaction with cytochrome P-450. Clearly, studies of this type require both care and caution when results are interpreted.

The recognition that cytochrome P-450 is a hemeprotein has prompted studies using a variety of physical techniques (28). One method for evaluating the interaction of substrate with P-450 has been the application of electron paramagnetic resonance (EPR) spectroscopy. Indeed, shortly after the recognition that P-450 was associated with liver microsomes and was functional in the oxidative metabolism of many drugs, Mason et al. (50), while studying the pigments of liver microsomes by EPR methods, identified an oxidation–reduction component which he termed FeX. Today we know that the FeX of Mason represents the substrate-free state of ferric cytochrome P-450.

The types of EPR spectra (presented as the first-derivative spectrum) one can observe for P-450 are shown in Fig. 7. The EPR spectrum is characterized by three absorbances typical of a "low-spin" hemeprotein, i.e., a hexacoordinate planar molecule with water as one of the ligands (60). Since the EPR spectrum is an indicator of the electron density distribution within the heme molecule, studies measuring the effect of agents that perturb this environment provide evidence of the influence of various chemicals at the "active site" of P-450. Most interesting is the observation that addition of a substrate capable of causing a type 1 optical spectral change (see Fig. 6) causes a loss of the EPR signals in the $g = 2$ region concomitant with the formation of an EPR signal at about $g = 8$. The latter is indicative of the formation of a "high-spin" ferric hemeprotein—a result consistent with the optical absorbance properties of the substrate-bound state of the hemeprotein.

The observation that a spin-state change accompanies the binding of the substrate to cytochrome P-450 strongly suggests that the substrate molecule is in closed proximity to the heme moiety. The fact that this is indeed the case has been shown by results using proton nuclear magnetic relaxation methods to probe the water environment in the neighborhood of the paramagnetic heme iron (27) and by use of a spin-labeled substrate molecule (a metyrapone analog) (29). It is now considered that the substrate molecule is captured in the hydrophobic pocket of the protein where the heme resides (concomitant with the displacement of a molecule of water) and approaches the "oxygen-activation site" to within a few Angstroms, where it is in the proper spatial environment for a stereospecific interaction with oxygen.

How the molecule of substrate is oriented relative to the plane of the heme of P-450 remains an unanswered question, although interesting speculations have been proposed (15). Studies on the interaction of a variety of different steroids with liver microsomal cytochrome P-450 have suggested that a unique spatial arrangement may exist whereby the site of heme-bound oxygen interaction with the substrate may be dictated by the "immobilization" of the substrate molecule. This hypothesis was tested by constructing molecular models of the heme using a variety of different substrates known to be metabolized by cytochrome P-450 (18). When a functional group on the substrate molecule was used as a point of interaction near the carboxyl groups of the heme (possibly as a result of the formation of a metal chelate), it was striking to note that the proper site of oxygen insertion into the substrate occurred at about 6 Å from the "fulcrum of the steering group."

Although this hypothesis is highly speculative, the importance of knowing the forces that dictate the pattern of products derived during metabolism of a chemical by different P-450s requires the need to propose concepts that then can be tested. Extension of this hypothesis to a consideration of chemicals, such as benzo(a)pyrene, in which no functional groups exist, requires the need to consider other directing forces (21). It has been proposed that π–π interactions of the resonant forces of the heme and polycyclic hydrocarbon serve to orient the substrate. It is interesting that recent studies using a variety of polycyclic hydrocarbons of differing size and structure have allowed the mapping of the "minimal" size of the heme environment in which such substrate molecules may reside for metabolism (44). Clearly, more information will be needed about the geometry of substrate interactions before one can predict the relative formation of a toxic versus an innocuous metabolite during the oxidative transformation catalyzed by cytochrome P-450.

Membrane Structure

The cytochromes P-450 of mammalian tissues are associated with membrane structures, either the endoplasmic reticulum or the mitochondria. Integration of P-450 and its requisite companion electron transfer proteins into a membrane structure may impose limitations on their mode of function and interaction. In addition, since such membranes are rich in phospholipids, and most of the substrates metabolized by P-450 are highly lipophilic, considerable interest has developed on the role of membrane structure relative to the metabolism of xenobiotics. An excellent review on the chemistry and properties of the microsomal membrane has recently been published (13).

Studies to examine the topology of microsomal electron transport proteins and the potential of an organized structure within the membrane milieu have provided interesting, albeit controversial, conclusions. Early observations had noted that the flavoprotein, NADPH–cytochrome P-450 reductase (then known as NADPH–cytochrome *c* reductase) as well as cytochrome b_5 were readily released from the membrane following incubation with proteolytic enzymes. These results suggested the asymmetric location of these proteins, i.e., exclusively residing in an exposed manner on the cytosol-bathed face of the endoplasmic reticulum (42). In contrast, a large portion of the microsomal cytochrome P-450 was resistant to the action of proteolytic enzymes, suggesting that it was more deeply sequestered in the membrane. The introduction of detergents as a means of isolating proteins from membranes soon revealed that both this flavoprotein and cytochrome b_5 are amphipathic proteins of larger molecular weight than the enzymes isolated by proteolysis (41,67). It is now accepted that these electron transport proteins are anchored to the membrane surface by a hydrophobic peptide tail.

Measurements on the content of liver microsomal proteins concerned with the function of cytochrome P-450 revealed that many more molecules of cytochrome P-450 are present than of the required flavoprotein reductase. Indeed, following induction of the microsomal electron transport system by treatment of animals with an agent such as phenobarbital, ratios as high as 20 to 40 molecules of P-450 per molecule of flavoprotein were noted (17). This posed the question of how a molecule of flavoprotein services by electron transfer the large excess of hemeprotein molecules present. Two alternatives were considered. First, the fluidity characteristics of the membrane allow the free and rapid mobility of the flavoprotein, whereby it traverses the surface of the membrane by a tortuous path as it seeks and careens from one P-450 molecule to another, delivering electrons needed for P-450 function (76). A second hypothesis has been proposed (62), that places the flavoprotein in close association with its P-450s as a multiprotein complex forming patches within the membrane. These hypotheses have been tested, and results have been presented in support of each, although a composite probably represents the actual situation, i.e., the transient formation of aggregates during the steady state of electron transport. A diagrammatic representation of the "organized complex" hypothesis in which the microsomal electron transport proteins appear as islands of flavoprotein surrounded by a periphery of P-450 molecules on the surface of the membrane is presented in Fig. 8. Some of the experimental evidence that serves as the foundation for the "limited mobility" model is as follows:

1. The unique temperature dependence for the enzymatic reduction of the membrane-bound cytochrome P-450 (62).
2. The apparent correlation of the magnitude of the biphasic kinetic characteristics of P-450 reduction with the existence of molecules of P-450 in close proximity to the flavoprotein with other molecules of P-450 further removed from this central core.
3. The limited ability to reduce the pool of cytochrome P-450 molecules when an inhibitor of the flavoprotein, such as the mercurial mersalyl, is present in the reaction mixture (23).

More recently, attention has been directed toward a better understanding of those factors that influence the interaction of a molecule of flavoprotein with a molecule of cytochrome P-450. It appears that the salt

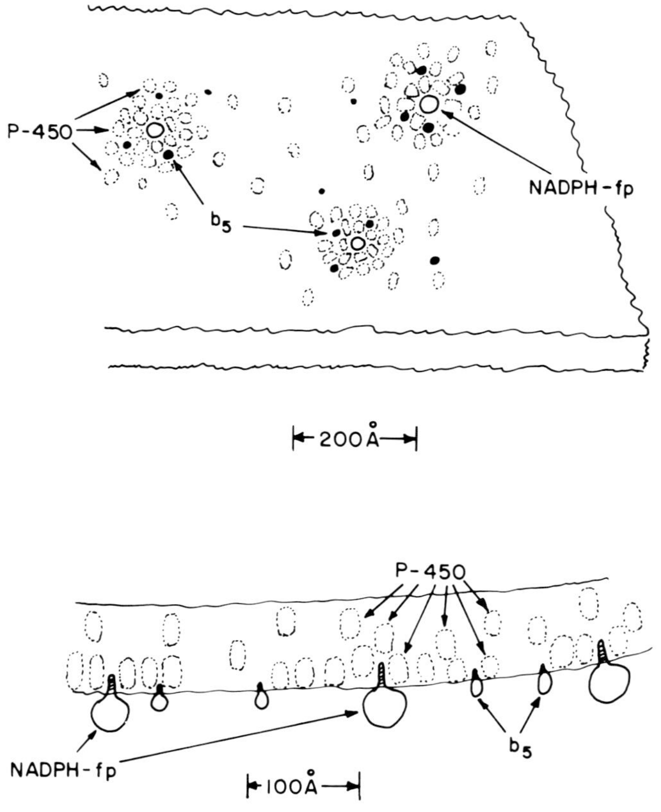

FIG. 8. A schematic representation of the organization of proteins associated with the endoplasmic reticulum of a liver cell. The **upper drawing** represents a visualization of the surface of the endoplasmic reticulum facing the cytosol of the cell. The **bottom drawing** represents a cross section through the membrane.

concentration in the reaction mixture is a major determinant. As shown in Fig. 9A, increasing concentrations of potassium chloride in the reaction mixture significantly stimulate the NADPH-dependent rate of the liver microsomal-dependent oxidation of ethylmorphine. Parallel studies to measure the kinetics of cytochrome P-450 reduction (Fig. 9B) show that the rate of electron transfer to the hemeprotein is significantly greater at high salt concentrations. These types of experiments suggest that the interaction of the flavoprotein with the hemeprotein is markedly influenced by ionic strength in such a manner that the limited number of flavoprotein molecules can dissociate more rapidly when initially captured by a P-450 desirous of its electron; i.e., their charge is modified at high salt concentrations.

Clearly, much more has to be learned about the role of the membrane and the associated topology of the enzymes in attenuating the reactions of cytochrome P-450. The need to know what controls P-450 during the metabolism of drugs and other xenobiotics is central to our knowledge of the pharmacologic effectiveness of a drug regimen. Current enthusiasm for studying the enzymatic properties of the isolated and purified flavoprotein and hemeprotein components of the microsomal electron transport system should not permit us to forget that the natural environment for this enzyme system is the milieu of the membrane and that

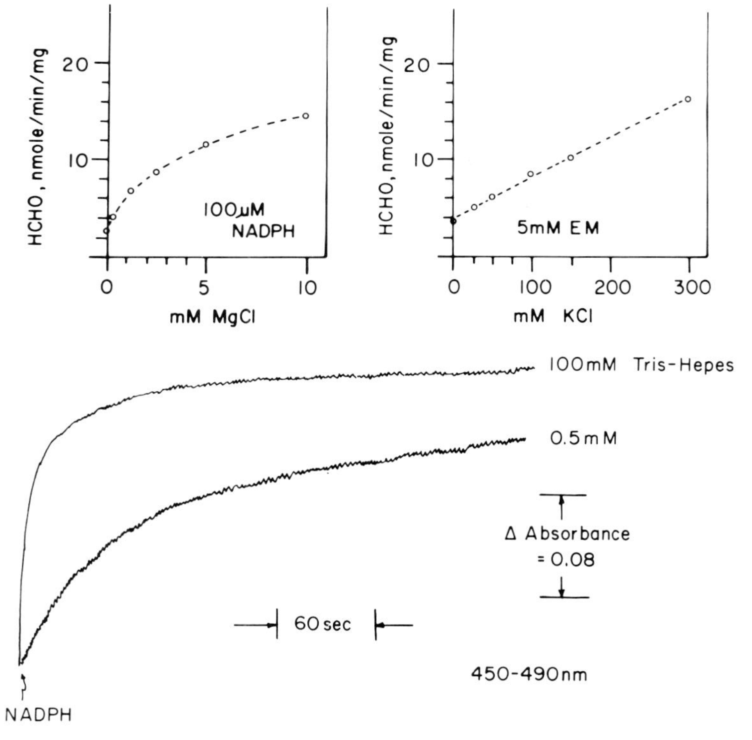

FIG. 9. The influence of salt concentration on the function of cytochrome P-450 in the metabolism of ethylmorphine and in the kinetics of reduction of the microsomal bound cytochrome P-450. **A:** The effect of varying concentrations of $MgCl_2$ and KCl on the rate of formaldehyde formation during the oxidative metabolism of ethylmorphine. **B:** The rate of reduction of microsomal cytochrome P-450 as determined using a stopped-flow apparatus in the presence of excess NADPH and carbon monoxide.

agents that perturb the composition and properties of the membrane may have a profound influence on the overall rate of drug metabolism.

P-450 as an Oxidase and/or Peroxidase (Peroxygenase)

The early observation (26) that hydrogen peroxide is produced during NADPH oxidation as catalyzed by liver microsomes, the so-called NADPH oxidase activity, has often been confirmed in recent years (38). The mechanism by which hydrogen peroxide is formed remains to be firmly established, although present evidence favors formation via a dismutation of the superoxide radical resulting from the decomposition of the one-electron reduced oxygen intermediate of P-450, oxycytochrome P-450. Although hydrogen peroxide may also be formed from the protonation of the two-electron reduced complex, peroxycytochrome P-450, no evidence has yet been presented to support this hypothesis. In both instances, the cycle of cytochrome P-450 function is abbreviated and functions as an energy dissipative pathway without the completion of the oxygenative metabolism of the substrate. Occasional reports also point to the possibility of hydrogen peroxide arising from the oxidation of the flavoprotein, NADPH–cytochrome P-450 reductase, or reduced cytochrome P-450. Although these reactions can be shown to occur, their rates are so small that they must be considered only minor contributors to the total amount of hydrogen peroxide formed.

It is of interest that some reports indicate that cytochrome P-450, after removal from the membrane environment for purification, has an enhanced rate of formation of hydrogen peroxide, suggesting that the integrity of the oxygen binding site on the heme may be less protected in the isolated hemeprotein. Also, a number of studies have shown the ability of some substrates to significantly enhance the rate of hydrogen peroxide formation, i.e., the uncoupler action of some substrates. Current studies (7) suggest that this finding may result in part from the role of oxycytochrome P-450 in hydrogen abstraction reactions.

A significant advancement for the understanding of cytochrome P-450 activity occurred when it was determined that many substrates could undergo oxidation when liver microsomes were incubated with an organic hydroperoxide such as cumene hydroperoxide or tertiary butyl peroxide. It is now accepted that cytochrome P-450 possesses peroxidatic activity (or peroxygenase activity). In addition, a number of secondary or tertiary amines can undergo a cytochrome P-450-directed dealkylation when hydrogen peroxide is used rather than organic peroxides. A number of studies have been carried out to determine if the intermediate formed between cytochrome P-450 and a peroxide is similar to the elusive peroxycytochrome P-450.

One means of visualizing these different types of reactions in the context of the cyclic function of cytochrome P-450 is illustrated in Fig. 10. The ability to separate the similarities or differences between the peroxygenase-type reaction and the oxygenase-type reaction remains an active area of investigation. Thus, from these studies, it appears that cytochrome P-450 can have multiple modes of action, depending on the substrate studied and the experimental conditions employed (oxygenase, oxidase, or peroxygenase). In many instances, the three activities of cytochrome P-450 may be occurring simultaneously, thereby leading to the variety of products often noted in attempts to establish a balance sheet between the amount of substrate metabolized and the concentration of products formed. Of key interest is the central role of oxycytochrome P-450 where it acts as a "branch point," leading to the operation of different pathways of P-450 function. Recent studies (7) on the role of liver cytochrome P-450 in the oxidation of polyunsaturated fatty acids suggest a role for the formation of "internal" fatty acid per-

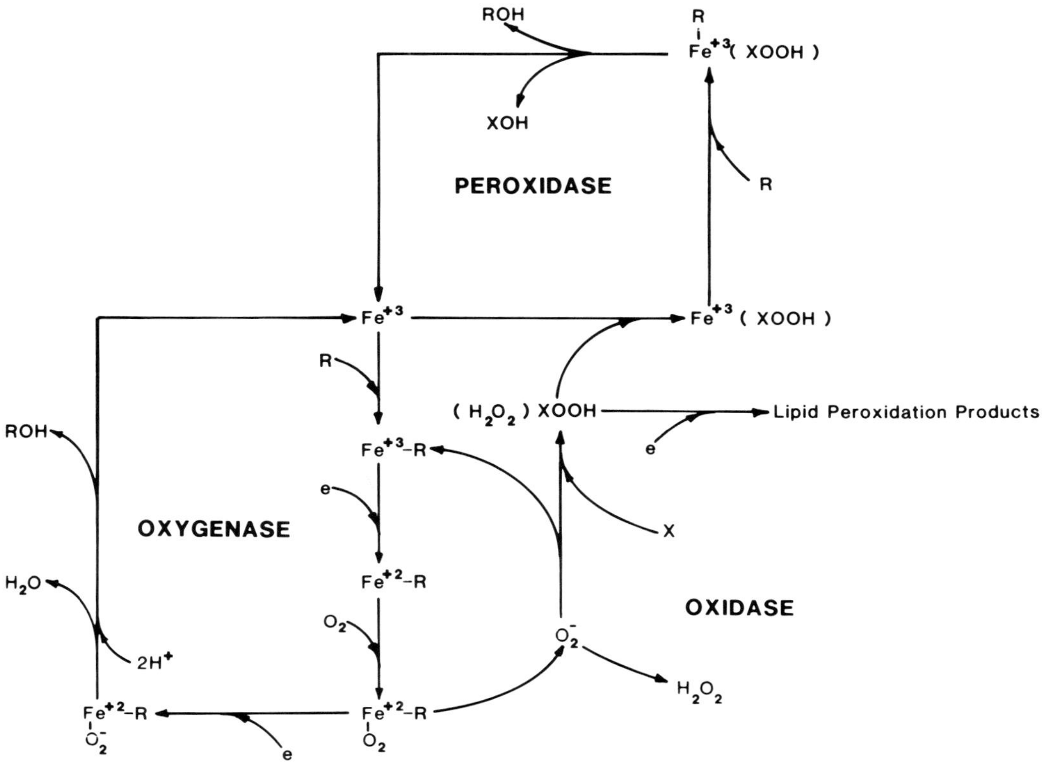

FIG. 10. A composite scheme showing the postulated function of cytochrome P-450 as it participates in oxygenase, oxidase, and peroxidase reactions.

oxides as concomitant contributors to the peroxygenase function of cytochrome P-450.

CONCLUSION

Less than 20 years have passed since the initial observation (16) that cytochrome P-450 can serve as the catalyst for many important cellular monooxygenase reactions. As frequently happens, an increase in interest and knowledge results in the ability to formulate and test many incisive questions. Today we stand on the crest of an exciting phase of science related to cytochrome P-450. In its short history, cytochrome P-450 has provided answers to many previously perplexing problems of biomedical science. Contributions to our knowledge of cellular toxicity, the synthesis of biologically important hormones, the efficacy of drug therapy, and the biotransformation of both exogenous (xenobiotic) and endogenous chemical species point to the early rewards associated with understanding of the key role played by this unique hemeprotein. Much more remains to be learned; new areas remain to be explored. The future is bright and full of untapped opportunities.

ACKNOWLEDGMENT

This work was supported in part by a grant from the National Institutes of Health (NIGMS 16488).

REFERENCES

1. Alvares, A. P., Schilling, G., Levin, W., and Kuntzman, R. (1967): Studies on the induction of CO-

binding pigments in liver microsomes by phenobarbital and 3-methylcholanthrene. *Biochem. Biophys. Res. Commun.*, 29:521–526.
2. Aoyama, T., Imai, Y., and Sato, R. (1982): Multiple forms of cytochrome P-450 from liver microsomes of drug-untreated rabbits: Purification and characterization. In: *Microsomes, Drug Oxidations and Drug Toxicities,* edited by R. Sato and R. Kato, pp. 83–85. Japan Scientific Societies Press, Tokyo and Wiley-Interscience, New York.
3. Aust, S. D., Roerig, D. L., and Pederson, T. C. (1972): Evidence for superoxide generation by NADPH-cytochrome *c* reductase of rat liver microsomes. *Biochem. Biophys. Res. Commun.*, 47:1133–1137.
4. Bidlack, W. R., Okita, R. T., and Hochstein, P. (1973): The role of NADPH-cytochrome b_5 reductase in microsomal lipid peroxidation. *Biochem. Biophys. Res. Commun.*, 53:459–465.
5. Bresnick, E., Brosseau, M., Levin, W., Reik, L., Ryan, D. E., and Thomas, P. E. (1981): Administration of 3-methylcholanthrene to rats increases the specific hybridizable mRNA coding for cytochrome P-450. *Proc. Natl. Acad. Sci. U.S.A.*, 78:4083–4087.
6. Bresnick, E., Vaught, J. B., Chuang, A. H. L., Stoming, T. A., Dockman, D., and Mukhtar, H. (1977): Nuclear aryl hydrocarbon hydroxylase and interaction of polycyclic hydrocarbons with nuclear components. *Arch. Biochem. Biophys.*, 181:257–269.
7. Capdevila, J., Chacos, N., Werringloer, J., Prough, R., and Estabrook, R. W. (1982): Liver microsomal cytochrome P-450 and the oxidative metabolism of arachidonic acid. *Proc. Natl. Acad. Sci. U.S.A.*, 78:5362–5366.
8. Chance, B., Saronio, C., and Leigh, J. S. (1975): Functional intermediates in the reaction of membrane-bound cytochrome oxidase with oxygen. *J. Biol. Chem.*, 250:9226–9237.
9. Conney, A. H. (1967): Pharmacological implications of microsomal enzyme induction. *Pharmacol. Rev.*, 19:317–366.
10. Coon, M. J., Chiang, Y. L., and French, J. S. (1979): Chemical characterization of the enzymes involved in drug metabolism. In: *The Induction of Drug Metabolism,* edited by R. W. Estabrook and E. Lindenlaub, pp. 201–211. F. K. Schattauer Verlag, Stuttgart.
11. Cooper, D. Y., Levin, S., Narashimhulu, S., Rosenthal, O., and Estabrook, R. W. (1965): Photochemical action spectrum of the terminal oxidase of mixed function oxidase systems. *Science,* 147:400–402.
12. Dailey, H. A., and Strittmatter, P. (1980): Characterization of the interaction of amphipathic cytochrome b_5 with stearyl coenzyme A desaturase and NADPH:cytochrome P-450 reductase. *J. Biol. Chem.*, 255:5184–5189.
13. Depierre, J. W., and Dalner, G. (1975): Structural aspects of the membrane of the endoplasmic reticulum. *Biochim. Biophys. Acta,* 415:411–472.
14. Dubois, R. N., and Waterman, M. R. (1979): Effect of phenobarbital administration to rats on the level of the *in vitro* synthesis of cytochrome P-450 directed by total rat liver RNA. *Biochem. Biophys. Res. Commun.*, 90:150–157.
15. Estabrook, R. W., Baron, J., Peterson, J., and Ishimura, Y. (1972): Oxygenated cytochrome P-450 as an intermediate in hydroxylation reactions. In: *Biological Hydroxylation Mechanisms, Biochemical Society Symposia: Number 34,* edited by G. S. Boyd and R. M. S. Smellie, pp. 159–186. Academic Press, London.
16. Estabrook, R. W., Cooper, D. Y., and Rosenthal, O. (1963): The light reversible carbon monoxide inhibition of the steroid C21-hydroxylase system of the adrenal cortex. *Biochem.*, 338:741–755.
17. Estabrook, R. W., Franklin, M., Baron, J., Shigematsu, A., and Hildebrandt, A. G. (1977): Properties of the membrane-bound electron transfer complex of the hepatic endoplasmic reticulum associated with drug metabolism. In: *Drugs and Cell Regulation: Organizational and Pharmacological Aspects on the Molecular Level,* edited by E. Mihich, pp. 227–257. Academic Press, New York.
18. Estabrook, R. W., Martinez-Zedillo, G., Young, S., Peterson, J. A., and McCarthy, J. (1975): The interaction of steroids with liver microsomal membrane P-450: A general hypothesis. *J. Steroid. Biochem.*, 6:419–425.
19. Estabrook, R. W., Peterson, J., Baron, J., and Hildebrandt, A. G. (1971): The spectrophotometric measurement of turbid suspensions of cytochromes associated with drug metabolism. In: *Methods in Pharmacology, Vol. 2, Physical Methods* edited by C. F. Chignell, pp. 303–350. Appleton-Century-Crofts, New York.
20. Estabrook, R. W., Suzuki, K., Mason, J. I., Baron, J., Taylor, W. E., Simpson, E. R., Purvis, J., and McCarthy, J. (1973): Adrenodoxin: An iron–sulfur protein of adrenal cortex mitochondria. In: *Iron–Sulfur Proteins, Vol. 1,* edited by W. Lovenberg, pp. 193–223. Academic Press, New York.
21. Estabrook, R. W., Werringloer, J., Capdevila, J., and Prough, R. A. (1978): The role of cytochrome P-450 and the microsomal electron transport system: The oxidative metabolism of benzo(a)pyrene. In: *Polycyclic Hydrocarbons and Cancer: Environment, Chemistry, and Metabolism, Vol. 1,* edited by H. V. Gelboin and P. O. P. Ts'o, pp. 285–320. Academic Press, New York.
22. Fong, K.-L., McCay, P. B., Poyer, J. L., Keele, B. B., and Misra, H. (1973): Evidence that peroxidation of lysosomal membranes is initiated by hydroxyl free radicals produced during flavin enzyme activity. *J. Biol. Chem.*, 248:7792–7797.
23. Franklin, M. R., and Estabrook, R. W. (1971): On the inhibitory action of mersalyl on microsomal drug oxidation: A rigid organization of the electron transport chain. *Arch. Biochem. Biophys.*, 143:318–329.
24. Fujii-Kuriyama, Y., Mizukami, Y., Tanaguchi, T., and Muramatsu, M. (1982): Molecular cloning of a complementary DNA of phenobarbital-inducible cytochrome P-450 mRNA from rat livers. In *Microsomes, Drug Oxidations and Drug Toxicities,* edited by R. Sato and R. Kato, pp. 589–596. Japan

Scientific Societies Press, Tokyo and Wiley-Interscience, New York.
25. George, P. (1965): The fitness of oxygen. In: *Oxidases and Related Redox Systems,* edited by T. E. King, H. S. Mason, and M. Morrison, pp. 3–33, John Wiley & Sons, New York.
26. Gillette, J. R., Brodie, B. B., and La Du, B. N. (1957): The oxidation of drugs by liver microsomes: On the role of TPNH and oxygen. *J. Pharmacol. Exp. Ther.,* 119:532–540.
27. Griffin, B. W., and Peterson, J. A. (1975): *Pseudomonas putida* cytochrome P-450. The effect of complexes of the ferric hemeprotein on the relaxation of solvent water protons. *J. Biol. Chem.,* 250:6445–6451.
28. Griffin, B. W., Peterson, J. A., and Estabrook, R. W. (1979): Cytochrome P-450: Biophysical properties and catalytic function. In: *The Porphyrins, Biochemistry, Part B, Vol. VII,* edited by D. Dolphin, pp. 333–375. Academic Press, New York.
29. Griffin, B. W., Smith, S. M., and Peterson, J. A. (1974): *Pseudomonas putida* cytochrome P-450. Binding of a spin-labeled analog of the inhibitor metyrapone. *Arch. Biochem. Biophys.,* 160:323–332.
30. Gunsalus, I. C., Lipscomb, J. D., Marshall, V., Frauenfelder, H., Greenbaum, E., and Munck, E. (1972): Structure and reactions of oxygenase active centres: Cytochrome P-450 and iron sulphur proteins in *Biological Hydroxylation Mechanisms, Biochemical Society Symposia: Number 34,* edited by G. S. Boyd and R. M. S. Smellie, pp. 135–158. Academic Press, London.
31. Gunsalus, I. C., Pederson, T. C., and Sligar, S. G. (1975): Oxygenase-catalyzed biological hydroxylations. *Annu. Rev. Biochem.,* 44:377–407.
32. Hall, P. F. (1980): The roles of cytochromes P-450 in the synthesis and metabolism of steroids. In: *Biochemistry, Biophysics and Regulation of Cytochrome P-450,* edited by J.-A. Gustafsson, J. Carlstedt-Duke, A. Mode, and J. Rafter, pp. 461–476. Elsevier/North Holland Biomedical Press, Amsterdam.
33. Hamilton, G. A. (1974): Chemical models and mechanism for oxygenases. In: *Molecular Mechanisms of Oxygen Activation,* edited by O. Hayaishi, pp. 405–451. Academic Press, New York.
34. Haugen, D. A., Van der Hoeven, T. A., and Coon, M. J. (1975): Purified liver microsomal cytochrome P-450: Separation and characterization of multiple forms. *J. Biol. Chem.,* 250:3567–3570.
35. Hayaishi, O., Katagiri, M., and Rothberg, S. (1955): Mechanism of the pyrocatechase reaction. *J. Am. Chem. Soc.,* 77:5450–5451.
36. Hayaishi, O. (1982): My life and oxygen—retrospective and perspective. In: *Oxygenases and Oxygen Metabolism,* edited by M. Nozaki, S. Yamamoto, Y. Ishimura, M. J. Coon, L. Ernster, and R. W. Estabrook, pp. 1–14. Academic Press, Tokyo.
37. Hildebrandt, A. G., and Estabrook, R. W. (1969): Spectrophotometric studies of cytochrome P-450 of liver microsomes after induction with phenobarbital and 3-methylcholanthrene. In: *Microsomes and Drug Oxidations,* edited by J. R. Gillette, A. H. Conney, G. J. Cosmides, R. W. Estabrook, J. R. Fouts, and G. J. Mannering, pp. 331–347. Academic Press, New York.
38. Hildebrandt, A. G., Speck, M., and Roots, I. (1973): Possible control of hydrogen peroxide production and degradation in microsomes during mixed function oxidation reactions. *Biochem. Biophys. Res. Commun.,* 54:968–975.
39. Hill, H. A. O., Roder, A., and Williams, R. J. P. (1970): Cytochrome P-450: Suggestions as to the structure and mechanism of action. *Naturwissenschaften,* 57:69–72.
40. Imai, Y., and Sato, R. (1966): Substrate interaction with hydroxylase system in liver microsomes. *Biochem. Biophys. Res. Commun.,* 22:620–626.
41. Ito, A., and Sato, R. (1968): Purification by means of detergents and properties of cytochrome b_5 from liver microsomes. *J. Biol. Chem.,* 243:4922–4930.
42. Ito, A., and Sato, R. (1969): Proteolytic microdissection of smooth-surfaced vesicles of liver microsomes. *J. Cell Biol.,* 40:179–189.
43. Iyanagi, T., and Mason, H. S. (1973): Some properties of hepatic reduced nicotinamide adenine dinucleotide phosphate–cytochrome *c* reductase. *Biochemistry,* 12:2297–2308.
44. Jerina, D. M. (1982): Polycyclic aromatic hydrocarbons as probes of the steric requirements of the active site of cytochrome P-450. In: *Microsomes, Drug Oxidations and Drug Toxicities,* edited by R. Sato and R. Kato, pp. 195–202. Japan Scientific Societies Press, Tokyo.
45. King, M. M., Lai, E. K., and McCay, P. B. (1975): Singlet oxygen production associated with enzyme-catalyzed lipid peroxidation in liver microsomes. *J. Biol. Chem.,* 250:6496–6502.
46. Leibman, K. C., Hildebrandt, A. G., and Estabrook, R. W. (1969): Spectrophotometric studies of interactions between various substrates in their binding to microsomal cytochrome P-450. *Biochem. Biophys. Res. Commun.,* 36:789–794.
47. Lu, A. Y. H., Strobel, H. W., and Coon, M. J. (1970): Properties of a solubilized form of the cytochrome P-450-containing mixed-function oxidase of liver microsomes. *Mol. Pharmacol.,* 6:213–220.
48. Mannering, G. J., Sladek, N. E., Parli, C. J., and Shoeman, D. W. (1969): Formation of a new P-450 hemoprotein after treatment of rats with polycyclic hydrocarbons. In: *Microsomes and Drug Oxidations,* edited J. R. Gillette, A. H. Conney, G. J. Cosmides, R. W. Estabrook, J. R. Fouts, and G. J. Mannering, pp. 303–326. Academic Press, New York.
49. Mason, H. S. (1957): Mechanisms of oxygen metabolism. In: *Advances in Enzymology, Vol. 19,* edited by F. F. Nord, pp. 79–233. Academic Press, New York.
50. Mason, H. S., Yamano, T., North, J.-C., Hashimoto, Y., and Sakagishi, P. (1965): The structure and oxidase function of liver microsomes. In: *Oxidases and Related Redox Systems, Vol. 2,* edited by T. E. King, H. S. Mason, and M. Morrison, pp. 879–903. John Wiley & Sons, New York.
51. Narasimhulu, S., Cooper, D. Y., and Rosenthal, O. (1965): Spectrophotometric properties of a triton

clarified steroid 21-hydroxylase system of adrenocortical microsomes. *Life Sci.,* 4:2101–2107.

52. Negishi, M., Swan, D. C., Enquist, L. W., and Nebert, D. W. (1981): Isolation and characterization of a cloned DNA sequence associated with the murine Ah locus and a 3-methylcholanthrene-induced form of cytochrome P-450. *Proc. Natl. Acad. Sci. U.S.A.,* 78:800–804.
53. Omura, T., and Sato, R. (1964): The carbon monoxide-binding pigment of liver microsomes. I. Evidence for its hemoprotein nature. *J. Biol. Chem.,* 239:2370–2378.
54. Omura, T., and Sato, R. (1964): The carbon monoxide-binding pigment of liver microsomes. II. Solubilization, purification and properties. *J. Biol. Chem.,* 239:2379–2385.
55. Omura, T., Sato, R., Cooper, D. Y., Rosenthal, O., and Estabrook, R. W. (1965): Functions of cytochrome P-450. *Fed. Proc.,* 24:1181–1189.
56. Oshino, N., Imai, Y., and Sato, R. (1971): A function of cytochrome b_5 in fatty acid desaturation by rat liver microsomes. *J. Biochem.,* 69:155–167.
57. Oshino, N., and Omura, T. (1973): Immunochemical evidence for the participation of cytochrome b_5 in microsomal stearyl-CoA desaturation reaction. *Arch. Biochem. Biophys.,* 157:395–404.
58. Park, S. S., Fujino, T., West, D., Guengerich, F. P., and Gelboin, H. V. (1982): Monoclonal antibodies inhibiting enzyme activity of cytochrome P-450 from 3-methylcholanthrene-treated rats. *Cancer Res.,* 42:1798–1808.
59. Peisach, J., and Blumberg, W. E. (1970): Electron paramagnetic resonance study of the high- and low-spin forms of cytochrome P-450 in liver and in liver microsomes from a methylcholanthrene-treated rabbit. *Proc. Natl. Acad. Sci. U.S.A.,* 67:172–179.
60. Peterson, J. A. (1979): The ligands of cytochrome P-450: Identification and role in the activation of dioxygen. In: *Biochemical and Clinical Aspects of Oxygen,* edited by W. S. Caughey, pp. 227–262. Academic Press, New York.
61. Peterson, J. A., and Griffin, B. W. (1972): Carbon monoxide binding by *Pseudomonas putida* cytochrome P-450. *Arch. Biochem. Biophys.,* 151:427–433.
62. Peterson, J. A., O'Keeffe, D. H., Werringloer, J., Ebel, R. E., and Estabrook, R. W. (1978): Patches and pockets: The microenvironments of a membrane bound hemeprotein. In: *Microenvironments and Metabolic Compartmentation,* edited by P. A. Srere and R. W. Estabrook, pp. 433–450. Academic Press, New York.
63. Remmer, H., Greim, H., Schenkman, J. B., and Estabrook, R. W. (1967): Methods for the elevation of hepatic microsomal mixed function oxidase levels and cytochrome P-450. In: *Methods in Enzymology,* Vol. 10, edited by R. W. Estabrook and M. E. Pullman, pp. 703–707. Academic Press, New York.
64. Remmer, H., and Merker, H. J. (1963): Drug induced changes in the liver endoplasmic reticulum associated with drug metabolizing enzyme. *Ann. N. Y. Acad. Sci.,* 142:1657–1658.
65. Remmer, H., Schenkman, J. B., Estabrook, R. W., Sasame, H., Gillette, J., Narasimhulu, S., Cooper, D. Y., and Rosenthal, O. (1966): Drug interaction with hepatic microsomal cytochrome. *Mol. Pharmacol.,* 2:187–190.
66. Slater, E. C., Van Gelder, B. F., and Minnaert, K. (1965): Cytochrome *c* oxidase. In: *Oxidases and Related Redox Systems,* edited by T. E. King, H. S. Mason and M. Morrison, pp. 667–700. John Wiley & Sons, New York.
67. Spatz, L., and Strittmatter, P. (1971): A form of cytochrome b_5 that contains an additional hydrophobic sequence of 40 amino acid residues. *Proc. Natl. Acad. Sci. U.S.A.,* 68:1042–1046.
68. Strittmatter, P. (1965): The reaction sequence in electron transfer in the reduced nicotinamide adenine dinucleotide–cytochrome b_5 reductase system. *J. Biol. Chem.,* 240:4481–4487.
69. Strittmatter, P., and Velick, S. F. (1957): The purification and properties of microsomal cytochrome reductase. *J. Biol. Chem.,* 223:785–799.
70. Thomas, P. E., Korzeniowski, D., Ryan, D., and Levin, W. (1979): Preparation of monospecific antibodies against two forms of rat liver cytochrome P-450 and quantitation of these antigens of microsomes. *Arch. Biochem. Biophys.,* 192:524–532.
71. Thomas, P. E., Lu, A. Y. H., Ryan, D., West, S. B., Kawalek, J., and Levin, W. (1976): Multiple forms of rat liver cytochrome P-450: Immunochemical evidence with the antibody against cytochrome P-448. *J. Biol. Chem.,* 251:1385–1391.
72. Thomas, P. E., Reik, L. M., Ryan, D. E., and Levin, W. (1981): Regulation of three forms of cytochrome P-450 and epoxide hydrolase in rat liver microsomes: Effect of age, sex, and induction. *J. Biol. Chem.,* 256:1044–1052.
73. Van der Hoeven, T. A., and Coon, M. J. (1974): Preparation and properties of partially purified cytochrome P-450 and reduced nicotinamide adenine dinucleotide phosphate–cytochrome P-450 reductase from rabbit liver microsomes. *J. Biol. Chem.,* 249:6302–6310.
74. Van der Hoeven, T. A., Haugen, D. A., and Coon, M. J. (1974): Cytochrome P-450 purified to apparent homogeneity from phenobarbital-induced rabbit liver microsomes: Catalytic activity and other properties. *Biochem. Biophys. Res. Commun.,* 60:569–575.
75. Vermilion, J. L., and Coon, M. J. (1974): Highly purified detergent-solubilized NADPH–cytochrome P-450 reductase from phenobarbital-induced rat liver microsomes. *Biochem. Biophys. Res. Commun.,* 60:1315–1322.
76. Yang, C. S., and Strickhart, F. S. (1975): Interactions between solubilized cytochrome P-450 and hepatic microsomes. *J. Biol. Chem.,* 250:7968–7972.
77. Yasukochi, Y., and Masters, B. S. S. (1976): Some properties of a detergent-solubilized NADPH–Cytochrome *c* (Cytochrome P-450) reductase purified by biospecific affinity chromatography. *J. Biol. Chem.,* 251:5337–5344.

Drug Metabolism and Drug Toxicity,
edited by J. R. Mitchell and M. G. Horning.
Raven Press, New York © 1984.

Role of Activated Oxygen in Chemical Toxicity

James S. Bus and James E. Gibson

Chemical Industry Institute of Toxicology, Research Triangle Park, North Carolina 27709

It has been recognized since the late 19th century that oxygen, which is essential for most living systems, is also inherently toxic (for reviews, see 8,25). In fact, long before this time, one of the two discoverers of oxygen, Joseph Priestly, suggested that "as a candle burns much faster in dephlogisticated than in common air, so we might, as may be said, live out too fast, and the animal powers be too soon exhausted in this pure kind of air" (51). In recent years, the toxicity of oxygen has been linked to its activation to reactive products such as the superoxide anion radical ($O_2^-\cdot$), hydrogen peroxide (H_2O_2), the hydroxyl radical ($OH\cdot$), and singlet oxygen ($^1O_2$). The purpose of this chapter is to describe several mechanisms by which the generation of activated oxygen is intimately associated with the toxicity of a variety of xenobiotics.

CHEMISTRY OF OXYGEN ACTIVATION

Chemistry of Oxygen Reduction

The formation of reactive products of oxygen is, for the most part, represented by one-electron transfer reactions to molecular oxygen (Fig. 1). The chemical properties of molecular oxygen make it well suited as a single-electron acceptor. Ground-state molecular oxygen has two unpaired electrons with parallel electronic spins, thus making a direct two-electron reduction kinetically unfavorable because of the requirement for reversal of one-electron spin. However, such kinetic constraints do not apply to sequential single-electron reductions of molecular oxygen, which result in formation of oxygen radicals (38).

Molecular oxygen can also be activated by electronic excitation of ground-state molecular oxygen, producing $^1O_2$. In $^1O_2$ formation, an electron of molecular oxygen is elevated to a higher orbital and inverted in its spin state. As a result of the removal of the spin restriction, $^1O_2$ is significantly more reactive to biological molecules than molecular oxygen. A common source of $^1O_2$ generation in biological systems is via photochemical oxidation reactions (23).

Reactions of $O_2^-\cdot$, H_2O_2, and $OH\cdot$

The superoxide anion radical functions both as an oxidant and as a reductant. This property is readily seen in the spontaneous dismutation reaction of $O_2^-\cdot$ (eq. 1), in which one molecule of $O_2^-\cdot$ is oxidized and another reduced. Despite the ability of $O_2^-\cdot$

$$O_2^-\cdot + O_2^-\cdot + 2H^+ \rightarrow H_2O_2 + O_2 \qquad (1)$$

to react directly with important biological substrates such as cytochrome *c* (48), it nonetheless appears that $O_2^-\cdot$ does not have sufficient reactivity to account for the variety of toxic consequences associated with generation of activated oxygen in biological systems (19).

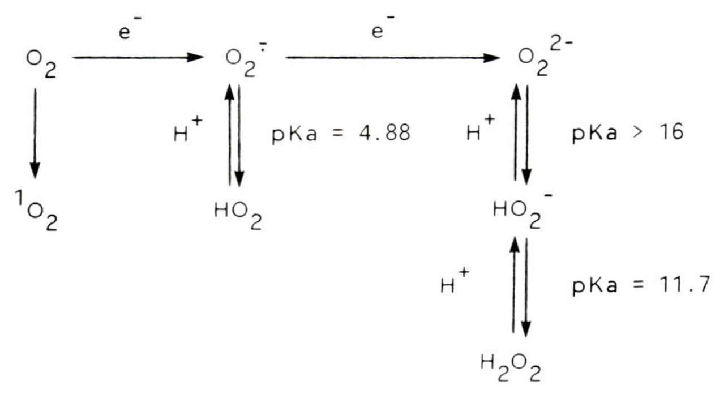

FIG. 1. Reduction products of molecular oxygen. In the presence of light and a photosensitizing agent, singlet oxygen ($^1O_2$) may be formed.

In 1934, Haber and Weiss proposed formation of $OH\cdot$, which is an extremely potent oxidant, by reaction of $O_2^-\cdot$ with the two-electron reduction product of oxygen, H_2O_2 (eq. 4). Although the occurrence of the Haber–Weiss reaction has been questioned because of its apparent slow reaction rate (65), several recent studies have suggested that the reaction may be catalyzed in biological systems by iron salts or other iron complexes (9,47,54; eq. 2–4). Because of the extreme reactivity of $OH\cdot$, several cellular macromolecules such as lipids,

$$O_2^-\cdot + Fe^{3+} \rightarrow O_2 + Fe^{2+} \qquad (2)$$

$$Fe^{2+} + H_2O_2 \rightarrow Fe^{3+} + OH\cdot + OH^- \qquad (3)$$

$$O_2^-\cdot + H_2O_2 \rightarrow O_2 + OH\cdot + OH^- \qquad (4)$$

nucleic acids, proteins, and polysaccharides are susceptible to $OH\cdot$ attack. In biological systems, the reactions of $OH\cdot$ are primarily characterized by hydrogen abstraction or addition reactions.

Reactions of $OH\cdot$ with unsaturated membrane lipids initiate the chain reaction process of lipid peroxidation (Fig. 2). The chain reaction process proceeds in three steps: initiation reactions by which lipid radicals are generated; propagation reactions in which more lipid radicals are formed; and termination reactions in which lipid free radicals

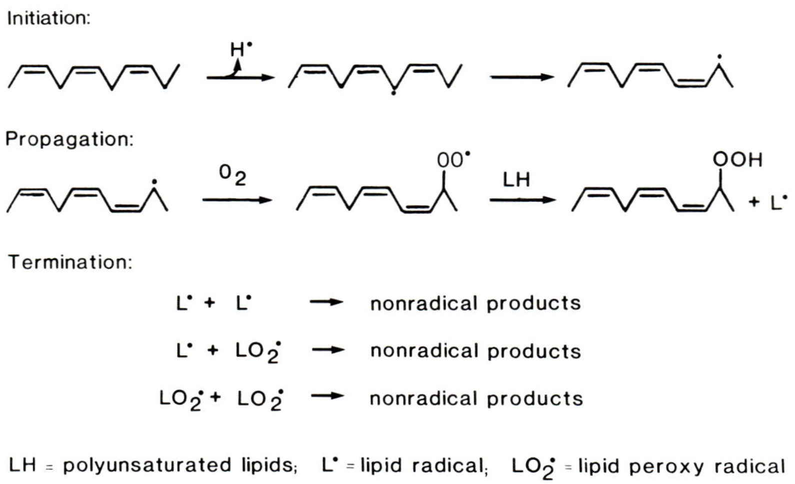

FIG. 2. Reactions in lipid peroxidation.

are consumed (6). The destruction of membrane lipids associated with peroxidation reactions results in loss of functional integrity of the membrane, leading to disturbances in cell function and, if these are too extensive, cell death.

Extensive studies evaluating the mechanisms of radiation-induced DNA damage have implicated OH· in DNA base and sugar phosphate damage (for reviews, see 64,65). Recent studies have demonstrated DNA strand scission following *in vitro* incubation of DNA with a superoxide-generating system (4) or potassium superoxide (42). In both studies, radical-scavenging experiments suggested OH· to be the intermediate responsible for DNA strand breakage. The toxic consequences of OH·-induced DNA damage, therefore, are clear: mutagenic, carcinogenic, and possibly teratogenic responses.

The reaction of OH· with proteins and polysaccharides also has been experimentally demonstrated. For example, the activity of lysozyme and ribonuclease was inhibited by radiation-mediated OH· generation, presumably because of OH· attack on amino acids at the active sites of the enzymes (65). McCord (45) found that both synovial fluid and purified hyaluronic acid were degraded when incubated *in vitro* with a superoxide-generating system. Inhibition of the polysaccharide degradation by the OH· radical scavenger mannitol suggested that OH· was the reactive oxygen species responsible for the depolymerization. This study is particularly interesting because it provides a mechanism by which granulocytes, which generate $O_2^-\cdot$ as an essential element of phagocytosis (1), may produce synovial fluid deterioration in inflammatory arthritic conditions.

Detection of $O_2^-\cdot$ and OH·

Detection of $O_2^-\cdot$ is generally accomplished by use of scavengers that are readily reduced or oxidized by $O_2^-\cdot$. The most common methods spectrophotometrically monitor $O_2^-\cdot$ reduction of cytochrome *c* or nitroblue tetrazolium, or $O_2^-\cdot$ oxidation of epinephrine to adrenochrome. The role of $O_2^-\cdot$ in mediating these reactions is confirmed by the ability of superoxide dismutase to inhibit the reduction or oxidation reaction (26). Superoxide and OH· radical generation may also be detected by spin trapping of the short-lived oxygen radicals, forming stable free radicals that can be quantitated by electron paramagnetic resonance (EPR) spectrometry (for review, see 20).

Hydroxyl radical generation is characterized by monitoring the liberation of ethylene from reaction of OH· with methional or 2-keto-4-thiomethylbutyric acid (15). Use of 2-keto-4-thiomethylbutyric acid is preferable because of its solubility advantages and lack of an unpleasant odor. The role of OH· in mediating ethylene liberation is confirmed by the ability of various OH· scavengers such as mannitol, ethanol, *n*-butanol, benzoate, and mono- and diethyl urea to inhibit the reaction.

BIOLOGICAL DEFENSES TO ACTIVATED OXYGEN

In aerobic biological systems $O_2^-\cdot$ is a product of many endogenous metabolic reactions (27). These include $O_2^-\cdot$ formed from autoxidations of hydroquinones, catecholamines, and thiols, and $O_2^-\cdot$ produced by catalytic activity of enzymes such as xanthine oxidase and aldehyde oxidase. In an aerobic environment, therefore, an essential element of survival is the ability of an organism to detoxify the products of univalent oxygen reduction. In view of the extremely detrimental consequences of $O_2^-\cdot$ production within cells, it is not surprising that a multitiered defense system exists to efficiently combat such fluxes. It will become clear from later discussion that these biological defense systems are also critical in controlling the toxic potential of $O_2^-\cdot$ produced during the metabolism of xenobiotics.

Superoxide Dismutases and Catalase

The first line of defense against the superoxide radical is a series of enzymes, the superoxide dismutases, that catalyze the dismutation of $O_2^- \cdot$ (eq. 5). The activity of superoxide dismutase,

$$O_2^- \cdot + O_2^- \cdot + 2H^+ \xrightarrow[]{\text{Superoxide dismutase}} H_2O_2 + O_2 \quad (5)$$

which was first described by McCord and Fridovich (48), has subsequently been found to be associated with three distinct metalloenzymes. Iron-containing and manganese-containing superoxide dismutase are most commonly found in prokaryotes, whereas the copper–zinc enzyme is characteristic of eukaryotes (27). Mitochondria of eukaryotes, however, contain only the manganoenzyme, with the copper–zinc enzyme found in the cytosol.

The biological importance of superoxide dismutase as a defense mechanism has been extensively characterized in several studies of bacterial oxygen toxicity. A mutant strain of *Escherichia coli* that had progressively decreased superoxide dismutase activity with growth at increasing temperatures also had progressively less tolerance to oxygen with increasing temperatures (46). In other studies, superoxide dismutase activity was increased in *E. coli* grown under hyperbaric oxygen (32). Growth of *E. coli* under nitrogen, however, which diminished superoxide dismutase activity, enhanced the susceptibility of the bacteria to hyperbaric oxygen toxicity. Indirect evidence for the necessity of superoxide dismutase for survival in an aerobic environment has been suggested from a survey of the distribution of enzyme activity in a wide range of bacteria (49). Aerobes were generally found to have the highest activity of superoxide dismutase; obligate anaerobes contained no activity. Intermediate activity was present in aerotolerant organisms, which have anaerobic metabolism even when grown in air. Thus, taken together, these studies and others (for review, see 27) provide strong evidence for the essential role of superoxide dismutase as a defense against superoxide-mediated toxicity.

The likelihood that the toxicity of $O_2^- \cdot$ is mediated via reaction with H_2O_2 with formation of $OH \cdot$ suggests that catalase is also an integral first-line oxidative defense mechanism. Catalase, by converting H_2O_2 to water and molecular oxygen, also removes a reactant necessary for $OH \cdot$ formation. Acting in concert with superoxide dismutase, therefore, catalase should minimize the potential for $OH \cdot$ formation. This phenomenon has, in fact, been observed. For example, liberation of ethylene from 2-keto-4-thiomethylbutyric acid induced by an $O_2^- \cdot$-generating system, xanthine oxidase metabolism of xanthine, was inhibited by superoxide dismutase or catalase (15).

Antioxidant Protection Against Lipid Peroxidation

Superoxide dismutase and catalase provide antioxidant protection by preventing formation of the potent oxidant, $OH \cdot$. In the case of $OH \cdot$ attack on membrane lipids, however, a second line of biological defenses is available to check the damaging chain reaction process of lipid peroxidation.

A primary mechanism by which lipoperoxidative reactions may be controlled is via intervention of antioxidants (Fig. 3). Two types of antioxidants function *in vivo:* water-soluble antioxidants such as ascorbic acid and reduced glutathione (GSH) and lipid-soluble antioxidants, which are exemplified by vitamin E (14). Antioxidants protect membrane unsaturated lipids by preferentially undergoing lipid radical-mediated hydrogen abstractions. By this process, further generation of lipid radicals is decreased.

The chain reaction process of lipid peroxidation may also be controlled by detoxification of lipid hydroperoxides, which, in the presence of transition metal ions, decompose to lipid radicals (Fig. 2). The reduction of lipid hydroperoxides to stable, nonradical-

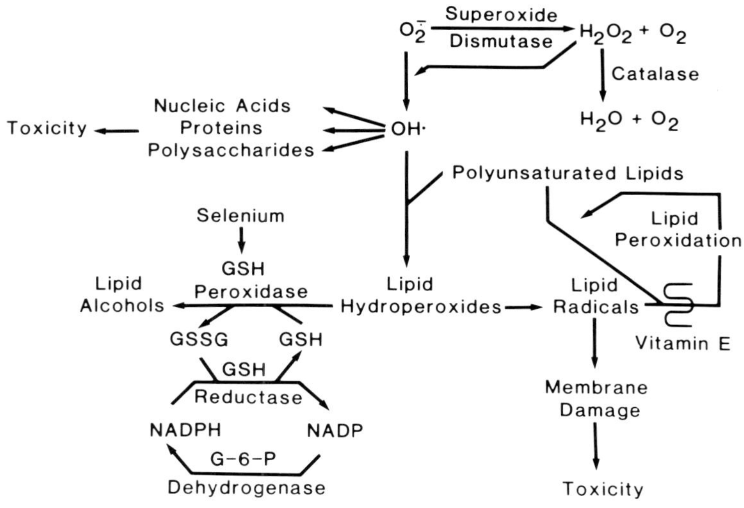

FIG. 3. Biochemical defense mechanisms that modulate toxic reactions initiated by superoxide radicals ($O_2^-\cdot$).

forming lipid alcohols is catalyzed by GSH peroxidase. Maintenance of the reducing equivalents required for the enzyme activity is accomplished by GSH reductase and the pentose shunt enzyme, glucose-6-phosphate (G-6-P) dehydrogenase (for review, see 6). Several GSH peroxidases have been identified. A cytosolic selenium-dependent enzyme catalyzes the reduction of H_2O_2 as well as a wide variety of organic hydroperoxides. A nonselenium-dependent GSH peroxidase that exhibits activity only with organic hydroperoxide substrates has been associated with both cytosolic and microsomal glutathione-*S*-transferases (7,52).

MECHANISMS OF XENOBIOTIC-MEDIATED ACTIVATED OXYGEN GENERATION

Formation of $O_2^-\cdot$ via Redox Cycling

In recent years, generation of $O_2^-\cdot$ has been suggested as a fundamental mechanism underlying the toxic action of a wide spectrum of chemicals (Table 1; for reviews, see 39,62). Two frequently encountered mechanisms by which metabolism of xenobiotics results in $O_2^-\cdot$ formation are single-electron redox cycling reactions and autoxidation reactions. Of the chemicals listed in Table 1,

TABLE 1. *Examples of chemicals whose toxicity may be mediated through generation of superoxide radicals*

Chemical	Toxicity	Ref.
Alloxan, dialuric acid	Pancreatic β-cell	(10)
Adriamycin, daunomycin	Heart	(28)
6-Hydroxydopamine	Adrenergic nerve terminals	(10)
Benzo(a)pyrenediones	Cancer(?)	(43)
β-Lapachone	Antimicrobial agent	(16)
Nitrofurantoin	Lung	(58)
Paraquat	Lung	(5)
Streptonigrin	Antitumor agent	(63)

those containing quaternary bipyridyl (paraquat), quinone [adriamycin, benzo(a)pyrenediones, β-lapachone, streptonigrin], or nitro groups (nitrofurantoin) generate $O_2^{-}\cdot$ by redox cycling. Autoxidation reactions account for $O_2^{-}\cdot$ formed from alloxan, dialuric acid, and 6-hydroxydopamine.

Paraquat

Paraquat is a broad-spectrum herbicide whose mammalian toxicity is characterized primarily by extensive lung injury (59). Both the herbicidal (17) and mammalian (5) toxicity of paraquat has been attributed to a single-electron reduction to the paraquat radical, which under aerobic conditions is immediately reoxidized to the parent molecule with concurrent $O_2^{-}\cdot$ formation (Fig. 4). In mammalian systems, paraquat has been shown to be reduced by microsomal NADPH cytochrome P-450 reductase, using NADPH as a source of reducing equivalents (5). Under aerobic conditions, reoxidation of the radical results in formation of $O_2^{-}\cdot$ as detected by a stimulation of epinephrine oxidation to adrenochrome (2).

Evidence for the role of $O_2^{-}\cdot$ in paraquat toxicity has been obtained from studies evaluating paraquat toxicity in bacteria. Incubation of paraquat with *E. coli* caused a rapid and significant increase in the biosynthesis of superoxide dismutase and also increased tolerance of the bacteria to hyperbaric oxygen exposure (35). *E. coli* containing high levels of superoxide dismutase were subsequently found to be considerably more resistant to paraquat-induced lethality than *E. coli* containing low levels of superoxide dismutase (36). Paraquat lethality was also completely dependent on the presence of oxygen and an adequate source of reducing equivalents, which emphasized the obligatory nature of redox cycling in paraquat toxicity. Similar phenomena were also observed in a subsequent study in which the mutagenicity and toxicity of paraquat in *Salmonella typhimurium* were examined (50). Both mutagenicity and toxicity were dependent on an adequate supply of electrons and oxygen and were moderated in bacteria containing elevated superoxide dismutase activity.

Evidence has also been developed to suggest that paraquat acts by an oxidant-related mechanism in animals. Incubations of paraquat with NADPH, NADPH–cytochrome P-450 reductase, and purified rat liver microsomal lipid stimulated lipid peroxidation in a concentration-dependent manner. The peroxidation was inhibited by both superoxide dismutase and a singlet-oxygen-trapping agent. The inhibition by the latter agent, however, was possibly a result of trapping of singlet oxygen produced during propagation reactions and not an inhibition of initiation reactions (5). Attempts to quantitate paraquat-induced lipid peroxidation in more complex *in vitro* systems (e.g., microsomes) have produced mixed results, with findings of both inhibition and stimulation of lipid peroxidation. A recent study (61), however, suggested that in order to detect paraquat-stimulated lipid peroxidation *in vitro,* precautions must be taken to ensure an adequate source of NADPH and a sufficient incubation time. Such conditions not only maximize paraquat redox cycling but may also allow a depletion of microsomal vitamin E to the point at which peroxidation can occur.

In vivo, paraquat lung toxicity in rats was significantly enhanced by simultaneous exposure to 100% oxygen (22) and decreased in mice placed in a 14% oxygen environment (53). Both of these reports support the re-

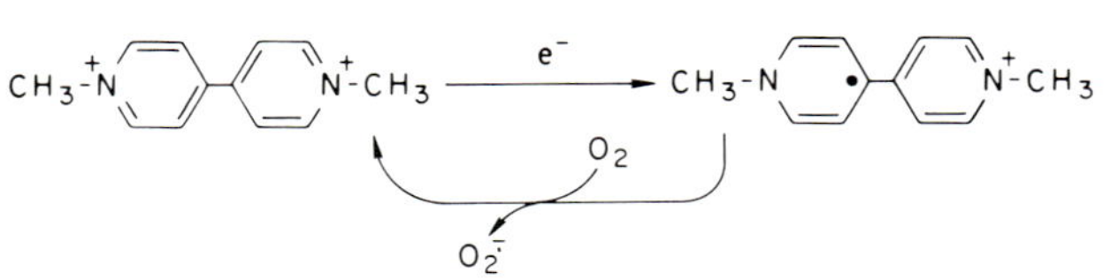

FIG. 4. Paraquat redox cycling.

quirement for oxygen in paraquat toxicity. Mice with decreased GSH peroxidase activity or vitamin E levels, obtained by feeding selenium- or vitamin E-deficient diets, were also found to be significantly less tolerant to paraquat-induced lethality (5). Conversely, pretreatment of rats with endotoxin and hyperoxia, a regimen that increases pulmonary superoxide dismutase, catalase, and GSH peroxidase activities, significantly increased tolerance to paraquat-induced lethality (24). These studies, therefore, are also consistent with the hypothesis of superoxide-mediated paraquat toxicity.

Although the complete mechanism of paraquat toxicity has yet to be described and likely involves additional cytotoxic events such as depletion of cellular NADPH (56) and formation of mixed disulfides (40), redox cycling with resultant $O_2^- \cdot$ generation appears to be an essential element in the toxicity of paraquat.

Nitrofurantoin

Therapeutic use of the urinary tract antibacterial drug nitrofurantoin produces both an acute and chronic pulmonary reaction in a limited number of patients. Although the lung toxicity was assumed to be of immunologic origin, demonstration of dose-related lung toxicity in rats indicated a possible nonimmunologic mechanism (2).

A study conducted by Mason and Holtzman (44) first suggested that nitrofurantoin was capable of single-electron redox cycling as described in equation 6. These investigators observed that lung microsomes catalyzed

$$\text{R-NO}_2 \xrightarrow[\text{Microsomes}]{\text{NADPH}} \text{R-NO}_2 \cdot \xrightarrow{O_2} \text{R-NO}_2 + O_2^- \cdot \quad (6)$$

an NADPH-dependent stimulation of oxygen consumption which was partially inhibited by superoxide dismutase. The superoxide dismutase inhibition of oxygen consumption was consistent with $O_2^- \cdot$ generation, since this enzyme catalyzes the conversion of two superoxide molecules to one molecule each of hydrogen peroxide and molecular oxygen. Lung microsomes generated the nitroanion radical only under anaerobic conditions, further suggesting the radical to be oxygen labile. Subsequent studies (58) confirmed that nitrofurantoin produced a large flux of $O_2^- \cdot$ (as measured by superoxide dismutase-inhibitable epinephrine oxidation) when incubated aerobically with rat lung microsomes and NADPH. Microsomal incubation of nitrofurantoin under anaerobic conditions greatly enhanced the covalent binding of nitrofurantoin, presumably because of stabilization of reduced nitro group intermediates (2).

The *in vivo* toxicity of nitrofurantoin parallels that of paraquat in two ways (3). Nitrofurantoin-induced lethality in rats was significantly elevated in animals fed vitamin E-deficient diets and also in rats exposed to 100% oxygen. Thus, the *in vivo* and *in vitro* similarities between nitrofurantoin and paraquat provide good evidence that these lung toxins may share a common toxic mechanism.

Streptonigrin

Redox cycling of toxic chemicals containing quinone structures is exemplified by the antibiotic streptonigrin. Early investigations of streptonigrin toxicity in *E. coli* demonstrated that, as for paraquat and nitrofurantoin, both oxygen and a source of electrons were necessary for lethality (63). Later studies found that streptonigrin could degrade DNA *in vitro* when incubated with a reductant and oxygen. Inhibition of the DNA degradation by superoxide dismutase subsequently implicated $O_2^- \cdot$ in this reaction (for review, see 26). The involvement of $O_2^- \cdot$ in streptonigrin toxicity was further supported by the observation that *E. coli* containing high levels of superoxide dismutase were more resistant to streptonigrin than *E. coli* containing low levels (26).

Formation of $O_2^-\cdot$ via Autoxidation Reactions

A second important mechanism by which $O_2^-\cdot$ is generated during the course of xenobiotic metabolism is via spontaneous autoxidation reactions. These reactions are most commonly encountered with chemicals containing polyhydroxyaromatic structural elements (e.g., catechols and hydroquinones). Two agents that are used as research tools in pharmacology and toxicology, 6-hydroxydopamine and alloxan, have served as useful models in evaluating the potential for autoxidation reactions to produce cell toxicity by $O_2^-\cdot$ formation.

An important factor in the toxicity of both 6-hydroxydopamine and alloxan is the specific accumulation of the toxic agent in cells exhibiting the toxic response. The diabetogenic agent alloxan is selectively accumulated by the insulin-producing β-cell of the pancreas (34). 6-Hydroxydopamine, which is preferentially toxic to sympathetic neurons, appears to be accumulated in the target cells by an amine transport system associated with the axonal membrane (57). Inhibition of the transport mechanism by various drugs prevented 6-hydroxydopamine toxicity, thereby emphasizing the important role of transport in the development of toxicity (12). It is interesting to note that the selective lung toxicity of paraquat is also associated with a transport-mediated accumulation in lung tissue (55). These observations raise the possibility that a concentration or retention of the oxidant agent in the target organ or cell may be needed to overwhelm the local oxidant defense mechanisms.

Formation of $O_2^-\cdot$ and H_2O_2 during the autoxidation of 6-hydroxydopamine has been proposed by Heikkila and Cohen (37) to occur in the following theoretical reaction sequence:

$$\text{6-OHDA} + O_2 \rightarrow SQ\cdot + O_2^-\cdot + H^+ \quad (7)$$

$$H^+ + \text{6-OHDA} + O_2^-\cdot \rightarrow SQ\cdot + H_2O_2 \quad (8)$$

$$SQ\cdot + O_2 \rightarrow Q + O_2^-\cdot + H^+ \quad (9)$$

$$SQ\cdot + O_2^-\cdot + H^+ \rightarrow Q + H_2O_2 \quad (10)$$

where 6-OHDA is 6-hydroxydopamine, SQ· is the semiquinone radical of 6-OHDA, and Q is the quinone of 6-OHDA. In this study, 6-hydroxydopamine autoxidation was monitored by quinone product formation and oxygen consumption. Superoxide dismutase inhibited both measures of autoxidation. This was consistent with the proposed reaction scheme, since superoxide dismutase would eliminate reactions 8 and 10 and reduce the overall rate of autoxidation to that of the rate-limiting step, reaction 7. The autoxidation of 6-hydroxydopamine was subsequently found to only slightly stimulate cytochrome *c* reduction (11). However, the weak action of this monitor of $O_2^-\cdot$ generation was attributed to the ability of 6-hydroxydopamine to directly scavenge $O_2^-\cdot$ itself (reaction 8).

Generation of $O_2^-\cdot$ by alloxan has been attributed to a two-electron reduction to dialuric acid, which autoxidizes back to alloxan with $O_2^-\cdot$ formation (10; Fig. 5). The reduction of alloxan to dialuric acid by ascorbic acid has been shown *in vitro* (13) and has also been postulated to occur via several nicotinamide nucleotide-linked enzymatic re-

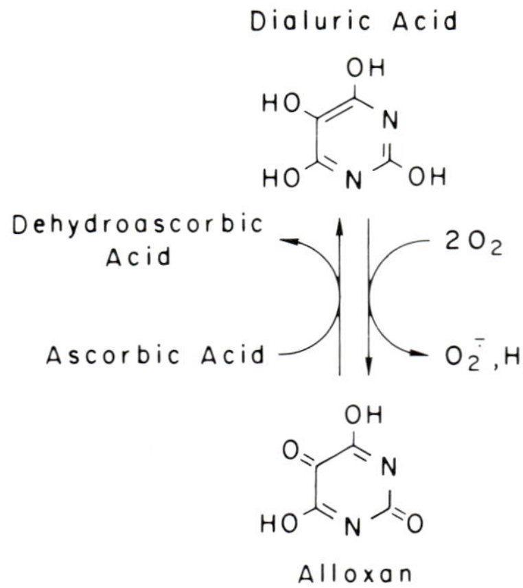

FIG. 5. Alloxan reduction to dialuric acid with subsequent autoxidation.

dox processes (30). It is likely that similar reductive mechanisms may also regenerate 6-hydroxydopamine from its oxidized quinone. Superoxide radical formation from dialuric acid autoxidation has been confirmed by a superoxide dismutase-inhibitable cytochrome *c* reduction (11).

Several studies have implicated OH· as the ultimate toxic species produced from 6-hydroxydopamine and alloxan metabolism. *In vitro,* 6-hydroxydopamine and dialuric acid stimulated ethylene production from methional. Inhibition by superoxide dismutase, catalase, or OH· scavengers suggested a metal ion-catalyzed Haber–Weiss reaction as the OH· source (11). In a more complex biological system, alloxan-induced inhibition of glucose-stimulated insulin release from isolated pancreatic islets was ameliorated by the OH· scavenger dimethylurea (21). *In vivo,* the toxicity of both agents has been diminished by treatment with OH· trappers. Pretreatment of mice with individual OH· scavengers prevented subsequent 6-hydroxydopamine toxicity to adrenergic neurons in the left atrium and iris, as determined by the ability of preparations of these tissues to accumulate tritiated norepinephrine *in vitro* (12). With alloxan, a series of urea derivatives prevented the diabetogenic toxicity in a manner that correlated with the capacity of the derivative to trap OH· (60). In addition, pretreatment of mice with a superoxide dismutase–polyethylene glycol complex, which significantly increases the serum half-life of the enzyme, markedly decreased the diabetogenic activity of alloxan (31). The protective effect of superoxide dismutase was attributed to decreased OH· generation resulting from O_2^-· formation. These data, therefore, provide strong evidence for the role of activated oxygen in toxicity of 6-hydroxydopamine and alloxan.

The autoxidation reactions of 6-hydroxydopamine (eqs. 7–10) illustrate an important concern that must be considered whenever these types of reactions are used to postulate O_2^-· formation as a toxic mechanism. Autoxidation reactions, and also redox cycling reactions, will result in formation of potentially toxic organic metabolites. Semiquinones, quinones, and nitroaromatic radicals all have the potential to alkylate tissue macromolecules under appropriate conditions. In the case of 6-hydroxydopamine, for example, the *p*-quinone oxidation product was considerably less effective as an inhibitor of a sulfhydryl-containing enzyme, DNA polymerase, than 6-hydroxydopamine itself. Since epinephrine, a potent O_2^-· and OH· scavenger, prevented the inhibition of the polymerase by 6-hydroxydopamine, O_2^-· generation was confirmed as the mechanism responsible for the inhibition (29).

In contrast to 6-hydroxydopamine, O_2^-· has been suggested to be a metabolic activator of the hepatotoxin α-methyldopa. The proposed reaction sequence was similar to that outlined in equations 8 through 10 (18). Incubation of radiolabeled α-methyldopa with rat liver microsomes and NADPH resulted in significant covalent binding to microsomal protein. The covalent binding was inhibited by superoxide dismutase O_2^-· scavengers such as epinephrine, glutathione, and carbon monoxide. These observations suggested that cytochrome P-450-mediated O_2^-· generation was responsible for oxidation of α-methyldopa to reactive semiquinone and/or quinone metabolites. Although it is possible that O_2^-· and H_2O_2 formed from oxidation of the semiquinone could in part be responsible for the toxicity, covalent binding of semiquinone and/or quinone oxidation products nonetheless appears a likely mechanism for α-methyldopa hepatotoxicity.

Formation of $^1O_2$ via Photochemical Oxidations

Singlet oxygen can be formed from photosensitized oxidations of xenobiotics. Xenobiotics capable of acting as photosensitizers include dyes such as methylene blue, rose bengal, or eosin and aromatic hydrocarbons such as rubrene (23). Photosensitizers absorb visible or near-ultraviolet light, producing both excited singlet and triplet excited states. Most photooxidation reactions proceed via the sensitizer triplet, which is much longer lived than the singlet. Singlet oxygen is formed from the interaction of a sensitizer triplet with ground-state molecular oxygen, regenerating ground-state sensitizer and $^1O_2$. A minor photooxidation pathway involves electron transfer to molecular oxygen, producing $O_2^- \cdot$ and an oxidized sensitizer (for review, see 23).

Singlet oxygen is extremely reactive. The consequences of $^1O_2$ generation in biological systems, therefore, encompass a spectrum of toxic injury similar to that seen with $O_2^- \cdot$. Singlet oxygen has been suggested as an initiator of lipid peroxidation (for review, see 6) and as an oxidant of amino acids and nucleic acids (23).

As with $O_2^- \cdot$, biological systems also possess an apparent defense mechanism that modulates potential $^1O_2$ toxicity. The carotenoid pigments, and in particular β-carotene, are capable of quenching $^1O_2$ without reaction. β-Carotene quenching of $^1O_2$ has been described as an energy transfer mechanism in which triplet carotene is produced and returned to ground state in a radiationless reaction (23). The importance of β-carotene as a defense mechanism has been described in a report by Krinsky (41). A mutant strain of bacteria lacking carotenoid pigments was found more susceptible to destruction by polymorphonuclear leukocytes than wild-type bacteria containing carotenoid pigments. The difference was attributed to the postulated ability of leukocytes to kill bacteria via $^1O_2$ generation.

CONCLUSIONS

The importance of activated oxygen in mediating xenobiotic toxicity is a phenomenon that has only recently been recognized. It is clear that the pioneering efforts of Fridovich in delineating the function of superoxide dismutase are responsible in a large degree for the rapid progress that has been made in recognizing the toxic potential of $O_2^- \cdot$. With this recognition, evaluation of the toxic mechanisms of a few model compounds has provided an excellent framework from which future mechanism studies can be constructed.

REFERENCES

1. Babior, B. M., Kipnes, R. S., and Curnette, J. T. (1973): Biological defense mechanisms. The production by leukocytes of superoxide, a potential bactericidal agent. *J. Clin. Invest.*, 52:741–744.
2. Boyd, M. R. (1980): Biochemical mechanisms in chemical-induced lung injury: roles of metabolic activation. *CRC Crit. Rev. Toxicol.*, 7:103–176.
3. Boyd, M. R., Catignani, G. L., Sasame, H. A., Mitchell, J. R., and Stiko, A. W. (1979): Acute pulmonary injury in rats by nitrofurantoin and modification by vitamin E, dietary fat and oxygen. *Am. Rev. Respir. Dis.*, 120:93–99.
4. Brawn, K., and Fridovich, I. (1981): DNA strand scission by enzymatically generated oxygen radicals. *Arch. Biochem. Biophys.*, 206:414–419.
5. Bus, J. S., and Gibson, J. E. (1976): Paraquat toxicity: Proposed mechanisms of toxicity involving lipid peroxidation. *Environ. Health Perspect.*, 16:139–146.
6. Bus, J. S., and Gibson, J. E. (1979): Lipid peroxidation and its role in toxicology. *Rev. Biochem. Toxicol.*, 1:125–149.
7. Chow, C. K. (1979): Nutritional influence on cellular antioxidant defense systems. *Am. J. Clin. Nutr.*, 32:1066–1081.
8. Clark, J. M., and Lambertsen, C. J. (1971): Pulmonary oxygen toxicity: a review. *Pharmacol. Rev.*, 23:37–133.
9. Cohen, G. (1977): In defense of Haber–Weiss. In: *Superoxide and Superoxide Dismutases,* edited by A. M. Michaelson, J. M. McCord, and I. Fridovich, pp. 317–321. Academic Press, London.
10. Cohen, G. (1978): The generation of hydroxyl radicals in biologic systems: toxicologic aspects. *Photochem. Photobiol.*, 28:669–675.
11. Cohen, G., and Heikkila, R. E. (1974): The generation of hydrogen peroxide, superoxide radical and hydroxyl radical by 6-hydroxydopamine, dialuric acid, and related cytotoxic agents. *J. Biol. Chem.*, 249:2447–2452.
12. Cohen, G., Heikkila, R. E., Allis, B., Cabbat, F., Dembiec, D., MacNamee, D., Mytilineou, C., and Winston, B. (1976): Destruction of sympathetic nerve terminals by 6-hydroxydopamine: protection by 1-phenyl-3-(2-thiazolyl)-2-thiourea, diethyldithiocarbamate, methimazole, cysteamine, ethanol and *n*-butanol. *J. Pharmacol. Exp. Ther.*, 199:336–352.
13. Deamer, D. W., Heikkila, R. E., Panganamala, R. V., Cohen, G., and Cornwell, D. G. (1971): The alloxan–dialuric acid cycle and the generation of

hydrogen peroxide. *Physiol. Chem. Phys.*, 3:426–430.

14. Demopoulos, H. P. (1973): The basis of free radical pathology. *Fed. Proc.*, 32:1859–1861.
15. Diguiseppi, J., and Fridovich, I. (1980): Ethylene from 2-keto-4-thiomethyl butyric acid: The Haber-Weiss reaction. *Arch. Biochem. Biophys.*, 205:323–329.
16. Docampo, R., Cruz, F. S., Boveris, A., Muniz, R. P. A., and Esquivel, D. M. S. (1979): β-Lapachone enhancement of lipid peroxidation and superoxide anion and hydrogen peroxide formation by sarcoma 180 ascites tumor cells. *Biochem. Pharmacol.*, 28:723–728.
17. Dodge, A. D. (1971): The mode of action of the bipyridylium herbicides, paraquat and diquat. *Endeavour*, 30:130–135.
18. Dybing, E., Nelson, S. D., Mitchell, J. R., Sasame, H. A., and Gillette, J. R. (1976): Oxidation of α-methyldopa and other catechols by cytochrome P-450-generated superoxide anion: Possible mechanism of methyldopa hepatitis. *Mol. Pharmacol.*, 12:911–920.
19. Fee, J. A., and Valentine, J. S. (1977): Chemical and physical properties of superoxide. In: *Superoxide and Superoxide Dismutases*, edited by A. M. Michaelson, J. M. McCord, and I. Fridovich, pp. 19–60. Academic Press, London.
20. Finkelstein, E., Rosen, G. M., and Rauckman, E. J. (1980): Spin trapping of superoxide and hydroxyl radical: practical aspects. *Arch. Biochem. Biophys.*, 200:1–16.
21. Fischer, L. A., and Hamburger, S. A. (1980): Dimethylurea: A radical scavenger that protects isolated pancreatic islets from the effects of alloxan and dihydroxyfumerate exposure. *Life Sci.*, 26:1405–1409.
22. Fisher, H. K., Clements, J. A., and Wright, R. R. (1973): Enhancement of oxygen toxicity by the herbicide paraquat. *Am. Rev. Respir. Dis.*, 107:246–252.
23. Foote, C. S. (1976): Photosensitized oxidation and singlet oxygen: consequences in biological systems. In: *Free Radicals in Biology, Vol. 2*, edited by W. A. Pryor, pp. 85–133. Academic Press, New York.
24. Frank, L. (1981): Prolonged survival after paraquat. Role of the lung antioxidant enzyme systems. *Biochem. Pharmacol.*, 30:2319–2324.
25. Frank, L., and Massaro, D. (1980): Oxygen toxicity. *Am. J. Med.*, 69:117–126.
26. Fridovich, I. (1974): Superoxide dismutase. *Adv. Enzymol.*, 41:35–97.
27. Fridovich, I. (1978): The biology of oxygen radicals. *Science*, 201:875–880.
28. Goodman, J., and Hochstein, P. (1977): Generation of free radicals and lipid peroxidation by redox cycling of adriamycin and daunomycin. *Biochem. Biophys. Res. Commun.*, 77:797–803.
29. Graham, D. G., Tiffany, S. M., Bell, W. R., Jr., and Gutnecht, W. F. (1978): Autoxidation versus covalent binding of quinones as the mechanism of toxicity of dopamine, 6-hydroxydopamine and related compounds towards C1300 neuroblastoma cells *in vitro*. *Mol. Pharmacol.*, 14:644–653.
30. Grankvist, K., Marklund, S., Sehlin, J., and Taljedal, I.-B. (1979): Superoxide dismutase, catalase and scavengers of hydroxyl radical protect against the toxic action of alloxan on pancreatic islet cells *in vitro*. *Biochem. J.*, 182:17–25.
31. Grankvist, K., Marklund, S., and Taljedal, I.-B. (1981): Superoxide dismutase is a prophylactic against alloxan diabetes. *Nature*, 294:158–160.
32. Gregory, E. M., and Fridovich, I. (1973): Oxygen toxicity and superoxide dismutase. *J. Bacteriol.*, 114:1193–1197.
33. Haber, F., and Weiss, J. (1934): The catalytic decomposition of hydrogen peroxide by iron salts. *Proc. R. Soc. Lond.* [*A*], 147:332–351.
34. Hammarstrom, L., and Ullberg, S. (1966): Specific uptake of labelled alloxan in the pancreatic islets. *Nature*, 212:708–710.
35. Hassan, H. M., and Fridovich, I. (1977): Regulation of the synthesis of superoxide dismutase in *E. coli*. *J. Biol. Chem.*, 252:7667–7672.
36. Hassan, H. M., and Fridovich, I. (1978): Superoxide radical and the enhancement of the toxicity of paraquat in *Escherichia coli*. *J. Biol. Chem.*, 253:8143–8148.
37. Heikkila, R. E., and Cohen, G. (1973): 6-Hydroxydopamine: Evidence for superoxide radical as an oxidative intermediate. *Science*, 181:456–457.
38. Hill, A. O. (1979): The chemistry of dioxygen and its reduction products. In: *Oxygen Free Radicals and Tissue Damage, Ciba Foundation Symposium 65*, edited by D. W. Fitzsimons, pp. 5–17. Excerpta Medica, Amsterdam.
39. Kappus, H., and Sies, H. (1981): Toxic drug effects associated with oxygen metabolism: Redox cycling and lipid peroxidation. *Experientia*, 37:1233–1241.
40. Keeling, P. L., Smith, L. L., and Aldridge, W. N. (1982): The formation of mixed disculphides in rat lung followed paraquat administration. Correlation with changes in intermediary metabolism. *Biochim. Biophys. Acta*, 716:249–257.
41. Krinsky, N. I. (1974): Singlet excited oxygen as a mediator of the antibacterial action of leukocytes. *Science*, 186:363–365.
42. Lesko, S. A., Lorentzen, R. J., and Ts'O, P. O. (1980): Role of superoxide in deoxyribonucleic acid strand scission. *Biochemistry*, 19:3023–3028.
43. Lorentzen, R. J., Lesko, S., McDonald, K., and Ts'O, P. O. (1979): Toxicity of metabolic benzo(a)pyrenediones to cultured cells and the dependence upon molecular oxygen. *Cancer Res.*, 39:3194–3198.
44. Mason, R. P., and Holtzman, J. L. (1975): Role of catalytic superoxide formation in the oxygen inhibition of nitroreductase. *Biochem. Biophys. Res. Commun.*, 67:1267–1274.
45. McCord, J. M. (1974): Free radicals and inflammation: Protection of synovial fluid by superoxide dismutase. *Science*, 185:529–531.
46. McCord, J. M., Beachamp, C. O., Goscin, S., Misra, H. P., and Fridovich, I. (1973): Superoxide and superoxide dismutases. In: *Oxidases and Related Redox Systems*, edited by T. E. King, H. S. Mason,

and M. Morrison, pp. 51–76. University Park Press, Baltimore.
47. McCord, J. M., and Day, E. D., Jr. (1978): Superoxide-dependent production of hydroxyl radical catalyzed by iron–EDTA complex. *FEBS Lett.*, 86:139–142.
48. McCord, J. M., and Fridovich, I. (1969): Superoxide dismutase: an enzymic function of erythrocuprein. *J. Biol. Chem.*, 244:6049–6055.
49. McCord, J. M., Keele, B. B., Jr., and Fridovich, I. (1971): An enzyme based theory of obligate anaerobiosis: The physiological function of superoxide dismutase. *Proc. Natl. Acad. Sci. U.S.A.*, 68:1024–1027.
50. Moody, C. S., and Hassan, H. M. (1982): Mutagenicity of oxygen free radicals. *Proc. Natl. Acad. Sci. U.S.A.*, 79:2855–2859.
51. Priestly, J. (1906): *The Discovery of Oxygen. Alembic Club Reprints, Part I, No. 7.* University of Chicago Press, Chicago.
52. Reddy, C. C., Tu, C.-P., and Burgess, J. R. (1981): Evidence for occurrence of selenium-independent glutathione peroxidase activity in rat liver microsomes. *Biochem. Biophys. Res. Commun.*, 101:970–978.
53. Rhodes, M. L., Zavalla, D. C., and Brown, D. (1976): Hypoxic protection in paraquat poisoning. *Lab. Invest.*, 35:496–500.
54. Rigo, A., Stevenato, R., Finazzi-Agro, A., and Rotilio, G. (1977): An attempt to evaluate the rate of the Haber–Weiss reaction by using ·OH radical scavengers. *FEBS Lett.*, 80:130–132.
55. Rose, M. S., Smith, L. L., and Wyatt, I. (1974): Evidence for energy-dependent accumulation of paraquat into rat lung. *Nature,* 252:314–315.
56. Rose, M. S., Smith, L. L., and Wyatt, I. (1976): The relevance of pentose phosphate stimulation in rat lung to the mechanism of paraquat toxicity. *Biochem. Pharmacol.*, 25:1763–1767.
57. Sachs, C., and Jonsson, G. (1975): Mechanisms of action of 6-hydroxydopamine. *Biochem. Pharmacol.*, 24:1–8.
58. Sasame, H. A., and Boyd, M. R. (1979): Superoxide and hydrogen peroxide production and NADPH oxidation stimulated by nitrofurantoin in lung microsomes: possible implications for toxicity. *Life Sci.*, 24:1091–1096.
59. Smith, P., and Heath, D. (1976): Paraquat. *CRC Crit. Rev. Toxicol.*, 4:411–445.
60. Tibaldi, J., Benjamin, J., Cabbat, F. S., and Heikkila, R. E. (1979): Protection against alloxan-induced diabetes by various urea derivatives: relationship between protective effects and reactivity with the hydroxyl radical. *J. Pharmacol. Exp. Ther.*, 211:415–418.
61. Trush, M. A., Mimnaugh, E. G., Ginsburg, E., and Gram, T. E. (1981): *In vitro* stimulation by paraquat of reactive oxygen-mediated lipid peroxidation in rat lung microsomes. *Toxicol. Appl. Pharmacol.*, 60:279–286.
62. Trush, M. A., Mimnaugh, E. G., and Gram, T. E. (1982): Activation of pharmacologic agents to radical intermediates. Implications for the role of free radicals in drug action and toxicity. *Biochem. Pharmacol.*, 31:3335–3346.
63. White, H. L., and White, J. R. (1968): Lethal action of metabolic effects of streptonigrin on *escherichia coli. Mol. Pharmacol.*, 4:549–565.
64. Willson, R. L. (1978): Free radicals and tissue damage: Mechanistic evidence from radiation studies. In: *Biochemical Mechanisms of Liver Injury,* edited by T. F. Slater, pp. 123–224. Academic Press, London.
65. Willson, R. L. (1979): Hydroxy radicals and biological damage *in vitro:* what relevance *in vivo?* In: *Oxygen Free Radicals and Tissue Damage, Ciba Foundation Symposium 65,* pp. 19–42. Excerpta Medica, Amsterdam.

Drug Metabolism and Drug Toxicity,
edited by J. R. Mitchell and M. G. Horning.
Raven Press, New York © 1984.

Metabolic Oxygenation of Organic Nitrogen and Sulfur Compounds

D. M. Ziegler

Clayton Foundation Biochemical Institute and Department of Chemistry, The University of Texas at Austin, Austin, Texas 78712

Foreign compounds bearing nucleophilic nitrogen or sulfur are frequently metabolized by oxygenation of the heteroatom. The nature and reactivity of the oxygenated products are quite diverse and, depending on the particular functional group and other substituents on or near the heteroatom, may be more or less chemically reactive than the parent compound. Properties of initial oxidation products can serve as a guide to physiological response, but reactions subsequent to the initial oxygenation are often responsible for toxic manifestations. Closely related compounds, oxygenated at virtually the same rates, often have very different pharmacological properties. Although information obtained from chemical model or *in vitro* studies must clearly be interpreted with caution, some knowledge of the physical and chemical properties of oxidation products is essential for assessing their potential toxicity. Therefore, the sections on metabolism of specific compounds are preceded by a brief description of the chemical properties of products formed by oxygenation of heteroatom, but the chemistry is restricted to those properties that are relevant to known biological reactions. More detailed descriptions of the chemical properties of *N*- or *S*-oxygenated functional groups can be found in standard references (10,55,56).

ORGANIC NITROGEN COMPOUNDS

The term *N*-oxidation is frequently used to denote addition of oxygen to nitrogen. However, this is technically incorrect, since oxidation at nitrogen refers to any reaction that leads to a greater formal positive charge on the nitrogen. Oxidation at nitrogen can occur in the absence of oxygen or precede addition of oxygen on a neighboring atom. It is therefore necessary to distinguish between oxidation and addition of oxygen. The term oxygenation (or hydroxylation) more accurately describes the latter process, and *N*-oxygenation or *N*-hydroxylation is used exclusively in this section to refer to reactions that lead to the formation of an N–O bond. This distinction appears necessary since metabolic *N*-oxidation of organic nitrogen compounds does not always produce *N*-oxygenated metabolites. In fact, *N*-oxygenated intermediates are rarely formed during oxidative metabolism of physiological amines. Metabolic *N*-oxygenation is largely restricted to xenobiotic compounds.

The metabolism of organic nitrogen compounds by *N*-oxygenation was discovered by Lintzel (41) who reported that trimethylamine administered to humans was largely excreted as trimethylamine *N*-oxide. Subsequent studies with more complex amines showed that *N*-oxygenation is a fairly general route for metabolism of nitrogen compounds, and metabolites produced by an oxidative attack on nitrogen are frequently detected both *in vivo* and *in vitro* (6,31). Interest in this pathway was further stimulated by the pioneering studies of the Millers (see 15) and Kiese (37) on the role of *N*-oxygenation in the metabolic activation of arylamines to more toxic and carcinogenic derivatives (58). The toxicity of a limited number of *N*-oxygenated functional groups has lead to the widespread assumption that *N*-oxygenation produces inherently more reactive metabolites. Although this is true for a few compounds, the vast majority of naturally occurring alkaloids and synthetic medicinal amines are converted to less reactive derivatives upon *N*-oxygenation.

Although metabolism of xenobiotics by *N*-oxygenation is generally accepted, there is less agreement as to the relative contribution of this route to overall metabolism. *N*-Oxygenation is usually considered to be of minor importance when alternate pathways are available. This conclusion is frequently based only on the nature of metabolic end products excreted by intact animals, and there is little question that for some compounds *N*-oxygenation is a minor route for disposition. However, disposition is the net result of formation, metabolism, and elimination—each governed by multiple factors. Since parameters controlling these processes are not known in detail, the relative contribution of a pathway to metabolism would be difficult to predict from metabolic end products excreted in urine or bile.

The contribution of heteroatom oxygenation is more accurately assessed from *in vitro* measurements. Thus, studies with microsomes and tissue homogenates suggest that this is a major route for metabolism of many amines, although considerable species differences have been reported (5,6). Disposition, as well as tissue levels, of *N*-oxygenated metabolites is frequently limited by reduction, and mechanisms for reduction are undoubtedly as important to overall metabolism as the more intensively studied mechanisms for oxidation. Although relatively few studies on reduction of *N*-oxygenated metabolites have appeared, the reduction of *N*-oxides and of hydroxylamines by liver microsomes (33,36) and by purified enzymes (30,35) has been described.

Enzymes Catalyzing *N*-Oxidation

Virtually all studies over the past two decades have concluded that *N*-oxygenation of xenobiotics is catalyzed by NADPH- and oxygen-requiring enzymes. This activity is most concentrated in the microsomal fraction of liver tissue, although it is also detectable in other organelles and in other tissues. The nature and number of *N*-oxidizing enzymes have been the subject of considerable debate (24), but it is now generally accepted that more than one monooxygenase is involved in microsomal catalyzed *N*-oxidation. Although the exact number is still not fully resolved, the oxidation of most functional groups bearing nitrogen is usually attributed either to the flavin-containing monooxygenase or to the cytochrome P-450-dependent family of monooxygenases. These monooxygenases have been purified to homogeneity, and their composition, properties, and general substrate specificities are described in recent reviews (13,61,63).

Many xenobiotic amines are substrates for both the flavin-containing and the cytochrome P-450-dependent monooxygenases. However, the final oxidation products obtained are usually different, and only rarely is the nitrogen of a specific compound *N*-oxygenated by both monooxygenases. This difference in oxidation products must reflect a difference in catalytic mechanism, and recent studies have shown that this is the case. The best current estimates indicate that oxidation of amines catalyzed by cytochrome P-450 occurs by a radical mechanism (59), whereas that of the flavin-containing monooxygenase is best described as ionic (63). A detailed analysis of enzyme reaction mechanisms is beyond the scope of this chapter, but some aspects relevant to *N*-oxidation are summarized below.

The oxidation of amines by a radical mechanism occurs in discrete steps. The initial attack involves abstraction of an electron from the heteroatom followed by radical rearrangement and subsequent oxygenation, as illustrated schematically in the following sequence of reactions.

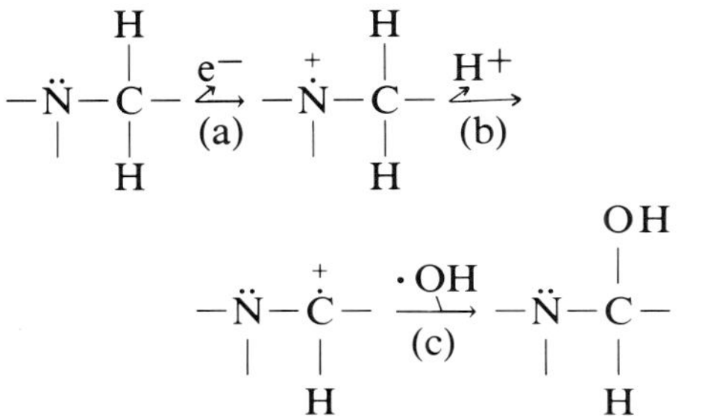

(1)

For simplicity, the nature of neither the oxidant (reaction 1a) nor the oxygenating species (reaction 1c) is specified, although the latter must add at the same redox state as the hydroxy radical. Oxygen at this redox state will add to the electron-deficient atom, and whether oxygenation occurs on the amine cation radical (aminium ion) or on the carbon radical depends solely on the rate of radical rearrangement (reaction 1b). Except for certain amines mentioned below, radical rearrangement is very fast for amines bearing a hydrogen on the α carbon. Therefore, it is apparent that oxidation of alkylamines by this mechanism leads to *C*-hydroxylation, and it is now almost universally accepted that cytochrome P-450 catalyzes *N*-dealkylation of aliphatic amines by rearrangement of the intermediate carbinolamine (the last product shown in the reaction sequence). It is also evident that cytochrome P-450 will catalyze *N*-oxygenation only of those nitrogen compounds that, after initial electron abstraction, cannot readily undergo radical rearrangement. As a first approximation, this would include nitrogen compounds such as arylamines, *N*-arylamides, carbamates, and other nitrogen compounds that lack a hydrogen on the α carbon. *N*-Oxygenation by cytochrome P-450 of certain members of these types of compounds has been fully documented. The presence or absence of a hydrogen on the α carbon is not, however, an infallible guide. For example, charge delocalization on an aminium ion by conjugation with an aromatic system limits *N*-oxygenation and promotes ring hydroxylation. In addition, radical rearrangement is quite restricted in some bicylic secondary amines, and *N*-oxygenation of norcocaine via cytochrome P-450 has been reported (51). However, cytochrome P-450-catalyzed *N*-oxygenation is restricted to relatively few types of compounds, and the vast majority of medicinal amines and naturally occurring alkaloids are not *N*-oxygenated by this monooxygenase.

The flavin-containing monooxygenase, on the other hand, catalyzes the direct insertion of oxygen without forming intermediate radicals. The mechanism of this enzyme is known in some detail (1,4,63), and there is little question that an enzyme-bound flavin hydroperoxide is the oxygenating intermediate. The mechanism is apparently quite similar to that for the oxygenation of nitrogen compounds by organic peroxides illustrated in reaction 2.

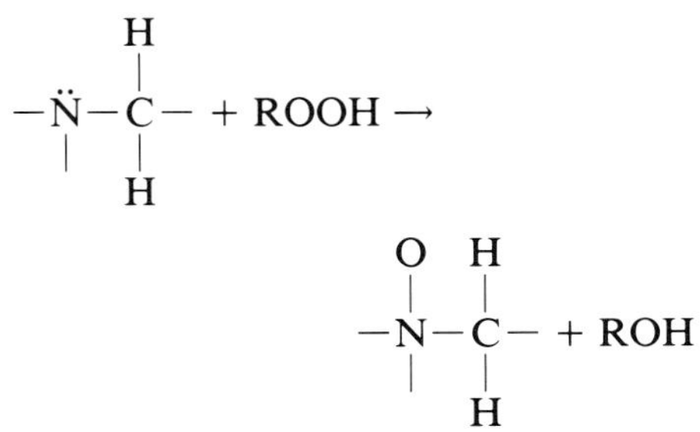

(2)

The reaction can be described as a direct two-electron oxidation of nitrogen without formation of intermediate radicals. The amine simply complexes with the hydroperoxide; this is followed by formation of the N–O bond and heterolytic cleavage of the hydroperoxide. With few exceptions, *N*-oxidation by this mechanism yields *N*-oxygenated products regardless of the nature of substituents on the nitrogen. Enzymatic *N*-oxygenation by this mechanism is only limited by the accessibility of the enzyme-bound hydroperoxide to the substrate. This is governed by steric factors not fully understood, but some structural features that prevent interaction of substrate with the enzyme will be mentioned in sections dealing with the metabolism of specific compounds.

Based on the preceding brief description of reaction mechanisms and on direct measurements, the more common types of functional groups *N*-oxygenated by microsomal monooxygenases are summarized in Table 1. It must be emphasized that the enzyme specificities are only a guide, and there are many exceptions. Nevertheless, an initial evaluation of the biochemical basis for *N*-oxygenation of a specific compound can often be made from the known specificities of these enzymes.

The specificities are based on information collected with purified enzymes as well as on studies carried out with microsomes. In the latter preparations, reactions catalyzed by different monooxygenases are readily distinguished by the use of differential inhibitors or by selective induction. Only the cytochrome P-450 system is induced by pretreating animals with foreign compounds, and this monooxygenase is also selectively inhibited by carbon monoxide and lipophilic primary alkylamines. The primary alkylamines are particularly useful diagnostic tools, since they not only inhibit the cytochrome P-450 system but also activate the flavin-containing monooxygenase.

TABLE 1. *Functional group specificities of major microsomal monooxygenases catalyzing N-oxygenation (61,63)*

	Monooxygenases	
Functional group	Cytochrome P-450	Flavin-containing
Amines		
Primary		
Alkyl	–[a]	–
Aryl	+	–[c]
Secondary		
Dialkyl	–[b]	+
Diaryl	+	–
Alkylaryl	–	+
Tertiary		
Trialkyl	–	+
Dialkylaryl	–	+
Aromatic heterocyclic	+	–
Amides		
N-Alkyl	–	–
N-Aryl	+	–
Hydrazines		
Monosubstituted	+	–[d]
1,2-Disubstituted	+	–[d]
1,1-Disubstituted	–[b]	+

[a] Except for phenteramine and a few other primary amines that do not contain a hydrogen on the α carbon.
[b] Some members of this class may be *N*-oxidized but the cytochrome–metabolite complex prevents turnover.
[c] Except for 2-napthylamine and possibly one or two others.
[d] Most members oxidized only at very high concentrations.

Metabolism

Amines

Hydroxylamines are the initial oxygenated products of primary and secondary amines as illustrated in the following reactions, where R can be either an alkyl (aliphatic) or aryl (aromatic) group.

$$RNH_2 \xrightarrow{[O]} RNHOH \quad (3)$$

$$RNHR \xrightarrow{[O]} RN(OH)R \quad (4)$$

Hydroxylamines are only slightly less basic than their parent amines, and those with lipophilic side chains are readily extracted into organic solvents from neutral or alkaline aqueous solutions. However, the stability of hydroxylamines as the free base is limited, especially in the presence of air or other oxidants. Alkylhydroxylamines are somewhat more stable in acid solutions. Arylhydroxylamines, on the other hand, decompose under acidic conditions, yielding aminophenols and a number of related products. The very reactive amine radical cation is an intermediate in the acid-catalyzed decomposition of arylhydroxylamines and may be responsible for toxicity of this class of hydroxylamines (34).

Hydroxylamines are also susceptible to reduction or further oxidation. Reduction generates the parent amine, but reduction does not present problems in the preparation or use of hydroxylamines. However, the facile oxidation of hydroxylamines and the number of possible products makes their quantitative determination both difficult and frustrating. The nature of the products depends on the number and type of substituents on the nitrogen, as illustrated in the following reactions.

$$\mathrm{ArNHOH} \xrightarrow{[\mathrm{O}]} \mathrm{ArN{=}O} \qquad (5)$$

$$\mathrm{RCH_2NHOH} \xrightarrow{[\mathrm{O}]} \mathrm{RCH{=}NOH} \qquad (6)$$

$$\mathrm{RCH_2\overset{\overset{\large OH}{|}}{N}R} \xrightarrow{[\mathrm{O}]} \mathrm{RCH{=}\overset{\overset{\large O}{|}}{N}R} \qquad (7)$$

Arylhydroxylamines are oxidized to nitroso derivatives (reaction 5), which can react with amines or unreacted hydroxylamine to form highly colored azo and azoxy compounds. Primary aliphatic hydroxylamines, on the other hand, are oxidized to oximes (reaction 6). Oximes are reasonably stable and are frequently the first products detected on direct chemical oxidation of primary aliphatic amines. Nitrones, formed on oxidation of disubstituted hydroxylamines with at least one aliphatic substituent (reaction 7), are much more reactive. Although both oximes and nitrones are subject to hydrolysis, the latter are unusually susceptible to nucleophilic attack and hydrolyze within minutes in aqueous solutions at room temperature as shown in the following reaction.

$$\mathrm{RCH{=}\overset{\overset{\large O}{|}}{N}R} \xrightarrow{\mathrm{H_2O}} \mathrm{RCHO + RNHOH} \qquad (8)$$

However, nitrones with an α-phenyl substituent (i.e., chlordiazepoxide, *N*-methylphenylnitrone) are quite stable.

Virtually all lipophilic primary arylamines are metabolized, at least to some extent, by *N*-oxygenation, as illustrated in Fig. 1 for aniline, the simplest member of the arylamines. The oxidation of aniline to the hydroxylamine is enzymatic, but its further oxidation to the nitroso derivative may be

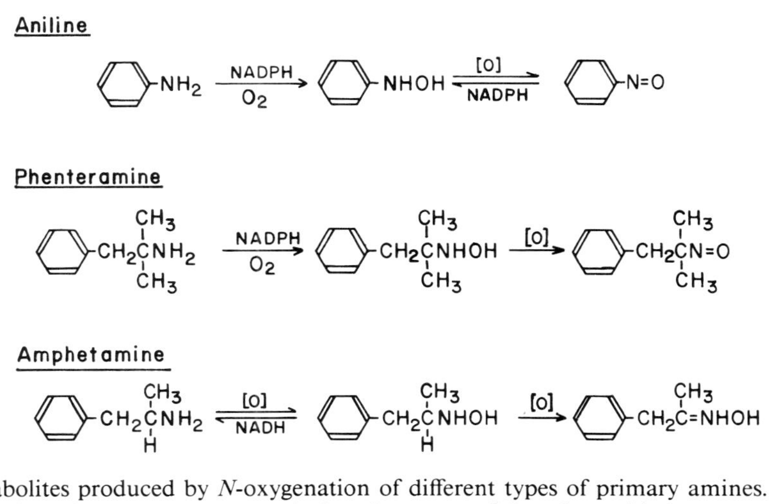

FIG. 1. Metabolites produced by *N*-oxygenation of different types of primary amines. Reactions requiring NADPH and oxygen are enzymatic, but the nature of the other oxidative steps are not known. (Data from refs. 61, 63.)

nonenzymatic. The *N*-hydroxylation of most primary arylamines is catalyzed by the cytochrome P-450-dependent monoxygenase. Some primary arylamines are also substrates for the flavin-containing monooxygenase, but these are limited to those like 2-napthylamine that readily form imine tautomers. Since the imine tautomer of most other arylamines is only a minor species under physiological conditions, the contribution of the flavin-containing monooxygenase to the oxidation of primary arylamines is probably minimal.

N-Hydroxyarylamines are almost without exception more toxic than their parent amines (38), and metabolic formation of hydroxylamines is usually considered a prerequisite for toxicity of primary arylamines. Hydroxylamines are usually not sufficiently reactive to combine with cellular macromolecules, but they yield potent electrophiles on further metabolic transformation. The toxicity and further metabolism of *N*-hydroxylarylamines are discussed in more detail by Thorgeirsson, *this volume.*

In contrast to primary arylamines, primary alkylamines are not usually metabolized by *N*-oxygenation. Phentermine and a few other primary alkylamines that do not have a hydrogen on the α carbon are exceptions. In this respect, these aliphatic amines resemble arylamines and, like the latter, will yield the nitroso derivative on sequential oxidation as shown in Fig. 1. The oxidation of phentermine to the intermediate hydroxylamine is enzymatic and is apparently catalyzed by the cytochrome P-450 system (12). The further oxidation of *N*-hydroxyphentermine may also be enzymatic, but this has not been definitely established. Metabolites that could arise from *N*-oxygenation of amphetamine are also shown in Fig. 1. Although the oxime has been detected in animals treated with amphetamine, the enzymatic basis for its formation is somewhat obscure. Significant oxygenation via cytochrome P-450 is unlikely, since amphetamine and other lipophilic primary alkylamines inhibit this system. This inhibition is caused by a metabolite that complexes strongly with the hemoprotein, preventing turnover (21).

The flavin-containing monooxygenase also does not catalyze *N*-oxygenation of primary alkylamines. Of the numerous primary alkylamines tested with the purified hog liver enzyme, not one is oxidized at a detectable rate. There is no satisfactory electronic basis for this lack of substrate activity towards primary amines, but studies with protein-free 4a-hydroperoxy flavin suggest the same type of specificity (1). Since the enzyme-bound 4a-hydroperoxide is the species responsible for the hydroxylation step, it appears that the functional group specificity of this enzyme resides, to a certain extent, in the nature of the prosthetic group hydroperoxide. Although nonenzymatic oxidation of primary alkylamines cannot be entirely excluded, the absence of a proven enzymatic basis suggests that, as a class, primary alkylamines are probably not metabolized by *N*-oxygenation.

On the other hand, secondary (disubstituted) amines are readily *N*-oxygenated both *in vivo* and *in vitro.* The enzymatic basis for *N*-oxygenation of both acyclic and cyclic secondary aliphatic amines is also well established. Many of a variety of lipophilic secondary amines free from carboxyl, phosphate, or other anionic groups are excellent substrates for the flavin-containing monooxygenase, and this enzyme is usually considered the principal catalyst for *N*-oxygenation of secondary aliphatic amines.

Sequential *N*-oxygenation of secondary amines followed by hydrolysis and reduction of intermediates can generate a large number of metabolites, as illustrated for the oxidative metabolism of methamphetamine (Fig. 2). Methamphetamine is presumably sequentially *N*-oxygenated to the very unstable *N*-hydroxyamine oxide. *N*-Hydroxyamine oxides dehydrate almost instantly to nitrones, and when both alkyl substituents possess hydrogens on the carbon α to the nitrogen, two different nitrones are formed. Hydrolysis of the nitrones (reaction 8) produces two alde-

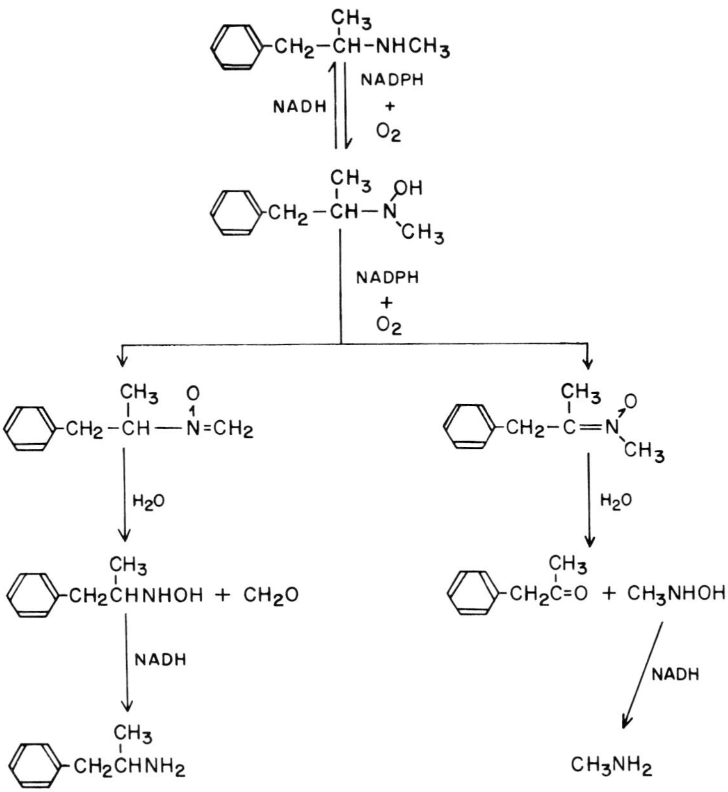

FIG. 2. Potential metabolites generated from sequential *N*-oxygenation of methamphetamine (14).

hydes and two *N*-hydroxyamines, as shown in Fig. 2. Reduction of the hydroxylamines by the microsomal NADH-dependent hydroxylamine reductase generates methylamine and amphetamine, and the enzymatic reduction of both of these hydroxylamines has been described (33). A similar reaction sequence could be written for any number of other secondary amines, and the oxidation of several medicinal amines by this mechanism has been reported (14). It should also be stressed that *N*-oxygenation of secondary amines, followed by reduction of the primary hydroxylamines formed on hydrolysis, gives the same products as those formed by oxidative *N*-dealkylation preceded by hydroxylation of the α carbon. Indeed, a substantial amount of formaldehyde formed in microsomal catalyzed oxidation of *N*-methyl secondary amines is produced by *N*-oxygenation of the nitrogen (50).

Although all of the reactions shown in Fig. 2 have been demonstrated *in vitro,* the contribution of this pathway to the metabolism of methamphetamine or of other secondary amines *in vivo* is not known. Reduction of the initial hydroxylamine would obviously limit generation of subsequent metabolites, and their tissue concentrations would be quite low. Furthermore, virtually nothing is known of the toxicity of nitrones or secondary aliphatic hydroxylamines. The toxicity of some *N*-alkylarylamines (i.e., *N*-methylaniline, *N*-methyl-*p*-aminoazobenzene) may be caused by metabolically produced nitrones, although these nitrones on hydrolysis produce arylhydroxylamines, which are known to be quite toxic. However, the physiological effects of aliphatic nitrones need more thorough investigation before their potential for cell damage can be evaluated.

In contrast to primary and secondary amines, *N*-oxygenation of tertiary aliphatic or heterocyclic aromatic amines produces stable amine oxides.

$$(R)_3N \xrightarrow{[O]} (R)_3N{-}O \xrightarrow{H^+} R_3\overset{+}{N}OH \qquad (9)$$

In aqueous solutions, the oxygen of amine oxides with one or more aliphatic substituents is protonated, and this class of *N*-oxide exists largely as the *N*-hydroxy ammonium salt. Although amine oxides are readily reduced by a variety of strong reducing agents, they are quite resistant to oxidation. Further reactions of amine oxides usually involve rearrangement or cleavage reactions in dehydrating solvents at elevated temperatures. Although these degradative reactions are not physiologically significant, they do limit detection and quantitative analysis of amine oxides by gas–liquid chromatography or mass spectroscopy.

Almost without exception, *N*-oxides of aliphatic tertiary amines are less toxic and pharmacologically less active than the parent amine. Since this is the most common nitrogen-containing functional group present in alkaloids and synthetic drugs, *N*-oxygenation represents a detoxification route for a large number of compounds. Amine oxides are sufficiently polar to clear the kidney, and tertiary amine oxides are frequently detected in the urine of animals treated with tertiary amines (31).

Aliphatic tertiary amines are particularly susceptible to metabolic *N*-oxygenation, and the reaction for a representative acyclic (chloropromazine) and cyclic (guanethidine) aliphatic tertiary amine is illustrated in Fig. 3. The oxidative attack on chloropromazine occurs exclusively on the side-chain nitrogen. Oxygenation of the phenothiazine ring nitrogen cannot be detected either *in vitro* or *in vivo.* Generally, in compounds with more than one nitrogen, the attack takes place on the more nucleophilic nitrogen. This is also evident for the *N*-oxygenation of guanethidine, in which only the ring nitrogen is oxidized. Metabolic *N*-oxygenation of guanidino groups apparently does not occur.

As indicated earlier, the *N*-oxygenation of aliphatic tertiary amines is catalyzed almost exclusively by the flavin-containing mono-

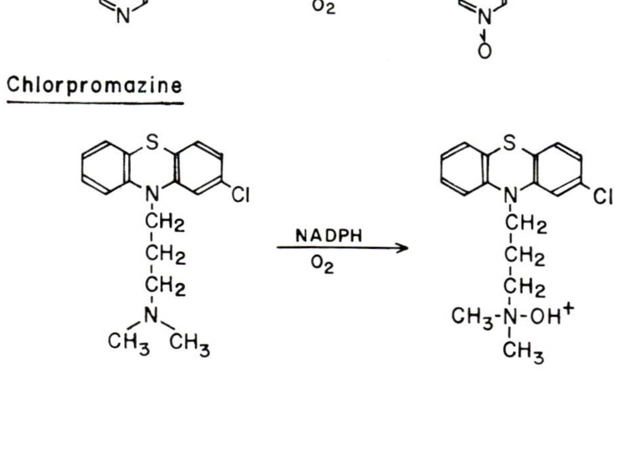

FIG. 3. Types of tertiary amines subject to metabolic *N*-oxygenation. (Data from refs. 24, 23.)

oxygenase. However, this enzyme does not catalyze *N*-oxidation of heterocyclic aromatic amines. Although the number of these compounds metabolized by *N*-oxygenation is limited, the oxidation of 3-methylpyridine (Fig. 3) has been described in reactions catalyzed by liver microsomes (24). The reaction is sensitive to inhibitors selective for the cytochrome P-450 system, and it would appear that *N*-oxygenation of aromatic heterocyclic amines is catalyzed by a cytochrome P-450-dependent monooxygenase. It should be stressed that even under the most favorable conditions, *N*-oxygenation of aromatic heterocyclic amines is very slow compared to other routes of metabolism. In contrast to aliphatic tertiary amines, *N*-oxygenation of aromatic heterocyclic tertiary amines is probably of little physiological significance.

Amides

Hydroxamic acids are the initial products of an oxidative attack on an amide nitrogen, and they may be considered as acyl derivatives of hydroxylamine. The acylhydroxylamines are an extremely diverse and complex group of chemical compounds. However, relatively few are formed (or have been detected) in biological systems. Most interest has focused on *N*-arylhydroxamic acids produced by oxidation of *N*-arylamides.

$$\mathrm{R\overset{\overset{\displaystyle O}{\|}}{C}{-}NHAr} \xrightarrow{[O]} \mathrm{R\overset{\overset{\displaystyle O}{\|}}{C}{-}\overset{\overset{\displaystyle OH}{|}}{N}{-}Ar} \qquad (10)$$

The arylhydroxamic acids retain some of the properties of hydroxylamines, but they are considerably more stable. Although they are readily reduced to amides by a variety of mild reducing agents, they are not as easily oxidized as hydroxylamines. Nevertheless, *N*-arylhydroxamic acids are quite reactive and will undergo complex rearrangements on warming in a number of solvents. They are particularly susceptible to *N–O* acyl transfer and to disproportionation. The *N–O* acyl derivatives are quite reactive, and the biological properties of these and other metabolites of amides are discussed in some detail by S. S. Thorgeirsson, *this volume.*

Hydrazines

Hydrazines are good reducing agents, easily oxidized by a variety of mild oxidizing agents. The oxidative attack occurs on the nitrogen, but the *N*-oxygenated intermediates have not been identified since they are extremely unstable. Their nature can only be inferred from the major reaction products.

Chemical oxidation of hydrazines may occur by one-, two-, or four-electron oxidations, and the products formed will, of course, depend on the extent of oxidation. Metabolic oxidation, however, occurs primarily by two-electron oxidations, so the following section is restricted to products arising from two-electron oxidation of hydrazines.

Hydrazines are probably first oxidized to diazenes (diimides), but the products formed depend on the number and nature of the substituents attached to the nitrogens.

$$\mathrm{RCH_2NHNH_2} \xrightarrow{[O]} \mathrm{RCH_2N{=}NH} \rightarrow \mathrm{RCH{=}N{-}NH_2} \qquad (11)$$

$$\mathrm{RCH_2NHNHR} \xrightarrow{[O]} \mathrm{RCH_2N{=}NR} \rightarrow \mathrm{RCH{=}N{-}NHR} \qquad (12)$$

$$\mathrm{RCH_2(R)NNH_2} \xrightarrow{[O]} \mathrm{RCH_2(R)\overset{+}{N}{=}NH} \xrightarrow{-(H^+)} \mathrm{RCH{=}N{-}NHR} \qquad (13)$$

The intermediate diazenes are tautomeric with the far more stable hydrazones and the latter compounds are usually the first stable derivatives obtained on oxidation of hydrazines. The oxidation of 1,1-disubstituted hydrazines (reaction 13) is undoubtedly more complex than shown. The postulated intermediate quaternary diazene is quite unstable and possibly rearranges through *N*- to *N'* migration of an alkyl group to 1,2-dialkyldiazene, and the latter rearranges to the hydrazone (39). Although hydrazones are fairly stable, in aqueous solutions they are in equilibrium with the corresponding aldehyde and hydrazine, as indicated in the following reaction.

$$RCH{=}N{-}NH_2 \xrightarrow{H_2O} RCHO + NH_2NH_2 \quad (14)$$

The oxidation of alkyl hydrazines can often be measured by following the formation of aldehyde.

As a group, the hydrazines are among the most toxic nitrogen-containing compounds known. This is especially true of simple industrial hydrazines, but some hydrazines employed in the therapy of depression had to be removed from the market because of the high incidence of hepatocellular damage and other toxic reactions.

The exact mechanisms responsible for toxicity of hydrazine and its derivatives are not known. Hydrazines can inhibit monoamine oxidase, and they also undergo a variety of biotransformations including reduction, acetylation, hydrolysis, and oxidation in addition to nonenzymatic Schiff's base formation with carbonyl compounds (32). The contribution of *N*-oxidation to the overall metabolism of hydrazines is also not known, but this route may be especially important for *N*-methylhydrazines.

Major metabolites produced by enzymatic *N*-oxidation of representative methylhydrazines are illustrated in Fig. 4. The oxidative metabolism of methylhydrazines is undoubtedly very complex, and only proven reactions are shown. The diazene is the first product formed on metabolic oxidation of all hydrazines, and further enzymatic, as well as nonenzymatic, reactions depend on the number and types of substituents on the nitrogen. For example, methane is a major product formed

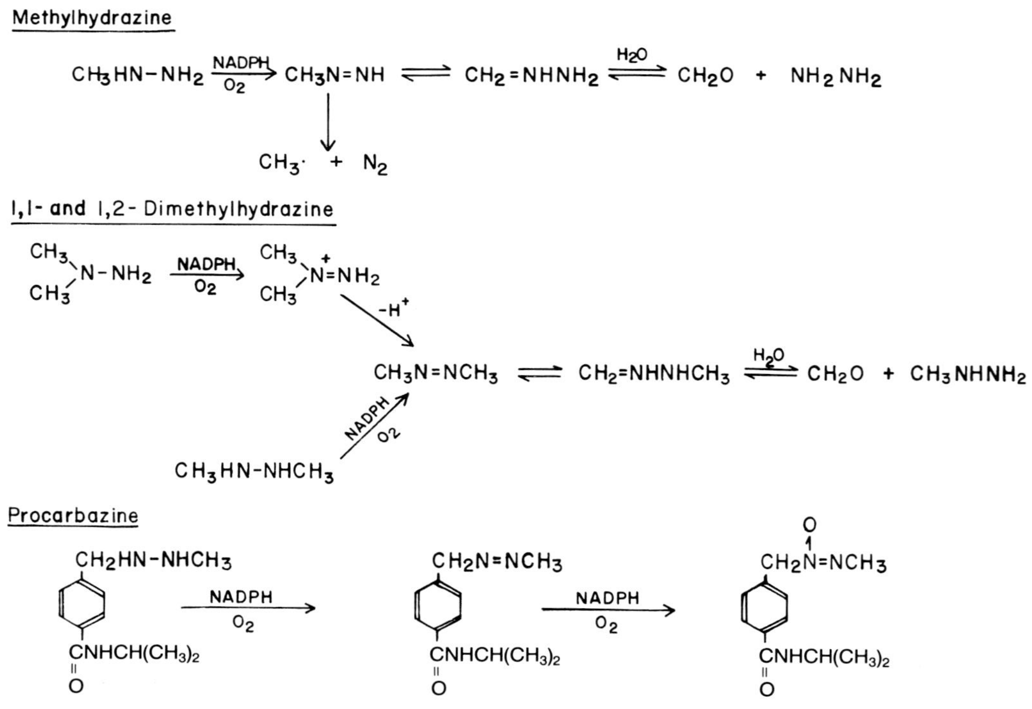

FIG. 4. Major metabolites generated on *N*-oxygenation of simple and complex hydrazines. (Data from ref. 48.)

during microsomal catalyzed oxidation of methyl hydrazine, but not of 1,1- or 1,2-disubstituted hydrazine (49). Methane probably arises from the methyl radical that may be formed, as indicated, by decomposition of methyldiazine, and the formation of radicals could be responsible for toxicity of monosubstituted hydrazines.

Methylhydrazine is also formed metabolically from 1,1- and 1,2-dimethylhydrazine through hydrolysis of the intermediate hydrazone produced by rearrangement of the respective diazenes. Although symmetrical and unsymmetrical hydrazines yield identical products on oxidation and hydrolysis, the initial oxidation is catalyzed by different enzymes. 1,2-Dimethylhydrazine, procarbizine, and other 1,2-substituted hydrazines are oxidized by the microsomal cytochrome P-450 system and by the mitochondrial monoamine oxidase (47,62). However, 1,1-disubstituted hydrazines form an inhibitory complex with cytochrome P-450, which limits their net metabolism by this enzyme (28). The most recent work indicates that oxidative metabolism of 1,1-disubstituted hydrazines is catalyzed exclusively by the flavin-containing monooxygenase (48). Differences in tissue distribution of these oxidative enzymes may, in part, account for some of the differences in toxicity of symmetrical and unsymmetrical hydrazines.

1,2-Disubstituted hydrazines are also capable of undergoing sequential oxidation to azoxy derivatives, as illustrated for the oxidation of procarbizine. The azoxy derivative of dimethyldiazine (azomethane) has also been detected in animals treated with 1,2-dimethylhydrazine (19). The azoxy metabolites are reactive and readily form covalent adducts with cellular macromolecules (60). However, as stated earlier, there may be several pathways for metabolic activation of hydrazines, and the relative importance of oxidation is not known.

ORGANIC SULFUR COMPOUNDS

The chemistry of sulfur rivals that of carbon in its complexity, and the number of different stable configurations of sulfur in organic compounds is large. Organic sulfur compounds can also exist in a wide range of oxidation states that exhibit marked differences in physical and chemical properties. The great diversity of organic sulfur compounds precludes an extensive review of all functional groups bearing this element. Only a few representative examples of foreign compounds known to undergo metabolic *S*-oxygenation are considered. However, this does not imply that functional groups omitted are not metabolized by *S*-oxygenation. Sulfur in most organic configurations is quite nucleophilic, and nucleophilic atoms are usually susceptible to metabolic oxidation. It is likely that as more compounds are examined, metabolism by oxidation at sulfur may prove to be a general route for metabolism of compounds bearing this element.

Enzymes Catalyzing *S*-Oxygenation

The molecular basis for *S*-oxygenation of xenobiotic compounds is not well defined, since relatively few studies have addressed this problem. Although *S*-oxygenation of foreign compounds by microsomes supplemented with NADPH and oxygen has been demonstrated repeatedly, the facile oxidation of sulfur compounds by hydrogen peroxide and other species of reduced oxygen frequently complicates interpretation of *in vitro* studies. Microsomes are known to generate copious quantities of superoxide anion and hydrogen peroxide that, along with lipid peroxides, readily oxidize nucleophilic sulfur compounds. Oxidations dependent on non-enzyme-bound reduced oxygen species are clearly nonenzymatic even though the oxidants may be generated enzymatically. The physiological significance of nonenzymatic oxidations is questionable, although in whole blood, radical-mediated oxidation of chlorpromazine has been demonstrated (57).

In general, the metabolism of chemically stable compounds depends on enzyme catalysis, and both the microsomal cytochrome P-450 system and the flavin-containing monooxygenase are often implicated in *S*-oxygenations catalyzed by microsomes. The oxidation of functional groups bearing sulfur with purified preparations of these monooxygenases has also been described (26,63), and there is no question that these microsomal enzymes can catalyze oxidation of nucleophilic sulfur compounds. However, a direct comparison of their substrate specificities for sulfur compounds has not been carried out, although from information currently available, it appears that the flavin-containing monooxygenase is the principal enzyme catalyzing oxidation of functional groups bearing sulfur.

In addition to catalysis by monooxygenases, the enzymatic oxidation of sulfides is also mediated by the prostaglandin cyclooxygenase hydroperoxidase (18). In tissues containing relatively high levels of prostaglandin synthetase activity, this peroxidase may provide a significant route for *S*-oxygenation of some sulfides. Whether the peroxidase can catalyze oxidation of other functional groups bearing sulfur is, however, not known.

The oxidation of sulfur in substrate analogs for a number of oxidative enzymes has also been described (44). The restricted substrate specificity of these enzymes usually limits the extent to which a molecule may be modified, and only closely related analogs are oxidized.

Metabolism

Thiols and Disulfides

Alkyl and aryl thiols are readily oxidized by mild oxidizing agents, and the rapid oxidation of thiols by air in alkaline solutions containing metal ions is well known. An oxidative attack on thiols produces very reactive sulfenic acids that usually react with excess thiol, yielding disulfides.

$$RSH \xrightarrow{[O]} RSOH \xrightarrow{RSH} RSSR + H_2O \qquad (15)$$

Disulfides, usually the first stable oxidation products of thiols, can be oxidized further to sulfonic acids through intermediate thiosulfenic and sulfinic acids

$$RSSR \xrightarrow{[O]} R\overset{O}{\overset{\|}{S}}SR \xrightarrow[H_2O]{[O]} RSO_2H \xrightarrow{[O]} RSO_3H \qquad (16)$$

This reaction is far more complex than indicated above, and the mechanism, as well as the extent, of the reaction depends on conditions used. The reaction can often be terminated at the sulfinic acid, but further oxidation to the sulfonic acid usually occurs with strong oxidizing agents. Sulfinic and sulfonic acids are reasonably stable compounds and readily form crystalline salts with inorganic cations.

Most alkyl and aryl thiols are quite toxic, but the reasons for their toxicity are not known. Although the formation of complexes with metalloenzymes is a likely cause, alkyl and aryl thiols are also rapidly oxidized to sulfenic acids by tissue homogenates. The sulfenic acids react almost instantly with thiols, yielding disulfides. Further enzymatic oxidation of disulfides can be demonstrated *in vitro,* but it is unlikely that this would occur *in vivo.* Metabolically generated alkyl sulfenic acids are preferentially reduced by glutathione, regenerating the alkyl thiol and glutathione disulfide as illustrated in Fig. 5. This cyclic oxidation followed by reduction could eventually deplete tissues of glycogen required for generation of NADPH and also seriously alter cellular redox potentials. Although cyclic oxidation and reduction of foreign thiols may be partly responsible for their toxicity, net metabolism by this route is unlikely, since it could occur only after glutathione depletion. *S*-Methylation followed by sulfoxygenation is usually the major route for disposition of lipophilic alkyl and aryl thiols (22).

The number of different enzymes catalyzing oxidation of lipophilic thiols is not known and is difficult to determine experimentally. As stated earlier, nonenzymatic oxidation of

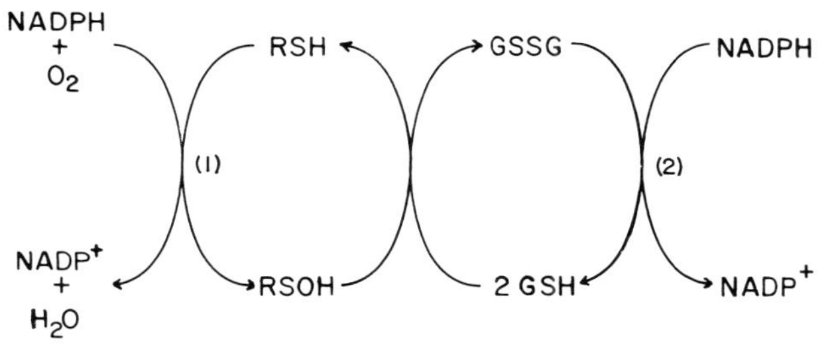

FIG. 5. Cyclic oxidation and reduction of thiols. Reaction catalysts: (1) microsomal monooxygenase(s); (2) glutathione reductase.

thiols by enzymatically generated hydrogen peroxide presents the most problems. At the present time, only the flavin-containing monooxygenase is known to catalyze oxidation of a large number of lipophilic thiols without the intervention of non-enzyme-bound reduced oxygen species. Furthermore, this enzyme can catalyze selective oxidation of xenobiotic thiols in the presence of physiological thiols such as glutathione or cysteine, which suggests that it is capable of oxidizing foreign thiols in whole cells.

Sulfides

The divalent sulfur atom of thioethers is one of the more common forms of this element in medicinal compounds, pesticides, and other xenobiotics. Sulfides are readily oxidized to sulfoxides, which can be further oxidized to sulfones.

$$\mathrm{RSR} \xrightarrow{[\mathrm{O}]} \mathrm{R\overset{\overset{\displaystyle O}{\|}}{S}R} \xrightarrow{[\mathrm{O}]} \mathrm{R\underset{\underset{\displaystyle O}{\|}}{\overset{\overset{\displaystyle O}{\|}}{S}}R} \qquad (17)$$

Both sulfoxides and sulfones are relatively stable and more polar than the parent sulfide. They are also usually less reactive than the parent sulfide, and *S*-oxygenation of this functional group is often a mechanism for detoxication. As a result of their stability and water solubility, sulfoxides and sulfones are the most common *S*-oxygenated metabolites detected in animals treated with sulfides.

Metabolic sulfoxidation is not restricted to a particular type of sulfide, as illustrated by some of the examples listed in Fig. 6. Cyclic as well as acyclic sulfides are oxidized. The presence of basic, acidic, or other complex functional groups does not prevent an oxidative attack on the thioether. It is evident that sulfides are especially prone to oxidation, even in compounds containing other nucleophilic centers.

All of the compounds listed in Fig. 6 are also metabolized to sulfones; however, the amount of sulfone formed both *in vivo* and *in vitro* is usually less than that of the sulfoxide, since increased polarity of the sulfoxide decreases binding to microsomal oxygenases. The amount of sulfoxide available for further oxidation in the intact animal is also limited by reduction. Reduction of sulfoxides is undoubtedly enzymatic, but few studies on mechanism have appeared.

The molecular mechanism for sulfide oxidation is not fully resolved. At least three different microsomal oxidative enzymes are known to catalyze *S*-oxidation of simple sulfides. Sulindac sulfide and some other compounds with anionic groups are preferentially oxidized by the prostaglandin synthetase peroxidase from ram seminal vesicle microsomes (18). However, in other tissues, this and other sulfides are largely oxidized by the flavin-containing monooxygenase or the cytochrome P-450 system. The oxygenation of sulindac sulfides and other achiral sulfides catalyzed by the flavin-containing monooxygenase is almost completely stereospecific (40). Thus, it is evident that oxygenation of sulfides by this enzyme is enzymatic, since stereospecific oxidation requires substrate binding to the asymmetric enzyme cavity. The oxidations of sulfides catalyzed by mi-

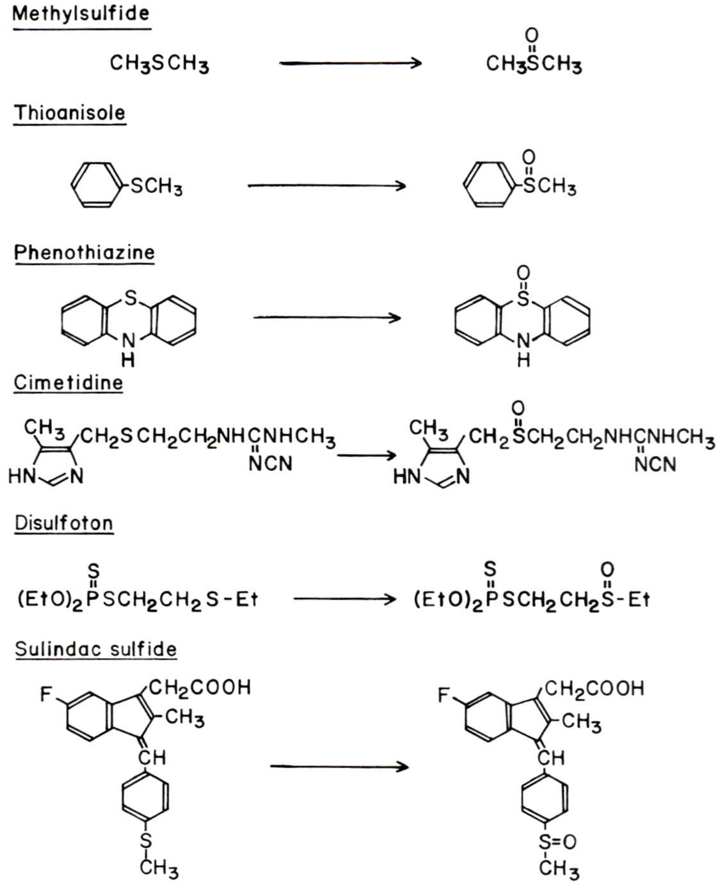

FIG. 6. Types of sulfides metabolized by sulfoxidation. (Data from refs. 18, 63.)

crosomes are frequently not chiral, which raises some question as to the nature of the oxygenation reaction. The lack of chirality suggests that an oxidant released into solution may be the oxidant, and until this problem is resolved, the role of enzymes other than the flavin-containing monooxygenase in the oxygenation of sulfides is difficult to assess.

Thioamides

Thioamides are easily oxidized to sulfoxides (sulfines), which, under more vigorous oxidation conditions, are further oxidized to iminosulfinic acids (sulfenes).

$$\overset{\displaystyle S}{\overset{\|}{RC}}-NH_2 \xrightarrow{[O]} \overset{\displaystyle S{=}O}{\overset{\|}{RC}}-NH_2 \xrightarrow{[O]} \overset{\displaystyle SO_2H}{\overset{|}{RC}}{=}NH \qquad (18)$$

Although some *N*-substituted derivatives are quite reactive, most unsubstituted thioamide sulfoxides are stable and can be isolated as crystalline solids. The dioxygenated product (sulfene) is, however, extremely reactive and only exists as a transient intermediate in solution. The sulfenes are moderate electrophiles, since the sulfinic acid group is a fairly good leaving group. In water, sulfenes hydrolyze almost immediately to amides and thiosulfate. The latter compound is a secondary product formed by disproportionation of the very unstable intermediate sulfoxylate (H_2O_2S)

$$\underset{|}{\overset{SO_2H}{}}\;RC{=}NH + \frac{1}{2}H_2O \rightarrow RC(=O){-}NH_2 + \frac{1}{2}H_2S_2O_3 \qquad (19)$$

The sulfenes will also react with such other nucleophiles as amines, yielding formamidines, but it is not known whether a nucleophilic attack on the sulfene is responsible for covalent binding of metabolically activated thioamides.

Thioamides are quite toxic to animals, and some are also carcinogenic. Thioacetamide, on chronic administration, produces liver tumors in rodents (20), and acute doses cause hepatic necrosis and damage to renal proximal tubules (2,3). The toxicity, and possibly the carcinogenicity, of thioamides is caused by their metabolic oxidation to sulfines (sulfoxides) and sulfenes. Although sulfoxides are more toxic than their parent thioamides (27,45), their deleterious properties are probably related to their further metabolism to sulfenes. This conclusion is supported by the observations of Cashman and Hanzlik (8) that the relative toxicities of different thiobenzamides are related to the rates at which they are metabolized to sulfenes.

The initial oxidative attack on thioamides is catalyzed almost exclusively by the flavin-containing monooxygenase. All thioamides free from anionic groups are rapidly *S*-oxygenated to sulfoxides, as illustrated in Fig. 7. Substituents on the thioamide will affect K_m but have little or no effect on maximum velocities. At saturation, all the thioamides listed are oxidized at the same rate in reactions catalyzed by the purified monooxygenase (63). Further oxidation of the sulfoxides to sulfenes can be detected, but the biochemical mechanism for the second oxidative step has not been satisfactorily resolved.

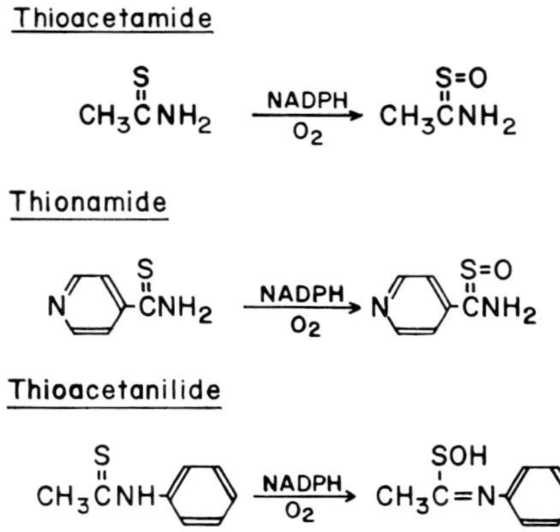

FIG. 7. Sulfoxides (sulfines) formed on enzymatic oxidation of thioamides. The properties of the *N*-arylthioamide (thioacetanilide) sulfoxide suggest that it exists largely as the iminosulfenic acid. (Data from ref. 27.)

Although the toxicity of most thioamides may be caused by their oxidation to sulfenes, this may not be entirely true of *N*-aryl thioamides. For example, the sulfoxide of thioacetanilide differs in chemical properties from that of an unsubstituted thioamide since it is readily reduced by glutathione. In this respect, thioacetanilide resembles the thiocarbamides, and one would anticipate that the toxic reactions of thioacetanilide are closer to those of the thiocarbamides than the thioamides.

Thiocarbamides

The thiocarbamides (thioureas) are similar in structure to thioamides, but the properties of the *S*-oxygenated derivatives are quite different. Thiocarbamides are readily oxidized to formamidine sulfonic acids through intermediate formamidine sulfenic and sulfinic acids.

$$RN{=}C(SH)NH_2 \xrightarrow{[O]} RN{=}C(SOH){-}NH_2 \xrightarrow{[O]} RN{=}C(SO_2){-}NH_2 \xrightarrow{[O]} RN{=}C(SO_3H){-}NH_2 \qquad (20)$$

TABLE 2. *Kinetic constants for sequential oxygenation of thiocarbamides*

Substrate	Kinetic constants (μM)[a] K_{m_1}	K_{m_2}
Thiourea	22	140
Ethylenethiourea	31	150
Phenylthiourea	5	30
Thiocarbanilide	6	7
Methimazole	6	22
2-Mecaptobenzimadazole	11	23

[a] K_{m_1} is the apparent Michealis constant for oxidation of the compound listed to the corresponding sulfenic acid. K_{m_2} is the constant for oxidation of the sulfenic acid to the sulfinic acid. Constants based on reaction velocity obtained with purified hog liver FAD-containing monooxygenase (46).

The first oxidation product, the formamidine sulfenic acid, is the most unstable and readily disproportionate on concentration (46). Like alkyl sulfenic acids, formamidine sulfenic acids are reduced by glutathione and other thiols.

The higher oxidation states are more stable, and a number of formamidine sulfinic and sulfonic acids are available as crystalline solids. However, in solution they are quite easily hydrolyzed to ureas. The sulfonic and, to a lesser degree, the sulfinic group can also be displaced by amines and other nucleophiles, and *N*-substituted guanidines are frequently synthesized by the reaction of formamidine sulfinic acids with amines as shown below.

$$\mathrm{R_1N{=}\overset{\displaystyle SO_2^-}{\overset{|}{C}}{-}NH_2 + RNH_2 \longrightarrow R_1N{=}\overset{\displaystyle NHR}{\overset{|}{C}}{-}NH_2 + \frac{1}{2}S_2O_3^{2-} + \frac{1}{2}H_2O} \qquad (21)$$

The reaction is base catalyzed, but rates at or near physiological pH are still detectable. Sulfinic acids generated metabolically are, therefore, sufficiently reactive to bind covalently to amino groups of proteins and other cellular macromolecules, and the toxicity of thiocarbamides has been known for some time.

At toxic doses, thiourea and its derivatives produce pulmonary edema and pleural effusion in susceptible animals (52). At one time it was thought that hydrogen sulfide liberated by reductive desulfuration was responsible, but more recent work has demonstrated that thiocarbamides are metabolized by sequential oxygenation of the sulfur to sulfinic acids through intermediate sulfenic acids (7,46). Both oxidative reactions are catalyzed almost exclusively by the flavin-containing monooxygenase, and the sequential oxygenation is unusual in that the K_ms of the sulfenic acids are only about 10-fold higher than the K_ms of the parent thiocarbamide (Table 2). This demonstrates that significant quantities of thiocarbamides administered to animals can be converted to sulfinic acids even though the first product, the formamidine sulfenic acid (like other sulfenic acids), is rapidly reduced by glutathione (Fig. 5). Although the latter reaction can explain the glycogen-depleting effects of thioureas (23), the formamidine sulfinic acids are probably the metabolites responsible for toxicity. Formamidine sulfinic acids can form covalent adducts with cellular macromolecules, probably by reacting with amino groups as illustrated in reaction 21. This reaction is consistent with the observation that the sulfur atom of thioureas is lost from thiocarbamide–protein adducts formed *in vivo* (29).

Mercaptobenzimadazoles are structurally similar to thiocarbamides and, like the latter, are rapidly metabolized to sulfinic acids. Kinetic constants for the two, listed in Table 2, show that the concentration of substrate required for half-maximal velocity for both oxidative steps is quite low, and mercaptoimadazoles are metabolized by essentially the same mechanism as the thioureas. However, imidazole sulfinic acids hydrolyze almost immediately to imidazole and sulfite by a mechanism quite different from that for the hydrolysis of formamidine sulfinic acids. This rather striking difference in properties of these sulfinic acids may be responsible for differences in teratogenicity of ethylenethiourea and 2-mercaptoimadazoles (53).

Thiocarbamates and Related Compounds

Thiocarbamates, like sulfides, can be oxidized to sulfoxides and sulfones by peracids.

$$\mathrm{RNH\overset{\overset{\displaystyle O}{\|}}{C}-S-R_1 \xrightarrow{[O]} RNH\overset{\overset{\displaystyle O}{\|}}{C}-\overset{\overset{\displaystyle O}{\|}}{S}=R_1 \xrightarrow{[O]}}$$

$$\mathrm{RNH\overset{\overset{\displaystyle O}{\|}}{C}-\underset{\underset{\displaystyle O}{\|}}{\overset{\overset{\displaystyle O}{\|}}{S}}-R_1} \qquad (22)$$

The *S*-oxygenated thiocarbamates differ considerably from thioether sulfoxides in that the hydrolytic stability of the former is greatly diminished. Thiocarbamate sulfones are especially susceptible to hydrolysis and usually decompose within minutes in alkaline aqueous solutions. Although thiocarbamate sulfoxides are somewhat more stable, they are quite susceptible to carbamylation by glutathione or other thiols, as indicated in reaction 23.

$$\mathrm{RNH\overset{\overset{\displaystyle O}{\|}}{C}-\overset{\overset{\displaystyle O}{\|}}{S}-R_1 + GSH \rightarrow RNH\overset{\overset{\displaystyle O}{\|}}{C}-SG + R_1SOH} \qquad (23)$$

S-Oxygenation to the sulfone followed by carbamoyl transfer to glutathione is an important route for detoxification of most thiocarbamate herbicides containing *S*-alkyl or *S*-benzyl substituents (9). However, sulfoxides of *S*-chloroallyl thiocarbamates also undergo an unusual sigmatropic rearrangement to an intermediate that releases 2-chloroacrolein on decomposition, as indicated in Fig. 8 (54). The latter compound is a potent mutagen, and its formation through spontaneous decomposition of the metabolically formed sulfoxide may account for the carcinogenicity of the *S*-chloroallyl thiocarbamates. In tissues, the sulfoxide would also be detoxified by carbamoyl transfer to glutathione, and cellular concentrations of 2-chloroacrolein would depend on relative rates of the two competing reactions shown in Fig. 8. This suggests that toxicity of *S*-chloroallyl thiocarbamates may be quite sensitive to the status of cellular glutathione.

The enzymatic basis for the metabolism of thiocarbamates is not known in detail. However, oxygenation of the sulfur is catalyzed by a microsomal oxygenase with the characteristics of the cytochrome P-450 system. Other enzymatic routes for oxygenation of thiocarbamates have not been described, and cytochrome P-450 may play a central role in initiating the metabolism of compounds bearing this functional group. Carbamoyl transfer subsequent to *S*-oxygenation is catalyzed by liver cytosol, presumably by a glutathione *S*-transferase, although this has not been verified by studies with purified preparations.

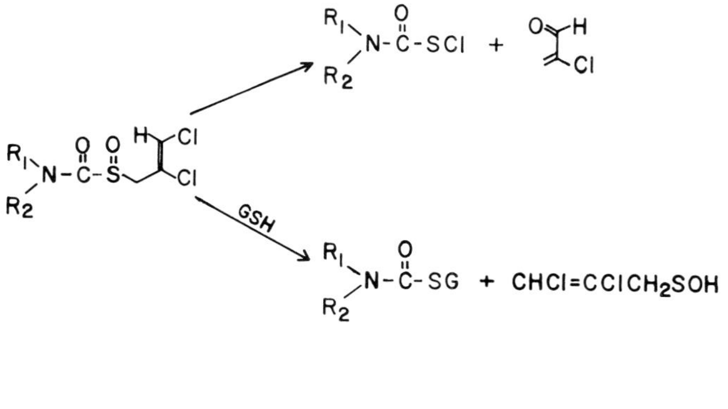

FIG. 8. Alternate routes for decomposition of *S*-alkylthiocarbamate sulfoxides. (Data from ref. 54.)

Carbon Disulfide

Carbon disulfide, the dithio analog of carbon dioxide, is an important industrial solvent. It is an extremely flammable liquid readily oxidized to carbon dioxide and sulfur dioxide by oxygen and other strong oxidizing agents. The toxicity of carbon disulfide is, at least in part, related to intracellular oxidation. The metabolism, examined in some detail by Neal and his associates (16,17) involves an initial oxidative desulfuration (reaction 24) followed by hydration and decomposition of the intermediate carbonyl sulfide (reaction 25).

$$CS_2 \xrightarrow[O_2]{NADPH} S{=}C{=}O + [S] \quad (24)$$

$$S{=}C{=}O + H_2O \rightleftharpoons H_2CO_2S \rightarrow H_2S + CO_2 \quad (25)$$

The oxidative desulfuration, catalyzed by cytochrome P-450, yields sulfur at the oxidation state of atomic sulfur in addition to carbonyl sulfide. The exact nature of the sulfur released is not known, but there is little question that sulfur at the redox state of atomic sulfur would be reduced to H_2S in the strong reducing environment present in cells.

Hydrogen sulfide is also generated by decomposition of monothiocarbonic acid formed by hydration of carbonyl sulfide. The hydration reaction, catalyzed by carbonic anhydrase (11), is quite rapid and can generate copious quantities of H_2S. The toxicity of hydrogen sulfide is well known, and the toxicity of carbon disulfide is undoubtedly related to the generation of this toxin by both initial oxidative desulfuration and subsequent hydrolysis of the intermediate carbonyl sulfide.

Phosphothionates

Phosphothionates are derivatives of phosphate esters in which one or more of the oxygens is replaced by sulfur. This type of functional group is present in a number of widely used pesticides, and their commercial importance has stimulated considerable work on their metabolism in mammals. Prior to 1970, it was assumed that phosphothionates were metabolized by esterase-catalyzed hydrolysis of one or more of the phosphate ester bonds. However, subsequent studies by Neal and his associates (42,43) clearly showed that this type of functional group is also metabolized by an initial oxidative attack on the thione sulfur.

The transformations of parathion shown in Fig. 9 summarize the generally accepted pathways for oxidative metabolism of phosphothionates. The oxidative attack is catalyzed by a microsomal cytochrome P-450-dependent monooxygenase. The initial product is presumably the sulfoxide which can undergo a number of rearrangement and decomposition reactions. Displacement of sulfur by oxygen and hydrolytic cleavage of one of the phosphate ester bonds are the prin-

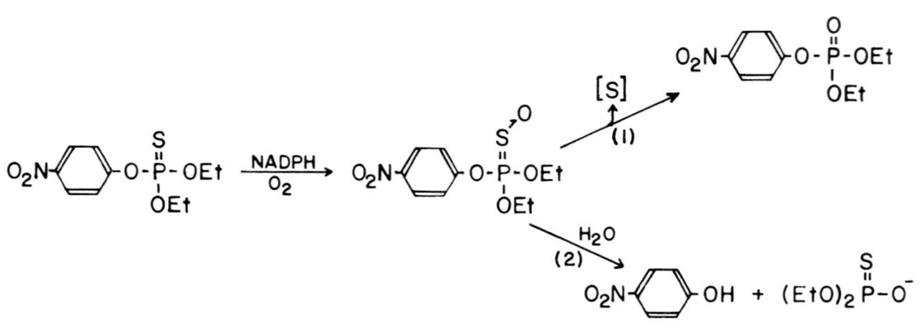

FIG. 9. Major metabolites formed on *S*-oxidation of parathion. The intermediate *S*-oxide formed enzymatically can decompose to more toxic metabolites (reaction 1) or to less reactive derivatives (reaction 2). Scheme based on information contained in Neal et al. (Data from refs. 42, 43.)

cipal reactions. Chemical model studies show that the oxygen replacement reaction usually predominates (43). The oxygen incorporated into the oxon product (paraoxon) comes from molecular oxygen and not from water. The chemical mechanism for rearrangement of the intermediate sulfoxide is not known, but sulfur replacement by oxygen, occurring through a three-membered cyclic resonance form similar to the oxythiranes, is most likely. Sulfur in this mechanism is displaced at the oxidation state of elemental sulfur, but release as free sulfur is highly unlikely. Concerted transfer to cellular nucleophiles is chemically more feasible. Regardless of mechanism, the released sulfur would be reduced to H_2S by glutathione. Rapid local generation of H_2S may be responsible for hepatotoxicity and destruction of cytochrome P-450 observed in animals treated with parathion. The oxon product, paraoxon, is also a potent anticholinesterase, and it is evident that *S*-oxidation of phosphothionates can lead to a number of toxic products.

REFERENCES

1. Ball, S., and Bruice, T. C. (1980): Oxidation of amine by a 4a-hydroperoxyflavin. *J. Am. Chem. Soc.,* 102:6498–6503.
2. Barker, E. A., and Smukler, E. A. (1972): Altered microsome function during acute thioacetamide poisoning. *Mol. Pharmacol.,* 8:318–326.
3. Barker, E. A., and Smukler, E. A. (1973): Nonhepatic thioacetamide injury: I. Thymic cortical necrosis. *Am. J. Pathol.,* 71:409–418.
4. Beaty, N., and Ballou, D. P. (1980): Transient kinetic study of liver microsomal FAD-containing monooxygenase. *J. Biol. Chem.,* 255:3817–3819.
5. Bickel, M. H. (1969): The pharmacology and biochemistry of *N*-oxides. *Pharmacol. Rev.,* 21:325–355.
6. Bickel, M. H. (1971): *N*-Oxide formation and related reactions in drug metabolism. *Xenobiotica,* 1:313–319.
7. Boyd, M. R., and Neal, R. A. (1976): Studies on the mechanism of toxicity and development of tolerance to the pulmonary toxin α-naphthylthiourea. *Drug Metab. Dispos.,* 4:314–321.
8. Cashman, J. R., and Hanzlik, R. P. (1981): Microsomal oxidation of thiobenzamide. A photometric assay for the flavin-containing monooxygenase. *Biochem. Biophys. Res. Commun.,* 98:147–153.
9. Casida, J. E., Kimmel, E. C., Ohkawa, H., and Ohkawa, R. (1975): Sulfoxidation of thiocarbamate herbicides and metabolism of sulfoxides in living mice and liver enzyme systems. *Biochem. Physiol.,* 5:1–11.
10. Capuzzi, G., and Modena, G. (1974): Oxidation of thiols. In: *The Chemistry of the Thiol Group,* edited by S. Patai, pp. 785–840. John Wiley & Sons, New York.
11. Chengelis, C. P., and Neal, R. A. (1979): Hepatic carbonyl sulfide metabolism. *Biochem. Biophys. Res. Commun.,* 90:993–999.
12. Cho, A. K., Lindeke, B., and Sum, C. Y. (1974): The *N*-hydroxylation of phentermine: Properties of the enzyme system. *Drug Metab. Dispos.,* 2:1–8.
13. Coon, M. J., and Persson, A. V. (1980): Microsomal Cyt. P-450: a central catalyst in detoxication reactions. In: *Enzymatic Basis of Detoxication,* edited by W. B. Jakoby, pp. 117–134. Academic Press, New York.
14. Coutts, R. T., and Beckett, A. H. (1977): Metabolic *N*-oxidation of primary and secondary medicinal amines. *Drug Metab. Rev.,* 6:41–104.
15. Cramer, J. W., Miller, J. A., and Miller, E. C. (1960): *N*-Hydroxylation: a new metabolic reaction observed in the rat with the carcinogen 2-acetylaminofluorene. *J. Biol. Chem.,* 235:885–888.
16. Dalvi, R. R., Hunter, A. L., and Neal, R. A. (1975): Toxicological implications of the mixed-function oxidase catalyzed metabolism of carbon disulfide. *Chem. Biol. Interact.,* 10:349–361.
17. Dalvi, R. R., Poore, R. E., and Neal, R. A. (1974): Studies of the metabolism of carbon disulfide by rat liver microsomes. *Life Sci.,* 14:1785–1796.
18. Egan, R. W., Gale, P. H., and Kuehl, F. A., Jr. (1979): Reduction of hydroperoxides in prostaglandin biosynthetic pathway by a microsomal peroxidase. *J. Biol. Chem.,* 254:3295–3302.
19. Fiala, E. S., Bobotas, G., Kulakis, C., and Weisburger, J. H. (1976): Separation of 1,2-dimethylhydrazine metabolites by high pressure liquid chromatography. *J. Chromatogr.,* 117:181–185.
20. Fitzhugh, O. A., and Nelson, A. A. (1948): Liver tumors in rats fed thiourea or thioacetamide. *Science,* 108:626–628.
21. Franklin, M. R. (1974): Complexes of metabolites of amphetamines with hepatic cytochrome P-450. *Xenobiotica,* 4:133–142.
22. Gillette, J. R., and Kamin, J. J. (1960): The enzymatic formation of sulfoxides: The oxidation of chlorpromazine and 4,4′-diaminodiphenyl sulfide by guinea pig liver microsomes. *J. Pharmacol. Exp. Ther.,* 130:262–267.
23. Giri, S. N., and Combs, A. (1970): Sulfur-containing compounds and tolerance in the prevention of certain metabolic effects of phenylthiourea. *Toxicol. Appl. Pharmacol.,* 16:709–717.
24. Gorrod, J. W. (1978): On the multiplicity of microsomal *N*-oxidase systems. In: *Mechanisms of Oxidizing Enzyme,* edited by T. P. Singer and R. N. Ondarza, pp. 189–197. Elsevier, Amsterdam.
25. Hajjar, N., and Hodgson, E. (1980): Mammalian hepatic microsomal FAD-dependent monooxygenase: Evidence for its role in the sulfoxidation of pesticides. *Science,* 209:1134–1136.

26. Halpert, J., Hammond, D., and Neal, R. A. (1980): Inactivation of purified rat liver cytochrome P-450 during metabolism of parathion. *J. Biol. Chem.*, 255:1080–1089.
27. Hanzlik, R. P., Cashman, J. P., and Traiger, G. J. (1980): Relative hepatotoxicity of thiobenzamides and thiobenzamide-*S*-oxides in the rat. *Toxicol. Appl. Pharmacol.*, 55:260–272.
28. Hines, R. N., and Prough, R. A. (1980): The characterization of an inhibitory complex formed with cytochrome P-450 and a metabolite of 1,1-disubstituted hydrazines. *J. Pharmacol. Exp. Ther.*, 214:80–86.
29. Hunter, A. L., Holscher, M. A., and Neal, R. A. (1977): Thioacetamide induced hepatic necrosis: I. Involvement of the mixed-function oxidase enzyme system. *J. Pharmacol. Exp. Ther.*, 200:439–448.
30. Iwasaki, K., Noguchi, H., Kato, R., Imai, Y., and Sato, R. (1977): Reduction of tertiary amine *N*-oxide by purified cytochrome P-450. *Biochem. Biophys. Res. Commun.*, 77:1143–1149.
31. Jenner, P. (1971): The role of nitrogen oxidation in the excretion of drugs and foreign compounds. *Xenobiotica,* 1:399–418.
32. Jauchau, M. R., and Horita, A. (1972): Metabolism of hydrazine derivatives of pharmacologic interest. *Drug Metab. Rev.*, 1:71–100.
33. Kadlubar, F. F., McKee, E. M., and Ziegler, D. M. (1973): Reduced pyridine nucleotide dependent *N*-hydroxyamine oxidase and reductase activities of hepatic microsomes. *Arch. Biochem. Biophys.*, 156:46–57.
34. Kadlubar, F. F., Miller, J. A., and Miller, E. C. (1976): Hepatic metabolism of N-hydroxy-N-methyl-4-aminoazobenzene and other *N*-hydroxy arylamines to reactive sulfuric acid esters. *Cancer Res.*, 36:2350–2359.
35. Kadlubar, F. F., and Ziegler, D. M. (1974): Properties of a NADH-dependent *N*-hydroxyamine reductase isolated from pig liver microsomes. *Arch. Biochem. Biophys.*, 162:83–92.
36. Kato, R., Iwasaki, K., and Naguchi, H. (1978): Reduction of tertiary amine *N*-oxides by cytochrome P-450. Mechanisms of the stimulation effect of flavins and methyl viologen. *Mol. Pharmacol.*, 14:654–664.
37. Kiese, M. (1966): The biochemical production of ferrihemoglobin forming derivatives from aromatic amines and mechanisms of ferrihemoglobin formation. *Pharmacol. Rev.*, 18:1091–1161.
38. Kiese, M. (1974): *Methemoglobinemia: A Comprehensive Treatise,* pp. 76–163. CRC Press, Cleveland.
39. Lemal, D. M., Menger, F., and Coata, E. (1964): The diazine–hydrazone rearrangement. *J. Am. Chem. Soc.*, 86:2395–2401.
40. Light, D. R., Waxman, D. J., and Walsh, C. (1982): Studies on the chirality of sulfoxidation catalyzed by bacterial flavoenzyme cyclohexanone monooxygenase and hog liver flavin adenine dinucleotide containing monooxygenase. *Biochemistry,* 21:2490–2498.
41. Lintzel, W. (1934): Untersuchungen uber trimethylammonium-basen. III. Trimethylammoniumbasen in menschlichen Harn. *Biochem. Z.*, 273:243–261.
42. Neal, R. A., Kamataki, T., Hunter, A. L., and Catignani, G. (1977): Monooxygenase catalyzed activation of thiono-sulfur containing compounds to reactive intermediates. In: *Microsomes and Drug Oxidations,* edited by V. Ullrich, A. Hildebrandt, J. Roots, R. W. Estabrook, and A. H. Conney, pp. 467–475. Pergamon Press, New York.
43. Neal, R. A., Kamataki, T., Lin, M., Ptashne, K. A., Dalvi, R. R., and Poore, R. E. (1977): Studies on the formation of reactive intermediates of parathion. In: *Biological Reactive Intermediates,* edited by D. Jollow, J. J. Kocsis, R. Snyder and B. Vainio, pp. 320–332, Plenum Press, New York.
44. Phillips, R. S., and May, S. (1981): Enzymatic sulphur oxygenation reactions. *Enzyme Microb. Technol.*, 3:8–18.
45. Porter, W. R., and Neal, R. A. (1978): Metabolism of thioacetamide and thioacetamide *S*-oxide by rat liver microsomes. *Drug Metab. Dispos.*, 6:379–388.
46. Poulsen, L. L., Hyslop, R. M., and Ziegler, D. M. (1979): *S*-Oxygenation of *N*-substituted thioureas catalyzed by the pig liver flavin-containing monooxygenase. *Arch. Biochem. Biophys.*, 198:78–88.
47. Prough, R. A., Coomes, M. W., Cummings, S. W., and Wiebkin, P. (1981): Metabolism of procarbazine. In: *Advances in Experimental Medicine and Biology,* edited by R. Synder, D. V. Parke, J. J. Kocsis, D. J. Jollow, G. G. Gibson, and C. M. Witmer, pp. 983–996. Plenum Press, New York.
48. Prough, R. A., Freeman, P. C., and Hines, R. N. (1981): The oxidation of hydrazine derivatives catalyzed by the purified liver microsomal FAD-containing monooxygenase. *J. Biol. Chem.*, 256:4178–4181.
49. Prough, R. A., Wittkop, J. A., and Reed, D. J. (1970): Further evidence on the nature of microsomal metabolism of procarbazine and related alkyl hydrazines. *Arch. Biochem. Biophys.*, 140:450–458.
50. Prough, R. A., and Ziegler, D. M. (1977): The relative participation of liver microsomal amine oxidase and cytochrome P-450 in *N*-demethylation reactions. *Arch. Biochem. Biophys.*, 180:363–373.
51. Rauckman, E. J., Rosen, G. M., and Cavagnaro, J. (1982): Norcocaine nitroxide—A potential hepotoxic metabolite of cocaine. *Mol. Pharmacol.*, 21:458.
52. Richter, C. P. (1952): The physiology and cytology of pulmonary edema and pleural effusion produced in rats by alpha-naphthyl thiourea. *J. Thoracic Cardiovasc. Surg.*, 23:66–91.
53. Ruddick, J. A., Newsome, W. H., and Nash, L. (1976): Correlation of teratogenicity and molecular structure: Ethylenethiourea and related compounds. *Teratology,* 13:263–266.
54. Schuphan, I., Rosen, J. D., and Casida, J. F. (1979): Novel activation mechanisms for the promutagenic herbicide Diallate. *Science,* 205:1013–1015.
55. Smith, P. A. S. (1966): *Open-Chain Nitrogen Compounds, Vol. II,* pp. 21–36. Benjamin, New York.
56. Sterling, C. J. M. (1974): The sulfinic acids and their derivatives. *Int. J. Sulfur Chem.*, 6:277–316.
57. Traficante, L. J., Sakalis, G., Sierkierski, J., Rotro-

sen, J., and Gershon, S. (1979): Rapid in vitro sulfoxidation of chlorpromazine by human blood: Inhibition by an endogenous plasma protein factor. *Life Sci.*, 24:337–346.
58. Weisburger, J. H., and Weisburger, E. K. (1973): Biochemical formation and pharmacological, toxicological and pathological properties of hydroxylamines and hydroxyamic acids. *Pharmacol. Rev.*, 25:1–66.
59. White, R. E., and Coon, M. J. (1980): Oxygen activation by cytochrome P-450. *Annu. Rev. Biochem.*, 49:315–56.
60. Wiebkin, P., and Prough, R. A. (1980): Oxidative metabolism of azoprocarbazine by rodent liver microsomes. *Cancer Res.*, 40:3524–3529.
61. Wislocki, P. G., Miwa, G. Y., and Lu, A. Y. H. (1980): Reactions catalyzed by the cytochrome P-450 system. In: *Enzymatic Basis of Detoxication, Vol. 1,* edited by W. B. Jacoby, pp. 135–182. Academic Press, New York.
62. Wittkop, J. A., Prough, R. A., and Reed, D. J. (1969): Oxidative demethylation of *N*-methylhydrazines by rat liver microsomes. *Arch. Biochem. Biophys.*, 134:308–315.
63. Ziegler, D. M. (1980): Microsomal flavin-containing monooxygenase: oxygenation of nucleophilic nitrogen and sulfur compounds. In: *Enzymatic Basis of Detoxication,* edited by W. B. Jakoby, pp. 201–227. Academic Press, New York.

Drug Metabolism and Drug Toxicity,
edited by J. R. Mitchell and M. G. Horning.
Raven Press, New York © 1984.

Biotransformation of Halogenated Hydrocarbons

[1]M. W. Anders

Department of Pharmacology, University of Minnesota, Minneapolis, Minnesota 55455

Halogenated hydrocarbons are a large group of chemicals of widely varying physical and chemical properties. Many halogenated hydrocarbons are manufactured in very large quantities and are used extensively in commerce and industry; it is estimated that the United States and world production of halocarbons exceeded 10 and 20 billion pounds, respectively, in 1973 (45). Such extensive production is sometimes accompanied by contamination of the ecosystem. Many halogenated hydrocarbons have been identified as contaminants of drinking water, and haloforms are formed during the chlorination of municipal drinking water supplies (42). The human health risk associated with exposure to halogenated hydrocarbons cannot be estimated accurately, but, because many halogenated chemicals are suspected mutagens (45), and some, e.g., vinyl chloride (86), are known human carcinogens, legitimate concern can be raised.

The toxicity of most halogenated hydrocarbons is dependent on metabolic activation, and this biotransformation is usually accompanied by dehalogenation. The toxicity of halogenated chemicals may be associated with biotransformation to stable, but toxic, metabolites. For example, dihalomethanes and haloforms are metabolized to carbon monoxide (3,83), and inorganic fluoride is formed as a metabolite of methoxyflurane (102). Biotransformation frequently yields highly reactive electrophilic metabolites as in the metabolism of chloroform to phosgene (118), of chlorinated ethylenes to oxiranes (15), and of *Z*-1,2-dichlorocyclohexane to a thiiranium ion (160).

The objective of this chapter is to summarize the existing body of knowledge concerning the biotransformation of halogenated hydrocarbons. Particular emphasis is given to the reaction mechanisms involved in the biotransformation of halogenated hydrocarbons.

Several reviews describing the metabolism and toxicity of halogenated hydrocarbons have been published (7,17,163,166). In addition, monographs concerned with the chemistry of the carbon–halogen bond (114) and the metabolism of volatile anesthetics (37) have appeared.

HALOGENATED ALKANES

Oxidative and Oxygenation Reactions[2]

The most important oxidative reaction of halogenated alkanes is C–H sigma bond ox-

[1] *Present address:* Department of Pharmacology, University of Rochester, Rochester, New York 14642.

[2] In this chapter, a distinction is made between oxidative and oxygenation reactions; in the former reaction, a change in the oxidation state of the organic molecule occurs, whereas in the latter reaction, an oxygen atom is incorporated into the metabolite although no change in oxidation state has necessarily taken place. Thus, the conversion of a simple alkyl halide (RCH_2X) to the corresponding alcohol (RCH_2OH) would be classified as an oxygenation, rather than an oxidative, reaction since the oxidation state of the carbon atom is unchanged. As an additional example, the conversion of chloroform (oxidation state = +2) to phosgene (oxidation state = +4)

idation. Direct oxidation of the halogen atom in alkyl halides has not been demonstrated in metabolic experiments, although stable hypervalent aryl iodides, e.g., iodoso- and iodoxybenzene, are well known (10); hypervalent alkyl iodides are unstable but may be formed as intermediates in some chemical reactions (29,129,165). Chlorosoalkanes ($RCl^{+}O^{-}$) have not been described and, indeed, would not be expected to exist because the oxidation potential of covalently bound chlorine is so high that oxidative reactions will only occur in other parts of the molecule (30). Thus, the suggestion that 1-chloroso-2-chloroethane may be formed as an intermediate in 1,2-dichloroethane metabolism is unlikely (53).

A general scheme for the oxidation or oxygenation of alkyl halides to alcohols, aldehydes, or acids is shown in Fig. 1. The first step in the reaction is a cytochrome P-450-dependent monooxygenation reaction yielding the intermediate *gem*-halohydrin [R-CH(OH)X; R-CX_2(OH)]; such intermediates are unstable and lose HX to form the aldehyde or acyl halide, which may undergo subsequent conversion to the alcohol or acid. It should be noted that the direct metabolic substitution of a hydroxyl group for a halide, the so-called "hydrolytic dehalogenation" (166), has not been unequivocally demonstrated but can be explained by the sequence:

$$\text{R-CH}_2\text{-X} \rightarrow \text{R-CH(OH)-X} \rightarrow \text{R-C(=O)H} \rightarrow \text{R-CH}_2\text{-OH}$$

Several lines of evidence support the reaction sequence shown in Fig. 1. First, the involvement of the microsomal cytochrome P-450-dependent polysubstrate monooxygenase system was proven by the finding that a purified and reconstituted monooxygenase system catalyzed the dechlorination of 1,1,2-trichloroethane (161). In addition, carbon monoxide, a specific inhibitor of cytochrome P-450-dependent monooxygenase reactions, inhibits the biotransformation of chloroform (120), fluroxene (68,70,99), 1,1,2-trichloroethane (161), 2,2,2-trifluoroethyl ethyl ether (68), enflurane (69), and methoxyflurane (69).

Inhibitors of the cytochrome P-450-dependent monooxygenase system also inhibit alkyl halide metabolism. For example, SKF 525-A (2-diethylaminoethyl-2,2-diphenylvalerate HCl) inhibits the microsomal metabolism of dihalomethanes (79) and haloforms (3) to carbon monoxide, of chloroform to carbon dioxide (85) and phosgene (120), of methoxyflurane to inorganic fluoride (40), and of fluroxene to 2,2,2-trifluoroethanol (99).

In addition, carbon tetrachloride treatment, which is known to lower hepatic cytochrome P-450 concentrations, decreases the metabolism of fluroxene (13) and halothane (133); however, halothane defluorination was not decreased in carbon tetrachloride-treated mice (50).

Many compounds have been shown to interact with oxidized cytochrome P-450 to produce characteristic difference spectra (95,139). A number of alkyl halides have been shown to produce typical type I (λ_{max} 385–390 nm, λ_{min} 418–427 nm) difference spectra including polyhalogenated methanes (41,106), ethanes (106,116), fluroxene (68), and 2,2,2-trifluoroethyl ethyl ester (68).

Finally, treatment of animals with many drugs has been shown to increase both the hepatic microsomal cytochrome P-450 content and rates of drug metabolism (38,112). Phenobarbital treatment leads to increased rates of metabolism of many halogenated alkanes, including the biotransformation of dihalomethanes (79) and haloforms (3) to carbon monoxide and the defluorination of anesthetic agents (1,50,103,104,135,162). Recent studies have shown that isoniazid,

or carbon dioxide (oxidation state = +4) is an oxidation, whereas the conversion of carbon tetrachloride (oxidation state = +4) to phosgene or carbon dioxide occurs without a change in oxidation state but with the incorporation of oxygen and would be described as an oxygenation reaction. For a discussion of oxidation states of organic molecules, the reader should consult an organic chemistry text such as Hendrickson et al. (58).

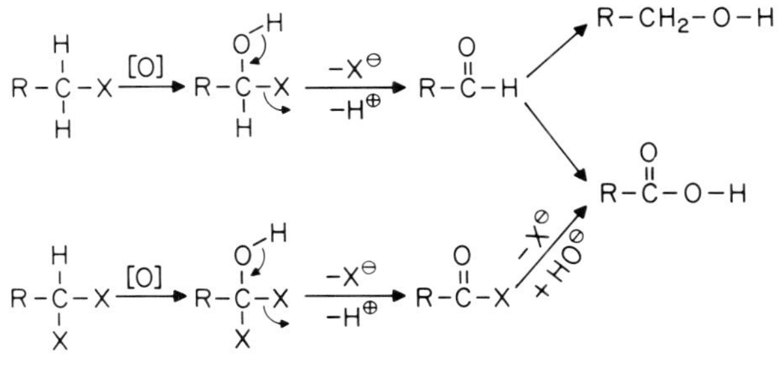

FIG. 1. Reaction mechanism for the metabolism of 1-haloalkanes and 1,1-dihaloalkanes to alcohols and acids. [O], cytochrome P-450-catalyzed oxidation.

but not phenobarbital, treatment increased the defluorination of enflurane, suggesting that isoniazid may represent a new class of enzyme inducer (134,135); the induction of unique forms of cytochrome P-450 appears to be a common phenomenon (112). Similarly, 2-propanol treatment of rats selectively induces the biotransformation of carbon tetrachloride to phosgene and increases the hepatotoxicity of carbon tetrachloride (56).

Reaction mechanism studies also support the metabolic scheme shown in Fig. 1. If C–H sigma bond cleavage is important, a deuterium isotope effect should be observed. For example, a large deuterium isotope effect ($V_{max_H}/V_{max_D} = 7.7$) is seen in the metabolism of dichloromethane to carbon monoxide (80). Similar results have been obtained in studies on the metabolism of haloforms to carbon monoxide (9,145) and phosgene (120), of methoxyflurane (62) and enflurane (23) to inorganic fluoride, and of halothane to bromide (142). Furthermore, if a cytochrome P-450-catalyzed oxidation or oxygenation is involved, the oxygen atom appearing in the product should be derived from dioxygen rather than from water; this is found in the metabolism of dichloromethane (80) and bromoform (145) to carbon monoxide and of chloroform (119) and carbon tetrachloride (81) to phosgene.

Although few detailed reaction mechanism studies have been conducted, C–H sigma bond oxidation is probably involved in the biotransformation of many halogenated alkanes (Table 1); the examples shown are limited to those in which metabolism was accompanied by dehalogenation and the metabolites were identified with reasonable certainty.

Reductive Reactions

Cytochrome P-450-Dependent Reductions

The first step in this reaction is a cytochrome P-450-dependent one-electron reduction to yield a radical intermediate ($R\text{-}\dot{C}X_2$) and inorganic halide. The radical may abstract a hydrogen atom to yield the reduced alkyl halide and, at the same time, initiate lipid peroxidative changes. The radical may also undergo a second one-electron reduction to yield a carbanionic intermediate ($R\text{-}CX_2^{\ominus}$), which may combine with a proton to yield the reduced alkyl halide or, alternatively, may undergo an α or β elimination to yield a carbene or alkene, respectively.

The best known example of a cytochrome P-450-dependent reduction of an alkyl halide is the biotransformation of carbon tetrachloride to chloroform. This reaction was first described by Butler (25). Subsequent studies have shown that the reaction is catalyzed by NADPH-dependent hepatic microsomal enzymes and is inhibited by carbon monoxide (131); these findings clearly implicate cytochrome P-450 in the reaction. A role for NADPH-cytochrome *c* reductase in the reduction of carbon tetrachloride to chloroform had been suggested earlier (144). The enzyme NADPH–cytochrome *c* reductase is probably not involved, since carbon monoxide, which does not inhibit NADPH–cytochrome *c* reductase, is an effective inhibitor of the reaction (131,169), and treatment of

TABLE 1. *Oxidative metabolism of halogenated alkanes*

Compound	Metabolites	Ref.
Dihalomethanes	Carbon monoxide	(80)
Haloforms	Carbon monoxide Dihalocarbonyl	(145) (96), (119), (145)
Chloramphenicol	Chloramphenicol oxamic acid [(1*R*, 2*R*)-1-nitrophenyl-1,3-propanediol-2-oxamic acid]	(121)
1,2-Dibromoethane	Bromoacetaldehyde	(60)
1,2-Dichloroethane	Chloroacetic acid	(174)
1,1,2-Trichloroethane	Chloroacetic acid	(173)
1,1,1-Trichloroethane	Trichloroacetic acid	(44)
1,1,2,2-Tetrachloroethane	Dichloroacetic acid, trichloroacetic acid, trichloroethanol, glyoxylic acid	(172)
1,1,1,2-Tetrachloroethane	Trichloroethanol, trichloroacetic acid	(66), (175)
	Urochloralic acid, trichloroacetic acid	(117), (153)
Pentachloroethane	Trichloroethanol, trichloroacetic acid	(176)
Halothane	Trifluoroacetic acid	(12), (36), (128), (168)
Methoxyflurane	Methoxydifluoroacetic acid, dichloroacetic acid Oxalic acid	(63) (177)
Fluroxene	Trifluoroethyl glucuronide, trifluoroacetic acid	(13), (49)
Enflurane	Difluoromethoxydifluoroacetic acid	(22), (107)

animals with cobaltous chloride, which reduces cytochrome P-450 levels but fails to alter NADPH–cytochrome *c* reductase levels, decreases carbon tetrachloride hepatotoxicity (147). Finally, purified reconstituted cytochrome P-450-dependent monooxygenase systems have been shown to catalyze the reduction of carbon tetrachloride to chloroform (169).

Recent studies on the mechanism of the reduction of carbon tetrachloride to chloroform indicate that the first step in the reaction is a one-electron reduction to yield the trichloromethyl radical ($\cdot CCl_3$) and inorganic chloride (Fig. 2, reaction 1). The trichloromethyl radical may abstract a hydrogen radical from proteins or lipids to yield chloroform (Fig. 2, reaction 3), which may be metabolized to phosgene. Alternatively, the trichloromethyl radical may undergo a second one-electron reduction to yield the trichloromethyl carbanion (Fig. 2, reaction 4); combination of the carbanion with a proton, which is known to be a very fast reaction (61), would yield chloroform. When the metabolism of carbon tetrachloride to chloroform was studied in the presence of deuterium oxide, little deuterochloroform formation was detected (4,82), suggesting that the trichloromethyl radical, rather than the trichloromethyl carbanion, is the important intermediate.

Other lines of evidence also support the concept that the trichloromethyl radical is an intermediate in carbon tetrachloride reduction. For example, hexachloroethane, which may arise by dimerization of trichloromethyl radicals, has been identified in the tissues of animals given carbon tetrachloride (11,46) and in incubation mixtures containing carbon tetrachloride (155); in the latter study, the amount of hexachloroethane formed was

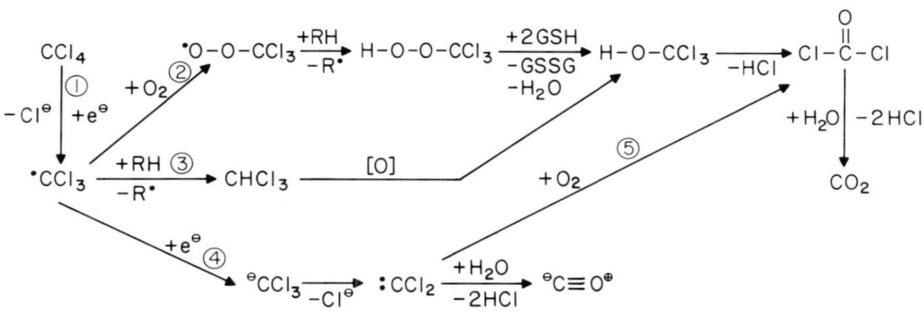

FIG. 2. Metabolic pathways for the metabolism of carbon tetrachloride. RH, unsaturated lipid; R·, lipid dienyl radical; GSH, glutathione; GSSG, glutathione disulfide; [O], cytochrome P-450-catalyzed oxidation.

near the limit of detection. Earlier reports on the direct identification of the trichloromethyl radical by electron spin resonance (ESR) (20,27) have been challenged (101, 138) and rebutted (28).

Subsequent studies reported the identification of the trichloromethyl radical by the ESR analysis of the spin-trapped radical (84,124); other workers suggested that the ESR spectrum identified as the spin-trapped trichloromethyl radical was, instead, consistent with a carbon-centered dienyl lipid radical adduct (74). Reinvestigation of the problem with [^{13}C]carbon tetrachloride yielded an ESR spectrum consistent with the formation of the ^{13}C-trichloromethyl radical spin-trap adduct and a spectrum different from that expected from a carbon-centered dienyl lipid radical or an oxygen-centered trichloromethylperoxy radical (125). Apart from the difficulties encountered in identifying unequivocally the trichloromethyl radical, the well-known ability of carbon tetrachloride to initiate lipid peroxidation is consistent with the generation of a free radical during carbon tetrachloride bioactivation (127,143). Very recent studies have shown that trichloromethyl radical–lipid adducts are formed when human cytochromes P-450 reconstituted in phospholipid vesicles are incubated with carbon tetrachloride (151); these results show clearly that the trichloromethyl radical is an intermediate in carbon tetrachloride metabolism.

In addition to initiating lipid peroxidation, the trichloromethyl radical may react with dioxygen to yield the trichloromethylperoxy radical (Fig. 2, reaction 2) (113), which may also serve as an initiator of lipid peroxidation or may undergo conversion to phosgene (97), a known metabolite of carbon tetrachloride (81,140). Carbon dioxide, a known metabolite of carbon tetrachloride (105,115,136), may arise from the hydrolysis of phosgene.

Carbon monoxide is also a known metabolite of carbon tetrachloride (4,55,171) and probably arises from the hydrolysis of dichlorocarbene formed by the two-electron reduction of carbon tetrachloride to the trichloromethyl carbanion followed by α elimination of chloride (Fig. 2, reactions 1 and 4). Dichlorocarbene may interact with reduced cytochrome P-450 to give rise to a characteristic Soret band (132,157,171). The dichlorocarbene–cytochrome P-450 complex may react with oxygen to yield phosgene (Fig. 2, reaction 5) (97).

Halothane also undergoes a cytochrome P-450-dependent reduction to yield 2-chloro-1,1,1-trifluoroethane and 2-chloro-1,1-difluoroethylene (93,110,141) (Fig. 3). Reaction mechanism studies suggest that the 2,2,2-trifluoro-1-chloroethyl radical is an intermediate in the formation of 2-chloro-1,1,1-trifluoroethane (82); furthermore, a radical formed during halothane metabolism *in vivo* has been spin trapped and detected by ESR (126). Moreover, when halothane

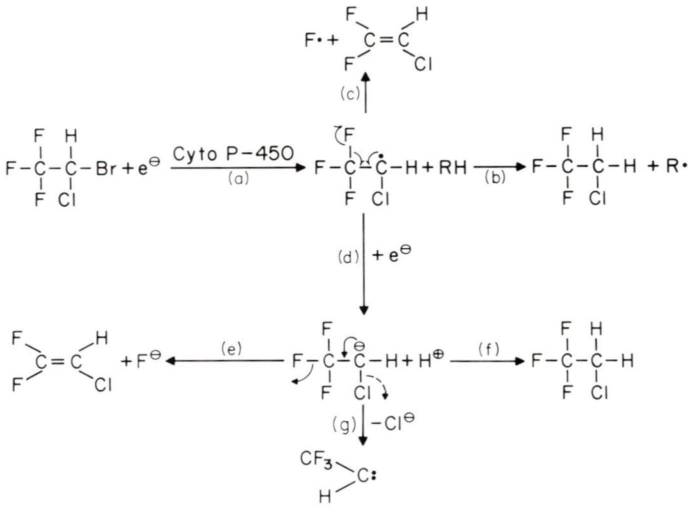

FIG. 3. Reaction mechanisms for the metabolism of halothane to 2-chloro-1,1,1-trifluoroethane and 2-chloro-1,1-difluoroethylene. RH, unsaturated lipid; R·, lipid dienyl radical.

was incubated with cytochromes P-450, NADPH–cytochrome *c* reductase, and cytochrome b_5 in phospholipid vesicles containing dioleoylphosphatidylcholine and egg phosphatidylethanolamine, a mixture of 9- and 10-(1-chloro-2,2,2-trifluoroethyl)-stearate was formed, showing that 1-chloro-2,2,2-trifluoroethyl radical is formed during halothane reduction (152).

Recent studies by Ahr et al. (5) show that 2-chloro-1,1-difluoroethylene is formed by a β elimination of fluoride from the 1-chloro-2,2,2-trifluoroethyl carbanion (Fig. 3, reaction e) rather than by the homolytic elimination of a fluorine radical from the 1-chloro-2,2,2-trifluoroethyl radical (Fig. 3, reaction c). The 2,2,2-trifluoro-1-chloroethyl carbanion can undergo an α elimination to give rise to trifluoromethylcarbene (Fig. 3, reaction g), which reacts with reduced cytochrome P-450 to produce a characteristic difference spectrum (98,155). The reductive metabolism of halothane to trifluoromethylcarbene becomes important at cellular oxygen concentrations lower than about 50 μM since dioxygen competes effectively with the carbene for cytochrome P-450 (111). The electronic spectrum of the cytochrome P-450–trifluoromethylcarbene complex has been calculated and agrees with the results obtained experimentally (92).

Additional examples of cytochrome P-450-dependent reductions of alkyl halides are shown in Table 2.

Glutathione-Dependent Reduction

A limited number of glutathione-dependent reductions of halogenated alkanes have been described. These reactions are probably

TABLE 2. *Cytochrome P-450-dependent reductive metabolism of halogenated alkanes*

Compound	Products	Ref.
Trichlorofluoromethane	Dichlorofluoromethane	(170)
Hexachloroethane	Pentachloroethane, tetrachloroethylene	(149)
Pentachloroethane	1,1,2,2-Tetrachloroethane, trichloroethylene	(149)
DDT	DDD	(164)

catalyzed by glutathione *S*-transferases, but studies with purified enzyme systems have not been reported.

The conversion of 1,2-dihaloethanes to ethylene is catalyzed by glutathione-dependent cytosolic enzymes (90). This reaction may proceed by a nucleophilic attack (S_N2) of glutathione on the 1,2-dihaloethane to yield *S*-(2-haloethyl)glutathione as an intermediate; thiol attack on the sulfur atom of the intermediate would give rise to ethylene and a disulfide (Fig. 4A). The observation that thiols react nonenzymatically with *S*-(2-chloroethyl)cysteine to yield ethylene supports the mechanism described above. Alternatively, glutathione may act as a base, and ethylene may be formed by an E2 elimination reaction from the 1,2-dihalothane (Fig. 4B).

Reaction mechanism studies on the metabolism of *vic*-dihaloalkanes to alkenes have been reported (91). The glutathione-dependent reduction of *meso*-2,3-dibromobutane and *erythro*-2-bromo-3-chlorobutane yielded predominately *E*-2-butene, and racemic 2,3-dibromobutane and *threo*-2-bromo-3-chlorobutane yielded predominately *Z*-2-butene. These results suggest that an enzyme-catalyzed E2 elimination reaction similar to that shown in Fig. 4B is involved. In contrast, *meso*-1,2-dideutero-1,2-dichloroethane yields exclusively *Z*-1,2-dideuteroethylene as a product. This result is consistent with an initial glutathione *S*-transferase-catalyzed nucleophilic attack of glutathione on the substrate to yield *S*-(1,2-dideutero-2-chloroethyl)glutathione; a second reaction of glutathione with the sulfur atom of the intermediate would yield *Z*-1,2-dideuteroethylene and glutathione disulfide as products (Fig. 4A). The intermediate *S*-(1,2-dideutero-2-chloroethyl)glutathione may also rearrange to form an episulfonium ion; such compounds are highly electrophilic and have been implicated as mutagenic metabolites of 1,2-dihaloethanes (159).

α-Haloketones undergo a glutathione-dependent reduction to the corresponding methyl ketones. For example, 2,2′,4′-trichloroacetophenone is metabolized to 2′,4′-dichloroacetophenone by glutathione-dependent cytosolic enzymes (18,64). *S*-(2,4-Dichlorophenacyl)glutathione, which is formed nonenzymatically by reaction of glutathione with 2,2′,4′-trichloroacetophenone, is the substrate for the enzyme. The reaction may involve an enzyme-catalyzed attack of glutathione on the sulfur atom of the substrate to yield glutathione disulfide and the 2,4-dichlorophenacyl carbanion; combination of the carbanion with a proton would give rise to 2′,4′-dichloroacetophenone.

Reactions Involving No Change in Oxidation State

Glutathione Conjugation

Conjugation of alkyl halides with glutathione is a common and important route of

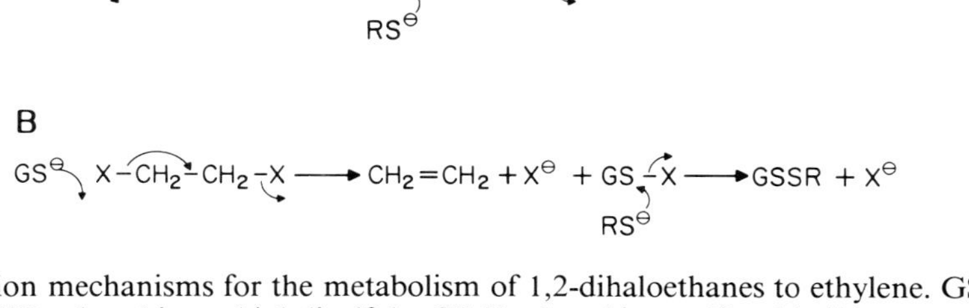

FIG. 4. Reaction mechanisms for the metabolism of 1,2-dihaloethanes to ethylene. GS^-, glutathione; RS^-, thiol; GSSR, glutathione thiol disulfide; GS-X, glutathionesulfenyl halide.

metabolism (31–33). The reaction is catalyzed by cytosolic glutathione *S*-transferases, a family of enzymes with broad and overlapping substrate specificities (54). The cytosolic transferases are widely distributed in the body, but are most abundant in the liver (33). Mitochondrial (78) and microsomal (47) glutathione *S*-transferases have also been described. Glutathione *S*-transferases catalyze the nucleophilic attack of glutathione on the electrophilic carbon of the haloalkane, and the enzyme enhances the nucleophilicity of the thiol group of glutathione (76). The glutathione *S*-transferase-catalyzed conjugation of (*R*)- and (*S*)-phenethyl chloride to yield *S*-(1-phenylethyl)glutathione has been shown to proceed with inversion of configuration, which is consistent with an S_N2 mechanism (94).

Many monohaloalkanes and monohaloalkenes serve as substrates for glutathione *S*-transferases and yield stable *S*-alkyl- or *S*-alkenyl-glutathione conjugates (35,72,75). In contrast, *vic*-dihaloalkanes yield unstable intermediates that are converted to alkenes (*vide supra*) or episulfonium (thiiranium) ions (158,160). *gem*-Dihaloalkanes also yield unstable intermediates that are converted to aldehydes. For example, dihalomethanes are metabolized by glutathione *S*-transferases to yield *S*-halomethylglutathione, which undergoes hydrolysis to *S*-hydroxymethylglutathione, the hemimercaptal of glutathione and formaldehyde, and yields formaldehyde on hydrolysis or is metabolized further to yield formic acid. Chloramphenicol is metabolized in a similar fashion to yield an aldehyde (100).

Perhalogenated alkenes may also serve as substrates for glutathione *S*-transferases. Chlorotrifluoroethylene has recently been shown to form a conjugate with glutathione, which was identified as *S*-(2-chloro-1,1,2-trifluoroethyl)glutathione (43). The reaction was catalyzed by both hepatic microsomal and cytosolic glutathione-dependent enzymes, but the former was much more active than the latter.

Dehydrohalogenation

Several examples of dehydrohalogenation have been reported. These include the biotransformation of hexachlorocyclohexene to pentachlorocycohexane (122,148), of DDT to DDE (19), of pentachloroethane to tetrachloroethylene (149), of 1,1,2,2-tetrachloroethane to trichloroethylene (172), and of carbromal to *Z*-2-ethylcrotonylurea (146). The enzymes catalyzing dehydrohalogenation reactions have not been characterized, although it is known that both cytosolic and microsomal enzymes requiring glutathione catalyze the dechlorination of α-hexachlorocyclohexane (77). When cytosolic enzymes are incubated with 3,4,6/5- and 3,6/4,5-pentachlorocyclohexene in the presence of glutathione, *S*-(dichlorophenyl)glutathione is formed (122).

HALOGENATED ALKENES

Halogenated alkenes are known to undergo cytochrome P-450-catalyzed epoxidation. The resulting epoxides are often highly reactive and have been implicated in the toxicity of many halogenated alkenes. The metabolism of halogenated alkenes has been reviewed (14,89).

Since the initial suggestion by Powell (123), a substantial body of literature has developed showing that trichloroethylene is metabolized to chloral hydrate via the intermediate formation of an epoxide. Butler (24) recognized that both chloral hydrate and trichloroethylene yield the same metabolites, namely, trichloroacetic acid, trichloroethanol, and urochloraclic acid. These findings suggest that the opening of the oxirane ring is accompanied by chlorine migration to yield chloral hydrate (Fig. 5). This was established by Daniel (41a) who found that the specific activities of ^{36}Cl-trichloroacetic acid and ^{36}Cl-trichloroethylene were approximately the same as the administered trichloroethylene. The formation of chloral hydrate as an intermediate in trichloroethylene

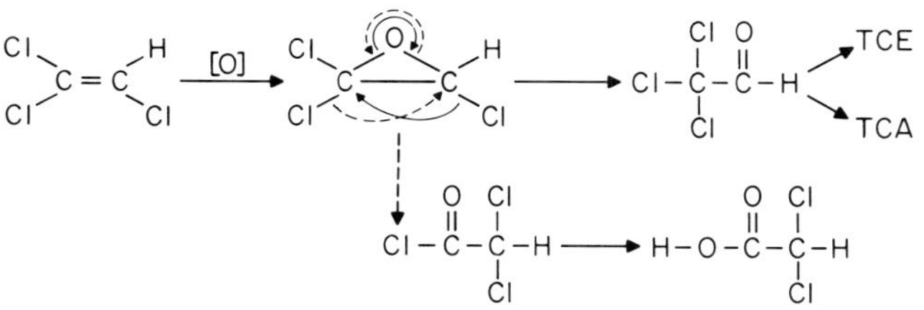

FIG. 5. Reaction mechanisms for the metabolism of trichloroethylene to trichloroacetaldehyde, trichloroethanol (TCE), and trichloroacetic acid (TCA) (*solid line*) and to dichloroacetic acid (*broken line*). [O], cytochrome P-450-catalyzed epoxidation.

metabolism was later established conclusively (26,65,87,88). Spectral evidence for the formation of trichloroethylene epoxide (2,2,3-trichlorooxirane) has been presented recently (156). Furthermore, the rearrangement of trichloroethylene epoxide to chloral hydrate may be catalyzed by Lewis acids such as cytochrome P-450 (14,15). Dichloroacetic acid is formed from trichloroethylene epoxide in chemical systems (59), but was not detected as a metabolite of trichloroethylene in the isolated, perfused rat liver (15). Hathway (57) has identified dichloroacetic acid as a metabolite of trichloroethylene in mice; conversion of trichloroethylene epoxide to dichloroacetic acid also requires a chlorine atom migration (Fig. 5). Carbon monoxide has been identified as a decomposition product of trichloroethylene epoxide in chemical systems (59) and as a metabolite of trichloroethylene in *in vitro* microsomal systems (150).

The formation of epoxide intermediates followed by rearrangement may be a general phenomenon in the metabolism of halogenated alkenes (14). Chloroacetylaldehyde is formed as a metabolite of vinyl chloride (51,52); this can be explained by rearrangement of vinyl chloride epoxide. 1,1-Dichloroethylene (vinylidene chloride) yields chloroacetic acid as a metabolite (73,130); opening of the oxirane ring and chlorine atom migration would yield chloroacetyl chloride which may undergo hydrolysis to chloroacetic acid. Both *E*- and *Z*-1,2-dichloroethylene yield dichloroethanol and dichloroacetic acid as metabolites in the isolated, perfused rat liver (15); again, opening of the oxirane ring and chlorine atom migration would account for the formation of these metabolites. Finally, tetrachloroethylene yields trichloroacetic acid as a metabolite (15,39,41a); this, too, can be explained by its conversion to the epoxide, rearrangement with chlorine atom migration to trichloroacetyl chloride, and hydrolysis.

Although chlorine migration may be a common occurrence in the metabolism of halogenated alkenes, Miller and Guengerich (108) have presented evidence indicating that trichloroethylene epoxide does not rearrange to chloral, a known metabolite of trichloroethylene, in the presence of cytochrome P-450. As an alternative mechanism, these authors have proposed that chlorine migration occurs within an oxygenated trichloroethylene–cytochrome P-450 transition-state complex to yield chloral.

The cytochrome P-450-dependent polysubstrate monooxygenase system is responsible for the epoxidation of halogenated alkenes; evidence includes subcellular location (65,87), cofactor requirements (65,87), enzyme induction (39,65,88,109), spectral interactions with cytochrome P-450 (39, 67,137,156), and inhibition by carbon monoxide (6,39).

ARYL HALIDES

Aryl halides, particularly polyhalogenated benzene derivatives, undergo glutathione *S*-transferase-catalyzed dehalogenation reactions. For example, 3,4-dichloronitrobenzene yields *S*-(2-chloro-4-nitrophenyl)-glutathione as a metabolite in mammals (16), birds (167), and insects (34) and is widely used in assaying glutathione *S*-transferase activity (54); bromsulfophthalein (BSP) undergoes a glutathione *S*-transferase-catalyzed

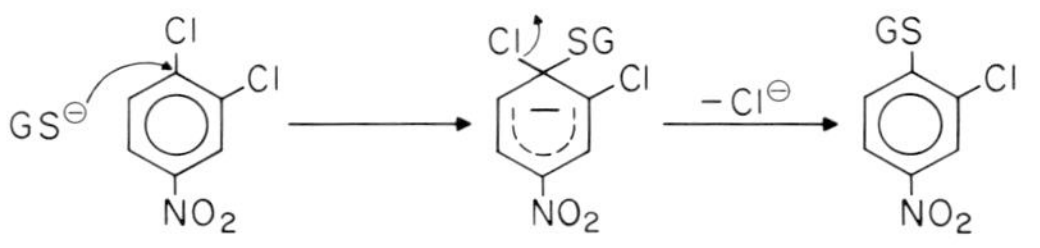

FIG. 6. Reaction mechanisms for the glutathione *S*-transferase-catalyzed formation of *S*-(2-chloro-4-nitrophenyl)glutathione. SG^-, glutathione.

debromination reaction to yield a glutathione conjugate (71) and is used to measure liver function. As in the case of alkyl halides, glutathione conjugation of aryl halides is the first enzymatic step in mercapturic acid formation.

The reaction mechanism for the dechlorination of 3,4-dichloronitrobenzene is shown in Fig. 6; the reaction presumably proceeds by the intermediate formation of a Meisenheimer complex (48).

Finally, the cytochrome P-450-catalyzed monooxygenation of iodobenzene has recently been reported (21). In this experiment, cytochrome P-450 preparations isolated from phenobarbital-treated rats catalyzed the equilibration of unlabeled iodosobenzene and [^{125}I]iodobenzene; cytochrome P-450 isolated from β-naphthoflavone-treated rats, horseradish peroxidase, and catalase failed to catalyze the reaction. Hypervalent states of alkyl and aryl iodides are well known (10); although hypervalent states of organochlorides have not been described, the formation of 1-chloroso-2-chloroethane (53) has been suggested as an intermediate in the metabolism of 1,2-dichloroethane.

REFERENCES

1. Adler, L., Brown, B. R., Jr., and Thompson, M. F. (1976): Kinetics of methoxyflurane biotransformation with reference to substrate inhibition. *Anesthesiology,* 44:380–385.
2. Ahmed, A. E., and Anders, M. W. (1978): Metabolism of dihalomethanes to formaldehyde and inorganic halide. II. Studies on the mechanism of the reaction. *Biochem. Pharmacol.,* 27:2021–2025.
3. Ahmed, A. E., Kubic, V. L., and Anders, M. W. (1977): Metabolism of haloforms to carbon monoxide. I. *In vitro* studies. *Drug Metab. Disp.,* 5:198–204.
4. Ahr, H. J., King, L. J., Nastainczyk, W., and Ullrich, V. (1980): The mechanism of chloroform and carbon monoxide formation from carbon tetrachloride by microsomal cytochrome P-450. *Biochem. Pharmacol.,* 29:2855–2861.
5. Ahr, H. J., King, L. J., Nastainczyk, W., and Ullrich, V. (1982): The mechanism of reductive dehalogenation of halothane by liver cytochrome P-450. *Biochem. Pharmacol.,* 31:383–390.
6. Allemand, H., Pessayre, D., Descatoire, V., Degott, C., Feldmann, G., and Benhamou, J. P. (1978): Metabolic activation of trichloroethylene into a chemically reactive metabolite toxic to the liver. *J. Pharmacol. Exp. Ther.,* 204:714–723.
7. Anders, M. W. (1982): Aliphatic halogenated hydrocarbons. In: *Metabolic Basis of Detoxification,* edited by W. B. Jakoby, J. R. Bend, and J. Caldwell, pp. 29–49. Academic Press, New York.
8. Anders, M. W., and Livesey, J. C. (1980): Metabolism of 1,2-dihaloethanes. In: *Banbury Report 5, Ethylene Dichloride: A Potential Health Risk?,* edited by B. Ames, P. Infante, and R. Reitz, pp. 331–341. Cold Spring Harbor Laboratory, Cold Spring Harbor, New York.
9. Anders, M. W., Stevens, J. L., Sprague, R. W., Shaath, Z., and Ahmed, A. E. (1978): Metabolism of haloforms to carbon monoxide. II. *In vivo* studies. *Drug Metab. Disp.,* 6:556–560.
10. Banks, D. F. (1966): Organic polyvalent iodine compounds. *Chem. Rev.,* 66:243–266.
11. Bini, A., Vecchi, G., Vivoli, G., Vannini, V., and Cessi, C. (1975): Detection of early metabolites in rat liver after administration of CCl_4 and $CBrCl_3$. *Pharmacol. Res. Commun.,* 7:143–149.
12. Blake, D. A., Barry, J. Q., and Cascorbi, H. F. (1972): Qualitative analysis of halothane metabolites in man. *Anesthesiology,* 36:152–154.
13. Blake, D. A., Rozman, R. S., Cascorbi, H. F., and Krantz, J. C., Jr. (1967): Anesthesia LXXIV: Biotransformation of fluroxene-I. Metabolism in mice and dogs *in vivo. Biochem. Pharmacol.,* 16:1237–1248.
14. Bonse, G., and Henschler, D. (1976): Chemical reactivity, biotransformation and toxicity of polychlorinated aliphatic compounds. *CRC Crit. Rev. Toxicol.,* 4:395–409.
15. Bonse, G., Urban, T., Reichert, D., and Henschler, D. (1975): Chemical reactivity, metabolic oxirane formation and biological reactivity in the isolated perfused rat liver preparation. *Biochem. Pharmacol.,* 24:1829–1834.
16. Booth, J., Boyland, E., and Sims, P. (1961): An enzyme from rat liver catalyzing conjugations with glutathione. *Biochem. J.,* 79:516–524.
17. Browning, E. (1965): *Toxicity and Metabolism of Industrial Solvents,* Elsevier, New York.
18. Brundin, A., Ratnayake, J. H., Sunram, J. M., and Anders, M. W. (1982): Glutathione-dependent reductive dehalogenation of 2,2′,4′-trichloroacetophenone to 2′,4′-dichloroacetophenone. *Biochem. Pharmacol.,* 31:3885–3890.
19. Bunyan, P. J., Page, J. M. J., and Taylor, A. (1966): *In vitro* metabolism of *p,p′*DDT in pigeon liver. *Nature,* 210:1048–1049.

20. Burdino, E., Gravela, E., Ugazio, G., Vannini, V., and Calligaro, A. (1973): Initiation of free radical reactions and hepatotoxicity in rats poisoned with carbon tetrachloride or bromotrichloromethane. *Agents Actions,* 4:244–253.
21. Burka, L. T., Thorsen, A., and Guengerich, F. P. (1980): Enzymatic monooxygenation of halogen atoms: Cytochrome P-450 catalyzed oxidation of iodobenzene by iodosobenzene. *J. Am. Chem. Soc.,* 102:7615–7616.
22. Burke, T. R., Jr., Branchflower, R. V., Lees, D. E., and Pohl, L. R. (1981): Mechanism of defluorination of enflurane. Identification of an organic metabolite in rat and man. *Drug Metab. Disp.,* 9:19–24.
23. Burke, T. R., Jr., Martin, J. L., George, J. W., and Pohl, L. R. (1980): Investigation of the mechanism of defluorination of enflurane in rat liver microsomes with specifically deuterated derivatives. *Biochem. Pharmacol.,* 29:1623–1626.
24. Butler, T. C. (1949): Metabolic transformations of trichloroethylene. *J. Pharmacol. Exp. Ther.,* 97:84–92.
25. Butler, T. C. (1961): Reduction of carbon tetrachloride *in vivo* and reduction of carbon tetrachloride and chloroform *in vitro* by tissues and tissue constituents. *J. Pharmacol. Exp. Ther.,* 134:311–319.
26. Byington, K. H., and Leibman, K. C. (1965): Metabolism of trichloroethylene in liver microsomes. II. Identification of the reaction product as chloral hydrate. *Mol. Pharmacol.,* 1:247–254.
27. Calligaro, A., and Vannini, V. (1975): Electron spin resonance study of homolytic cleavage of carbon tetrachloride in rat liver: Trichloromethyl free radicals. *Pharmacol. Res. Commun.,* 7:323–329.
28. Calligaro, A., and Vannini, V. (1976): Reply to the comments of K. M. Sancier concerning the communication: "Electron spin resonance study of homolytic cleavage of carbon tetrachloride in rat liver: Trichloromethyl free radicals." *Pharmacol. Res. Commun.,* 8:431–434.
29. Cambie, R. C., Lindsay, B. G., Rutledge, P. S., and Woodgate, P. D. (1978): Oxidative displacement of iodine from vicinal iodocarboxylates and alkyl iodides. *J. Chem. Soc. Commun.,* 919.
30. Casanova, J., and Eberson, L. (1973): Electrochemistry of the carbon–halogen bond. In: *The Chemistry of the Carbon-Halogen Bond,* edited by S. Patai, pp. 979–1047. John Wiley & Sons, New York.
31. Chasseaud, L. F. (1973): The nature and distribution of enzymes catalyzing the conjugation of glutathione with foreign compounds. *Drug Metab. Rev.,* 2:185–220.
32. Chasseaud, L. F. (1976): Conjugation with glutathione and mercapturic acid excretion. In: *Glutathione: Metabolism and Function,* edited by I. M. Arias and W. B. Jakoby, pp. 77–114. Raven Press, New York.
33. Chasseaud, L. F. (1979): The role of glutathione and glutathione *S*-transferases in the metabolism of chemical carcinogens and other electrophilic agents. *Adv. Cancer Res.,* 29:175–274.
34. Clark, A. G., Darby, F. J., and Smith, J. N. (1967): Species differences in the inhibition of glutathione *S*-aryltransferase by phthaleins and dicarboxylic acids. *Biochem. J.,* 103:49–54.
35. Climie, I. J. G., Hutson, D. H., Morrison, B. J., and Stoydin, G. (1979): Glutathione conjugation in the detoxication of (*Z*)-1,3-dichloropropene (a component of the nematocid D-D) in the rat. *Xenobiotica,* 9:149–156.
36. Cohen, E. N., Trudell, J. R., Edmunds, H. N., and Watson, E. (1975): Urinary metabolites of halothane in man. *Anesthesiology,* 43:392–401.
37. Cohen, E. N., and Van Dyke, R. A. (1977): *Metabolism of Volatile Anesthetics.* Addison-Wesley, Reading, Massachusetts.
38. Conney, A. H. (1967): Pharmacological implications of microsomal enzyme induction. *Pharmacol. Rev.,* 19:317–366.
39. Costa, A. K., and Ivanetich, K. M. (1980): Tetrachloroethylene metabolism by the hepatic microsomal cytochrome P-450 system. *Biochem. Pharmacol.,* 29:2863–2869.
40. Cousins, M. J., Mazze, R. I., Kosek, J. C., Hitt, B. A., and Love, F. V. (1974): The etiology of methoxyflurane nephrotoxicity. *J. Pharmacol. Exp. Ther.,* 190:530–541.
41. Cox, P. J., King, L. J., and Parke, D. V. (1976): The binding of trichlorofluoromethane and other haloalkanes to cytochrome P-450 under aerobic and anaerobic conditions. *Xenobiotica,* 6:363–375.
41a. Daniel, J. W. (1963): The metabolism of ^{36}Cl-labelled trichloroethylene and tetrachloroethylene. *Biochem. Pharmacol.,* 12:795–802.
42. Deinzer, M., Schaumburg, F., and Klein, E. (1978): Environmental health sciences center task force review on halogenated organics in drinking water. *Environ. Health Perspect.,* 24:209–239.
43. Dohn, D. R., and Anders, M. W. (1982): The enzymatic reaction of chlorotrifluoroethylene with glutathione. *Biochem. Biophys. Res. Commun.,* 109:1339–1345.
44. Eben, A., and Kimmerle, G. (1974): Metabolism, excretion and toxicology of methylchloroform in acute and subacute exposed rats. *Arch. Toxikol.,* 31:233–242.
45. Fishbein, L. (1976): Industrial mutagens and potential mutagens. I. Halogenated aliphatic derivatives. *Mutat. Res.,* 32:267–308.
46. Fowler, J. S. L. (1969): Carbon tetrachloride metabolism in the rabbit. *Br. J. Pharmacol.,* 37:733–737.
47. Friedberg, T., Bentley, P., Stasiecki, P., Glatt, H. R., Raphael, D., and Oesch, F. (1979): The identification, solubilization, and characterization of microsome-associated glutathione *S*-transferases. *J. Biol. Chem.,* 254:12028–12033.
48. Gan, L. H. (1977): Kinetic studies of the reactions of glutathione with aromatic compounds. *Aust. J. Chem.,* 30:1475–1479.
49. Gion, H., Yoshimura, N., Holaday, D. A., Fiserova-Bergerova, V., and Chase, R. E. (1974): Biotransformation of fluroxene in man. *Anesthesiology,* 40:553–562.
50. Gorsky, B. H., and Cascorbi, H. F. (1979): Halo-

thane hepatotoxicity and fluoride production in mice and rats. *Anesthesiology,* 50:123–125.

51. Green, T., and Hathway, D. E. (1975): The biological fate in rats of vinyl chloride in relation to its oncogenicity. *Chem. Biol. Interact.,* 11:545–562.
52. Green, T., and Hathway, D. E. (1977): The chemistry and biogenesis of the *S*-containing metabolites of vinyl chloride in rats. *Chem. Biol. Interact.,* 17:137–150.
53. Guengerich, F. P., Crawford, W. M., Jr., Domoradzki, J. Y., Macdonald, T. L., and Watanabe, P. G. (1980): *In vitro* activation of 1,2-dichloroethane by microsomal and cytosolic enzymes. *Toxicol. Appl. Pharmacol.,* 55:303–317.
54. Habig, W. H., Pabst, M. J., and Jakoby, W. B. (1974): Glutathione *S*-transferases. The first enzymatic step in mercapturic acid formation. *J. Biol. Chem.,* 249:7130–7139.
55. Harris, R. N., and Anders, M. W. (1980): Metabolism of carbon tetrachloride to carbon monoxide and carbon dioxide. *Fed. Proc.,* 39:611.
56. Harris, R. N., and Anders, M. W. (1981): 2-Propanol treatment induces selectively the metabolism of carbon tetrachloride to phosgene: Implications for carbon tetrachloride hepatotoxicity. *Drug Metab. Disp.,* 9:551–556.
57. Hathway, D. E. (1980): Consideration of the evidence for mechanisms of 1,1,2-trichloroethylene metabolism, including new identification of its dichloroacetic acid and trichloroacetic acid metabolites in mice. *Cancer Lett.,* 8:263–269.
58. Hendrickson, J. B., Cram, D. J., and Hammond, G. S. (1970): *Organic Chemistry,* 3rd ed., pp. 739–744. McGraw-Hill, New York.
59. Henschler, D., Hoos, W. R., Fetz, H., Dallmeier, E., and Metzler, M. (1979): Reactions of trichloroethylene epoxide in aqueous systems. *Biochem. Pharmacol.,* 28:543–548.
60. Hill, D. L., Shih, T. W., Johnston, T. P., and Struck, R. F. (1978): Macromolecular binding and metabolism of the carcinogen 1,2-dibromoethane. *Cancer Res.,* 38:2438–2442.
61. Hine, J., Peek, R. C., Jr., and Oakes, B. D. (1954): The kinetics of the base-catalyzed deuterium exchange of chloroform in aqueous solution. *J. Am. Chem. Soc.,* 76:827–829.
62. Hitt, B. A., Mazze, R. I., and Denson, D. D. (1979): Isotopic probe of the mechanism of methoxyflurane defluorination. *Drug Metab. Dispos.,* 7:446–447.
63. Holaday, D. A., Rudofsky, S., and Treuhaft, P. S. (1970): The metabolic degradation of methoxyflurane in man. *Anesthesiology,* 33:579–593.
64. Hutson, D. H., Holmes, D. S., and Crawford, M. J. (1976): The involvement of glutathione in the reductive dechlorination of a phenacylhalide. *Chemosphere,* 5:79–84.
65. Ikeda, M., Miyake, Y., Ogata, M., and Ohmori, S. (1980): Metabolism of trichloroethylene. *Biochem. Pharmacol.,* 29:2983–2992.
66. Ikeda, M., and Ohtsuji, H. (1972): Comparative study of the excretion of Fujiwara reaction-positive substances in urine of rats and rodents given trichloro- or tetrachloro-derivatives of ethane and ethylene. *Br. J. Ind. Med.,* 29:99–104.
67. Ivanetich, K. M., Aronson, I., and Katz, I. D. (1977): The interaction of vinyl chloride with rat hepatic microsomal cytochrome P-450 *in vitro. Biochem. Biophys. Res. Commun.,* 74:1411–1418.
68. Ivanetich, K. M., Bradshaw, J. J., Marsh, J. A., and Kaminsky, L. S. (1976): The interaction of hepatic microsomal cytochrome P-450 with fluroxene (2,2,2-trifluoroethyl vinyl ether) *in vitro. Biochem. Pharmacol.,* 25:779–784.
69. Ivanetich, K. M., Lucas, S. A., and Marsh, J. A. (1979): Enflurane and methoxyflurane. Their interaction with hepatic cytochrome P-450 *in vitro. Biochem. Pharmacol.,* 28:785–792.
70. Ivanetich, K. M., Marsh, J. A., Bradshaw, J. J., and Kaminsky, L. S. (1975): Fluroxene (2,2,2-trifluoroethyl vinyl ether) mediated destruction of cytochrome P-450 *in vitro. Biochem. Pharmacol.,* 24:1933–1936.
71. Javitt, N. B. (1976): Biochemical probes for the study of binding and conjugation of glutathione *S*-transferases. In: *Glutathione: Metabolism and Function,* edited by I. M. Arias and W. B. Jakoby, pp. 309–314. New York, Raven Press.
72. Johnson, M. K. (1966): Studies on glutathione *S*-alkyltransferase of the rat. *Biochem. J.,* 98:44–56.
73. Jones, B. K., and Hathway, D. E. (1978): The biological fate of vinylidene chloride in rats. *Chem. Biol. Interact.,* 20:27–41.
74. Kalyanaraman, B., Mason, R. P., Perez-Reyes, E., Chignell, C. F., Wolf, C. R., and Philpot, R. M. (1979): Characterization of the free radical formed in aerobic microsomal incubations containing carbon tetrachloride and NADPH. *Biochem. Biophys. Res. Commun.,* 89:1065–1072.
75. Kaye, C. M., Clapp, J. J., and Young, L. (1972): The metabolic formation of mercapturic acids from allyl halides. *Xenobiotica,* 2:129–139.
76. Keen, J. H., Habig, W. H., and Jakoby, W. B. (1976): Mechanism for the several activities of glutathione *S*-transferases. *J. Biol. Chem.,* 251:6183–6188.
77. Kraus, P. (1975): Biodegradation of alpha-hexachlorocyclohexane. VI. The dechlorination of α-hexachlorocyclohexane by microsomes and cytosol of rat liver. *Naunyn Schmiedebergs Arch. Pharmacol.,* 291:79–87.
78. Kraus, P. (1980): Resolution, purification and some properties of three glutathione transferases from rat liver mitochondria. *Hoppe Seylers Z. Physiol. Chem.,* 361:9–15.
79. Kubic, V. L., and Anders, M. W. (1975): Metabolism of dihalomethanes to carbon monoxide. II. *In vitro* studies. *Drug Metab. Dispos.,* 3:104–112.
80. Kubic, V. L., and Anders, M. W. (1978): Metabolism of dihalomethanes to carbon monoxide. III. Studies on the mechanism of the reaction. *Biochem. Pharmacol.,* 28:3189–3194.
81. Kubic, V. L., and Anders, M. W. (1980): Metabolism of carbon tetrachloride to phosgene. *Life Sci.,* 26:2151–2155.
82. Kubic, V. L., and Anders, M. W. (1980): Mechanism of the microsomal reduction of carbon tet-

rachloride and halothane. *Chem. Biol. Interact.*, 34:201–207.
83. Kubic, V. L., Anders, M. W., Engel, R. R., Barlow, C. M., and Caughey, W. S. (1974): Metabolism of dihalomethanes to carbon monoxide. I. *In vivo* studies. *Drug Metab. Dispos.*, 2:53–57.
84. Lai, E. K., McCay, P. B., Noguchi, T., and Fong, K. L. (1979): *In vivo* spin-trapping of trichloromethyl radicals formed from CCl_4. *Biochem. Pharmacol.*, 28:2231–2235.
85. Lavigne, J. G., and Marchand, C. (1974): The role of metabolism in chloroform hepatotoxicity. *Toxicol. Appl. Pharmacol.*, 29:312–326.
86. Lee, C. C., Bhandari, J. C., Winston, J. M., House, W. B., Dixon, R. L., and Woods, J. S. (1978): Carcinogenicity of vinyl chloride and vinylidene chloride. *J. Toxicol. Environ. Health*, 4:15–30.
87. Leibman, K. C. (1965): Metabolism of trichloroethylene in liver microsomes. I. Characteristics of the reaction. *Mol. Pharmacol.*, 1:239–246.
88. Leibman, K. C., and McAllister, W. J., Jr. (1967): Metabolism of trichloroethylene in liver microsomes. III. Induction of the enzymic activity and its effect on excretion of metabolites. *J. Pharmacol. Exp. Ther.*, 157:574–580.
89. Leibman, K. C., and Ortiz, E. (1977): Metabolism of halogenated ethylenes. *Environ. Health Perspect.*, 21:91–97.
90. Livesey, J. C., and Anders, M. W. (1979): *In vitro* metabolism of 1,2-dihaloethanes to ethylene. *Drug Metab. Dispos.*, 7:199–203.
91. Livesey, J. C., Anders, M. W., Langvardt, P. W., Putzig, C. L., and Reitz, R. H. (1982): Stereochemistry of the glutathione-dependent biotransformation of *vicinal*-dihaloalkanes to alkenes. *Drug Metab. Disp.*, 10:201–204.
92. Loew, G., and Goldblum, A. (1980): Electronic spectrum of model cytochrome P450 complex with postulated carbene metabolite of halothane. *J. Am. Chem. Soc.*, 102:3657–3659.
93. Maiorino, R. M., Sipes, I. G., Gandolfi, A. J., and Brown, B. R., Jr. (1979): Quantitative analysis of volatile halothane metabolites in biological tissues by gas chromatography. *J. Chromatogr.*, 164:63–72.
94. Mangold, J. B., and Abdel-Monem, M. M. (1980): Stereoselectivity of the glutathione *S*-transferase catalyzed conjugation of aralkyl halides. *Biochem. Biophys. Res. Commun.*, 96:333–340.
95. Mannering, G. J. (1971): Microsomal enzyme systems which catalyze drug metabolism. In: *Fundamentals of Drug Metabolism and Drug Disposition,* edited by B. N. LaDu, H. G. Mandel, and E. L. Way, pp. 206–252. Williams & Wilkins, Baltimore.
96. Mansuy, D., Beaune, P., Cresteil, T., Lange, M., and Leroux, J. P. (1977): Evidence for phosgene formation during liver microsomal oxidation of chloroform. *Biochem. Biophys. Res. Commun.*, 79:513–517.
97. Mansuy, D., Fontecave, M., and Chottard, J. C. (1980): A heme model study of carbon tetrachloride metabolism: Mechanisms of phosgene and carbon dioxide formation. *Biochem. Biophys. Res. Commun.*, 95:1536–1542.
98. Mansuy, D., Nastainczyk, W., and Ullrich, V. (1974): The mechanism of halothane binding to cytochrome P450. *Naunyn Schmiedebergs Arch. Pharmacol.*, 285:315–324.
99. Marsh, J. A., Bradshaw, J. J., Sapeika, G. A., Lucas, S. A., Kaminsky, L. S., and Ivanetich, K. M. (1977): Further investigations on the metabolism of fluroxene and the degradation of cytochromes P-450 *in vitro. Biochem. Pharmacol.*, 26:1601–1606.
100. Martin, J. L., George, J. W., and Pohl, L. R. (1980): Glutathione-dependent dechlorination of chloramphenicol by cytosol of rat liver. *Drug Metab. Dispos.*, 8:93–97.
101. Mason, R. P. (1979): Free radical metabolites of foreign compounds and their toxicological significance. *Rev. Biochem. Toxicol.*, 1:151–200.
102. Mazze, R. I., Cousins, M. J., and Kosek, J. C. (1972): Dose-related methoxyflurane nephrotoxicity in rats: A biochemical and pathological correlation. *Anesthesiology,* 36:571–587.
103. Mazze, R. I., and Hitt, B. (1978): Effects of phenobarbital and 3-methyl-cholanthrene on anesthetic defluorination in Fischer 344 rats. *Drug Metab. Dispos.*, 6:680–681.
104. Mazze, R. I., Hitt, B. A., and Cousins, M. J. (1974): Effect of enzyme induction with phenobarbital on the *in vivo* and *in vitro* defluorination of isoflurane and methoxyflurane. *J. Pharmacol. Exp. Ther.*, 190:523–529.
105. McCollister, D. D., Beamer, W. H., Atchison, G. J., and Spencer, H. C. (1951): The absorption, distribution and elimination of radioactive carbon tetrachloride by monkeys upon exposure to low vapor concentrations. *J. Pharmacol. Exp. Ther.*, 102:112–124.
106. McLean, A. E. M. (1967): Effect of hexane and carbon tetrachloride on microsomal cytochrome (P450). *Biochem. Pharmacol.*, 16:2030–2033.
107. Miller, M. S., and Gandolfi, A. J. (1980): Enflurane biotransformation in humans. *Life Sci.*, 27:1465–1468.
108. Miller, R. E., and Guengerich, F. P. (1982): Oxidation of trichloroethylene by liver microsomal cytochrome P-450: Evidence for chlorine migration in a transition state not involving trichloroethylene oxide. *Biochemistry,* 21:1090–1097.
109. Moslen, M. T., Reynolds, E. S., and Szabo, S. (1977): Enhancement of the metabolism and hepatotoxicity of trichloroethylene and perchloroethylene. *Biochem. Pharmacol.*, 26:369–375.
110. Mukai, S., Morio, M., Fujii, K., and Hanaki, C. (1977): Volatile metabolites of halothane in the rabbit. *Anesthesiology,* 47:248–251.
111. Nastainczyk, W., Ullrich, V., and Sies, H. (1978): Effect of oxygen concentration on the reaction of halothane with cytochrome P450 in liver microsomes and isolated perfused rat liver. *Biochem. Pharmacol.*, 27:387–392.
112. Nebert, D. M., Eisen, H. J., Negishi, M., Lang, M. A., Hjelmeland, L. M., and Okey, A. B. (1981): Genetic mechanisms controlling the induction of

polysubstrate monooxygenase (P-450) activities. *Annu. Rev. Pharmacol. Toxicol.*, 21:431–462.

113. Packer, J. E., Slater, T. F., and Willson, R. L. (1978): Reactions of the carbon tetrachloride-related peroxy free radical ($CCl_3O_2\cdot$) with amino acids: Pulse radiolysis evidence. *Life Sci.*, 23:2617–2620.
114. Patai, S. (1973): *The Chemistry of the Carbon–Halogen Bond.* John Wiley & Sons, New York.
115. Paul, B. B., and Rubinstein, D. (1963): Metabolism of carbon tetrachloride and chloroform by the rat. *J. Pharmacol. Exp. Ther.*, 141:141–148.
116. Pelkonen, O., and Vainio, M. (1975): Spectral interactions of a series of chlorinated hydrocarbons with cytochrome P-450 of liver microsomes from variously-treated rats. *FEBS Lett.*, 51:11–14.
117. Phu Lich, N., Cluet, J. L., and Dutertre-Catella, H. (1971): 1,1,1,2-Tetra-chloroethane metabolism. *C. R. Acad. Sci. [D] (Paris)*, 272:1173–1176.
118. Pohl, L. R. (1979): Biochemical toxicology of chloroform. *Rev. Biochem. Toxicol.*, 1:79–107.
119. Pohl, L. R., Bhooshan, B., Whittaker, N. F., and Krishna, G. (1977): Phosgene: A metabolite of chloroform. *Biochem. Biophys. Res. Commun.*, 79:684–691.
120. Pohl, L. R., and Krishna, G. (1978): Deuterium isotope effect in bioactivation and hepatotoxicity of chloroform. *Life Sci.*, 23:1067–1072.
121. Pohl, L. R., Nelson, S. D., and Krishna, G. (1978): Investigation of the mechanism of the metabolic activation of chloramphenicol by rat liver microsomes. Identification of a new metabolite. *Biochem. Pharmacol.*, 27:491–496.
122. Portig, J., Kraus, P., Stein, K., Koransky, W., Noack, G., Gross, B., and Sodomann, S. (1979): Glutathione conjugate formation from hexachlorocyclohexane and pentachlorocyclohexene by rat liver *in vitro*. *Xenobiotica*, 9:353–378.
123. Powell, J. F. (1945): Trichloroethylene: Absorption, elimination and metabolism. *Br. J. Ind. Med.*, 2:142–145.
124. Poyer, J. L., Floyd, R. A., McCay, P. B., Janzen, E. G., and Davis, E. R. (1978): Spin-trapping of the trichloromethyl radical produced during enzymic NADPH oxidation in the presence of carbon tetrachloride or bromotrichloromethane. *Biochim. Biophys. Acta*, 539:402–409.
125. Poyer, J. L., McCay, P. B., Lai, E. K., Janzen, E. G., and Davis, E. R. (1980): Confirmation of assignment of the trichloromethyl radical spin adduct detected by spin trapping during ^{13}C-carbon tetrachloride metabolism *in vitro* and *in vivo*. *Biochem. Biophys. Res. Commun.*, 94:1154–1160.
126. Poyer, J. L., McCay, P. B., Weddle, C. C., and Downs, P. E. (1981): *In vivo* spin-trapping of radicals formed from halothane. *Biochem. Pharmacol.*, 30:1517–1519.
127. Recknagel, R. O., and Glende, E. A., Jr. (1973): Carbon tetrachloride hepatotoxicity: An example of lethal cleavage. *CRC Crit. Rev. Toxicol.*, 2:263–297.
128. Rehder, K., Forbes, J., Alter, H., Hessler, O., and Stier, A. (1967): Halothane biotransformation in man: A quantitative study. *Anesthesiology*, 28:711–715.
129. Reich, H. J., and Peake, S. L. (1978): Hypervalent organoiodine chemistry: *Syn* elimination of alkyl iodoso compounds. *J. Am. Chem. Soc.*, 100:4888–4889.
130. Reichert, D., and Bashti, N. (1976): Metabolism and disposition of 1,1-dichloroethylene in the isolated perfused liver of the rat. *Naunyn Schmiedebergs Arch. Pharmacol.* [*Suppl.*], 293:R255.
131. Reiner, O., Athanassopoulos, S., Hellmer, K. H., Murray, R. E., and Uehleke, H. (1972): Bildung von Chloroform aus Tetrachlorkohlenstoff in Lebermikrosomen, Lipidperoxidation und Zerstörung von Cytochrom P-450. *Arch. Toxicol.*, 29:219–233.
132. Reiner, O., and Uehleke, H. (1971): Binding von Tetrachlorkohlenstoff an reduziertes mikrosomales Cytochrom P-450 und an Häm. *Hoppe Seylers Z. Physiol. Chem.*, 352:1048–1052.
133. Reynolds, E. S., and Moslen, M. T. (1975): Metabolism of (^{14}C-1)-halothane *in vivo*—Effects of multiple halothane anesthesia, phenobarbital and carbon tetrachloride pretreatment. *Biochem. Pharmacol.*, 24:2075–2081.
134. Rice, S. A., Sbordone, L., and Mazze, R. I. (1980): Metabolism by rat hepatic microsomes of fluorinated ether anesthetics following isoniazid administration. *Anesthesiology*, 53:489–493.
135. Rice, S. A., and Talcott, R. E. (1979): Effects of isoniazid treatment on selected hepatic mixed-function oxidases. *Drug Metab. Dispos.*, 7:260–262.
136. Rubinstein, D., and Kanics, L. (1964): The conversion of carbon tetrachloride and chloroform by rat liver homogenates. *Can J. Biochem.*, 42:1577–1585.
137. Salmon, A. G. (1976): Cytochrome P-450 and the metabolism of vinyl chloride. *Cancer Lett.*, 2:109–114.
138. Sancier, K. M. (1976): Reply to "Electron spin resonance study of homolytic cleavage of carbon tetrachloride in rat liver: Trichloromethyl free radicals." *Pharmacol. Res. Commun.*, 8:429–430.
139. Schenkman, J. B., Sligar, S. G., and Cinti, D. L. (1981): Substrate interaction with cytochrome P-450. *Pharmacol. Ther.*, 12:43–71.
140. Shah, H., Hartman, S. P., and Weinhouse, S. (1979): Formation of carbonyl chloride in carbon tetrachloride metabolism by rat liver *in vitro*. *Cancer Res.*, 39:3942–3947.
141. Sharp, J. H., Trudell, J. R., and Cohen, E. N. (1979): Volatile metabolites and decomposition products of halothane in man. *Anesthesiology*, 50:2–8.
142. Sipes, I. G., Gandolfi, A. J., Pohl, L. R., Krishna, G., and Brown, B. R., Jr. (1980): Comparison of the biotransformation and hepatotoxicity of halothane and deuterated halothane. *J. Pharmacol. Exp. Ther.*, 214:716–720.
143. Slater, T. F. (1972): *Free Radical Mechanisms in Tissue Injury.* Pion, London.
144. Slater, T. F., and Sawyer, B. C. (1971): The stim-

ulatory effect of carbon tetrachloride on peroxidative reactions in rat liver fractions *in vitro*. Interaction sites in the endoplasmic reticulum. *Biochem. J.*, 123:815–821.

145. Stevens, J. L., and Anders, M. W. (1979): Metabolism of haloforms to carbon monoxide. III. Studies on the mechanism of the reaction. *Biochem. Pharmacol.*, 28:3189–3194.

146. Sticht, G., and Käferstein, M. (1973): Untersuchungen zur Metabolisierung von Bromharnstoffderivaten. *Arzneim. Forsch.*, 23:1021–1023.

147. Suarez, K. A., and Bhonsle, P. (1976): The relationship of cobaltous chloride-induced alterations of hepatic microsomal enzymes to altered carbon tetrachloride hepatotoxicity. *Toxicol. Appl. Pharmacol.*, 37:23–27.

148. Tanaka, K., Kurihara, N., and Nakajima, M. (1979): Oxidative metabolism of lindane and its isomers with microsomes from rat liver and house fly abdomen. *Pest. Biochem. Physiol.*, 10:96–103.

149. Town, C., and Leibman, K. C. (1979): *In vitro* dechlorination of polychlorinated ethanes by rat homogenates. *Fed. Proc.*, 38:538.

150. Traylor, P. S., Nastainczyk, W., and Ullrich, V. (1977): Conversion of trichloroethylene to carbon monoxide by microsomal cytochrome P450. In: *Microsomes and Drug Oxidations*, edited by V. Ullrich, I. Roots, A. Hildebrandt, R. W. Estabrook, and A. H. Conney, pp. 615–621. Pergamon Press, New York.

151. Trudell, J. R., Bösterling, B., and Trevor, A. J. (1982): Reductive metabolism of carbon tetrachloride by human cytochromes P-450 reconstituted in phospholipid vesicles: Mass spectral identification of trichloromethyl radical bound to dioleoyl phosphatidylcholine. *Proc. Natl. Acad. Sci. U.S.A.*, 79:2678–2682.

152. Trudell, J. R., Bösterling, and Trevor, A. J. (1982): Reductive metabolism of halothane by human and rabbit cytochrome P-450. Binding of 1-chloro-2,2,2-trifluoroethyl radical to phospholipids. *Mol. Pharmacol.*, 21:710–717.

153. Truhaut, R., and Phu Lich, N. (1973): Metabolic transformations of 1,1,1,2-tetrachloroethane in rats, guinea pigs and rabbits. *J. Eur. Toxicol.*, 6:211–217.

154. Uehleke, H., Hellmer, K. H., and Tabarelli, S. (1973): Binding of ^{14}C-carbon tetrachloride to microsomal proteins *in vitro* and formation of $CHCl_3$ by reduced liver microsomes. *Xenobiotica*, 3:1–11.

155. Uehleke, H., Hellmer, K. H., and Tabarelli-Poplawski, S. (1973): Metabolic activation of halothane and its covalent binding to liver endoplasmic proteins *in vitro*. *Naunyn Schmiedebergs Arch. Pharmacol.*, 279:39–52.

156. Uehleke, H., Tabarelli-Poplawski, S., Bonse, G., and Henschler, D. (1977): Spectral evidence for 2,2,3-trichloro-oxirane formation during microsomal trichloroethylene oxidation. *Arch. Toxicol.*, 37:95–105.

157. Ullrich, V., and Schnabel, K. H. (1971): Formation and binding of carbanions by cytochrome P-450 of liver microsomes. *Drug. Metab. Dispos.*, 1:176–182.

158. van Bladeren, P. J., Breimer, D. D., Rotteveel-Smijs, G. M. T., de Jong, R. A. W., Buijs, W., van der Gen, A., and Mohn, G. R. (1980): The role of glutathione conjugation in the mutagenicity of 1,2-dibromoethane. *Biochem. Pharmacol.*, 29:2975–2982.

159. van Bladeren, P. J., Breimer, D. D., van Huijgevoort, J. A. T. C. M., Vermeulen, N. P. E., and van der Gen, A. (1981): The metabolic formation of *N*-acetyl-*S*-2-hydroxyethyl-L-cysteine from tetradeutero-1,2-dibromoethane. Relative importance of oxidation and glutathione conjugation *in vivo*. *Biochem. Pharmacol.*, 30:2499–2502.

160. van Bladeren, P. J., van der Gen, A., Breimer, D. D., and Mohn, G. R. (1979): Stereoselective activation of vicinal dihalogen compounds to mutagens by glutathione conjugation. *Biochem. Pharmacol.*, 28:2521–2524.

161. Van Dyke, R. A., and Gandolfi, A. J. (1975): Characteristics of a microsomal dechlorination system. *Mol. Pharmacol.*, 11:809–817.

162. Van Dyke, R. A., and Wood, C. L. (1973): Metabolism of methoxyflurane: Release of inorganic fluoride in human and rat hepatic microsomes. *Anesthesiology*, 39:613–618.

163. von Oettingen, W. F. (1955): *The Halogenated Aliphatic, Olefinic, Cyclic, Aromatic, and Aliphatic-Aromatic Hydrocarbons Including the Halogenated Insecticides, Their Toxicity and Potential Dangers*, Public Health Service Publication No. 414. U.S. Government Printing Office, Washington.

164. Walker, C. H. (1969): Reductive dechlorination of *p,p'*-DDT by pigeon liver microsomes. *Life Sci.*, 8:1111–1115.

165. Wallmeier, H., and Kutzelnigg, W. (1979): Nature of the semipolar XO bond: Comparative *ab initio* study of H_3NO, H_2NOH, H_3PO, H_2POH, $H_2P(O)F$, H_2SO, HSOH, HClO, ArO, and related molecules. *J. Am. Chem. Soc.*, 101:2804–2814.

166. Williams, R. T. (1959): *Detoxification Mechanisms*. John Wiley & Sons, New York.

167. Wit, J. G., and Leeuwangh, P. (1969): Mercapturic acid formation and enzyme-catalyzed conjugations with glutathione in pigeons. *Biochim. Biophys. Acta*, 177:329–335.

168. Witte, L., Nau, H., Fuhrhop, J. H., Doenicke, A., and Grote, B. (1977): Quantitative analysis of trifluoroacetic acid in body fluids of patients treated with halothane. *J. Chromatogr.*, 143:329–334.

169. Wolf, C. R., Harrelson, W. G., Jr., Nastainczyk, W. M., Philpot, R. M., Kalyanaraman, B., and Mason, R. P. (1980): Metabolism of carbon tetrachloride in hepatic microsomes and reconstituted monoxygenase systems and its relationship to lipid peroxidation. *Mol. Pharmacol.*, 18:553–558.

170. Wolf, C. R., King, L. J., and Parke, D. V. (1978): The anaerobic dechlorination of trichlorofluoromethane by rat liver preparations *in vitro*. *Chem. Biol. Interact.*, 21:277–288.

171. Wolf, C. R., Mansuy, D., Nastainczyk, W., Deutschmann, G., and Ullrich, V. (1977): The reduction of polyhalogenated methanes by liver microsomal cytochrome P450. *Mol. Pharmacol.,* 13:698–705.

172. Yllner, S. (1971): Metabolism of 1,1,2,2-tetrachloroethane-^{14}C in the mouse. *Acta Pharmacol. Toxicol. (Kbh.),* 29:499–512.

173. Yllner, S. (1971): Metabolism of 1,1,2-trichloroethane-1,2-^{14}C in the mouse. *Acta Pharmacol. Toxicol. (Kbh.),* 30:248–256.

174. Yllner, S. (1971): Metabolism of 1,2-dichloroethane-^{14}C in the mouse. *Acta Pharmacol. Toxicol. (Kbh.),* 30:257–265.

175. Yllner, S. (1971): Metabolism of 1,1,1,2-tetrachloroethane in the mouse. *Acta Pharmacol. Toxicol. (Kbh.),* 29:471–480.

176. Yllner, S. (1971): Metabolism of pentachloroethane in the mouse. *Acta Pharmacol. Toxicol. (Kbh.),* 29:481–489.

177. Yoshimura, N., Holaday, D. A., and Fiserova-Bergerova, V. (1976): Metabolism of methoxyflurane in man. *Anesthesiology,* 44:372–379.

Drug Metabolism and Drug Toxicity,
edited by J. R. Mitchell and M. G. Horning.
Raven Press, New York © 1984.

Studies on Drug Metabolism and Drug Toxicity in Isolated Mammalian Cells

Martyn T. Smith and Sten Orrenius

Department of Forensic Medicine, Karolinska Institutet, S-104 01 Stockholm, Sweden

During the last few years suspensions of freshly isolated mammalian cells, including hepatocytes, intestinal epithelial cells, and kidney epithelial cells, have become increasingly used as an experimental model for studies on the metabolism of various drugs and other xenobiotics and on their toxicity (42,65,76,110). The viability of the freshly isolated cells is usually excellent, and they catalyze the various phase I and phase II reactions involved in drug biotransformation (Fig. 1) at rates comparable to those observed *in vivo* or with isolated perfused organs (5).

The isolated epithelial cells also retain most of the other biochemical properties of the *in vivo* system and do not dedifferentiate during the relatively short incubation periods used in most studies. This means that a high level of organization is maintained, making it possible to study the relationship between normal cellular metabolism and drug biotransformation. For example, the generation and supply of cofactors required for drug metabolism and competition between drug metabolism and other metabolic processes for these cofactors can easily be studied. Perfused organ systems are cumbersome for such studies because of the difficulty in obtaining repeated tissue samples and because subfractions of the tissue cannot be obtained rapidly. In contrast, a suspension of cells from a single liver can be divided into several flasks and can therefore be examined under a wide variety of experimental manipulations. In addition, the time course of metabolite changes can be readily studied, and the

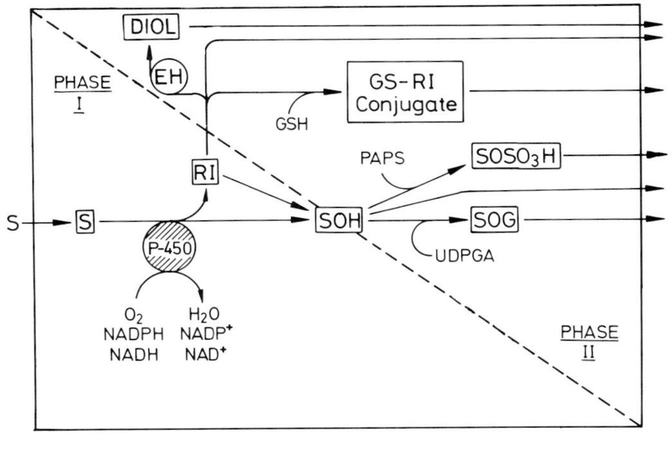

FIG. 1. Schematic representation of drug biotransformation by phase I (oxidation) and phase II (conjugation) reactions in hepatocytes. S, substrate; SOH, hydroxylated product; RI, reactive intermediate; EH, epoxide hydrolase; GSH, glutathione, reduced form; SG, glutathione conjugate; SOG, glucuronide; PAPS, 3′-phosphoadenosine-5′-phosphosulfate; UDPGA, uridine-5′-diphosphoglucuronic acid. Diols may be excreted either directly or as conjugates.

cells can be rapidly separated into several subcellular fractions. For studies of oxygen dependence, tissue oxygen gradients are eliminated, which allows direct observation of oxygen delivery on a cellular basis.

Possibly the major advantage of the isolated-cell model system resides, however, in its accessibility to studies of sequences of reactions. This is especially important for the elucidation of the role of various conjugation reactions, notably the formation of glucuronide, sulfate, and glutathione conjugates (Fig. 1). The substrates of these reactions are often formed by preceding cytochrome P-450-linked monooxygenation reactions and can be toxic reactive metabolites of the original drug substrate (Fig. 1) (57,109). The activating role of cytochrome P-450 monooxygenation and the protective role of the various conjugation reactions, especially conjugation with glutathione, can therefore be studied simultaneously in isolated cells, making them extremely useful in studies on drug toxicity, since the balance between activating and protective systems appears to be of primary importance in determining the extent of cell damage as a result of toxic injury (57,96,97,109). Moreover, the toxicity of a large number of foreign compounds is thought to occur via the generation of harmful side products such as active oxygen species and not directly by the formation of potentially toxic metabolites (10,12,45). We hope to show in this chapter that isolated cells may also be useful in studies on this particular type of toxicity and in evaluating the relative importance of specific events that result in toxic cell injury.

Two further advantages of using the isolated cell system as an experimental model in studies on drug toxicity are as follows. First, it is relatively simple to directly correlate biochemical changes with morphological alterations in the structure of the cells by using a combination of biochemical techniques and both light and electron microscopy. Furthermore, since isolated cells can be rapidly separated into the various subcellular fractions, the subcellular compartmentation of detoxication reactions can easily be studied. This is an area of increasing importance in studies on drug biotransformation and drug toxicity (79), because toxic metabolites generated in one cellular compartment may depend on enzymes present in another compartment for inactivation. Coordination of the various metabolic pathways located in different compartments is therefore essential for the survival of the cell as well as of the organism.

However, it should be realized that suspensions of isolated mammalian cells are not a completely ideal experimental model and that this model system does, of course, have certain limitations, which will be discussed later in this chapter. Despite these limitations, isolated mammalian cells are widely used today in studies of intermediary metabolism as well as drug biotransformation. In this chapter, we hope to show how the use of isolated cells has recently led to a much better understanding of several aspects of drug metabolism and drug toxicity and to speculate on how this model may be used in future studies aimed at elucidating the biochemical mechanisms involved in drug-induced cell toxicity.

PREPARATION AND CHARACTERISTICS OF ISOLATED CELLS

The most extensively used cell preparation is that of rat hepatocytes, originally developed in the late 1960s (4,32) and subsequently modified by several research groups. The procedure currently used in our laboratory was designed for drug metabolism studies (65) and involves perfusion of the liver through the hepatic portal vein with a calcium-free Hanks' balanced salt solution containing EGTA and albumin to remove blood cells and extracellular calcium, followed by a second perfusion with Hanks' medium containing collagenase, dispersion of the liver, and washing of the cells at least twice with Kreb–Henseleit buffer. Relatively high yields of viable single hepatocytes with a spherical appearance are produced by this procedure (Figs. 2 and 3), and the preparation is essentially free of nonparenchymal cells. A schematic representation of the perfusion apparatus used in this procedure is shown in Fig. 4.

Modifications of the above procedure have been used to obtain isolated cell suspensions for drug metabolism studies from small intestine (25,103) and kidney (44,74). We are

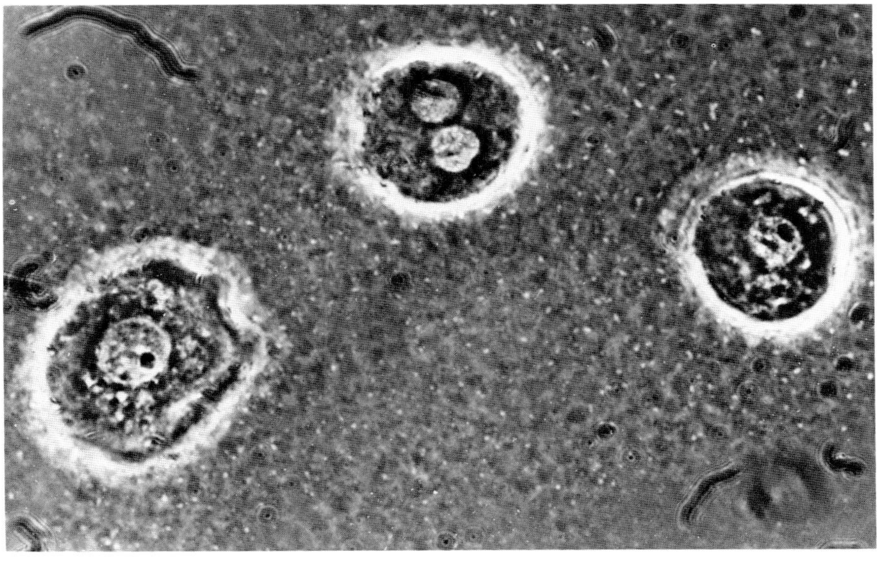

FIG. 2. Photomicrograph showing freshly isolated hepatocytes with distinct plasma membranes and regular granularity of the cytoplasm. Phase contrast microscopy, ×260.

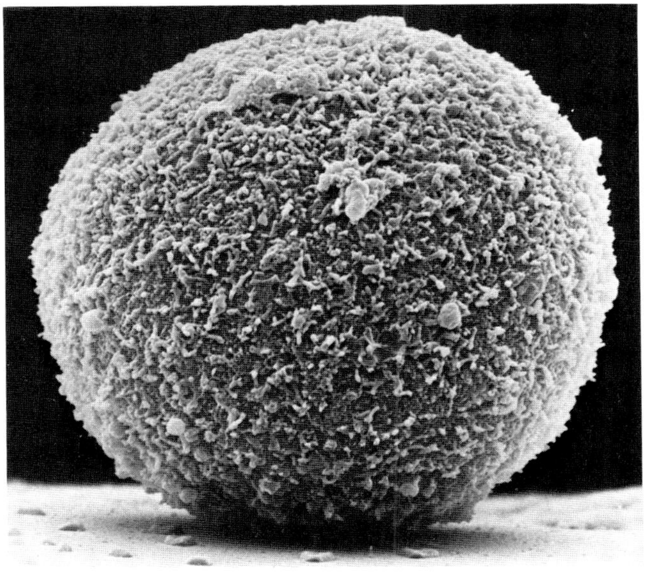

FIG. 3. Scanning electron micrograph of a freshly isolated hepatocyte from a phenobarbital treated rat. Magnification ×2,880. Standard processing procedures were used, involving glutaraldehyde and osmium fixation followed by critical-point drying. A Jeol Model JSM 35 SEM was used.

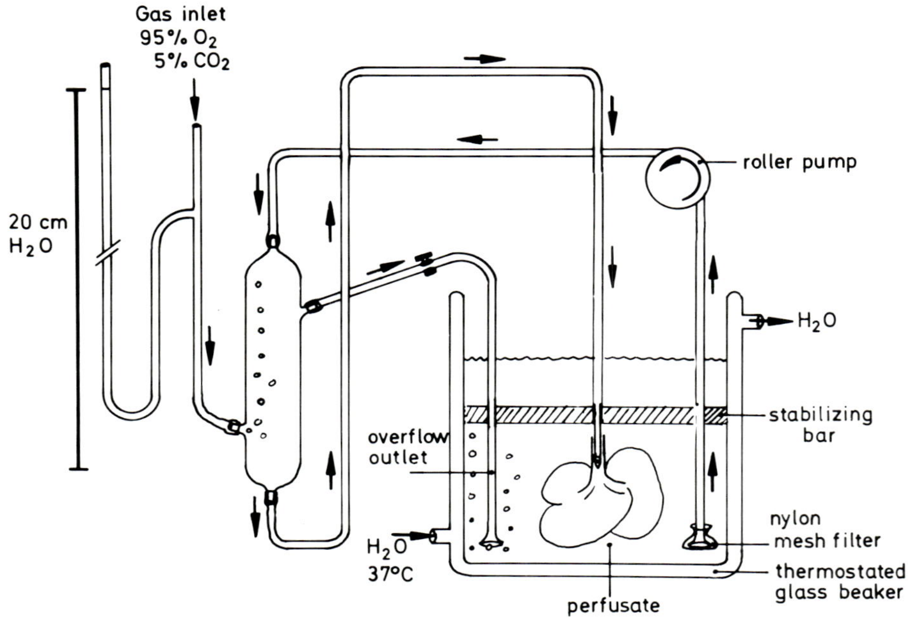

FIG. 4. Schematic drawing of the apparatus used for preparing isolated hepatocytes.

also presently perfecting techniques for the rapid isolation of rat lung and heart cells with high viability and in yields suitable for drug metabolism and toxicity studies. Some of the properties of cell suspensions freshly isolated from different rat tissues are outlined in Table 1. These methods have also been successfully applied for cell isolation from the tissues of other species, including the mouse (59), guinea pig (13), and dog (6).

Incubations are started immediately after isolation of the cells and are performed in rotating round-bottom flasks (31,65) using a final cell concentration of 1 to 3 × 10^6 cells/ml. The isolated cells maintain metabolic integrity for several hours of incubation and can be prepared under sterile conditions for the establishment of primary cultures. The cytochrome P-450 content of isolated liver cells is constant for at least 4 hr but declines during longer incubation (43). The glutathione level in hepatocytes is stable provided that either cysteine or methionine is present in the medium (108). Addition of other amino acids or carbohydrates to the medium is usually not necessary if cells from fed an-

TABLE 1. *Characteristics of cell suspensions freshly isolated from rat liver, small intestine, and kidney*[a]

	Liver	Small intestine	Kidney
Yield (cells/g tissue)	~5 × 10^7	~6 × 10^6	~10^7
Trypan blue exclusion frequency (%)	>95	>90	>90
NADH exclusion frequency (%)	>90	>85	>85
Cytochrome P-450 (nmole/10^6 cells)	~0.25	~0.03	~0.07
GSH (nmole/10^6 cells)	~50	~10	~30
Endogenous respiration (nmole O_2/10^6 cells per min)	~15	~10	~25

[a] Data compiled from Stohs et al. (103), Moldéus et al. (65), Jones et al. (38,44), and Ormstad et al. (74).

imals are used for experiments lasting up to 2 to 3 hr unless a particular metabolic stress is created. Cells from starved animals are more dependent on sources of extracellular metabolites and have therefore been used in studies on the supply of reducing equivalents and metabolic intermediates (54a,63,116). During the incubation of freshly isolated hepatocytes, levels of ATP, ADP, AMP, NADH, and NADPH and rates of glucose synthesis, albumin synthesis, and endogenous respiration remain constant for up to 4 hr and are similar to values obtained for intact or isolated perfused liver (39).

The pretreatment of animals with various agents has been used to obtain isolated cells, especially hepatocytes, with altered metabolic activities. Phenobarbital, 3-methylcholanthrene, β-naphthoflavone, and ethanol have all been used to increase the concentrations of various forms of cytochrome P-450 (43,65). Clofibrate has been administered to increase the content of peroxisomes (43); a selenium-deficient diet and aminotriazole pretreatment have been used to decrease the levels of glutathione peroxidase and catalase, respectively (37); and diethyl maleate pretreatment has been employed to lower the glutathione content of liver and kidney cells (44,45,65,109). Incubations of isolated cells in different media such as sulfate-free Krebs–Henseleit buffer (61) and Krebs–Henseleit buffer with varying concentrations of calcium (2,99) have also been used to study specific aspects of drug metabolism and drug toxicity. In general, with the proper selection of conditions, these manipulations can be made so that there is no significant effect on the viability of the cells.

APPLICATIONS OF ISOLATED CELLS IN STUDIES ON DRUG METABOLISM

As we briefly indicated above, suspensions of freshly isolated cells are now frequently used in biochemical studies. A wide variety of new techniques have therefore been developed and successfully employed in studies in gluconeogenesis, glycolysis, protein, lipid, fatty acid and urea syntheses, ketone body production, protein metabolism, drug and carcinogen metabolism, membrane transport, and response to hormones (42,105). In this part of the discussion, we only describe how some of these techniques have been used to study drug metabolism and the factors regulating this metabolism in isolated cells. However, new applications for isolated cells in such studies are constantly being found as new techniques emerge for investigating the relationships between normal cellular biochemistry and drug metabolism.

Hemoprotein Quantitation

A large proportion of the oxidative metabolism occurring within intact cells is dependent, either directly or indirectly, on hemoproteins present in the mitochondria (cytochrome $b_{561} + b_{566}$, $c + c_1$, $a + a_3$), endoplasmic reticulum (cytochromes P-450 and b_5), and peroxisomes (catalase). It was therefore necessary to develop relatively simple methods for the quantitation of these hemoproteins in isolated cells. In principle, they may be quantitated using established optical spectroscopic methods (11,18). However, several modifications have recently been introduced for the accurate determination of hemoproteins in isolated cells (43), and the effect of various pretreatments on the concentration of several hemoproteins has been assessed (37,43). The results outlined in Table 2 exemplify this by showing concentrations of several hemoproteins in hepatocytes isolated from rats subjected to different pretreatments.

Development of techniques for the accurate determination of cytochrome P-450 in isolated cells was, of course, of primary importance for studies on drug metabolism. Such methods have recently been developed (43) on the basis of either the original procedure of Omura and Sato (73) or differential reduction techniques (21,78). In liver cells

TABLE 2. *Hemoprotein concentrations[a] in hepatocytes isolated from rats pretreated with various agents*

Component	Control	Pheno-barbital	3-Methyl-cholanthrene	Ethanol	Amino-triazole	Clofibrate
Catalase	0.22	0.20	0.21	0.17	0.02	0.27
Cytochrome $a + a_3$	0.18	0.20	0.16	0.09	0.17	0.20
Cytochromes $b_{561} + b_{566}$	0.14	0.17	0.16	0.13	0.17	
Cytochromes $c + c_1$	0.17	0.20	0.17	0.19	0.19	
Cytochrome P-450	0.26	0.90	0.84	0.40	0.16	
Cytochrome b_5	0.09	0.29	0.24	0.09	0.10	

[a] Values shown are expressed as nmole/10^6 cells and were compiled from Jones et al. (37,43).

from animals pretreated with phenobarbital or 3-methylcholanthrene to increase the hepatic cytochrome P-450 concentration, application of the former method (CO difference spectrum of the reduced forms) results in only a 2 to 3% underestimation of the cytochrome P-450 content. However, in hepatocytes from untreated animals, or in other isolated cell types, the relatively large negative absorbance at 445 nm of the CO difference spectrum of reduced cytochrome *c* oxidase results in at least a 10% underestimation of cytochrome P-450. Consequently, accurate determination of cytochrome P-450 concentration in these cells requires the use of a differential reduction technique.

The cytochrome b_5 concentration in isolated hepatocytes can be determined from the *t*-butylhydroperoxide difference spectrum obtained in the presence of a mitochondrial uncoupler such as carbonyl cyanide *p*-trifluoromethoxyphenylhydrazone (FCCP) (43). Under these conditions, the mitochondrial cytochromes are oxidized and therefore do not contribute to the absorbance change on addition of *t*-butylhydroperoxide. The principal absorbance change results from the oxidation of cytochrome b_5 by *t*-butylhydroperoxide. The facility of this oxidation appears to depend on electron flow through cytochrome P-450, and this approach seems to be reliable only for hepatocytes in which the cytochrome P-450 content has been increased by phenobarbital or 3-methylcholanthrene treatment. With control hepatocytes, or intestinal and kidney cells, this procedure always gives an underestimation of cytochrome b_5 content (38,43,74). Under these conditions, an alternative approach is to use a combination of methylviologen and oxygen as the oxidizing agent. The methylviologen-induced difference spectrum of renal cells in the presence of FCCP gives a characteristic oxidized-minus-reduced difference spectrum of cytochrome b_5 and allows a more accurate determination of its concentration in these cells.

Spectral studies of cytochrome P-450 in isolated cells are complicated by the presence of this hemoprotein in the mitochondrial compartment as well as in the endoplasmic reticulum. Subfractionation studies of isolated intestinal cells have allowed indentification of at least three forms of cytochrome P-450 (38). One form is found in the mitochondrial fraction, is not inducible by 3-methylcholanthrene, and does not metabolize benzo(a)pyrene. Two forms are present in the microsomal fraction, one that is present in control animals and metabolizes benzo(a)pyrene at a slow rate and one that is inducible by 3-methylcholanthrene and metabolizes benzo(a)pyrene at a rapid rate.

Altered levels of cytochrome P-450 caused by various agents have been reported in isolated liver cells for both *in vivo* and *in vitro* treatments. The most thoroughly studied inducer has been phenobarbital, which results in a four- to fivefold increase in cytochrome P-450 content in hepatocytes after repeated administration to rats *in vivo.* This increase has long been recognized to be caused by a proliferation of the endoplasmic reticulum within the cells as well as by an increase in the specific membrane content of cytochrome P-450 (17). Pretreatment of rats with 3-methylcholanthrene causes a similar increase in hepatocyte cytochrome P-450 level, whereas chronic ethanol treatment results in only about 50% increase on a cellular basis (43).

A decrease in cellular cytochrome P-450 concentration during establishment of primary cultures of hepatocytes has been reported (27) and also occurs in liver cells maintained in suspension for more than 4 to 5 hr (43). Loss of other cytochromes accompanied the loss of cell viability measured by trypan blue exclusion or NADH penetration, but the decrease in the levels of cytochromes P-450 and b_5 was more rapid. This loss was partially blocked by cycloheximide and was enhanced by inclusion of cobalt in the medium, as reported for the primary cultures. However, there was an overriding loss of cell viability (~30% loss) over the period from 6 to 10 hr of incubation that made suspensions of isolated hepatocytes a poor model for study of these changes in different hemoprotein concentrations.

Drug Uptake and Interaction with Cytochrome P-450

Direct spectrophotometry of isolated cells in suspension has provided a useful means of studying drug interactions with cytochrome P-450 in intact cells. Type I spectral changes have been observed when isolated hepatocytes were incubated with several different compounds (64,114), but studies on other cell types have been less successful, primarily because of the lower concentrations of cytochrome P-450 in extrahepatic tissues. The formation of type I spectral changes with cytochrome P-450 was used by Moldéus and his associates (64) as a measure of the uptake of hexobarbital, lidocaine, and nortriptyline by isolated hepatocytes. Drug uptake occurred rapidly in control cells but was even faster in hepatocytes from phenobarbital-treated rats. Additional studies (114) showed that the rate of hexobarbital uptake increased with temperature in a manner compatible with that expected from passive diffusion.

These and other results led to the conclusion that hexobarbital is taken up by a passive diffusion process. This hypothesis is further supported by the observation that the apparent K_m values for both alprenolol [1-(2-allylphenoxy)-3-isopropylaminopropanol] and hexobarbital metabolism by liver cells are similar to those observed with liver microsomes. However, other drugs, such as bromosulfophthalein and rifampicin, are taken up into isolated hepatocytes by energy-requiring carrier-mediated processes (94,115), and the results of Laperche and co-workers (51) have demonstrated that several different carriers may be involved.

Isolated hepatocytes also provide a suitable model in which to examine various cytochrome P-450–product complexes, including those formed with amphetamine derivatives (29). These relatively stable complexes are catalytically inactive and are characterized by absorption maxima in the 450-nm region. If formed *in vivo,* they may inhibit cytochrome P-450-dependent reactions by converting it to an inactive form. Formation of such complexes in isolated hepatocytes is, however, much slower and less extensive than in liver microsomes (29). A comparison of complex formation in liver microsomes and hepatocytes after addition of amphetamine derivatives suggests that conjugation with glutathione may protect the intact cell against the conversion of its cytochrome P-450 to the inactive complex. Inactivation of cytochrome P-450 by this mechanism may therefore only occur *in vivo* under conditions in which GSH is depleted.

Drug-induced spectral changes therefore offer a useful tool for study of drug uptake and interaction with cytochrome P-450 in intact cells. However, it is necessary to distinguish between spectral changes caused by interaction with cytochrome P-450 and those caused by interaction of drugs with other hemoproteins in the cells. Drugs that act as inhibitors of electron transport or uncouple oxidative phosphorylation may cause spectral changes as a result of effects on the oxidation–reduction state of the mitochondrial cytochromes. Similarly, agents such as *t*-butylhydroperoxide and methylviologen result in oxidation of cytochrome b_5. Other changes can be observed to result in variations in the steady-state concentration of the primary hydrogen peroxide–catalase complex (Compound I), which occur on addition of suitable hydrogen donors such as ethanol, methanol, or formic acid to hepatocytes (45). Further, drugs that result in formation of formaldehyde can also cause these spectral changes through generation of formic acid which binds to hemoproteins. Finally, conversion of catalase to the secondary H_2O_2 complex (Compound II) has also been detected in suspensions of isolated hepatocytes following addition of α-methyldopa (40). The formation of this complex, which is also catalytically inactive, is dependent on the rate of intracellular H_2O_2 production as well as on the α-methyldopa concentration.

Supply of Cosubstrates for Drug Metabolism

The factors regulating drug metabolism in intact cells, including cosubstrate supply, have recently been extensively reviewed (110), and in this section we only concentrate on how isolated cells have contributed to our understanding of this particular aspect of drug metabolism.

The oxidation–reduction state of NADP in the cytoplasm of rat hepatocytes is heavily biased towards the reduced form (Table 3), but there are many uses for this NADPH, including drug monooxygenation, and it must be constantly synthesized in order to maintain the cytosolic NADPH/($NADP^+$ + NADPH) ratio. In liver cells from well-fed animals, glycogen forms a large substrate reserve for the NADPH-generating pentose shunt dehydrogenases, and the cytosolic NADPH/($NADP^+$ + NADPH) ratio remains constant even during relatively high rates of drug monooxygenation, such as during alprenolol metabolism in hepatocytes from phenobarbital-treated rats (Table 3). However, in the starved, glycogen-depleted state, isolated hepatocytes are unable to maintain their cytosolic NADPH/($NADP^+$ + NADPH) ratio during high rates of drug monooxygen-

TABLE 3. *Effect of different pretreatments and agents on level of reduced NADPH*[a] *during alprenolol metabolism in isolated hepatocytes*[b]

Additions	Starved: Control	Starved: Phenobarbital treated	Fed, phenobarbital treated
None	0.69	0.51	0.75
Alprenolol, 75 μM	0.72	0.37	0.74
Lactate, 10 mM	0.80	0.83	0.81
Lactate + alprenolol	0.79	0.74	0.77
Glucose, 10 mM	0.79	0.67	0.78
Glucose + alprenolol	0.82	0.68	0.70
Rotenone, 25 μM	0.41	0.21	0.75
Rotenone + glucose	0.51	0.22	0.74

[a] Data are expressed as NADPH/($NADP^+$ + NADPH).
[b] Data from Moldéus et al. (63) and recent unpublished experiments.

ation, and the availability of NADPH for drug metabolism may become rate limiting (Table 3) (110).

The addition of either lactate or glucose to the medium restores the cytosolic NADPH/($NADP^+$ + NADPH) ratio to its usual level (Table 3) and stimulates the rate of drug monooxygenation in liver cells from starved, phenobarbital-treated animals (63,65). These results suggest that in the glycogen-depleted state, the NADPH for drug monooxygenation is generated via energy-dependent mitochondrial shuttle mechanisms. This hypothesis is further supported by the fact that inhibitors of mitochondrial respiration, such as rotenone and antimycin A, lower the cytosolic NADPH/($NADP^+$ + NADPH) ratio and inhibit drug metabolism in isolated hepatocytes from starved animals (Table 3). When glycogen is present, however, it appears that the pentose shunt dehydrogenases are capable of maintaining the supply of NADPH for drug monooxygenation in the absence of this mitochondrial supply (Table 3).

Further studies on the supply of reducing equivalents for drug metabolism therefore seem warranted, especially in light of the contributions of Ernster and his colleagues on the energy-dependent transhydrogenase (90,91). Moreover, the use of isolated cells in combination with recently developed quantitative cytochemical techniques (100, 101) may reveal a great deal of information about the utilization of NADPH in different biochemical pathways within the cell, and especially about competition between drug metabolism and other pathways of NADPH utilization.

The oxygen dependence of monooxygenase reactions has been shown to be similar to that observed for microsomal metabolism (39). The results of this study indicated that although there appears to be a marked gradient of oxygen into the mitochondrial membrane under hypoxic conditions, there is at most a minimal gradient to the endoplasmic reticulum. Thus, since hexobarbital and alprenolol metabolism is oxygen dependent below 20 to 35 μM, and the normal concentration of oxygen in tissues is within this range, the metabolism of certain drugs may be impaired during hypoxia (36).

Sequential Metabolism of Drugs in Isolated Cells

In 1977, Billings and her associates reported that freshly isolated liver cells catalyze the various phase I and phase II reactions involved in drug metabolism at rates comparable to those observed *in vivo* or with the isolated perfused liver (5). Moreover, studies in our laboratory have shown that the phase I and phase II metabolism of several different drugs occurs at similar rates in isolated hepatocytes and liver microsomes (1,65).

Using alprenolol, benzo(a)pyrene, and 7-ethoxycoumarin as substrates, Moldéus and his associates (65) were able to compare the rate of oxidation of these three compounds in isolated hepatocytes and liver microsomes. Alprenolol was chosen as a substrate because it is rather rapidly metabolized and shows a high affinity for cytochrome P-450 (7). This latter property enabled a substrate disappearance method to be used to measure its metabolism. A similar technique was also used for assaying benzo(a)pyrene metabolism (112). Although objections may be raised against substrate disappearance measurements of phase I drug metabolism, difficulties in assaying metabolite formation in isolated cells often leave no alternative, especially in hepatocytes, where the primary products are further metabolized in phase II reactions.

The rate of oxidation of the three substrates was linear with time for at least 1 hr in isolated hepatocytes without any addition of cofactors. When compared to the rates found with isolated microsomes supplemented with an NADPH-generating system, the oxidation of benzo(a)pyrene and 7-ethoxycoumarin was found to be somewhat slower in the hepatocytes, whereas alprenolol metabolism was slightly faster (Table 4). In liver cells isolated from phenobarbital-treated rats, the metabolism of both alprenolol and 7-ethoxycoumarin was increased, and for 7-ethoxycoumarin, this increase was more than 10-fold (Table 4). Benzo(a)pyrene metabolism was not affected by this treatment but was enhanced six- to sevenfold in liver cells from 3-methylcholanthrene-treated rats. In general, the changes in the rates of oxidation caused by phenobarbital and 3-methylcholanthrene administration were the same in isolated liver cells and microsomes (Table 4).

Similarly, analysis of the rates of glucuronidation of several substrates, including 4-methylumbelliferone and harmol, indicates that the activities observed with isolated hepatocytes are not significantly different from those obtained with nonactivated microsomes (Table 5) (1). Glucuronidation rates observed after activation of microsomal UDP-glucuronosyltransferase (53,113) may thus be artificially high and lack physiological significance.

One of the major advantages of freshly isolated cells as an experimental model is the ability to study sequences of reactions catalyzed by enzymes located in different cellular compartments. For example, the cytochrome P-450-linked phase I metabolism of 7-ethoxycoumarin results in the formation of the dealkylated product 7-hydroxycoumarin. This metabolite is then subsequently conjugated in a phase II reaction to form either a sulfate or a glucuronide. The results shown in Tables 4 and 6 clearly show that both phenobarbital and 3-methylcholanthrene pretreatments lead to a severalfold increase in the rate of oxidative dealkylation of this drug in isolated hepatocytes. However, no similar enhancement of the rate of conjugate formation is found after these treatments (Table 6). Such treatments may therefore lead to the accumulation of oxidized, nonconjugated metabolites of many similar drugs within the liver cells. Hence, induction of the rate of cytochrome P-450-linked drug oxidation but not of subsequent conjugate formation could cause increased drug hepatotoxicity, since formation of glucuronide, sulfate, and glutathione conjugates of oxidized drug products is generally associated with decreased toxicities of these species, although there are a few notable exceptions to this rule (14, 56,85).

The availability of isolated cells from various tissues has allowed comparative studies to be made of drug biotransformation in dif-

TABLE 5. *Rate of glucuronidation[a] in hepatocytes and microsomes from control rats[b]*

Substrate	Cells	Microsomes
4-Methylumbelliferone	5.01 ± 0.64	5.30 ± 0.08
Harmol	4.33 ± 0.46	4.96 ± 0.52

[a] Rate expressed in nmole/mg microsomal protein per min.
[b] Data from Andersson et al. (2).

TABLE 4. *Rate of cytochrome P-450-linked drug metabolism in rat hepatocytes and liver microsomes[a]*

	Microsomes			Hepatocytes		
Substrate	Control	PB	3-MC	Control	PB	3-MC
Benzo(a)pyrene	1.0	0.3	2.8	0.5	0.1	1.7
Alprenolol	2.0	1.1	0.7	2.4	0.9	0.7
7-Ethoxycoumarin	0.6	2.6	5.3	0.4	1.0	2.0

[a] Values are expressed as nmole substrate metabolized per min per nmole cytochrome P-450. Pretreatments: PB, phenobarbital (0.1%) in drinking water for 7 days; 3-MC, 20 mg/kg body weight 3-methylcholanthrene injected daily for 3 days. Data from Moldéus et al. (65).

TABLE 6. *Oxidative deethylation and conjugation of 7-ethoxycoumarin and 7-hydroxycoumarin, respectively, in isolated rat hepatocytes*[a]

Treatment	Deethylation (nmole 7-hydroxycoumarin formed/min/10^6 cells)	Conjugation (nmole conjugate formed/min/10^6 cells)	Deethylation/ conjugation
None	0.08	0.17	0.44
Phenobarbital	0.94	0.23	4.08
3-Methylcholanthrene	1.25	0.33	3.78
Phenobarbital + 3-methylcholanthrene	2.15	0.23	9.35

[a] Data from Moldéus et al. (67).

ferent cell types. The metabolism of a large number of drugs has been examined (cf. 110), and it is quite clear that the metabolism of most foreign compounds occurs at a much slower rate in cells from extrahepatic tissues. This is exemplified by the results outlined in Table 7, which show that the metabolism of paracetamol (acetaminophen) takes place at a rate approximately 40 times faster in isolated rat hepatocytes than it does in cells isolated from rat kidney or small intestine. However, subsequent metabolism of the conjugates formed also appears to be unevenly distributed or compartmentalized within the organism (cf. 79).

By using sequential incubations of different isolated cells, it has been possible to reconstitute the entire biotransformation pathway for the conversion of paracetamol to its mercapturic acid derivative (26,41,66). In liver cells, paracetamol is oxidized by the cytochrome P-450-linked monooxygenase system to an electrophilic product that reacts with acid-soluble thiols (95% reduced glutathione in the liver) to form a conjugate (Table 7; Fig. 5). The glutathione conjugate is normally released from the liver into the bile but is recovered in the medium of liver cell incubations. Removal of the liver cells from the suspension by centrifugation, followed by subsequent addition of either isolated kidney or intestinal cells, results in the rapid conversion of the glutathione conjugate to the cysteine derivative (Fig. 5). The cysteine derivative is finally acetylated in kidney cells to form the mercapturic acid derivative (Fig. 5). Figure 6 illustrates the tissue localization of the major metabolic steps involved in the conversion of paracetamol to its mercapturic acid derivative.

APPLICATIONS OF ISOLATED CELLS IN STUDIES ON DRUG TOXICITY

Suspensions of freshly isolated cells are an extremely useful model for studies on drug toxicity because they are capable of meta-

TABLE 7. *Paracetamol metabolite formation in isolated liver, kidney, and small intestine cells from the rat*[a]

Cell type	Glucuronide conjugate	Sulfate conjugate	Thiol conjugates	Total conjugates
Liver	76.6	48.0	8.4	134.0
Kidney	1.4	0.9	0.4	2.7
Small intestine	2.6	0.2	0.3	3.1

[a] Values are expressed as nmole conjugate formed/10^6 cells per hour. Data from Moldéus (59), Grafström et al. (25), and Jones et al. (44).

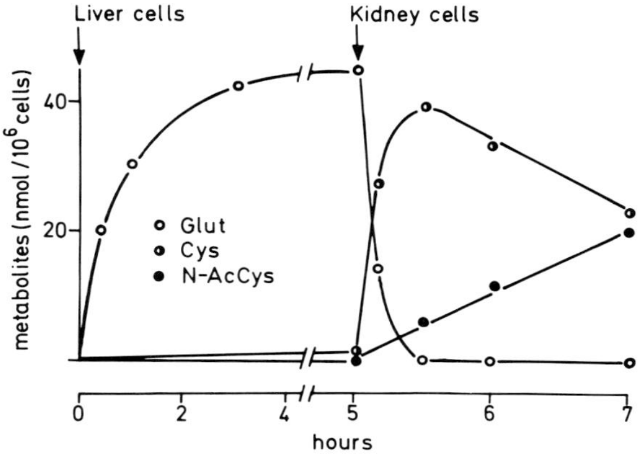

FIG. 5. Sequential metabolism of paracetamol (acetaminophen) by isolated liver and kidney cells. Paracetamol-glutathione was formed during incubation of isolated liver cells with paracetamol. Liver cells were then removed by centrifugation, and kidney cells added as indicated. Data from Moldéus et al. (66).

bolic activation and/or inactivation of a variety of toxic agents and, at the same time, serve as a sensitive indicator system for various toxic effects.

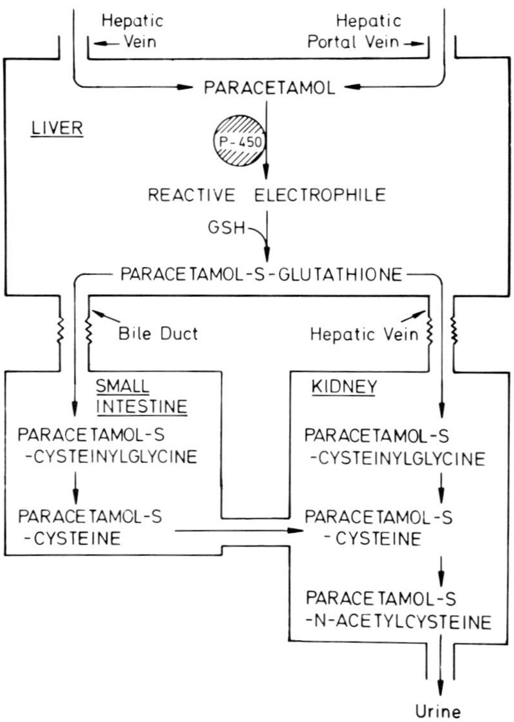

FIG. 6. Tissue localization of major reactions involved in the conversion of paracetamol to its corresponding mercapturic acid derivative.

Measurement of Toxic Effects

The plasma membrane has often been implicated as the primary target in the pathogenesis of toxic cell death (see 19), and in many studies it has been shown that a gradual increase in plasma membrane permeability occurs as a result of cellular injury (81,93,109). The permeability of the plasma membrane is therefore routinely used as an index of cell viability, and its usefulness has been clearly established (93). Fortunately, the plasma membrane permeability of isolated cells in suspension is readily determined by using the trypan blue exclusion test (65) or by measuring the latency of cytosolic enzymes (31,65). Moreover, these assays are extremely sensitive and can be performed on very small samples (<50 μl) of isolated cell suspensions. It is therefore possible to directly correlate changes in biochemical parameters with cell viability during the toxic exposure of isolated cells to a drug. Isolated cells may thus be used to evaluate the importance of widely different biochemical events in the toxicity of a specified drug (98,99,109).

Although changes in plasma membrane permeability are easy to monitor and are normally used as a measure of cytotoxicity in suspensions of isolated cells, it is important to note that other toxic effects can also be investigated in this model system. For example, the alkylation of low-molecular nucleophiles, such as reduced glutathione, nicotinamide nucleotides, and coenzyme A, and high-molecular nucleophiles, such as proteins and nucleic acids, is relatively easy to investigate, as is the binding of toxic electrophilic metabolites to these nucleophiles (9,107–109). The alkylation of these low- and high-molecular nucleophilic compounds could lead to the depletion of cofactors and cosubstrates required for important metabolic reactions in the cell and to the inhibition and denaturation of important enzymes (23,30,109). The relative importance of such alkylating events in the cytotoxicity of several different compounds is discussed later in this chapter.

Lipid peroxidation is also considered to be an important event in the cytotoxicity of several different compounds including carbon tetrachloride (86) and bromotrichloromethane (49), but its role in the toxic effects of other compounds, including paraquat and anthracycline cytostatics, remains a highly controversial matter (10,68,71,95,102). The biochemical consequences of lipid peroxidation are well known and include membrane damage, enzyme inhibition, release of lysosomal enzymes, and protein–protein cross linking (10,52,118).

The role of lipid peroxidation in the cytotoxicity of drugs and xenobiotics, however, has been difficult to evaluate, largely because it is so difficult to measure low levels of lipid peroxidation in living systems and in complex *in vitro* experimental systems. For example, the thiobarbituric acid assay of malondialdehyde formation is a reliable index of lipid peroxidation in isolated subcellular fractions but is less suitable for the measurement of lipid peroxidation *in vivo* and in complex model systems because malondialdehyde is metabolized by mitochondria present in intact cells and also interacts with many cellular components. This makes the assay insensitive, and failure to detect malondialdehyde *in vivo* or in complex *in vitro* systems, such as isolated cells, cannot be taken as reflecting an absence of lipid peroxidation.

In the last few years, however, the measurement of hydrocarbon gas evolution has shown itself to be a reliable and sensitive index of lipid peroxidation *in vivo* (46,89,92), and very recently this technique has been adapted for use with complex *in vitro* experimental systems, including suspensions of isolated cells (98) and the isolated perfused liver (69). Later in this chapter we discuss how these recent developments can help the biochemical toxicologist to evaluate the importance of lipid peroxidation in the toxicity of a variety of xenobiotics.

As outlined briefly above, the compartmentation of detoxication reactions is becoming an area of intense research interest in drug metabolism and drug toxicity (79), and isolated cells provide an almost ideal experimental model for studies on compartmentation at the subcellular level. Freshly isolated cells can be rapidly fractionated into the various subcellular fractions using either digitonin or cavitation techniques (119) or a combination of the two (70). The intracellular distribution of ATP, ADP, AMP, NADP(H), NAD(H), reduced and oxidized glutathione, and even small ions such as Ca^{2+} can therefore be investigated (70,119). Changes in the intracellular distribution of these small molecules and ions may be one of the earliest responses of the cell to toxic injury and could upset a large number of cellular homeostatic mechanisms. The importance of such events in the toxicity of a variety of different drugs and other xenobiotics is presently the subject of intense research activity in our laboratory.

In the final part of this chapter, we wish to summarize the results of a series of experiments performed with isolated rat hepatocytes and a variety of potentially toxic drugs. This summary may serve to illustrate how the biochemical measurement of toxic effects in isolated cells and its correlation with morphological changes have contributed towards a better understanding of the mechanisms involved in drug-induced toxicity.

Studies on Bromobenzene Toxicity

Bromobenzene is a widely studied hepatotoxic agent that produces pericentral or centrilobular liver necrosis when administered in sufficient doses to laboratory animals (48,88). Hepatocytes isolated from phenobarbital-treated rats metabolize bromobenzene to a reactive intermediate, which has been tentatively identified as bromobenzene 3,4-epoxide (35). This metabolite, which is formed in a cytochrome P-450-dependent reaction, may subsequently rearrange nonenzymatically to yield the corresponding phenol, act as a substrate for epoxide hydrolase to produce a *trans*-dihydrodiol, or react with reduced glutathione (GSH) to form the corresponding conjugate. The latter reaction, which may occur both enzymatically and nonenzymatically, is the main pathway for inactivation of the epoxide. Thus, in the absence of glutathione, the reactive intermediate can accumulate intracellularly and interact with various low-molecular and macromolecular nucleophiles. The final result of these interactions is cell death.

Figure 7 shows that the formation of water-soluble metabolites of bromobenzene by hepatocytes isolated from phenobarbital-treated rats is associated with a decrease in the intracellular level of GSH. However, the total depletion of GSH did not occur because GSH was constantly resynthesized from precursor amino acids in the medium (see 108). Moreover, the incubation of these cells with bromobenzene was not associated with accelerated cell damage, as indicated by the low rate of NADH penetration (Fig. 7). When rats were treated with phenobarbital and diethyl maleate (DEM), however, the isolated hepatocytes were extremely susceptible to bromobenzene toxicity (Fig. 7). The DEM pretreatment is a standard procedure to lower tissue GSH levels (8), and Fig. 7 shows that hepatocytes from phenobarbital- and DEM-treated rats are not capable of retaining a sufficient level of GSH during bromobenzene metabolism by resynthesis of the thiol, although they are able to replenish their depleted GSH when incubated in the presence of precursor amino acids in the absence of bromobenzene (87,106).

Thus, bromobenzene-induced cell damage is observed only in the GSH-depleted state and is counteracted by facilitated GSH resynthesis. In liver, the intracellular concentration of cysteine is low and rate limiting for GSH biosynthesis (87). The presence of cysteine or methionine in the medium facilitates GSH biosynthesis by providing intracellular cysteine; methionine yields cysteine via the cystathionine pathway. The results outlined

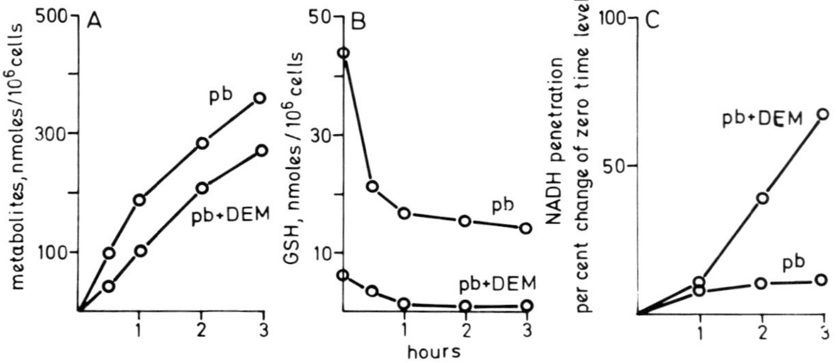

FIG. 7. Bromobenzene metabolites (**A**), GSH level (**B**), and NADH penetration (**C**) in hepatocytes isolated from phenobarbital- or phenobarbital- and DEM-treated rats. Data from Thor et al. (107).

in Table 8 show that both cysteine and methionine protect isolated hepatocytes from the toxic effects of bromobenzene. Moreover, the effect of the glutathione biosynthesis inhibitor methionine sulfoximine (82) (Table 8) indicated that protection by methionine and cysteine is in fact exerted via GSH synthesis and not by a direct effect of either of the two amino acids (108).

A decreased level of cellular GSH is a constant and early effect of bromobenzene metabolism by hepatocytes. The decrease in GSH is followed by lowered levels of various coenzymes including NAD(H), NADP(H), and free and bound coenzyme A (Fig. 8). This effect is particularly pronounced in the GSH-depleted state, and the available evidence suggests that it may be caused by direct alkylation of the coenzymes by reactive bromobenzene metabolites (106).

Accumulation of bromobenzene metabolites strongly bound to cellular protein occurs in parallel to the effect on soluble nucleophiles (109). This binding could be related to the inhibition of certain cytosolic enzymes, notably glucose-6-phosphate dehydrogenase (G-6-PDH) and glutathione (GSSG) reductase, whereas other enzyme activities, such as the activities of lactate dehydrogenase (LDH) and isocitrate dehydrogenase (IDH), were less affected or completely unaffected by bromobenzene metabolism (Fig. 9A). When the purified enzymes were incubated with liver microsomes, NADPH, and bromobenzene, a similar pattern of response was observed (Fig. 9B). The inhibitory effect of bromobenzene metabolism on G-6-PDH and GSSG reductase activities is probably related to an effect of reactive metabolites on free thiol groups required for enzyme activity. Electrophilic metabolites, including epoxides, have previously been found to inhibit enzyme activity by direct interaction with SH groups on the enzyme protein.

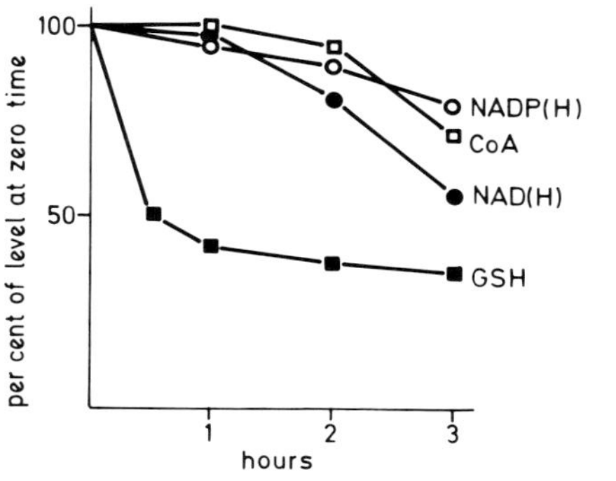

FIG. 8. Levels of GSH, NAD(H), NADP(H), and coenzyme A in hepatocytes isolated from a phenobarbital-treated rat incubated with bromobenzene (0.6 mM). From Thor and Orrenius (109).

TABLE 8. *Cysteine and methionine protect hepatocytes against bromobenzene toxicity by facilitated glutathione synthesis*[a]

Addition	Percent trypan blue uptake after 2.5 hr incubation
None	20
Bromobenzene (0.6 mM)	47
Methionine sulfoximine (5 mM)	21
Bromobenzene + cysteine (0.5 mM)	20
Bromobenzene + cysteine + methionine sulfoximine	40
Bromobenzene + methionine (0.5 mM)	25
Bromobenzene + methionine + methionine sulfoximine	40

[a] Data from Thor et al. (109).

The metabolism of bromobenzene in isolated hepatocytes also alters the biochemical properties of the plasma membrane. For example, the uptake of certain amino acids, notably methionine, is inhibited during bromobenzene metabolism in isolated hepatocytes (108), possibly as a result of inhibition of the Mg^{2+}-dependent Na^+, K^+-stimulated ATPase present in the hepatocyte plasma membrane (109). There is also a dramatic loss of normal permeability barriers, as indicated by increased trypan blue, NADH, and succinate penetration (Fig. 10A,B,D) and leakage of intracellular potassium (Fig. 10C). However, the recent proposal that the loss of the plasma membrane permeability

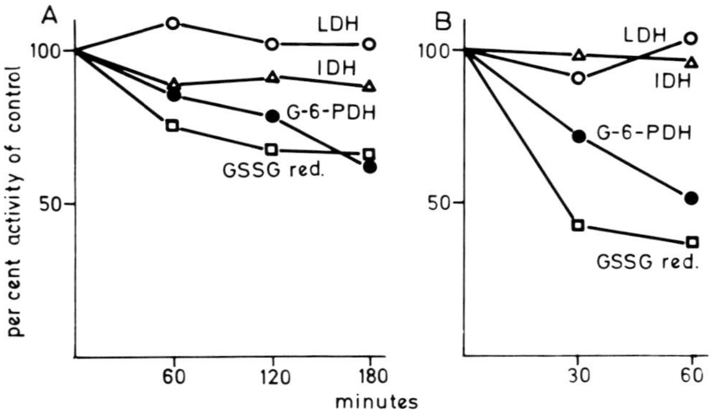

FIG. 9. Effect of bromobenzene metabolism on the activities of various cytosolic enzymes in (**A**) the cytosolic fraction of disrupted hepatocytes from phenobarbital- and DEM-treated rats and (**B**) on samples of the purified enzymes. Data from Thor and Orrenius (109).

barrier to extracellular Ca^{2+} ions is the final common pathway in toxic cell death by widely differing compounds (93) does not seem to hold true for bromobenzene hepatotoxicity or for other forms of toxic cell death in freshly isolated liver cells (99). In contrast, removal of Ca^{2+} ions from the incubation medium made isolated hepatocytes more susceptible to the toxic effects of bromobenzene (Table 9). Moreover, bromobenzene, carbon tetrachloride, and the direct alkylating agent ethylmethanesulfonate were

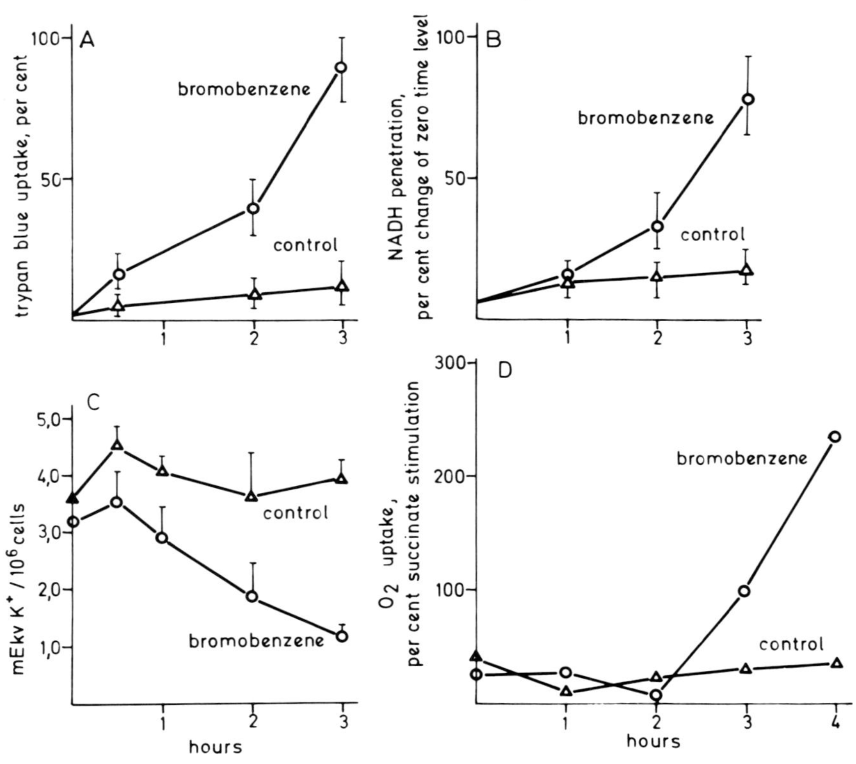

FIG. 10. Effect of bromobenzene metabolism on the viability of hepatocytes isolated from phenobarbital- and DEM-treated rats as determined by (**A**) trypan blue uptake, (**B**) NADH penetration, (**C**) loss of intracellular potassium, and (**D**) succinate penetration. Data from Thor and Orrenius (109).

TABLE 9. *Bromobenzene hepatocytotoxicity is not dependent on extracellular calcium*[a]

Addition	Percent dead cells after 4 hr incubation	
	Ca^{2+} present	Ca^{2+} absent
None	21.5 ± 3.5	31.7 ± 4.7
Bromobenzene (0.6 mM)	35.2 ± 4.3	88.0 ± 3.5

[a] Isolated hepatocytes from phenobarbital-treated male rats were incubated in the absence and presence of 2.6 mM Ca^{2+} in Krebs–Henseleit buffer. The percentage of dead cells was determined by trypan blue uptake after 4 hr incubation. Values represent means (±SEM) of four separate experiments. Data from Smith et al. (99).

all highly toxic to isolated liver cells suspended in Ca^{2+}-free buffer containing the Ca^{2+}-specific chelator EGTA, indicating that toxic liver cell injury caused by these compounds is not dependent on an influx of extracellular Ca^{2+} (99).

The metabolism of bromobenzene also causes alterations in the morphology of isolated hepatocytes. Freshly isolated hepatocytes incubated in the absence of bromobenzene have a normal, rounded appearance and a regular, villous surface structure with numerous microspikes (see Fig. 3). The loss of these microvilli and the development of a smooth surface with occasional blebbing of the plasma membrane are early signs of bromobenzene toxicity (Fig. 11A) and are followed by the formation of blebs of increased size (Fig. 11B). Eventually, the plasma membrane of the hepatocytes breaks down, and the dead cells have a fragmented appearance (Fig. 11C). The formation of blebs at the hepatocyte surface probably reflects a change in cytoskeletal structure, because substances that interact directly with the hepatocyte cytoskeleton, such as cytochalasins B and D and phalloidin, produce blebs of similar appearance to those seen with bromobenzene (83) (Fig. 12). As yet, however, we have found no evidence that bromobenzene metabolites interact directly with cytoskeletal proteins, but recently we observed that intracellular calcium homeostasis is altered during the metabolism of bromobenzene in isolated hepatocytes (34).

Since Ca^{2+} and its associated binding proteins play such a pivotal role in regulating cytoskeletal structure and function, it is probable that a change in intracellular Ca^{2+} distribution is responsible for the bromobenzene-induced bleb formation. More specifically, it appears that the depletion of GSH is followed by the mobilization and loss of Ca^{2+} from an extramitochondrial source, which then brings about the formation of surface blebs (34). The precise mechanism by which the release of Ca^{2+} from extramitochondrial stores causes the formation of blebs in the plasma membrane is presently under investigation but could involve an initial rise in the cytosolic Ca^{2+} concentration.

We hope that these studies with bromobenzene and isolated hepatocytes illustrate the potential usefulness of isolated cells in studies on drug toxicity. Their use has enabled us to clarify several of the potentially cytotoxic effects of bromobenzene metabolism. However, the question of whether or not the cell death is the result of a complex summation of these and possibly other effects or is simply the result of a "critical" injury is not yet clear and hence must remain the subject of further investigation.

Studies of the Acute Toxicity of Other Foreign Compounds

The cytotoxic effects of bromobenzene in isolated hepatocytes are similar to those observed with paracetamol, but there are several distinct differences. For example, paracetamol cytotoxicity is not observed in isolated rat hepatocytes even after induction with phenobarbital or ethanol, but in isolated mouse hepatocytes, paracetamol-induced cell damage can occur (59,62). Moreover, paracetamol toxicity is enhanced in hepatocytes isolated from either phenobarbital- or 3-methylcholanthrene-pretreated mice,

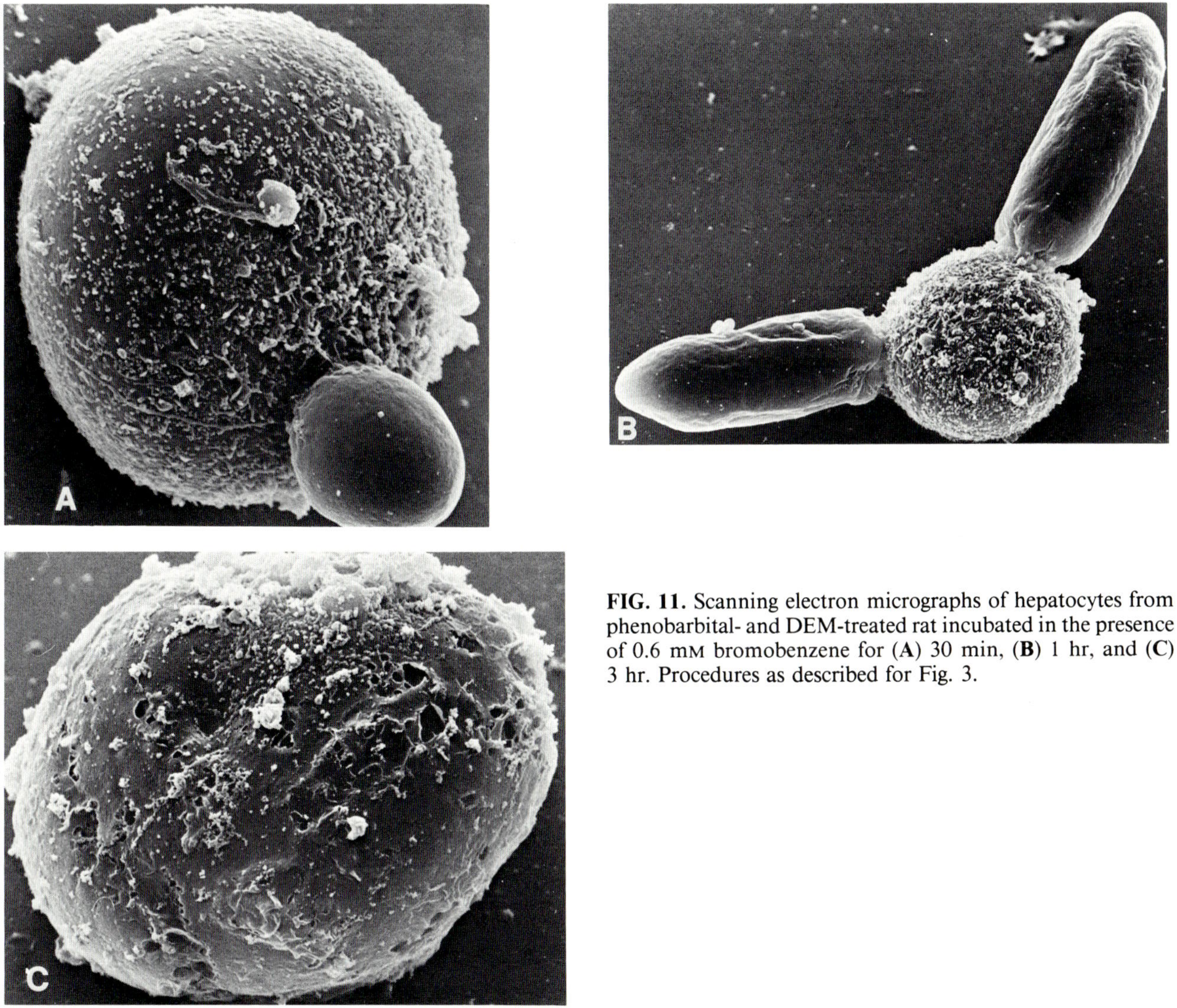

FIG. 11. Scanning electron micrographs of hepatocytes from phenobarbital- and DEM-treated rat incubated in the presence of 0.6 mM bromobenzene for (**A**) 30 min, (**B**) 1 hr, and (**C**) 3 hr. Procedures as described for Fig. 3.

whereas only phenobarbital, but not 3-methylcholanthrene, pretreatment increases the cytotoxicity of bromobenzene (35,60,80). The prior depletion of intracellular glutathione is, however, absolutely required for both paracetamol and bromobenzene to elicit their cytotoxic effects, and the inclusion of GSH precursor amino acids in the incubation medium prevents paracetamol toxicity in isolated mouse hepatocytes, most probably by facilitating GSH resynthesis (59,60). Other aspects of paracetamol metabolism and toxicity in isolated cells have also recently been reviewed (60).

In contrast to bromobenzene and paracetamol, the cytotoxicity of carbon tetrachloride in isolated hepatocytes is not preceded by a dramatic depletion of intracellular glutathione (80). This suggests that mechanisms other than the alkylation of intracellular nucleophiles are responsible for the toxic effects of carbon tetrachloride, and the available evidence indicates that carbon tetrachloride exerts its hepatotoxic effect by initiating lipid peroxidation (86).

However, as discussed previously in this chapter, there are several problems associated with the measurement of lipid peroxidation in isolated cells and a general lack of sensitive methods. We therefore recently performed a comparative study of five different techniques for the measurement of lipid peroxidation in isolated hepatocytes, using carbon tetrachloride as a model substrate (98). The results of this study are summarized in Fig. 13 and show that ethane production and chemiluminescence are much more sensitive indices of lipid peroxidation in isolated hepatocytes than malondialdehyde formation. Using these techniques, we were then able to show that lipid peroxidation occurs at a very early stage and prior to cell death in carbon tetrachloride hepatocytotoxicity (Fig. 14A,C) but at a much later stage, and only after glutathione depletion and cell death, in bromobenzene hepatocytotoxicity (Fig. 14B,D). Lipid peroxidation therefore appears to be an important event in carbon tetrachloride cytotoxicity but only a subsequent event of the cytotoxic effects of bromobenzene (98). These findings are in agreement with the conclusions of previous workers (3,58) and show that the use of sensitive indices of lipid peroxidation such as ethane production and chemiluminescence in isolated cells can yield valuable information regarding the primary toxic effects of drugs and other foreign compounds. These methods are now being applied in studies on the toxic effects of xenobiotics such as paraquat and adriamycin, where the role of lipid peroxidation remains unclear.

In this discussion we have, so far, concentrated mainly on the acute toxic effects of drugs and foreign compounds, but isolated mammalian cells also provide a useful model for studies on the chronic effects of foreign compounds that are not necessarily associated with their acute toxicity. For example, the role of metabolic activation in the carcinogenic effects of the polycyclic aromatic hydrocarbon benzo(a)pyrene has been extensively studied in isolated hepatocytes (9,33). Figure 15 shows that the overall metabolism of benzo(a)pyrene in hepatocytes involves a series of consecutive reactions including monooxygenation, hydration, and conjugation as well as reactions associated with the repair of modified DNA. In the intact cell, the balance between activation and deactivation processes will therefore determine the intracellular concentrations of metabolites that can be further activated to DNA-binding products. The isolated hepatocyte offers an excellent model for observing these processes individually or in concert. Moreover, coincubation of isolated hepatocytes with other cell types has shown that DNA-binding metabolites formed within the hepatocytes can be excreted and transferred to cells of a different type, such as fibroblasts, where they can exert their DNA-modifying effects (72).

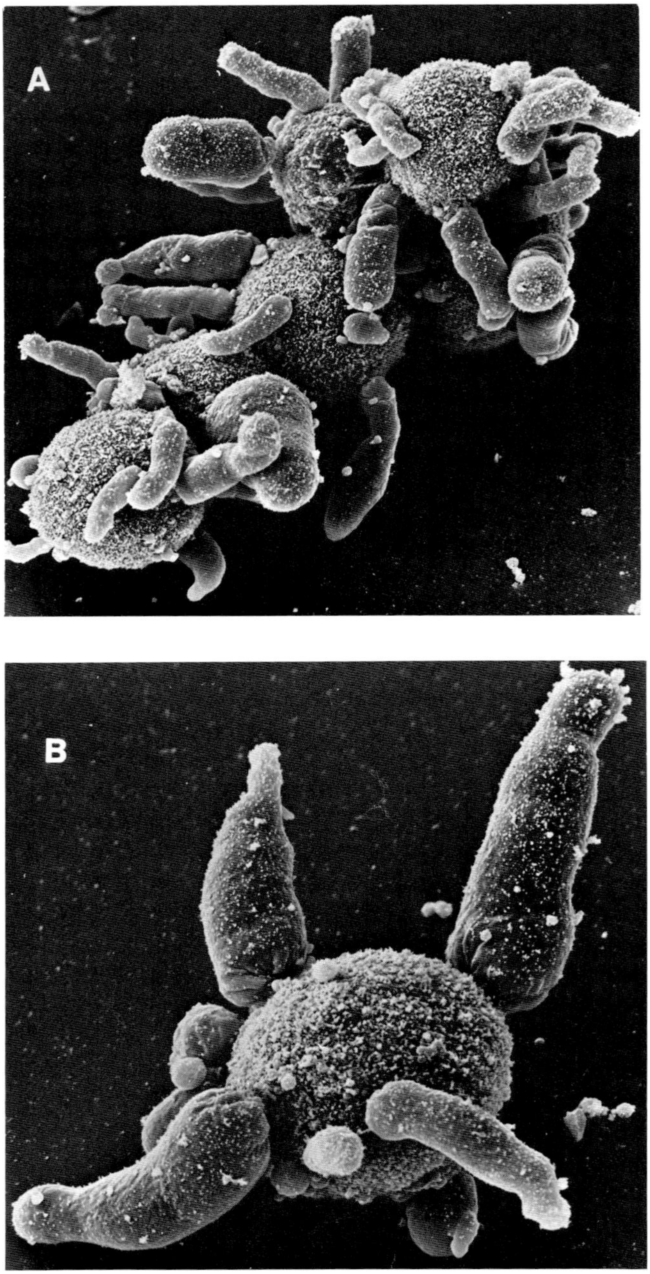

FIG. 12. Scanning electron micrographs of hepatocytes isolated from phenobarbital-treated rat incubated in the presence of cytochalasin B (10 μg/ml) for 5 min. **A:** A single hepatocyte. **B:** Aggregated hepatocytes. **C** (*facing page*): The "pinching off" of a large bleb. Procedures as described for Fig. 3.

Formation of Toxic Side Products During Drug Metabolism

During the metabolism of a wide variety of foreign compounds, various potentially toxic side products are formed. For example, the oxidative demethylation of drugs by the cytochrome P-450 system yields formaldehyde, which is a highly toxic compound (47,117). However, in isolated hepatoctyes, formaldehyde is not detectable during oxidative demethylation (16), presumably be-

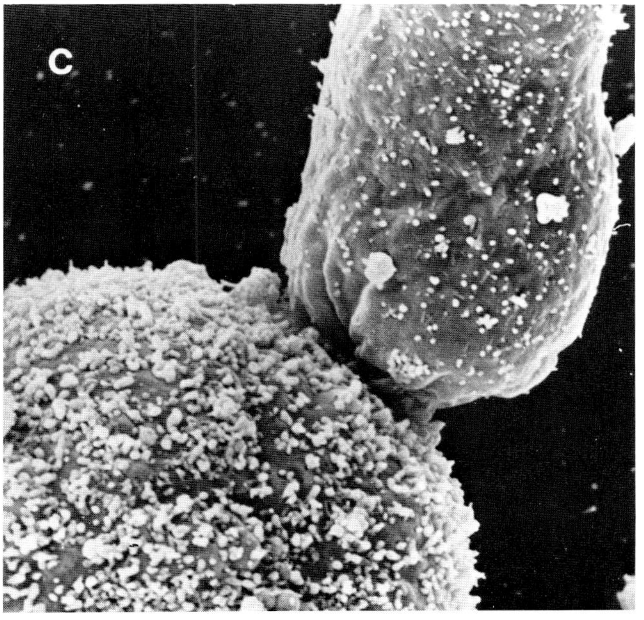

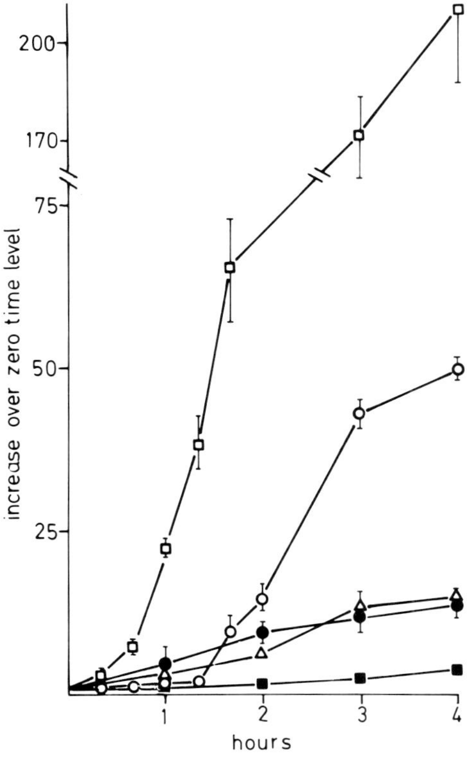

FIG. 13. Comparison of the sensitivity of different assays of CCl_4-induced lipid peroxidation in hepatocytes isolated from phenobarbital-treated rat. Malondialdehyde production (●); fluorescent products (■); chemiluminescence (○); ethane production (□); pentane production (△). Data from Smith et al. (98).

cause it is rapidly oxidized by formaldehyde dehydrogenases, producing formic acid, which is then further oxidized to H_2O and CO_2 (75). Although several aldehyde dehydrogenases may be involved in formaldehyde oxidation (54,104), the depletion of cellular glutathione by pretreatment with DEM decreases the rate of formic acid production in isolated hepatocytes (45). Thus, most of the formaldehyde produced during oxidative demethylation appears to be oxidized by the GSH-dependent formaldehyde dehydrogenase present in rat and human liver (24,45,111). Moreover, because of the rapid nonenzymatic reaction of formaldehyde with GSH, this enzyme system may be viewed as essential to prevent the loss of GSH as a result of *S*-hydroxymethylglutathione formation in the detoxication of formaldehyde (45).

The toxicological implications of the formation of active forms of oxygen during drug

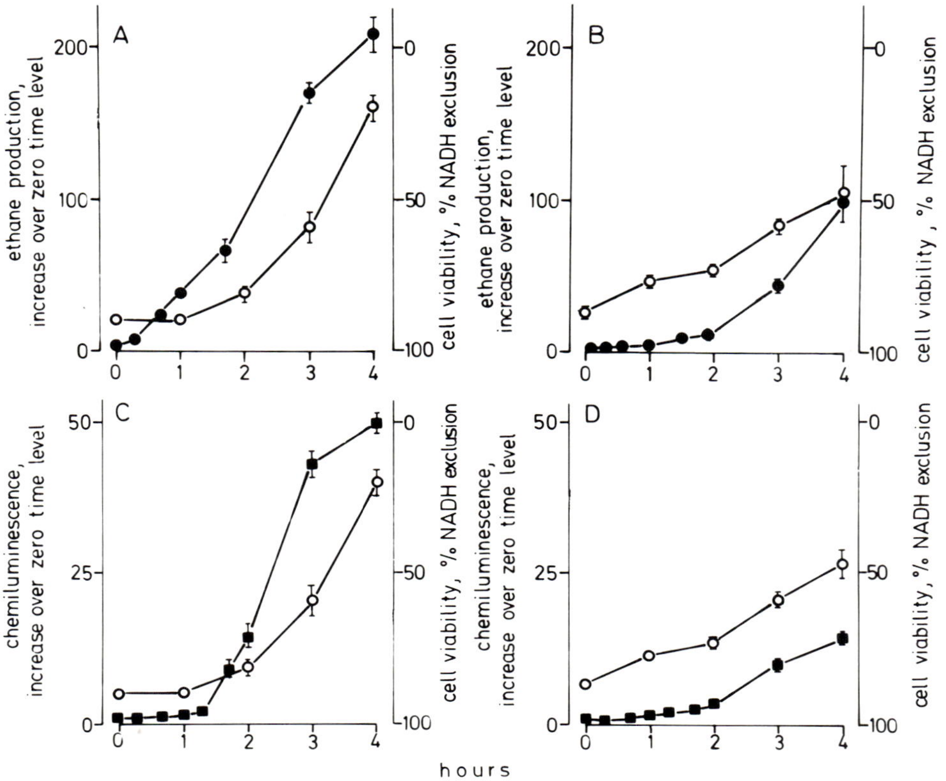

FIG. 14. Relationship between lipid peroxidation and the toxicity of carbon tetrachloride (**A, C**) and bromobenzene (**B, D**) in isolated hepatocytes from phenobarbital-treated rat. Increases in ethane production (●) and chemiluminescence (■) over the zero-time level were used as the indices of lipid peroxidation. Cell viability (○) was measured by the NADH penetration assay. Data from Smith et al. (98).

treatment have recently received increased attention. Superoxide radical ($O_2^- \cdot$), hydrogen peroxide (H_2O_2), hydroxyl radical ($OH \cdot$), and singlet oxygen ($^1\Delta g\ O_2$) are all reactive forms of oxygen that may cause cell toxicity when present at sufficiently high concentrations. Since these species are reactive, and because there are ubiquitous enzyme systems to decompose them (20), evidence for their formation in intact cells following drug administration is frequently only indirect. However, techniques for the measurement of increased hydrogen peroxide formation in isolated hepatocytes following drug administration have recently been developed (37,45). It is therefore possible to study the relationship between H_2O_2 production and drug toxicity using this system.

Incubation of liver microsomes with NADPH has long been known to result in formation of H_2O_2 (22). More recently, microsomal H_2O_2 production has been shown to be affected by cytochrome P-450 inducers and by the presence of various drug substrates in the microsomal incubation (28), and available evidence indicates that it is the result of autooxidation of cytochrome P-450 and is mediated by release of superoxide from the cocomplex of the hemoprotein (50).

Studies of ethylmorphine metabolism in hepatocytes suggested that drug oxidation can also be associated with stimulated H_2O_2

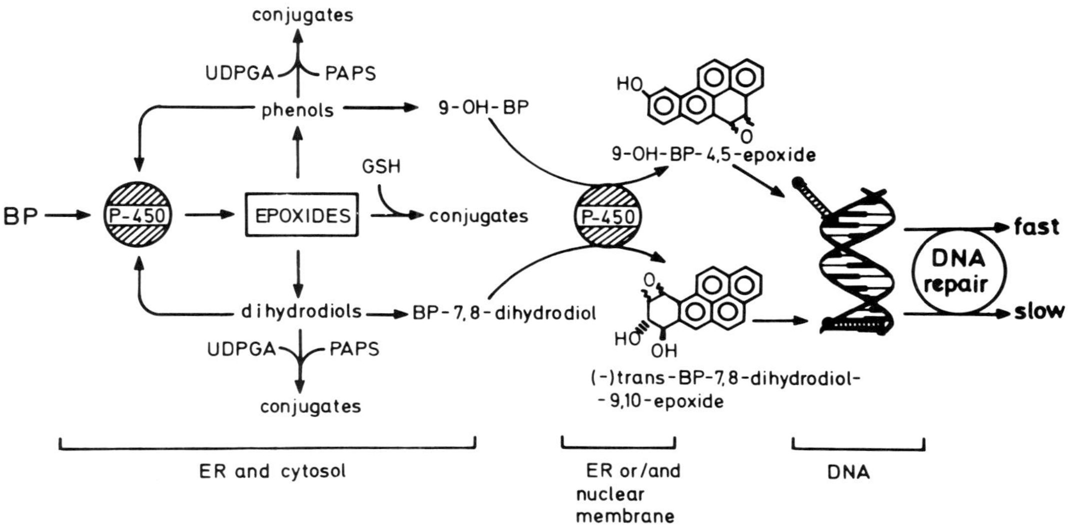

FIG. 15. Possible mechanisms involved in the formation and regulation of DNA-binding products of benzo(a)pyrene in hepatocytes isolated from 3-methylcholanthrene-treated rats. BP, benzo(a)pyrene; UDPGA, uridine-5′-diphosphoglucuronic acid; PAPS, 3′-phosphoadenosine-5′-phosphosulfate; GSH, reduced glutathione; ER, endoplasmic reticulum. Data from S. Orrenius et al., ref. 80, with permission.

generation in the intact cell (45). Thus, incubation of hepatocytes from phenobarbital-treated rat with ethylmorphine resulted in oxidation of intracellular GSH and release of glutathione disulfide into the medium. When cells depleted of glutathione by pretreatment of the animal with diethylmaleate (65) were used for incubation, titration with methanol revealed that a relatively larger fraction of catalase was present as the primary H_2O_2 complex, Compound I, when ethylmorphine or related drugs were present in the medium (45).

These early observations have recently been extended into a more detailed study of H_2O_2 generation and catabolism in hepatocytes (37). In this investigation, ethylmorphine and glycolate have been used to stimulate H_2O_2 generation in different cellular compartments, and the contribution of catalase and glutathione peroxidase to the metabolism of endogenously generated H_2O_2 has been compared (Fig. 16). The results of this study support the conclusion that in hepatocytes the relative contributions of catalase and glutathione peroxidase in the decomposition of endogenously generated H_2O_2 are determined by the subcellular distributions of the enzymes (37). Thus, the glutathione peroxidase/GSSG reductase system (Fig. 16) is quantitatively more important in the metabolism of H_2O_2 generated in the endoplasmic reticulum during drug metabolism (37). However, under conditions of limiting NADPH supply or high H_2O_2 production, the contribution of catalase will be enhanced.

The mechanism underlying the release of glutathione disulfide into the medium as a result of stimulation of the glutathione peroxidase reaction has also recently been studied in isolated hepatocytes (15), and it appears that the lack of NADPH is not the only reason for the release of GSSG by hepatocytes. The other factors involved are presently under detailed investigation.

Failure to metabolize the H_2O_2 produced during drug metabolism could obviously lead to conditions of oxidative stress within the hepatocytes. One of the implications of this

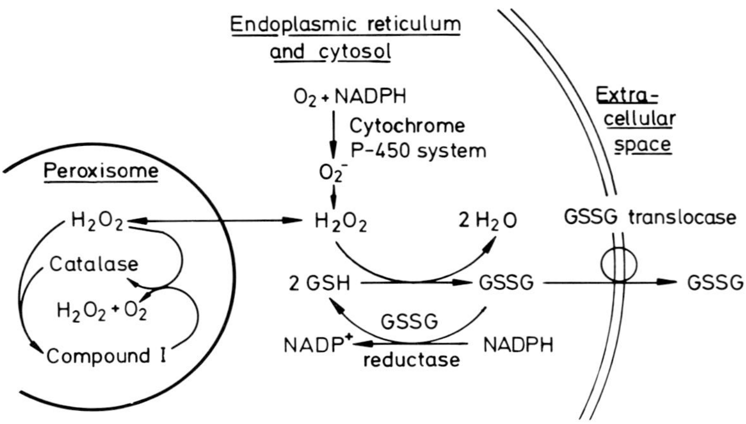

FIG. 16. Formation and catabolism of hydrogen peroxide in isolated hepatocytes.

may be an increased rate of lipid peroxidation, because H_2O_2 is known to initiate a free-radical chain reaction leading to lipid peroxidation in the presence of superoxide radical ($O_2^- \cdot$) and certain metals (84). However, in a recent study, no increase in ethane, chemiluminescence, or malondialdehyde production was observed during incubation of hepatocytes with ethylmorphine and aminopyrine at concentrations known to stimulate H_2O_2 production (98). The results of this study also showed, however, that these drugs are powerful inhibitors of lipid peroxidation in isolated hepatocytes as well as in liver microsomes (55,77), probably as a result of their antioxidant properties (55), and this may therefore have prevented any lipid peroxidation from occurring as a result of H_2O_2 accumulation. Other drugs that stimulate H_2O_2 production by the cytochrome P-450 system but lack antioxidant properties may therefore cause toxicity by increased formation of reactive oxygen species including H_2O_2.

CONCLUSION

Isolated mammalian cells have become an extremely useful experimental model for the study of many different aspects of drug metabolism and drug toxicity. In particular, improved methodology has allowed the direct quantitation of various hemoproteins and detailed analysis of interactions between drugs and cytochrome P-450 in intact cells. The generation of cosubstrates for drug biotransformation is also readily studied and appears to be one of the areas that can be favorably approached in future studies with isolated cells. Recent studies employing model toxins, such as bromobenzene and carbon tetrachloride, and isolated cells have also been described in detail in this presentation, and it is hoped that these studies illustrate the usefulness of the isolated cell model in studies of drug toxicity. It should be borne in mind, however, that suspensions of isolated cells are not necessarily an ideal experimental model in every situation. One important consideration that is often overlooked is that in such a preparation the spatial heterogeneity of the cells is not the same as in the whole organ. This can be particularly important in studies on cells from complex organs such as the kidney, where the metabolic zonation of biochemical reactions probably plays a significant role.

Despite such limitations, freshly isolated cells are widely used today in studies of cellular metabolism as well as drug biotransformation and toxicity. Moreover, as further progress is made in the development of techniques for studies on intact cells, it is quite clear that such preparations will become increasingly used in areas in which isolated cells constitute a good experimental model.

REFERENCES

1. Andersson, B., Berggren, M., and Moldéus, P. (1978): Conjugation of various drugs in isolated hepatocytes. *Drug. Metab. Dispos.*, 6:611–616.
2. Andersson, B., Jones, D. P., and Orrenius, S. (1979): Effect of calcium ions on ethanol oxidation and drug glucuronidation in isolated hepatocytes. *Biochem. J.*, 184:709–711.
3. Anundi, I., Högberg, J., and Stead, A. H. (1979): Glutathione depletion in isolated hepatocytes; its relation to lipid peroxidation and cell damage. *Acta Pharmacol. Toxicol.*, 45:45–51.
4. Berry, M. N., and Friend, D. S. (1969): High-yield preparation of isolated rat liver parenchymal cells; a biochemical and fine structural study. *J. Cell Biol.*, 43:506–520.
5. Billings, R. E., McMahon, R. E., Ashmore, J., and Wagle, S. R. (1977): The metabolism of drugs in isolated rat hepatocytes. A comparison with *in vivo* drug metabolism and drug metabolism in subcellular liver fractions. *Drug. Metab. Dispos.*, 5:518–526.
6. Bolcsfoldi, G., Johansson, M., Andersson, B., and Moldéus, P. (1981): Biotransformation of xenobiotics in isolated dog hepatocytes. *Acta Pharmacol. Toxicol. (Kbh.)*, 48:227–232.
7. Borg, K. O., Eklund, B., Skåneberg, I., and Wallborg, M. (1974): Metabolism of alprenolol in liver microsomes, perfused liver and conscious rat. *Acta Pharmacol. Toxicol. (Kbh.)*, 35:169–174.
8. Boyland, E., and Chasseaud, L. F. (1967): Enzyme-catalyzed conjugations of glutathione with unsaturated compounds. *Biochem. J.*, 104:95–102.
9. Burke, M. D., Vadi, H., Jernström, B., and Orrenius, S. (1977): Metabolism of benzo(a)pyrene with isolated hepatocytes and the formation and degradation of DNA-binding derivatives. *J. Biol. Chem.* 252:6424–6431.
10. Bus, J. S., and Gibson, J. E. (1979): Lipid peroxidation and its role in toxicity. In: *Reviews in Biochemical Toxicology, Vol. 1*, edited by E. Hodgson, J. R. Bend, and R. M. Philpot, pp. 125–149. Elsevier-North Holland, Amsterdam.
11. Chance, B. (1957): Techniques for the assay of the respiratory enzymes. *Methods Enzymol.*, 4:273–329.
12. Cohen, G., and Heikkila, R. E. (1974): The generation of hydrogen peroxide, superoxide radical and hydroxyl radical by 6-hydroxydopamine, dialuric acid and related cytotoxic agents. *J. Biol. Chem.*, 249:2447–2452.
13. Dawson, J. R., and Bridges, J. W. (1979): Xenobiotic metabolism by isolated intestinal epithelial cells from guinea pigs. *Biochem. Pharmacol.*, 28:3299–3305.
14. De Baun, J. R., Miller, E. C., and Miller, J. A. (1970): *N*-Hydroxy-2-acetylaminofluorene sulphotransferase. Its probable role in carcinogenesis and in protein-(methionyl-*S*-yl) binding in rat liver. *Cancer Res.*, 30:577–595.
15. Eklöw, L., Thor, H., and Orrenius, S. (1981): Formation and efflux of glutathione disulphide studied in isolated rat hepatocytes. *FEBS Lett.*, 127:125–128.
16. Erickson, R. R., and Holtzman, J. L. (1976): Kinetic studies on the metabolism of ethylmorphine by isolated hepatocytes from adult rats. *Biochem. Pharmacol.*, 25:1501–1506.
17. Ernster, L., and Orrenius, S. (1965): Substrate-induced synthesis of the hydroxylating enzyme system of liver microsomes. *Fed. Proc.*, 24:1190–1199.
18. Estabrook, R. W., Peterson, J., Baron, J., and Hildebrandt, A. (1972): In: *Methods in Pharmacology, Vol. 2*, edited by C. F. Chignell, pp. 303–350. Appleton-Century-Crofts, New York.
19. Farber, J. L., and El-Mofty, S. L. (1975): The biochemical pathology of liver cell necrosis. *Am. J. Pathol.*, 81:237–250.
20. Fridovich, I. (1974): Superoxide dismutase. *Adv. Enzymol.*, 41:35–97.
21. Ghazarian, J. G., Jefcoate, C. R., Knutson, J. C., Orme-Johnson, W. H., and De Luca, H. F. (1974): Mitochondrial cytochrome P-450: Component of chick kidney 25-hydroxycholecalciferol-1 alpha-hydroxylase. *J. Biol. Chem.*, 249:3026–3033.
22. Gillette, J. R., Brodie, B. B., and La Du, B. N. (1957): The oxidation of drugs by liver microsomes: on the role of TPNH and oxygen. *J. Pharmacol. Exp. Ther.*, 119:532–540.
23. Gillette, J. R., Mitchell, J. R., and Brodie, B. B. (1974): Biochemical basis for drug toxicity. *Annu. Rev. Pharmacol.*, 14:271–288.
24. Goodman, J. I., and Tephly, T. R. (1971): A comparison of rat and human liver formaldehyde dehydrogenase. *Biochim. Biophys. Acta*, 252:489–505.
25. Grafström, R., Moldéus, P., Andersson, B., and Orrenius, S. (1979): Xenobiotic metabolism by isolated rat small intestinal cells. *Med. Biol.*, 57:287–293.
26. Grafström, R., Ormstad, K., Moldéus, P., and Orrenius, S. (1979): Paracetamol metabolism in the isolated perfused rat liver with further metabolism of a biliary paracetamol conjugate by the small intestine. *Biochem. Pharmacol.*, 28:3573–3579.
27. Guzelian, P. S., and Bissell, D. M. (1976): Effect of cobalt on synthesis of heme and cytochrome P-450 in the liver. Studies of adult rat hepatocytes in primary monolayer culture and *in vivo*. *J. Biol. Chem.*, 251:4421–4427.
28. Hildebrandt, A., Tjoe, M., and Roots, I. (1975): Monooxygenase-linked hydrogen peroxide production and degradation in liver microsomal fractions. *Biochem. Soc. Transact.*, 3:807–811.
29. Hirata, M., Högberg, J., Thor, H., and Orrenius, S. (1977): Cytochrome P-450 product complexes produced by amphetamine derivatives: A compar-

ative study with isolated liver microsomes and hepatocytes. *Acta Pharmacol. Toxicol. (Kbh.),* 41:177–189.

30. Högberg, J., Ekström, T., Anundi, I., and Kristoferson, A. (1980): Metabolism of toxic substances in isolated hepatocytes. *Toxicology,* 17:113–118.
31. Högberg, J., and Kristoferson, A. (1977): A correlation between glutathione levels and cellular damage in isolated hepatocytes. *Eur. J. Biochem.,* 74:77–82.
32. Howard, R. B., and Pesch, L. A. (1968): Respiratory activity of intact isolated parenchymal cells from rat liver. *J. Biol. Chem.,* 243:3105–3109.
33. Jernström, B., Guenthner, T., Dock, L., Svensson, S.-Å., and Orrenius, S. (1980): Biotransformation of benzo(a)pyrene to DNA-binding products by isolated hepatocytes. In: *Microsomes, Drug Oxidations and Chemical Carcinogenesis, Vol. 2,* edited by M. J. Coon, A. H. Conney, R. W. Estabrook, H. V. Gelboin, J. R. Gillette, and P. J. O'Brien, pp. 1053–1064. Academic Press, New York.
34. Jewell, S. A., Bellomo, G., Thor, H., Orrenius, S., and Smith, M. T. (1982): Bleb formation in hepatocytes during drug metabolism is caused by disturbances in thiol and calcium ion homeostasis. *Science,* 217:1257–1259.
35. Jollow, D. J., Mitchell, J. R., Zampaglione, N., and Gillette, J. R. (1974): Bromobenzene-induced liver necrosis. Protective role of glutathione and evidence for 3,4-bromobenzene oxide as the hepatotoxic metabolite. *Pharmacology,* 11:151–169.
36. Jones, D. P. (1981): Hypoxia and drug metabolism. *Biochem. Pharmacol.,* 30:1019–1023.
37. Jones, D. P., Eklöw, L., Thor, H., and Orrenius, S. (1981): Metabolism of hydrogen peroxide in isolated hepatocytes: Relative contributions of catalase and glutathione peroxidase in decomposition of endogenously generated H_2O_2. *Arch. Biochem. Biophys.,* 210:505–516.
38. Jones, D. P., Grafström, R., and Orrenius, S. (1980): Quantitation of hemoproteins in rat small intestinal mucosa with identification of mitochondrial cytochrome P-450. *J. Biol. Chem.,* 255:2383–2390.
39. Jones, D. P., and Mason, H. S. (1978): Gradients of O_2 concentration in hepatocytes. *J. Biol. Chem.,* 253:4874–4880.
40. Jones, D. P., Meyer, D. B., Andersson, B., and Orrenius, S. (1981): Conversion of catalase to the secondary catalase–peroxide complex (Compound II) by α-methyldopa. *Mol. Pharmacol.,* 20:159–164.
41. Jones, D. P., Moldéus, P., Stead, A. H., Ormstad, K., Jörnvall, H., and Orrenius, S. (1979): Metabolism of glutathione and a glutathione conjugate by isolated kidney cells. *J. Biol. Chem.,* 254:2787–2792.
42. Jones, D. P., and Orrenius, S. (1981): Reactions related to monooxygenase functions in isolated cells. In: *Mitochondria and Microsomes,* edited by C. P. Lu, G. Schatz, and G. Dallner, pp. 749–772. Addison-Wesley, Reading, Massachusetts.
43. Jones, D. P., Orrenius, S., and Mason, H. S. (1979): Hemoprotein quantitation in isolated hepatocytes. *Biochim. Biophys. Acta,* 576:17–29.
44. Jones, D. P., Sundby, G.-B., Ormstad, K., and Orrenius, S. (1979): Use of isolated kidney cells for study of drug metabolism. *Biochem. Pharmacol.,* 28:929–935.
45. Jones, D. P., Thor, H., Andersson, B., and Orrenius, S. (1978): Detoxification reactions in isolated hepatocytes. *J. Biol. Chem.,* 253:6031–6037.
46. Kappus, H., Köster, U., Köster-Albrecht, D., Kieczka, H., and Remmer, H. (1978): Lipid peroxidation induced by ethanol and halogenated hydrocarbons *in vivo* as measured by ethane exhalation. In: *Functions of Glutathione in Liver and Kidney,* edited by H. Sies and A. Wendel, pp. 176–182. Springer-Verlag, New York.
47. Kini, M. M., and Cooper, J. R. (1962): Biochemistry of methanol poisoning. 4. The effect of methanol and its metabolites on retinal metabolism. *Biochem. J.,* 82:164–172.
48. Koch-Weser, D., de la Huerga, J., Yesinick, D., and Popper, H. (1953): Hepatic necrosis due to bromobenzene as an example of conditioned amino acid deficiency. *Metabolism,* 2:248.
49. Köster-Albrecht, D., Kappus, H., and Remmer, H. (1978): Lipid peroxidation and cell damage in isolated hepatocytes due to bromotrichloromethane. *Toxicol. Appl. Pharmacol.,* 46:499–505.
50. Kuthan, H., Tsuji, H., Graf, H., Ullrich, V., Werringloer, J., and Estabrook, R. W. (1978): Generation of superoxide anion as a source of hydrogen peroxide in a reconstituted monooxygenase system. *FEBS Letts.,* 91:343–345.
51. Laperche, Y., Graillot, C., Arondel, J., and Bethelot, P. (1979): Uptake of rifampicin by isolated rat liver cells. Interaction with sulphobromophthalein uptake and evidence for separate carriers. *Biochem. Pharmacol.,* 28:2065–2069.
52. Lewis, S. E., and Wills, E. D. (1962): The destruction of -SH groups of proteins and amino acids by peroxides of unsaturated fatty acids. *Biochem. Pharmacol.,* 11:901–912.
53. Lueders, K. K., and Kuff, E. L. (1967): Spontaneous and detergent activation of a glucuronyltransferase *in vitro. Arch. Biochem. Biophys.,* 120:198–203.
54. Marjanen, L. A. (1973): Comparison of aldehyde dehydrogenases from cytosol and mitochondria of rat liver. *Biochim. Biophys. Acta,* 327:238–246.

54a. Miejer, A. J., Gimpel, J. A., Deleeuw, G., Tischler, M. E., Tager, J. M., and Williamson, J. R. (1978): Interrelationships between gluconeogenesis and ureogenesis in isolated hepatocytes. *J. Biol. Chem.,* 253:2308–2320.

55. Miles, P. R., Wright, J. R., Bowman, L., and Colby, H. D. (1980): Inhibition of hepatic microsomal lipid peroxidation by drug substrates without drug metabolism. *Biochem. Pharmacol.,* 29:565–570.
56. Miller, J. A. (1970): Carcinogenesis by chemicals: An overview. *Cancer Res.,* 30:559–576.
57. Mitchell, J. R., Nelson, S. D., Thorgeirsson, S. S., McMurty, R. J., and Dybing, E. (1976): Metabolic activation: Biochemical basis for many drug-induced liver injuries. In: *Progress in Liver Diseases, Vol. 5,* edited by H. Popper and F. Schaffner, pp. 259–279. Grune & Stratton, New York.
58. Mitchell, J. R., Smith, C. V., Lauterberg, B. H., and Horning, E. C. (1974): In: *Proceedings 30th*

Annual Meeting of the American Association for Study of Liver Diseases, Chicago.
59. Moldéus, P. (1978): Paracetamol metabolism and toxicity in isolated hepatocytes from rat and mouse. *Biochem. Pharmacol.,* 27:2859–2863.
60. Moldéus, P. (1981): Use of isolated cells in the study of paracetamol metabolism and toxicity: Capacity of conjugative pathways and glutathione homeostasis. In: *Drug Reactions and the Liver: Mechanisms and Measures for Control,* edited by M. Davis, J. M. Tredger, and R. Williams, pp. 144–156. Pitman Press, Bath.
61. Moldéus, P., Andersson, B., and Gergely, V. (1979): Regulation of glucuronidation and sulfate conjugation in isolated hepatocytes. *Drug Metab. Dispos.,* 7:416–419.
62. Moldéus, P., Andersson, B., Norling, A., and Ormstad, K. (1980): Effect of chronic ethanol administration on drug metabolism in isolated hepatocytes with emphasis on paracetamol activation. *Biochem. Pharmacol.,* 29:1741–1745.
63. Moldéus, P., Grundin, R., Vadi, H., and Orrenius, S. (1974): A study of drug metabolism linked to cytochrome P-450 in isolated rat liver cells. *Eur. J. Biochem.,* 46:351–360.
64. Moldéus, P., Grundin, R., von Bahr, C., and Orrenius, S. (1973): Spectral studies on drug cytochrome P-450 interaction in isolated rat liver cells. *Biochem. Biophys. Res. Commun.,* 55:937–944.
65. Moldéus, P., Högberg, J., and Orrenius, S. (1978): Isolation and use of liver cells. *Methods. Enzymol.,* 52:60–71.
66. Moldéus, P., Jones, D. P., Ormstad, K., and Orrenius, S. (1978): Formation and metabolism of a glutathione-*S*-conjugate in isolated rat liver and kidney cells. *Biochem. Biophys. Res. Commun.,* 83:195–200.
67. Moldéus, P., Thor, H., Högberg, J., and Orrenius, S. (1977): Drug metabolism and toxicity studied in isolated rat liver cells. In: *Clinical Toxicology, Vol. 18,* edited by W. A. M. Duncan and B. J. Leonard, pp. 75–84. Excerpta Medica, Amsterdam.
68. Muliawan, H., Scheulen, M. E., and Kappus, H. (1980): Acute adriamycin treatment of rats does not increase ethane expiration. *Res. Commun. Chem. Pathol. Pharmacol.,* 30:509–519.
69. Müller, A., Graf, P., Wendel, A., and Sies, H. (1981): Ethane production by isolated perfused rat liver. A system to study metabolic effects related to lipid peroxidation. *FEBS Lett.,* 126:241–244.
70. Murphy, E., Coll, K., Rich, T. L., and Williamson, J. R. (1980): Hormonal effects on calcium homeostasis in isolated hepatocytes. *J. Biol. Chem.,* 255:6600–6607.
71. Myers, C. E., McGuire, W. P., Liss, R. H., Ifrim, I., Grotzinger, K., and Young, R. C. (1977): Adriamycin: the role of lipid peroxidation in cardiac toxicity and tumor response. *Science,* 197:165–167.
72. Nordenskjöld, M., Svensson, S.-Å., Jernström, B., Moldéus, P., Dock, L., and Söderhäll, S. (1981): Studies on the *in vitro* transfer of DNA binding benzo(a)pyrene metabolites from rat hepatocytes to human fibroblasts. *Carcinogenesis,* 2:1151–1160.
73. Omura, T., and Sato, R. (1964): The carbon monoxide-binding pigment of liver microsomes. I. Evidence for its hemoprotein nature. *J. Biol. Chem.,* 239:2370–2378.
74. Ormstad, K., Orrenius, S., and Jones, D. P. (1981): Preparation and characteristics of isolated kidney cells. *Methods Enzymol.,* 77:137–146.
75. Oro, J., and Rappoport, D. A. (1959): Formate metabolism by animal tissues. II. The mechanism of formate oxidation. *J. Biol. Chem.,* 234:1661–1665.
76. Orrenius, S., Andersson, B., Jernström, B., and Moldéus, P. (1978): Isolated hepatocytes as an experimental tool in the study of drug conjugation reactions. In: *Conjugation Reactions in Drug Biotransformation,* edited by A. Aitio, pp. 273–282. Elsevier-North Holland, Amsterdam.
77. Orenius, S., Dallner, G., and Ernster, L. (1964): Inhibition of the TPNH-linked lipid peroxidation of liver microsomes by drugs undergoing oxidative demethylation. *Biochem. Biophys. Res. Commun.,* 14:329–334.
78. Orrenius, S., Ellin, Å., Jakobsson, S. J., Thor, H., Cinti, D. L., Schenkman, J. B., and Estabrook, R. W. (1973): The cytochrome P-450-containing monooxygenase system of rat kidney cortex microsomes. *Drug Metab. Dispos.,* 1:350–357.
79. Orrenius, S., and Sies, H. (1982): Compartmentation of detoxication reactions. In: *Metabolic Compartmentation,* edited by H. Sies, pp. 485–520. Academic Press, London.
80. Orrenius, S., Thor, H., and Jernström, B. (1980): The influence of inducers on drug-metabolizing enzyme activity and on formation of reactive drug metabolites in the liver. *Environmental Chemicals, Enzyme Function and Human Disease, Ciba Foundation Symposium 76,* pp. 25–42. Excerpta Medica, Amsterdam.
81. Orrenius S., Thor, H., Rajs, J., and Berggren, M. (1976): Isolated rat hepatocytes as an experimental tool in the study of cell injury. Effect of anoxia. *Forens. Sci.,* 8:255–263.
82. Palekar, A. G., Tate, S. S., and Meister, A. (1975): Decrease in glutathione levels of kidney and liver after injection of methionine sulfoximine into rats. *Biochem. Biophys. Res. Commun.,* 62:651–657.
83. Prentki, M., Chaponnier, C., Jeanrenaud, B., and Gabbiani, G. (1979): Actin microfilaments, cell shape, and secretory processes in isolated rat hepatocytes. Effect of phalloidin and cytochalasin D. *J. Cell Biol.,* 81:592–607.
84. Pryor, W. A. (1978): The formation of free radicals and the consequence of their reactions *in vivo. Photochem. Photobiol.,* 28:787–801.
85. Rannug, U., Sundvall, A., and Ramel, C. (1978): The mutagenic effect of 1,2-dichloroethane on *Salmonella typhimurium.* I. Activation through conjugation with glutathione. *Chem. Biol. Interact.,* 20:1–16.
86. Recknagel, R. O., and Glende, E. A. (1973): Carbon tetrachloride hepatotoxicity: An example of lethal cleavage. *Crit. Rev. Toxicol.,* 2:263–297.
87. Reed, D. J., and Orrenius, S. (1977): The role of methionine in glutathione biosynthesis by isolated hepatocytes. *Biochem. Biophys. Res. Commun.,* 77:1257–1264.
88. Reid, W. D., Christie, B., Krishna, G., Mitchell,

J. R., Moskowitz, J., and Brodie, B. B. (1971): Bromobenzene metabolism and hepatic necrosis. *Pharmacology,* 6:41–55.

89. Riely, C. A., Cohen, G., and Liebeman, M. (1974): Ethane evolution. A new index of lipid peroxidation. *Science,* 183:208–210.
90. Rydström, J., da Cruz, A. T., and Ernster, L. (1970): Factors governing the kinetics and steady state of the mitochondrial nicotinamide nucleotide transhydrogenase system. *Eur. J. Biochem.,* 17:56–62.
91. Rydström, J., da Cruz, A. T., and Ernster, L. (1971): Steady-state kinetics of mitochondrial nicotinamide nucleotide transhydrogenase. 2. The energy-linked reaction. *Eur. J. Biochem.,* 23:212–219.
92. Sagai, M., and Tappel, A. L. (1978): Effect of vitamin E on carbon tetrachloride-induced lipid peroxidation as demonstrated by *in vivo* pentane production. *Toxicol. Lett.,* 2:149–155.
93. Schanne, F. A. X., Kane, A. B., Young, E. E., and Farber, J. L. (1979): Calcium dependence of toxic cell death: A final common pathway. *Science,* 206:700–702.
94. Schwenk, M., Burr, R., Schwarz, L., and Pfaff, E. (1976): Uptake of bromosulphophthalein by isolated liver cells. *Eur. J. Biochem.,* 64:189–197.
95. Shu, H., Talcott, R. E., Rice, S. A., and Wei, E. T. (1979): Lipid peroxidation and paraquat toxicity. *Biochem. Pharmacol.,* 28:327–331.
96. Slater, T. F. (1978): In: *Biochemical Mechanisms of Liver Injury,* edited by T. F. Slater, pp. 1–44. Academic Press, London.
97. Smith, M. T., Loveridge, N., Wills, E. D., and Chayen, J. (1979): The distribution of glutathione in the rat liver lobule. *Biochem. J.,* 182:103–108.
98. Smith, M. T., Thor, H., Hartzell, P., and Orrenius, S. (1982): The measurement of lipid peroxidation in isolated hepatocytes. *Biochem. Pharmacol.,* 31:19–26.
99. Smith, M. T., Thor, H., and Orrenius, S. (1981): Toxic injury to isolated hepatocytes is not dependent on extracellular calcium. *Science,* 213:1257–1259.
100. Smith, M. T., and Wills, E. D. (1980): A comparison of biochemical and cytochemical methods for studying the utilization of NADPH in rat liver. *Proc. R. Microsc. Soc.,* 15:114–115.
101. Smith, M. T., and Wills, E. D. (1981): Effect of dietary lipid and phenobarbitone on the production and utilization of NADPH in the liver. A combined biochemical and quantitative cytochemical study. *Biochem. J.,* 200:691–699.
102. Steffen, C., Muliawan, H., and Kappus, H. (1980): Lack of *in vivo* lipid peroxidation in experimental paraquat poisoning. *Naunyn Schmiedebergs Arch. Pharmakol.,* 310:241–243.
103. Stohs, S. J., Grafström, R. C., Burke, M. D., and Orrenius, S. (1977): Benzo(a)pyrene metabolism in isolated rat intestinal epithelial cells. *Arch. Biochem. Biophys.,* 179:71–80.
104. Strittmatter, P., and Ball, E. G. (1955): Formaldehyde dehydrogenase, a glutathione-dependent enzyme system. *J. Biol. Chem.,* 213:445–461.
105. Tager, J. M., Söling, H. D., and Williamson, J. R. (1976): *The Use of Isolated Liver Cells and Kidney Tubules in Metabolic Studies.* North-Holland, Amsterdam.
106. Thor, H., Moldéus, P., Hermanson, R., Högberg, J., Reed, D. J., and Orrenius, S. (1978): Metabolic activation and hepatotoxicity. Toxicity of bromobenzene in hepatocytes isolated from phenobarbital and diethyl maleate treated rats. *Arch. Biochem. Biophys.,* 188:122–129.
107. Thor, H., Moldéus, P., Kristoferson, A., Högberg, J., Reed, D. J., and Orrenius, S. (1978): Metabolic activation and hepatotoxicity. Metabolism of bromobenzene in isolated hepatocytes. *Arch. Biochem. Biophys.,* 188:114–121.
108. Thor, H., Moldéus, P., and Orrenius, S. (1979): Metabolic activation and hepatotoxicity. Effect of cysteine, *N*-acetylcysteine, and methionine on glutathione biosynthesis and bromobenzene toxicity in isolated rat hepatocytes. *Arch. Biochem. Biophys.,* 192:405–413.
109. Thor, H., and Orrenius, S. (1980): The mechanism of bromobenzene-induced cytotoxicity studied with isolated hepatocytes. *Arch. Toxicol.,* 44:31–43.
110. Thurman, R. G., and Kauffman, F. C. (1980): Factors regulating drug metabolism in intact hepatocytes. *Pharmacol. Rev.,* 31:229–251.
111. Uotila, L., and Koivusalo, M. (1974): Formaldehyde dehydrogenase from human liver. Purification, properties and evidence for the formation of glutathione thiol esters by the enzyme. *J. Biol. Chem.,* 249:7653–7663.
112. Vadi, H., Moldéus, P., Capdevilla, J., and Orrenius, S. (1975): The metabolism of benzo(a)pyrene in isolated rat liver cells. *Cancer Res.,* 35:2083–2091.
113. Vessey, D. A., and Zakim, D. (1971): Regulation of microsomal enzymes by phospholipids. II. Activation of uridine diphosphate-glucuronyltransferase. *J. Biol. Chem.,* 246:4649–4656.
114. van Bahr, C., Vadi, H., Grundin, R., Moldéus, P., and Orrenius, S. (1974): Spectral studies on the rapid uptake and subsequent binding of drugs to cytochrome P-450 in isolated rat liver cells. *Biochem. Biophys. Res. Commun.,* 59:334–339.
115. von Bezooijen, C. F. A., Grell, T., and Knook, D. L. (1976): Bromosulphophthalein uptake by isolated liver parenchymal cells. *Biochem. Biophys. Res. Commun.,* 69:354–361.
116. Weigl, K., and Sies, H. (1977): Drug oxidations dependent on cytochrome P-450 in isolated hepatocytes. *Eur. J. Biochem.,* 77:401–408.
117. Werringloer, J. (1978): Assays of formaldehyde generated during microsomal oxidation reactions. *Methods Enzymol.,* 52:297–302.
118. Wills, E. D., and Wilkinson, A. E. (1966): Release of enzymes from lysosomes by irradiation and the relation of lipid peroxide formation to enzyme release. *Biochem. J.,* 99:657–666.
119. Zuurendonk, P. F., Tischler, M. E., Akerboom, T. P. M., van der Meer, R., Williamson, J. R., and Tager, J. M. (1979): Rapid separation of particulate and soluble fractions from isolated cell preparations. *Methods Enzymol.,* 56:207–223.

Drug Metabolism and Drug Toxicity,
edited by J. R. Mitchell and M. G. Horning.
Raven Press, New York © 1984.

Xenobiotic Metabolism by Extrahepatic Tissues: Relationship to Target Organ and Cell Toxicity

John R. Bend and Cosette J. Serabjit-Singh

Laboratory of Pharmacology, National Institute of Environmental Health Sciences, National Institutes of Health, Research Triangle Park, North Carolina 27709

Historically, most studies of xenobiotic metabolism have focused on mammalian liver because this organ generally contains the highest concentration (both specific and total) of enzymes involved in chemical biotransformation. Preparation of subcellular fractions from liver is easy when compared to extrahepatic tissues such as skin, lung, or gut mucosa. Furthermore, there are only a few cell types in liver, with hepatocytes predominating, and these different cell types can now be readily separated from each other by enzyme digestion coupled with differential centrifugation or elutriation.

Extrahepatic metabolism usually does not play a major role in the total metabolism of xenobiotics; this role is reserved for the liver. There are, of course, exceptions to this generalization. For example, kidney is the major site of mitochondrial glycine *N*-acyltransferase activity (94), and consequently, the renal contribution to *in vivo* conversion of benzoic acid to hippuric acid is quantitatively important. Over the last decade, there has been increasing interest in the ability of extrahepatic tissues to metabolize both endogenous and exogenous substrates, but primarily from the standpoint of understanding relationships between xenobiotic metabolism and target organ and cell toxicity.

With the development of sensitive (histochemical, fluorescence, radiochemical) assays, cytochrome P-450-dependent monooxygenase activity has been reported in virtually every mammalian organ adequately tested, including lung (143), kidney (147), placenta (101), small intestine (202), skin (68), adrenal (109), testis (126), ovary (123), eye (177), pancreas (91), mammary gland (34), aorta walls (103), brain (169), nasal epithelial membranes (40), colon (192), salivary glands, prostate, heart, lymph nodes, spleen, thymus, and thyroid (35,201,202). Similarly, most enzymes involved in hydrolytic and conjugation pathways for xenobiotic substrates, such as UDP-glucuronosyltransferase (1), the glutathione transferases (93), and epoxide hydrolase (142), are widely distributed in extrahepatic tissues.

Thus, current interest is focused on the physiological function of extrahepatic metabolism of both endogenous and exogenous substrates, as extrahepatic tissues, or, more accurately, certain populations of cells in these tissues, are frequently sites for chemical-mediated toxicity (e.g., necrosis, chemical carcinogenesis). The importance of extrahepatic xenobiotic biotransformation is obvious, especially to biochemists, cancer biologists, pharmacologists, pathologists, and toxicologists. In this regard, there are many questions that remain to be answered. These include the relationships between cell-selective or cell-specific toxicity in organs with pronounced cellular heterogeneity and the ability of individual cell types in that organ to metabolize (both activate and detoxify) chemicals, the contribution of hepatic metabolism of chemicals to target organ toxicity in extrahepatic sites and the ability of one extrahepatic organ to affect toxicity in another, and the contribution of extrahepatic metabolism to total *in vivo* metabolism. In addition, the effects of previous or concomitant exposure to other chemicals (e.g., inducers or inhibitors of drug-metabolizing enzymes) on specific xenobiotic metabolizing enzymes (e.g., individual cytochrome P-450 isozymes) and the effects exerted, in turn, on target organ/cell toxicity are important.

For chemical carcinogens, the cell selectivity/specificity of metabolite–DNA adduct formation and repair in extrahepatic tissues after *in vivo* treatment is of interest. The relative contribution of cytochrome P-450-dependent monooxygenase activity, of prostaglandin synthetase-dependent monooxygenase activity, and of flavin-containing monooxygenase activity for the metabolic activation and detoxication of chemicals that are substrates for these pathways in cells that contain all three enzyme activities is also a problem which should be investigated.

The scientific literature describing the metabolism of chemicals by, and the toxicity of chemicals to, extrahepatic tissues is extensive. In this chapter, recent articles are cited to provide a reference point for the interested reader. These include an excellent general review on the microsomal cytochrome P-450-dependent monooxygenases of extrahepatic tissues (30) and more specialized reviews of xenobiotic metabolism by lung (23–25,72,157,183), kidney (4,87,96,108), intestine (209), skin (19), placenta (102), adrenal (37), ovary and testis (81), eye (178), extrahepatic glucuronide conjugation (2), extrahepatic glutathione transferases (31,93), extrahepatic *N*-acetyltransferases and *N*-deacetylases (203), and the metabolism of chemicals by gastrointestinal microflora (69,172). We discuss an integrated experimental approach used in our laboratory and others for studying the metabolism of xenobiotics in extrahepatic tissues and for determining mechanistic aspects of the relationships between chemical metabolism and target organ/cell toxicity in these organs. We illustrate the important points with recent literature citations whenever possible and delineate the disadvantages as well as the advantages of each experimental system. The organization is such that we proceed from the most complicated experimental system for deriving information about extrahepatic xenobiotic metabolism, the whole animal, via several intermediary steps, to homogeneous enzymes purified from extrahepatic tissues. At the outset, we point out that extrapolation of information obtained with highly purified proteins back to the *in vivo* situation is often complicated.

EXPERIMENTAL SYSTEMS WITH INTACT CELLULAR STRUCTURE

There are several aspects of xenobiotic metabolism and the relationships between this metabolism and target organ toxicity that make studies in systems with intact cellular architecture a requirement for elucidating mechanisms of *in vivo* metabolism and toxicity. First, the biotransformation of a chemical usually requires the sequential involvement of several enzymatic pathways that frequently differ in subcellular localizations; the interactions of the various pathways can best be studied prior to cell disruption. Second, individual cell types can serve as sensitive indices for chemical-mediated toxicity, and these indices can be pathological, biochemical, or physiological. Finally, cells may contain metabolically important enzymatic pathways that, in the absence of the appropriate cofactor or subcellular fraction, are not active *in vitro*.

Intact Animals

Almost all studies of extrahepatic metabolism are indirect. For example, a chemical requiring metabolism for the formation of a reactive, toxic metabolite, such as acetaminophen, carbon tetrachloride (CCl_4),[1] or 4-ipomeanol, is routinely administered to an animal, and various tissues are sampled for evidence of pathological damage and/or for covalent reactions between various macromolecules (protein, RNA, DNA, phospholipid) and radiolabeled metabolites. It is common to test the effects of compounds known to induce or inhibit various metabolic pathways, especially the cytochrome P-450-dependent monooxygenase system, on the chemical-mediated event being studied.

In a series of comprehensive investigations, Boyd and his colleagues have used this approach to demonstrate that 4-ipomeanol (1-[3-furyl]-4-hydroxypentanone) causes necrosis of pulmonary nonciliated bronchiolar epithelial (Clara) cells in several mammalian species (22,25), that substantial amounts of 4-ipomeanol-derived radioactivity are typically bound to lung proteins (27), that piperonyl butoxide, an inhibitor of the cytochrome P-450-dependent metabolic activation of 4-ipomeanol, dramatically decreases the amount of radioactivity covalently bound to both lung and liver *in vivo* (26), and, from autoradiography, that 4-ipomeanol is covalently bound preferentially to the Clara cells of the terminal airways in lung (22). Collectively, these data are consistent with metabolic activation of 4-ipomeanol to a highly reactive intermediate by the Clara cell of the lung. This has now been demonstrated in Clara cells isolated from rabbit lung through collaborative studies with our laboratory (48), and alveolar type II cells were also shown to metabolize 4-ipomeanol. The characteristic that makes 4-ipomeanol such a valuable experimental tool for identifying extrahepatic cell types that activate the chemical is that the reactive metabolite(s) formed is very unstable and selectively (maybe even specifically) covalent binds in the cell type where it is formed, subsequent, of course, to GSH depletion.

In a similar vein, Davidson and Eastham (41) first reported that acetaminophen (4-hydroxyacetanilide) induces degenerative changes in both proximal and distal tubules of human kidney in addition to causing hepatotoxicity. Subsequently, it was reported that acetaminophen produces proximal tubular necrosis in Fischer-344 rats and that pretreatment with 3-MC reduces the nephrotoxicity (124). At larger doses of acetaminophen, the kidney GSH content is reduced by approximately 50%, and radioactivity derived from acetaminophen becomes covalently bound to renal protein (134). It appears likely that a reactive metabolite of acetaminophen is formed in tubular kidney cells, exerting a nephrotoxic effect. More recent studies have shown that *p*-aminophenol is a potent cortical nephrotoxicant and that it can be generated from acetaminophen by rat kidney (141).

It is now known that many chemical carcinogens require metabolic activation *in vivo* to an electrophilic species, termed the ultimate carcinogen. This ultimate carcinogen binds covalently to DNA, and, for several classes of chemical carcinogens, this appears to be a requisite step in tumorigenesis. Con-

---

[1] List of abbreviations: 2-AAF, 2-acetylaminofluorene; ACE, angiotensin-converting enzyme; ACTH, adrenocorticotrophic hormone; AHH, aryl hydrocarbon hydroxylase; BP, benzo(a)pyrene; BPDEI, (±)-7β,8α-dihydroxy-9α,10α-epoxy-7,8,9,10-tetrahydrobenzo(a)pyrene; BPDEII, (±)-7β,8α-dihydroxy-9β,10β-epoxy-7,8,9,10-tetrahydrobenzo(a)pyrene; 4,5-BPO, benzo(a)pyrene 4,5-oxide; CCl_4, carbon tetrachloride; CYS-A, 3-(cystein-*S*-yl)acetaminophen; DEN, *N*-nitrosodiethylamine; DMBA, 7,12-dimethylbenz(a)anthracene; 1,2-DMH, 1,2-dimethylhydrazine; DMN, *N*-nitrosodimethylamine; GSH, glutathione; HPLC, high-performance liquid chromatography; LH, luteinizing hormone; 3-MC, 3-methylcholanthrene; N-AC-A, *N*-acetyl-3-(cystein-*S*-yl)acetaminophen; α-NF, α-naphthoflavone; β-NF, β-naphthoflavone; NMEA, *N*-nitrosomethylethylamine; NNMU, *N*-nitroso-*N*-methylurea; NPD, *N*-nitrosopyrrolidine; PAGE, polyacrylamide gel electrophoresis; PAH, polycyclic aromatic hydrocarbon; PB, phenobarbital; PCB, polychlorinated biphenyl; PNP, *p*-nitrophenol; PNPG, *p*-nitrophenyl glucuronide; PNPS, *p*-nitrophenyl sulfate; SADR, specific activity difference ratio; SDS, sodium dodecyl sulfate; SO, styrene 7,8-oxide; SO-GSH, [^{14}C]styrene 7,8-oxide–glutathione conjugates; TCDD, 2,3,7,8-tetrachlorodibenzo-*p*-dioxin.

sequently, the tissue and cellular distribution of the various metabolite–DNA adducts, their chemical identification (because not all chemical metabolite–DNA adducts are associated with tumorigenesis), and the ability of various tissues and cells to remove DNA adducts and to repair damaged DNA are areas of active investigation. Pegg (153) has recently written an extensive review that, among other things, discusses the alkylation of DNA following *in vivo* exposure to several carcinogenic nitrosamines. Nitrosamines, which require metabolism for activation, preferentially alkylate DNA in tissues and cells that contain the activating enzymes. For example, DNA alkylation is observed in liver, kidney, esophagus, and lung of rats following intravenous administration of DMN or DEN (52,151,154), and each of these tissues has the ability to metabolically activate these compounds (132,152).

TABLE 1. *Major DNA adducts*[a] *in liver, lung, and forestomach of A/HeJ and ICR/Ha mice 48 hr after* in vivo *treatment with* ^{3}*H-benzo(a)pyrene (6 mg/mouse)*[b]

Mouse strain	Specific activity (pmole/mg DNA) of BPDEI and BPDEII adducts[c]		
	Liver	Lung	Fore-stomach
A/HeJ	5.5[d]	4.7	3.4
ICR/Ha	0.44	0.42	0.43

[a] DNA was isolated from lung, liver, and forestomach and was enzymatically digested, and the resulting deoxyribonucleosides were chromatographed by HPLC. The specific activity of the adducts was calculated from HPLC chromatograms.

[b] Data from Anderson et al. (16) and Ioannou et al. (89, 90).

[c] Deoxyguanosine adducts of (±) − 7β,8α-dihydroxy-9α,10α-epoxy-7,8,9,10-tetrahydrobenzo(a)pyrene (BPDEI) and (±) − 7β,8α-dihydroxy-9β-10β-epoxy-7,-8,9,10-tetrahydrobenzo(a)pyrene (BPDEII).

[d] Experiments were carried out at least in duplicate, with 25 to 50 mice per data point.

Anderson and his colleagues at NIEHS (6,89,90) have performed similar experiments with A/HeJ and ICR/Ha mice after *in vivo* treatment with BP. The results of initial experiments demonstrated that the major DNA adduct in liver, lung, and forestomach after enzymatic hydrolysis of the DNA to deoxyribonucleosides is BPDEI bound to deoxyguanosine, although there are considerable amounts (5–20% of BPDEI) of BPDEII bound to deoxyguanosine present as well. The relative amounts of total BPDEI– and BPDEII–deoxyguanosine adducts present in three tissues of the two mouse species 48 hr after oral administration of BP (6 mg/mouse) are illustrated in Table 1. Specific DNA alkylation is about the same in all three tissues of each species but about 10-fold higher in A/HeJ then in ICR/Ha mice. This is interesting because BP-induced pulmonary adenomas occur at approximately 10-fold higher frequency in A/HeJ than in ICR/Ha mice at similar BP doses (200). That factors other than DNA alkylation by BPDEI are involved in tumorigenesis is clearly demonstrated by the fact that liver of A/HeJ mice is refractory to BP-mediated neoplasia. However, there seems to be some relationship between specific DNA alkylation by BPDEI and carcinogenic risk in those tissues that are susceptible to neoplasia. Thus, treatment of A/HeJ mice with butylated hydroxyanisole under conditions that markedly reduce (50%) the incidence of pulmonary adenomas (200) also markedly decreases (about 50%) specific DNA alkylation by BPDEI and BPDEII (6).

It might be assumed that, as is apparently the case with DMN and DEN (153), specific alkylation of DNA by BPDEI and BPDEII would be highest in those tissues that are relatively high in cytochrome P-450-dependent monooxygenase activity. Recent experiments by S. J. Stowers and M. W. Anderson (*unpublished observations*) suggest that this might not be the case, however (Table 2). Brain and muscle, tissues almost totally deficient in monooxygenase activity, show much more specific DNA alkylation (50% liver values) by BPDEI and BPDEII than expected. This suggests that metabolites such as BPDEI, which are unstable in aqueous media, may be transported from one tissue to another in a stabilized form, probably bound to protein

TABLE 2. *Deoxyguanosine adducts of BPDEI and BPDEII[a] in DNA isolated from various tissues of A/HeJ mice 48 hr after* in vivo *treatment with ^{3}H-benzo(a)pyrene (6 mg/mouse)[b]*

Tissue	Specific activity (pmol/mg DNA) of deoxyguanosine adducts: BPDEI	BPDEII
Liver	5.8	1.0
Lung	5.8	0.8
Forestomach	5.8	0.3
Kidney	3.9	0.7
Brain	3.2	0.4
Muscle	3.2	0.3
Colon	3.0	0.3

[a] Experimental details and nomenclature as given in Table 1.
[b] Data from S. J. Stowers and M. W. Anderson (*unpublished*).

or lipid, or, alternatively, that extrahepatic tissues deficient in activating systems are also deficient in those metabolic pathways that detoxify PAH metabolites that bind to DNA. In any event, it is obvious that DNA alkylation by carcinogen metabolites and repair of DNA damage should be studied at the cellular level in extrahepatic tissues, as has recently been accomplished in liver (16,118). This is an area that our laboratory is currently investigating in Clara cells and alveolar type II cells isolated from lungs after *in vivo* treatment with carcinogens.

A biochemical approach has also been successfully used to monitor extrahepatic tissues or cells for chemical-mediated damage. Concentrations of serum enzymes are determined before and after chemical administration to the test species; enzyme activities should also be measured in tissues to determine if enzyme release into the serum is organ specific. In the context of the present discussion, this approach is particularly attractive for enzymes that are predominantly localized in extrahepatic cells. Recently, Hollinger (84) measured the activity of ACE, which is concentrated in pulmonary endothelial cells (76), in serum 24 hr after the oral administration of CCl_4 to Swiss–Webster mice. There is a dose–response relationship between serum levels of ACE and the dose of CCl_4 administered, and the increase in serum ACE correlates with a reduction in pulmonary, but not renal or hepatic, ACE activity. The data are consistent with the elevation of serum ACE being caused by CCl_4-mediated toxicity in the pulmonary endothelial cell, resulting in the eventual release of ACE. The obvious next step is to determine whether CCl_4 biotransformation is required, whether it is occurring within the endothelial cell, or whether a toxic metabolite is being transported to these cells. Carbon tetrachloride is also known to damage pulmonary alveolar type II cells (32) and Clara cells (28), both of which are deficient in ACE activity.

Although most *in vivo* procedures used to study the extrahepatic contribution to total xenobiotic metabolism are indirect, there is one refreshing exception. Diamond and Quebbemann (51) have developed a specific activity difference ratio (SADR) technique that allows the simultaneous *in vivo* quantitation of sulfate and glucuronide conjugates that are formed in the kidneys of chickens and excreted directly into the urine during the intravenous perfusion of phenolic substrates. This procedure can also be adapted to other chemicals as long as the metabolites can be recovered from or analyzed in urine. A wing vein and a saphenous leg artery are cannulated while the chicken is under local anesthesia, and precautions are taken to guarantee total collection of urine. ^{14}C-*p*-Nitrophenol (PNP), *p*-nitrophenyl sulfate (PNPS), and *p*-nitrophenyl glucuronide (PNPG), each at a rate of 100 nmole/kg per min, were infused into the systemic circulation via the wing vein, and the ^{14}C-labeled material in the plasma and excreted in the urine was analyzed. The specific activity of the ^{14}C-PNPS in the urine is higher than that of the same conjugate in plasma, suggesting that the kidneys synthesize PNPS and that at least some of the conjugate synthesized in kidney is excreted in urine. In contrast, a negligible amount of PNPG is synthesized in the kidney (Table 3). These experiments demonstrated that at least 38% of the total PNPS excreted in chicken urine is synthesized by the kidney. A more recent study from this laboratory using the SADR technique (50) demonstrated that the administration of salicylate (150 mg/kg, twice daily for 5 days) to chickens selectively enhances renal glucuronide conjugation with PNP or catechol as substrate without affecting formation of the sulfate conjugate of either substrate in kidney. This SADR technique may soon be exploited to delineate the renal contribution to the *in vivo* metabolism of various nephrotoxins.

An *in vivo* approach is also often used to elucidate the contribution of intestinal microflora to chemical metabolism and toxicity. It utilizes germ-free or antibiotic-treated animals. Remel et al. (164) demonstrated an important role for intestinal microflora of the rat in the enterohepatic circulation of warfarin in such a system, and Levin and Dent (117) showed that sterilization of the gut diminishes the urinary excretion of *p*-hydroxyacetanilide by 94% in the same species without affecting the excretion of *m*- and *p*-nitrophenol, oxidative metabolites of *p*-nitrobenzene formed predominantly in liver. Germ-free animals are preferable to those that have been administered antibiotics to reduce the gut flora, however, as antibiotics interfere with xenobiotic metabolism. Thus, neomycin treatment markedly decreases the rate of excretion of urinary metabolites of propham (isopropyl *N*-phenylcarbamate) in the rat, although it does not alter total urinary excretion of metabolites or the metabolic profile (17). More recently, Remel et al. (164) reported that the volume of distribution of warfarin is significantly decreased in rats treated by oral intubation with a combination of neomycin, bacitracin, and tetracycline.

Because antibodies have been prepared against homogeneous enzymes purified from extrahepatic tissues (e.g., rabbit pulmonary cytochrome P-450 isozymes) or from liver (e.g., NADPH–cytochrome P-450 reductase), it has become possible to determine the cellular distribution of certain xenobiotic-metabolizing enzymes in sections prepared from whole tissue. Serabjit-Singh et al. (176) used an antibody against form 2 of rabbit cytochrome P-450 to demonstrate that this P-450 isozyme is localized in the apices of nonciliated bronchiolar epithelial (Clara) cells of the rabbit by both immunofluorescence and antibody peroxidase–antiperoxide techniques. Dees et al. (42) used an immunofluorescence procedure to study the distribution of NADPH–cytochrome P-450 reductase in liver, lung, and kidney of Sprague–Dawley rats and minipigs before and after administration of PB. In rat kidney, positive fluorescence is confined to the cortex and outer

TABLE 3. *Conjugation of* p-*nitrophenol (PNP) with glucuronide (G) and sulfate (S)* in vivo *during infusion of* ^{14}*C-PNP, PNPG, and PNPS (100 nmole each/min/kg chicken)*

Metabolite	Rate of synthesis (nmole/min/kg/kidney) Renal	Nonrenal	% Renal contribution
PNPS	27.1 ± 5.7[a]	46.2 ± 4.4	38.2 ± 0.05
PNPG	−0.1 ± 0.2	0.6 ± 0.1	

[a] Mean ± SD, $N = 7$.

Adapted from Diamond and Quebbeman (51).

stripe of the medulla; all segments of the proximal tubule are also stained, and there is no difference between untreated and PB-treated rats. In lungs, positive staining is present in bronchi and bronchioles and in an unidentified cell type in lung parenchyma. Minipig lungs show a similar distribution of the enzyme.

It is obvious that this experimental approach offers excellent potential for elucidation of the cellular and, with electron microscopy, the subcellular localization of xenobiotic-metabolizing enzymes. It allows study of the relationships between cell-specific chemical insult and cell-specific content of the individual cytochrome P-450 isozymes involved in metabolic activation and/or detoxication of the chemical. In this respect, chemical modulation (i.e., induction or repression) of individual P-450 isozymes will be a powerful experimental tool (discussed in more detail below). It must be kept in mind, however, that an immunochemical staining reaction cannot always be equated with biochemical function, especially in a multicomponent system such as the cytochrome P-450-dependent monooxygenases.

Morphological analysis of tissue sections, preferably from the same animal used for biochemical measurements, can also be very valuable in certain studies of xenobiotic metabolism by extrahepatic tissues. Consider, for example, the question of perinatal development of cytochrome P-450-dependent monooxygenase activity in rabbit lung. Since this enzyme system is localized in the endoplasmic reticulum, the time of appearance, increase in numbers, and maturation of cells rich in endoplasmic reticulum is of relevance. A recent study (160) demonstrated that by 4 weeks of age, a time when specific pulmonary monooxygenase activity is attaining adult levels (62), Clara cells first resemble those of adult animals, containing abundant apical agranular endoplasmic reticulum. Other conclusions from this study were that rabbit Clara cells are immature at birth, that large amounts of cytoplasmic glycogen are present in undifferentiated Clara cells, and that Clara cell differentiation occurs between 3 and 4 weeks of age.

In concluding this section on *in vivo* techniques for studying xenobiotic metabolism by extrahepatic tissues and the relationships between such metabolism and target organ/cell toxicity, it is obvious that experimental approaches are becoming more sophisticated and that important questions that could only be asked a few years ago can now be answered.

Isolated Perfused Organs

Isolated, perfused organ preparations offer several advantages over *in vitro* or *in vivo* systems for the study of xenobiotic metabolism by extrahepatic tissues; there are also disadvantages associated with their use. The advantages include the following: (a) cellular structure remains intact, preserving sequential metabolic pathways localized in different subcellular compartments; (b) metabolism of xenobiotics can be studied in the absence of other tissues, particularly the liver, that mask the contribution of extrahepatic organs to total metabolism; (c) certain complicating factors inherent in *in vivo* experiments are eliminated in perfused organs including the concentration of substrate reaching the extrahepatic tissue and redistribution to and metabolism by other tissues; (d) blood samples or perfusion medium may be readily obtained for analysis of both the xenobiotic and its metabolites; and (e) cell-free perfusion media can be employed that allow easy recovery of test compound, its metabolites, and endogenous chemicals and macromolecules. Disadvantages include the following: (a) perfusion experiments can be performed only for a limited period; (b) perfused organs are an imperfect model for *in vivo* conditions because of the lack of neural and hormonal control; (c) artificial, cell-free perfusion media are routinely used in place of blood; and (d) comprehensive analysis of total metabolites from all compartments in the system is required to guarantee accurate interpretation of experimental data. This means that both polar and nonpolar biotransformation products must be quantified in the perfusion medium and in the tissue at the end of the experiment. Such detailed analyses are very time consuming. However, done properly, experiments with isolated perfused organs can provide important information concerning xenobiotic metabolism and relationships between metabolism and target organ/cell toxicity. We next discuss several perfusion systems that are available and which have been used for studies of xenobiotic metabolism. These include perfused lung, kidney, testis, and *in situ* small intestine preparations.

Isolated Perfused Lung

Some recent reviews are available concerning the use of the isolated perfused lung for studies of xenobiotic metabolism and biochemical toxicology (168,183,184). Perfused lung preparations retain the organ in a breathing, viable state; and test chemicals may be conveniently added to either the circulation or into the trachea by inhalation or instillation.

Our laboratory has investigated the metabolism of benzo(a)pyrene 4,5-oxide (4,5-BPO), a stable K-region arene oxide, in the isolated perfused rabbit lung (185). Sixty minutes after addition of 4,5-BPO (5 μmole) to the recirculating perfusate of rabbit lung, most of the substrate is metabolized. Approximately two-thirds of the oxide is enzymatically conjugated with GSH by the cytosolic GSH transferases, and the remaining substrate is converted to *trans*-benzo(a)pyrene-4,5-dihydrodiol by epoxide hydrolase. The diol metabolite is not further conjugated with glucuronide or sulfate but is concentrated within the lung. On the other hand, the GSH conjugates of 4,5-BPO show no tendency to accumulate in lung, diffusing freely into the perfusion medium. Similar experiments were conducted in the perfused rat liver for comparison (181). Binding of 4,5-BPO-derived radioactivity to RNA and DNA is about 10-fold higher in the lung at equivalent arene oxide doses, and this is consistent with the much more rapid metabolism of liver. (An equivalent dose of 4,5-BPO is completely metabolized within 5 min.)

We have also performed single-pass perfusion experiments with 4,5-BPO to determine the ability of rabbit lungs to remove this substrate from the circulation (182). Clearance concepts initially developed to describe the elimination of xenobiotics by liver and kidney were used to calculate the pulmonary extraction of 4,5-BPO. The experimentally determined extraction ratio, 0.64 ± 0.04 (mean $\pm$ SD, $N = 3$), demonstrated that the lung removed a large percentage of circulating 4,5-BPO during a single pass through the tissue. Given that the entire cardiac output passes through the pulmonary capillary bed, this tissue will play a significant role in removing and metabolizing any polycyclic arene oxide formed in the liver and released into the circulation.

More recently, we (186) used isolated perfused lung and liver preparations to study relationships between *p*-xylene metabolism and the selective destruction of pulmonary cytochrome P-450. Patel et al. (149) reported that *p*-xylene administration to rabbits or rats causes a loss of pulmonary, but not hepatic, cytochrome P-450. These authors postulated that the liver releases *p*-tolualdehyde, which is further metabolized by a cytochrome P-450-dependent reaction in lung to a chemical moiety that destroys P-450 (150). We found that perfusion of rabbit lungs with either *p*-xylene or *p*-tolualdehyde (0.5 mM in perfusate) for 60 min results in a significant destruction of pulmonary cytochrome P-450 (up to 30%). This suggested that hepatic metabolism of *p*-xylene is not mandatory for the *in vivo* *p*-xylene effect. Subsequent experiments supported this assumption.

The metabolism of [^{3}H]*p*-xylene was studied in both perfused lung and perfused liver preparations, as illustrated in Table 4. The

TABLE 4. *Total metabolites formed from* p-*xylene (100 μmole) by perfused rabbit lungs and liver over 60 min*[a]

	Lung		Liver	
Metabolite	Perfusion medium	Lung	Perfusion medium	Liver
p-Methylbenzyl alcohol	32.1 ± 3.3[b]	0.2 ± 0.3	<0.02	<0.01
p-Toluic acid	6.2 ± 2.4	1.5 ± 1.0	4.4 ± 3.5	2.0 ± 0.3
2,5-Dimethylphenol	0.9 ± 0.2	<0.1	ND[c]	ND
p-Toluric acid	ND	ND	69.1 ± 5.6	6.2 ± 2.6
p-Tolualdehyde	ND	ND	ND	ND

[a] Adapted from Smith et al. (186).
[b] Micromoles metabolite (mean ± SD, $N = 3$).
[c] None detected.

metabolites were separated by HPLC and quantitated radiometrically. Rabbit livers do not release detectable amounts of *p*-tolualdehyde. However, perfused lungs produce 2,5-dimethylphenol, a metabolite not produced by perfused liver, which is the rearrangement product of the unstable 3,6-dimethylbenzene 1,2-oxide (106). This suggests an alternative mechanism for the selective destruction of pulmonary cytochrome P-450 via the unstable arene oxide. However, the presence of *p*-toluic acid as a minor metabolite of *p*-xylene in rabbit lungs also indicates that *p*-tolualdehyde is produced intracellularly in the Clara cell or the alveolar type II cell and that it may be rapidly converted to a reactive metabolite before leaving the cell. This is consistent with the aldehyde dehydrogenase activity of rabbit liver exerting a protective role for hepatic cytochrome P-450 by the rapid conversion of *p*-tolualdehyde to *p*-toluic acid. The deficiency of aldehyde dehydrogenase in lung appears to preclude its playing a major detoxication role there. Consequently, there may be two metabolic pathways contributing to the *p*-xylene-mediated selective destruction of cytochrome P-450 in rabbit lung. This is consistent with the observation that both *p*-methylbenzyl alcohol and 2,5-dimethylphenol are oxidative metabolites of *p*-xylene in reconstituted monooxygenase systems containing cytochrome P-450 form 2 or form 5, the major P-450 isozymes present in rabbit lung microsomes (186). We are further investigating the relationships between alkylbenzene metabolism and cytochrome P-450 destruction, and experiments in perfused rabbit lungs are an important part of this initiative.

Isolated Perfused Kidney

Perfused kidney preparations have been used only recently for studying the metabolism, transport, and urinary excretion of xenobiotics. One of the major advantages of this preparation is that renal excretion mechanisms, including filtration, secretion, and reabsorption, are similar to those that occur *in vivo.* Ross et al. (167) and Newton and Hook (140) have recently described the perfused rat kidney model in detail, including a discussion of the advantages and limitations of this system.

As previously mentioned, acetaminophen causes acute renal tubular necrosis in the Fischer-344 rat, and this lesion is restricted to the pars recta of the proximal renal tubule (124). Consequently, it is not surprising that the metabolism of acetaminophen has been studied in the perfused kidney (61,139,167). The urinary metabolites excreted by the perfused kidneys include 4-hydroxyacetanilide sulfate, 4-hydroxyacetanilide glucuronide, a mercapturic acid derivative, presumably *N*-acetyl-3-(cystein-*S*-yl)acetaminophen (N-

AC-A) based on the identification of 3-(glutathione-*S*-yl)acetaminophen as a biliary metabolite of acetaminophen in rats (83), and the corresponding cysteine conjugate, 3-(cysteine-*S*-yl)acetaminophen (CYS-A). The sulfate and glucuronide conjugates arise directly from acetaminophen; N-AC-A and CYS-A are degradation products of the GSH adduct formed from the reaction of this tripeptide with *N*-acetyl-*p*-benzoquinoneimine, a reactive metabolite produced from acetaminophen by cytochrome P-450-dependent monooxygenases [see review by Hinson (82)] and prostaglandin synthetase (128).

The rate of urinary excretion of these various acetaminophen metabolites and of unchanged drug following perfusion of kidney with several different concentrations of acetaminophen is shown in Table 5. These data demonstrate conclusively that oxidative metabolism of acetaminophen occurs, although conjugation with sulfate and glucuronide and excretion of unchanged substrate predominate over thioether (N-AC-A and CYS-A) metabolites (61). The covalent binding of acetaminophen-derived radioactivity to renal protein was also found to increase with the concentration of acetaminophen in the perfusion medium (6 ± 1 nmole/hr per g wet weight at 3.4 mM versus 87 ± 19 at 24.7 mM, mean ± SEM, $N = 4$), which is consistent with renal oxidative activity.

Newton et al. (139) also found evidence for cytochrome P-450-dependent oxidation of acetaminophen. Treatment of rats with a polybrominated biphenyl mixture, an inducer of the monooxygenase system, or piperonyl butoxide, an inhibitor of this system, enhances or decreases, respectively, the ability of acetaminophen to deplete renal GSH. Furthermore, urinary excretion of N-AC-A is increased approximately fourfold in kidneys from rats treated with polybrominated biphenyls. An interesting aspect of this study is that the acetaminophen-mediated GSH depletion in the renal papilla may have been catalyzed by prostaglandin synthetase and not cytochrome P-450. This seems likely because the papilla (inner medulla and papilla) of rat kidney does not contain detectable cytochrome P-450, and the GSH depletion observed in perfused kidneys from control rats is the same as that in kidneys from rats treated with polybrominated biphenyls or piperonyl butoxide. In this context, the inner medulla of the rabbit contains appreciable prostaglandin synthetase activity (210).

Our laboratory (189) used the isolated perfused rat kidney preparation to study the metabolism and excretion of the GSH conjugates of [^{14}C]styrene 7,8-oxide ([^{14}C]SO-GSH). Approximately 20% of the radioactivity derived from ^{14}C-SO-GSH (26.8 μmole) is excreted in the urine of the perfused kidney over 2 hr; HPLC analysis showed that more than 60% of the urinary activity is SO-cys-

TABLE 5. *Urinary excretion of acetaminophen and its metabolies by the perfused rat kidney*[a]

Acetaminophen in perfusate (mM)	Amount excreted (nmole/hr/g wet wt kidney)[b]			
	Acetaminophen	ACET-S[c]	ACET-G[d]	*N*-AC-ACET + CYS-ACET[e]
2.4 ± 0.2 (4)[f]	7,090 ± 1,250	124 ± 28	33 ± 28	33 ± 8
3.4 ± 0.4 (6)	10,050 ± 1,751	77 ± 23	60 ± 12	38 ± 6
10.8 ± 0.6 (4)	27,668 ± 2,868	ND[g]	ND	51 ± 4
24.7 ± 1.4 (4)	119,109 ± 16,920	ND	ND	16 ± 3

[a] Adapted from Emslie et al. (61).
[b] During 60 min of perfusion.
[c] 4-Hydroxyacetanilide sulfate.
[d] 4-Hydroxyacetanilide glucuronide.
[e] *N*-Acetyl-3(cysteine-*S*-yl)-4-hydroxyacetanilide and 3-(cysteine-*S*-yl)-4-hydroxyacetanilide.
[f] Mean ± SEM (*N*).
[g] Not determined.

teine adducts, 30% is SO-*N*-acetylcysteine adducts, with only traces of SO-GSH and SO-cysteinylglycine being present. The homogenized kidney contains 8% of the total radioactivity at the end of the experiment, and more than 85% of this occurs as SO-cysteine conjugates. There is one major difference between the results obtained with the perfused kidney and those from *in vivo* studies of the metabolism and urinary excretion of [^{14}C]SO-GSH in the rat. The ratio of SO-*N*-acetylcysteine:SO-cysteine is 30:1 in intact animals but only 1:2 in the isolated kidney. This indicates that our isolated kidney preparation does not retain the *N*-acetylation capacity found in the intact rat.

Ormstad and her colleagues have studied several aspects of GSH metabolism in the isolated perfused rat kidney because this organ is known to have a major role in the metabolism of plasma GSH (125). Glutathione oxidase activity is observed in the perfused kidney only with extracellular GSH (144,145), indicating that renal GSH oxidase activity is localized in the basal plasma membrane of tubular cells, facing the capillary bloodstream. On the other hand, γ-glutamyltransferase-mediated degradation occurs only with GSH in the tubular fluid, consistent with renal localization of this enzyme in the brush border membranes of the tubular epithelium.

The studies discussed above delineate the types of experiments that can be performed in perfused kidneys. The utility of this system for investigating the metabolism and excretion of chemicals toxic to the kidney guarantees that it will be frequently utilized in the future.

Isolated Perfused Testis

There are very few studies of xenobiotic metabolism in perfused testis, but the system offers considerable potential for genotoxic chemicals. With a preparation similar to that described by VanDemark and Ewing (197), Lee and Nagayama (115) demonstrated that BP is converted to the normal myriad of oxidative metabolites during single-pass perfusion through rat testis and that most (76%) of the radioactivity remains in the aqueous phase after extraction. Unfortunately, the water-soluble metabolites were not identified individually or even by chemical class, making meaningful interpretation of the data difficult. However, nonpolar metabolites in both the tissue and the perfusate were analyzed by HPLC at the termination of the experiment. Perfusion of testes removed from rats treated with TCDD (10 μg/kg, 72 hr prior to death) shows a small but statistically significant increase (1.5-fold) in the total BP metabolism occurring over 60 min relative to testes from control rats; polar metabolites account for 74% of total metabolism in perfused testes from TCDD-treated rats.

More recently, the metabolism of 4,5-BPO was studied in perfused rat testis (114). The polar metabolite(s), formed subsequent to an enzyme-catalyzed reaction between the arene oxide and GSH, predominates both in the effluent (6.9-fold; mean of three trials) and in the tissue (18.4-fold; mean of three trials) when testis is perfused in single-pass experiments with media containing 5×10^{-6} M 4,5-BPO. Benzo(a)pyrene 4,5-dihydrodiol accounts for only 7% of the total metabolites produced. This is consistent with the relative amounts of GSH transferase and epoxide hydrolase activity in rat testis (136), each determined *in vitro* with 4,5-BPO as substrate: 20.1 $\pm$ 1.1 nmole/min per mg cytoplasmic protein for the transferase versus 0.77 $\pm$ 0.06 nmol/min per mg microsomal protein for epoxide hydrolase (mean $\pm$ SD, $N = 8$). The studies mentioned here demonstrate the potential, more than anything else, of the perfused testis preparation for studies of xenobiotic metabolism.

In Situ *Perfusion of Small Intestine*

Although methods are available for the vascular perfusion of entire rat small intestine, the methodology is difficult; moreover, a glucocorticoid and norepinephrine must be added to the perfusate to overcome the effects of denervation (207). For these reasons, a simpler system was developed that allows vascular perfusion of rat small intestinal segments *in situ* (205,207). The venous effluent is collected, and arterial, lymphatic, and neural connections remain intact. Blood is replaced by continuous infusion with heparinized blood from donor rats. Xenobiotics can be introduced either into the closed intestinal segment, or the distal end of the intestinal segment can be cannulated, allowing perfusion through the intestinal loop. Samples for xenobiotic and metabolite analysis can be removed from the lumen of the intestine, from the lymphatic drainage, and from both the arterial and venous circulation, allowing determination of arteriovenous differences. Windmueller and Spaeth (206) have successfully utilized this preparation to study luminal and atrial substrates as energy sources for small intestine.

Xenobiotic metabolism has also been investigated in this system. Bock and Winne (21) demonstrated that 1-naphthol is converted almost exclusively to its glucuronide after instillation into the intestinal lumen and that the majority of this conjugate is present in venous blood (3.5-fold as much as in the lumen). On the other hand, when 1-naphthol glucuronide is introduced into the lumen, the majority of the conjugate remains in the intestine (threefold more than in venous blood). On perfusion of the small intestine with 1-naphthol (65 μM; 0.1 ml/min), more than 90% of the phenol absorbed from the lumen is glucuronidated at a rate of 6.7 nmole/min per g tissue. Similar studies were also performed with acetaminophen and morphine (100). They demonstrated that conjugation of acetaminophen by the rat intestine is minor, and no evidence is presented for oxidative metabolism, although this was not specifically studied. Morphine is absorbed only slowly from the lumen, but approximately equal amounts of unchanged drug and conjugates appear in venous blood.

There is one excellent drug metabolism study in the *in situ* perfused rat small intestine that illustrates the potential of this preparation (29). The metabolism and absorption of the phenothiazine drug perazine (10-[3 - (4 - methyl - 1 - piperazinyl)propyl]-phenothiazine) were investigated. Both parent drug and its metabolites were quantitated in plasma and red cells of venous blood, in the intestinal lumen, and in the intestinal wall. Of the total perazine-derived radioactivity administered, 56.9 $\pm$ <2% is excreted in venous blood, 15.9 $\pm$ 1.2% is in the intestinal wall at the end of the experiment (60 min), and 15.0 $\pm$ 2.4% (mean $\pm$ SEM, N = 7) is in the intestinal lumen. The major metabolites in plasma are 3-hydroxyperazine glucuronide and perazine sulfoxide; red cells contain perazine sulfoxide in addition to desmethyl perazine. Desmethyl perazine is primarily localized in the intestinal wall, emphasizing the importance of studying this cellular compartment. Small amounts of 3-hydroxyperazine glucuronide and desmethyl perazine are found in the lumen along with traces of perazine *N*-oxide. Unchanged perazine was the major radioactive compound in blood, lumen, and tissue.

Given the excellent reproducibility that was achieved from one perfused gut preparation to another in this perazine study and the ease with which the rat intestine autoperfusion system can be set up (207), more extensive use should be made of this preparation for investigating xenobiotic biotransformation by intact intestine and for studying relationships between metabolism and target cell toxicity in this tissue.

Freshly Isolated Cells

Suspensions of isolated hepatocytes are widely used for investigating xenobiotic metabolism and its relationship to chemical toxicity (65,130), and detailed procedures for the preparation of these cells are available (64,129). In biochemical toxicology, hepatocytes serve as an intermediate between the intact animal and the perfused liver on one hand and subcellular fractions or purified enzymes prepared from homogenized liver on the other. Advantages of hepatocytes, relative to disrupted systems, are that they contain a full complement of enzymes and cofactors present in intact tissue, that sequential metabolic pathways for xenobiotics retain their integrity, that damage to the cells can serve as a sensitive toxicological end point, and that all cells are exposed approximately equally to added chemicals. The same arguments can be made for cells isolated from extrahepatic tissues. In addition, there is one further important advantage. The isolation and enrichment of cell populations of a single type allow one to localize different metabolic pathways to different cell types and also to study xenobiotic biotransformation at the cellular level. This is especially important in organs of high cellular heterogeneity such as the lung or kidney.

Pulmonary Cells

Over the last few years, Fouts and his colleagues have developed procedures for isolating and enriching populations of viable alveolar type II cells and nonciliated bronchiolar epithelial (Clara) cells from rabbits (44,45,47) and rats (98,99). These particular cell types were selected for isolation because they are quantitatively important in terms of their endoplasmic reticulum content, the major site for cytochrome P-450-dependent monooxygenase activity in rabbit lung (86).

As the methodology for isolation of type II and Clara cells from rabbits and rats has been described in detail elsewhere (46,99), it is described only briefly here. Rabbit lungs are thoroughly perfused *in situ* with buffer to remove blood while they are ventilated with air through a cannula inserted into the trachea.

Following thorough perfusion, the lungs are removed intact and are flushed five times with cold buffer via the trachea to remove macrophages. Then, a solution of protease I is instilled into the trachea. The trachea is closed off, and the lungs are incubated in a beaker of buffer at 37°C for 15 min. The trachea and large bronchi are removed, and the lungs are placed in a small beaker in ice and chopped into 1-mm pieces with scissors. The mince is suspended in cold buffered F12K growth medium containing 0.5% BSA. The remainder of the cell separation procedure utilizes this buffer and is performed in an ice bath.

Initial separation of alveolar type II and Clara cells is by centrifugal elutriation. Alveolar type II cells, which are smaller and elutriate earlier than Clara cells, are further enriched by density-gradient centrifugation in metrizamide or Percoll®. The final type II cell preparation is enriched to an average purity of 80%.

Further purification of Clara cells, subsequent to elutriation, is achieved by Percoll® discontinuous density-gradient centrifugation. The final fraction has a cell population containing approximately 70% Clara cells.

Modification of the procedures used for rabbits allows the preparation of populations of alveolar type II cells of 80% purity and of Clara cells of 40 to 60% purity from rats (99).

Cell identification is carried out by light and electron microscopy. Alveolar type II cells are identified by the characteristic lamellar bodies (Fig. 1), which are visualized after staining with the modified Papanicolaou stain without acid alcohol (106a). Clara cells are identified under the light microscope by nitro blue tetrazolium staining (47). Clara cells stain purple (dark in Fig. 2), whereas other cells appear blue or light pink (light in Fig. 2).

The viability of freshly isolated cells is determined by exclusion of trypan blue dye and by comparing cytochrome P-450-dependent monooxygenase activities in the presence and absence of exogenous NADPH (NADPH does not cross intact cell membranes). Routinely, the viability of the isolated type II and Clara cells is greater than 90%.

As proteolytic enzymes are used to release these epithelial cells from the basement

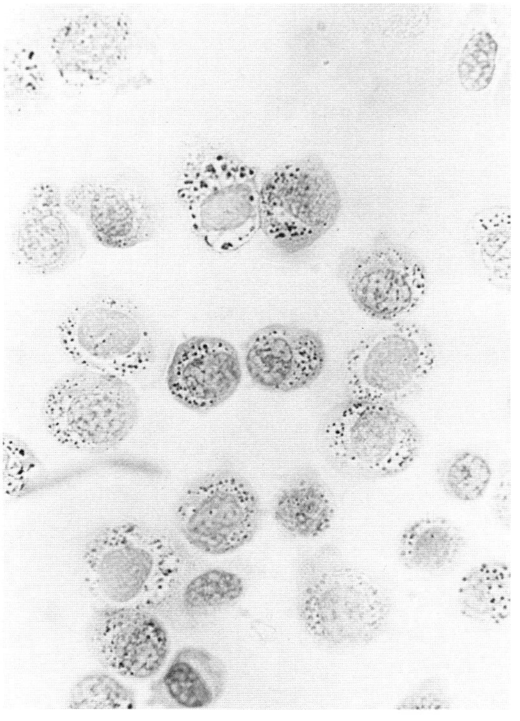

FIG. 1. Alveolar type II cells isolated from rabbit lungs. Following isolation of type II cells, a 0.1-ml aliquot was cytocentrifuged onto a slide, allowed to air dry, and stained (modified Papanicolaou stain). Inclusion particles are lamellar bodies, characteristic of type II cells. Magnification, 695×. (Courtesy of T. R. Devereux and K. G. Jones.)

membrane, there is always the possibility of selective destruction of xenobiotic-metabolizing enzymes during cell preparation. Protease I is a potent inhibitor of pulmonary P-450-dependent monooxygenase activity if it enters the cells. This factor must be taken into consideration when comparing specific enzyme activities in the isolated cells or in subcellular fractions prepared from these cells to activities observed in perfused lung or subcellular fractions prepared from homogenized lung.

Several studies of xenobiotic metabolism have been performed with enriched populations of type II and Clara cells from rabbit lung with sonicated cells or with subcellular fractions prepared from sonicated cells. Alveolar macrophage fractions are frequently included in these experiments because, as our laboratory noted several years ago, they are very low in cytochrome P-450-dependent monooxygenase activity (85).

Alveolar type II cells were shown to contain 7-ethoxycoumarin *O*-deethylase and BP hydroxylase activities (P-450-dependent reactions) as well as *N,N*-dimethylaniline *N*-oxidase activity (a flavin-containing monooxygenase-catalyzed reaction). On the other hand, type II cells display only a trace of coumarin hydroxylase activity (44,45). Coumarin hydroxylation is selectively enhanced in populations of Clara cells, however, relative to monooxygenase activities with the other substrates. Specific epoxide hydrolase activity (0.59 nmole/min per mg protein) in sonicated fractions of enriched Clara cells (60%) is also much higher than in similar fractions of cells enriched (80%) in alveolar type II cells (0.06 nmole/min per mg protein) with 4,5-BPO as substrate (18).

In a collaborative study with Boyd and his colleagues at NCI, we showed that both Clara cells and alveolar type II cells of the rabbit metabolize 4-ipomeanol (48). Covalent binding of radioactivity derived from ^{3}H-4-ipomeanol to proteins in isolated cells is almost totally prevented by piperonyl butoxide, an inhibitor of cytochrome P-450-dependent monooxygenase activity. As expected, no covalent binding of tritium to protein of alveolar macrophages is observed in the absence or presence of piperonyl butoxide. The maximal rates of covalent binding of substrate to protein are much greater in Clara cells (135 pmole/min per 10^6 cells) than in type II cells (13 pmole/min per 10^6 cells), consistent with the *in vivo* necrosis of Clara cells but not alveolar type II cells on 4-ipomeanol administration to the rabbit (59). Subsequent investigations in reconstituted monooxygenase systems containing either cytochrome P-450, form 2, or cyto-

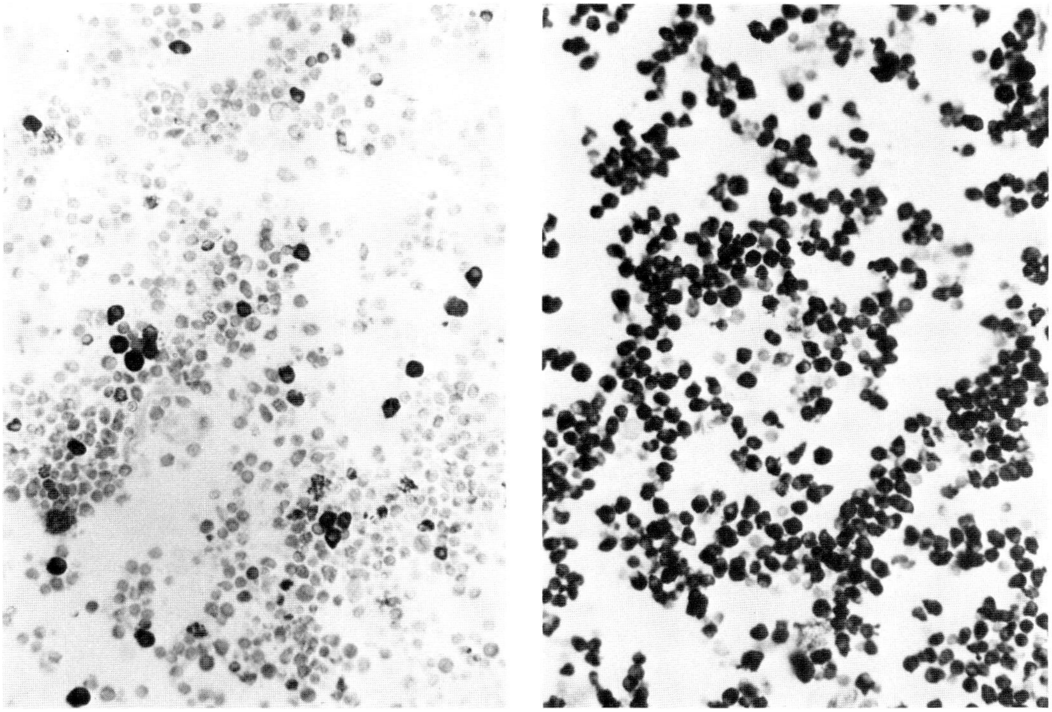

FIG. 2. Purification of Clara cells from rabbit lungs. Air-dried smears of cells were stained with nitro blue tetrazolium. Clara cells stain dark; others remain light. **Left:** cell digest prior to cell separation (approximately 5% Clara cells). **Right:** after purification of Clara cells (70–80%). Magnification, 176×. (Courtesy of T. R. Devereux and K. G. Jones.)

chrome P-450, form 5, the two major rabbit pulmonary cytochrome P-450 isozymes, showed that 4-ipomeanol is converted to a reactive metabolite by both forms of cytochrome P-450 (208). Earlier studies had shown that both P-450 isozymes are present in alveolar type II cells and Clara cells (49).

One deficiency of the rabbit pulmonary monooxygenase system for studies of chemical toxicity is that it does not respond dramatically to cytochrome P-450-inducing agents. For this reason, rat lung cells offer certain advantages in some experiments because their P-450 isozyme content can be markedly altered. Recently, we completed a study in which the effect of treating rats with β-NF was tested on the activities of several metabolic pathways in alveolar type II cells and Clara cells isolated from lung (98). As shown in Table 6, enzyme activities are all markedly higher in fractions enriched in Clara cells than in fractions enriched in alveolar type II cells (from sixfold for UDP-glucuronosyltransferase to >75-fold for epoxide hydrolase). β-NF causes significant induction of 7-ethoxycoumarin *O*-deethylase and BP hydroxylase activities in both type II and Clara cells, whereas glucuronosyltransferase activity is only significantly increased in type II cells; β-NF has no effect on GSH transferase or epoxide hydrolase activity in either cell type. From these data, it seems possible that induction of cytochrome P-450-dependent monooxygenase activity in rat lung by PAH-type inducers may alter the cell-selective or -specific toxicity of chemicals

TABLE 6. *Effect of β-naphthoflavone (β-NF) treatment on several xenobiotic-metabolizing enzyme activities in viable lung cells of the rat*[a]

	Specific activity (pmole/min per 10^6 cells)			
	Alveolar type II cells[b]		Clara cells[c]	
Enzyme activity[d]	Control	β-NF treated[e]	Control	β-NF treated
7-Ethoxycoumarin *O*-deethylase	0.7 ± 0.2[f]	3.0 ± 1.1[g]	13.3 ± 4.6	27.7 ± 3.5[h]
Aryl hydrocarbon hydroxylase	≤0.02	0.62 ± 0.27[i]	0.14 ± 0.03	4.9 ± 1.0[i]
UDP-glucuronosyltransferase[j]	32 ± 10	101 ± 9[g]	189 ± 54	255 ± 68
Glutathione transferase[k]	36 ± 28	38 ± 21	630 ± 47	575 ± 41
Epoxide hydrolase[k]	<2	<2	154 ± 19	114 ± 69

[a] Adapted from Jones et al. (98).
[b] Alveolar type II cell fractions were 80% pure, with no detectable Clara cells.
[c] Clara cell fractions were 50% pure and had less than 1% cross contamination with type II cells.
[d] Enzyme assays were performed with sonicated cells.
[e] Rats were treated with β-NF (50 mg/kg) i.p. 48 hr prior to death.
[f] Mean ± SD for 3 to 10 different experiments. Lung cells were pooled from 8 rats for each experiment.
[g] Significantly different from control values, unpaired *t*-test. $p < 0.01$.
[h] $p < 0.05$.
[i] $p < 0.001$.
[j] 4-Methylumbelliferone was the substrate.
[k] Benzo(a)pyrene 4,5-oxide was the substrate.

metabolized via reactive epoxides in lung by changing the relationship between metabolic activation pathways and detoxication pathways to a different degree in different cells.

The experiments discussed here demonstrate the utility of enriched populations of freshly isolated cells from mammalian lung in biochemical toxicology studies. However, it must be emphasized that our laboratory isolates only three of the 40 or so cell types in lung. Future efforts will include the adaptation of methods to isolate additional cell types from the respiratory tract including tracheal, endothelial, and alveolar type I cells, which are important in xenobiotic transformation or as targets for chemical-mediated toxicology. In this context, methods for the isolation of tracheal (70), type I (158), and endothelial cells (76) have recently been reported.

Renal Cells

Orrenius and his colleagues (97,146) and Fry et al. (67) have developed methods for isolating cells from the rat kidney and then used the cells for studying xenobiotic metabolism and biochemical toxicology. Orrenius' preparation contains mainly spherical cells of which 70 to 80% are believed to be of proximal tubular origin, as judged by light microscopy. The methodology used for the isolation and characterization of these cell preparations has been described in detail (97,146) and is not repeated here.

Acetaminophen is converted to its sulfate and glucuronide conjugates, but at rates only about 5% those found in hepatocytes (97). The *N*-acetylcysteine and cysteine conjugates are the only thioether metabolites of acetaminophen found in renal cells, consistent with high γ-glutamyltransferase activity and dipeptidase activity in rat kidney. The rate of formation of total thioether metabolites in renal cells is only about 50% that found in isolated hepatocytes per nanomole of cytochrome P-450. Treatment of rats with 3-MC increases the rate of formation of total thioether metabolites from acetaminophen in renal cells by approximately threefold, suggesting that the cytochrome P-450-dependent monooxygenase system is induced. Similar results were reported by Fry and Perry (66), who found that kidney cortex cells isolated from rats treated with Aroclor 1254® have elevated 7-ethoxycoumarin *O*-deethylase activities (6.4-fold) relative to cells from untreated rats (Table 7). On the other hand, this PCB mixture had no inductive effect on sulfotransferase or glucuronosyltransferase activity with 7-hydroxycoumarin.

Various aspects of GSH biosynthesis and turnover and of the formation and degradation of GSH adducts of xenobiotics have also been studied in renal cells. For example, Moldéus et al. (130a) observed that the decrease of intracellular GSH that occurs in rat kidney cells in the absence of a sulfur donor is prevented by cysteine because of rapid synthesis of GSH. Cystine is rapidly reduced in the renal cells to cysteine.

Methionine does not prevent loss of intracellular GSH, and only a low amount of ^{35}S from methionine is incorporated into cellular GSH. Glutathione conjugates of xenobiotics were also found not to accumulate in incubation medium containing renal cells. Rather, they are further metabolized to the corresponding cysteinylglycine, cysteine, and *N*-acetylcysteine derivatives (95), reminiscent of what happens in perfused kidney.

The separation of renal cells into populations enriched in a single cell type will allow an even more complete understanding of the cell selectivity of xenobiotic metabolism and chemical-mediated target organ toxicity in kidney.

Testicular Cells

Hall et al. (77) described a method to separate interstitial cells and spermatogenic cells from the rat testis. We utilized their procedure to study the activities of a few xenobiotic-metabolizing enzymes in these two different cell compartments of testis (136). The interstitial cell fractions obtained were contaminated with 5% mature sperm and approximately 25% other spermatogenic cells. However, there were no interstitial cells contaminating the spermatogenic cell fraction. As seen in Table 8, AHH activity and cytochrome P-450 content of microsomes prepared from interstitial cells are about twofold greater than those in microsomes from spermatogenic cells; in contrast, specific microsomal epoxide hydrolase and cytosolic glutathione transferase activities are twice those found in the interstitial cells. This differential distribution of enzyme activities is of some interest. We also found significant GSH transferase, but not epoxide hydrolase, activity in rat and mouse sperm and human semen (135). Thus, mammalian germ cells have certain detoxication mechanisms for reactive xenobiotic metabolites.

TABLE 7. *Effect of Aroclor 1254® treatment on several xenobiotic-metabolizing activities in viable kidney cells of the rat*[a]

	Specific activity (pmole/min/mg cell protein)	
Enzyme activity	Control	Aroclor 1254® treated[b]
7-Ethoxycoumarin *O*-deethylase	2.9 ± 1.7 (8)[c]	18.6 ± 12.5 (8)[d]
UDP-glucuronosyltransferase[e]	160.4 ± 42.0 (4)	131.2 ± 37.3 (4)
Sulfotransferase[e]	12.8 ± 2.9 (4)	13.4 ± 5.2 (4)

[a] Adapted from Fry and Perry (66).
[b] Rats were injected i.p. with 500 mg/kg Aroclor 1254® 5 days before death.
[c] Mean ± SD (*N*).
[d] Significantly different from control, $p < 0.01$.
[e] 7-Hydroxycoumarin was the substrate.

TABLE 8. *Distribution of several xenobiotic-metabolizing enzymes between interstitial and spermatogenic cells isolated from rat testis*[a]

	Specific activity (nmole/min/mg protein) or content	
Enzyme activity	Interstitial cells	Spermatogenic cells
Glutathione transferase[b]	65.3 ± 4.8[c]	119.4 ± 6.8
Epoxide hydrolase[b]	1.1 ± 0.3	2.4 ± 0.5
Aryl hydrocarbon hydroxylase	0.006 ± 0.001	0.003 ± 0.0003
Cytochrome P-450[d]	0.17, 0.22[e]	0.08, 0.09[e]

[a] Adapted from Mukhtar et al. (136). Microsomes and microsomal supernatant fractions were prepared from the cells and used as the source of enzyme activity.
[b] Styrene 7,8-oxide was substrate.
[c] Mean ± SD (N = 3).
[d] Nanomoles/mg protein.
[e] Individual values for two experiments.

Small Intestinal Cells

The epithelium of the small intestine is composed of several distinct cell types but consists principally of the absorptive (villous) cells, which are located at the tips of the villi, and the crypt cells, which proliferate rapidly and are precursors of the villous cells. These cells can be isolated by enzymatic, vibrational, and chelation–elution methods, and detailed procedures are available (107,159).

Intestinal epithelial cells have been used for several studies of xenobiotic metabolism. Stohs et al. (191) isolated metabolically active epithelial cells from rat intestine that were 90 to 95% viable immediately after cell preparation and showed that cells from animals treated with 3-MC metabolize BP at 30-fold the rate for intestinal cells from control animals. Metyrapone and SKF 525-A both inhibited BP metabolism in cells from untreated rats, whereas α-NF increased the rate of formation of fluorescent metabolites. In intestinal cells isolated from 3-MC-treated rats, α-NF is a potent inhibitor of BP metabolism, indicating the presence of a different form or forms of cytochrome P-450 in these cells. The authors also noted that 4,5-BPO is metabolized slowly because of the low epoxide hydrolase activity in the intestinal cells.

Bridges and his colleagues have also studied the metabolism of several xenobiotics in viable (85–95%) intestinal mucosal cells isolated from rat (179) and guinea pig (41a). Rat intestinal cells have sulfotransferase and UDP-glucuronsyltransferase activities (with phenol, 1-naphthol, or 7-hydroxycoumarin as substrate), *N*-acetyltransferase activity (with aniline as substrate), and cytochrome P-450-dependent monooxygenase activity (with 7-ethoxycoumarin as substrate), but no detectable glycine *N*-acyltransferase activity (with benzoic acid as substrate). Intestinal cells isolated from PB- or 3-MC-treated rats have rates of 7-ethoxycoumarin *O*-deethylation that are about twofold higher than those in cells isolated from untreated rats (179). One advantage for the isolation of intestinal epithelial cells from guinea pigs is minimal interference from mucus, which is plentiful in the rat (41a). Guinea pig intestinal cells also have sulfotransferase, UDP-glucuronsyltransferase, and cytochrome P-450-dependent monooxygenase activities.

There is also a study that describes the cell-selective induction of UDP-glucuronosyltransferase activity in intestine by TCDD administration (173). Tip (differentiated) and crypt (undifferentiated) cells were isolated separately from rat duodenum at various times after TCDD treatment. The separation of the two cell types was monitored by electron microscopy and marker enzymes (alkaline phosphatase, acid phosphatase, and DNA synthesis). Basal UDP-glucuronsyltransferase activities are twofold greater in the differentiated than the undifferentiated cells (13 and 6.5 nmole/min per mg protein for tip and crypt cells, respectively). On the other hand, TCDD selectively induces transferase activity in the undifferentiated cells (200% versus 50%, 24 hr after treatment). This report suggests that biochemically characterized tip and crypt cells are useful tools for investigating target-cell toxicity and metabolism in the two major cell types of small intestine.

Skin Cells

Fouts and his colleagues have adapted procedures developed for the separation of lung cells (see above) to skin cells of female hairless mice (HRS/J strain) and have begun xenobiotic metabolism studies with the enriched skin-cell populations. The initial method involved enzymatic digestion with trypsin (38), but disadvantages of the procedure include the low viability of the isolated cell digest (about 30%) and the fact that basal cells are more resistant to proteolytic damage than the more differentiated cells. Nonetheless, the cells isolated can be further separated by metrizamide or Percoll® gradient centrifugation into fractions enriched in different cell types. In one fraction, sebaceous (differentiated) cells account for 80% of the population, and in another 50% are basal (undifferentiated) cells. Benzo(a)pyrene hydroxylase (3.2-fold), 7-ethoxycoumarin *O*-deethylation (sixfold), UDP-glucuronsyltransferase (2.9-fold), and glutathione transferase (3.5-fold) activities (nmole/min per mg DNA) are all higher in the fraction enriched in sebaceous cells. In this study, cells were sonicated and supplemented with the required cofactor or cosubstrate prior to assay. Treatment of hairless mice by topical administration of β-NF (1.25 mg/mouse) results in the induction of 7-ethoxycoumarin *O*-deethylase and BP hydroxylase activities in cell populations enriched in sebaceous cells (about 10-fold and twofold, respectively) and basal cells (approximately 16-fold and fourfold, respectively). Thus, cytochrome P-450-dependent monooxygenase activity is preferentially increased in the undifferentiated versus the differentiated cells of mouse skin by β-NF.

More recently, pronase has replaced trypsin for enzymatic digestion (162). This results in markedly increased viability (75%) of skin epidermal cells in the initial cell digest. Viability is unchanged over a 5-hr period after isolation if cells are kept on ice, a total of 7 hr from the time the mice are killed. 7-Ethoxycoumarin *O*-deethylase and NADPH–cytochrome P-450 reductase activities also remain stable over this time period. The cell digest is separated into fractions by centrifugal elutriation. Epidermal cells in later stages of differentiation are collected in later cell elutriator fractions; the average volume of the cells in each fraction and the relative amount of cytoplasm, estimated by morphological appearance and the determination of DNA-to-protein ratios (Table 9), increase progressively. Fraction E-2 is composed mostly of basal cells, identified morphologically as small cells with a nucleus constituting more than 70% of the cell diameter. Monooxygenase activities are higher in the more differentiated keratinocytes than in basal cells, consistent with the earlier study (38).

Coomes et al. (39) have also studied the overall metabolism of 7-ethoxycoumarin in intact epidermal cells from hairless mice. 7-Ethoxycoumarin is deethylated at a rate of 3 pmole/min per 10^6 cells and converted to glucuronide and sulfate conjugates (total) at a rate of 1 pmole/min per 10^6 cells. The rate of cytochrome P-450-dependent monooxygenase activity in disrupted cells with added NADPH is similar to, but lower than, the rate in whole cells. Induction with β-NF causes a fivefold increase of 7-ethoxycoumarin *O*-deethylase activity and a twofold

TABLE 9. *Some characteristics of epidermal cell fractions isolated from hairless mice and enriched in different cell types by elutriation*[a]

Fraction	7-Ethoxycoumarin *O*-deethylase (pmole/min/mg DNA)	Milligrams protein/ mg DNA	Average cell volume (μm^3)
E-2	77 ± 83[b]	43 ± 27[c]	271 ± 57[b]
E-4	105 ± 77	33 ± 11	293 ± 84
E-6	138 ± 57	39 ± 15	506 ± 183
E-7	208 ± 88[d]	55 ± 15	481 ± 143[d]

[a] Adapted from Pohl et al. (162).
[b] Mean ± SD, $N = 4$.
[c] Mean ± SD, $N = 5$.
[d] Significantly different than E-2 value by one-sided test, $p < 0.05$.

increase in both the rate of glucuronidation and the intracellular concentration of UDP-glucuronic acid.

The epidermal cells described here should prove valuable for studies of xenobiotic metabolism and toxicity in skin. With this tissue, the availability of such a system is especially important, because skin is very difficult to disrupt.

Needless to say, fresh cells from other extrahepatic tissues that are sites for chemical-mediated toxicity or for the action of pharmacologically active agents—e.g., adrenal, ovary, eye, ear, nose, trachea, pancreas (170), bladder, stomach, colon, brain, spleen, heart, mammary gland, lymph nodes, bone marrow—can also be isolated and selectively enriched with regard to individual cell type by existing or adaptation of existing methodology. Isolated cells from these tissues will facilitate investigation of the specific role of individual extrahepatic cell types in chemical metabolism and toxicity. A dramatic increase in the number of such endeavors is expected in the next decade. Consequently, it may be worthwhile to consider briefly some problems associated with the use of freshly isolated cells for such studies. First, the use of mixed cell populations is of limited value, especially if the cells are not characterized and identified morphologically. Enzymatic digestion, which is almost always used to release cells from the basement membrane, may cause selective degradation of certain xenobiotic biotransformation pathways or of enzymes required for the biosynthesis of essential cofactors and cosubstrates.

Thus, rates of metabolism obtained in isolated cells must be compared to those determined under optimal conditions with subcellular fractions prepared by conventional tissue homogenization and, preferably, also to rates determined in perfused organs. This will at least indicate dramatic losses of activity in the cell populations. The procedures required for isolation of enriched cell populations from extrahepatic tissues are labor intensive, and the yields of specific cell types are often too low to allow comprehensive metabolic studies with cells from the same animal or group of animals. Moreover, considerable experience is required to routinely isolate suitable numbers of cells in high purity. Even so, freshly isolated cells have one major advantage for studies of xenobiotic metabolism relative to cells in culture: they retain their state of differentiation. This is very important because dedifferentiation that occurs as cells enter culture is known to affect the amount of cytochrome P-450 and its associated monooxygenase activity in hepatocytes (180) as well as in extrahepatic tissues, such as skin (20) and lung (R. Wu and T. R. Devereux, *unpublished data*). Cytochrome P-450 isozymes appear to be affected selectively during dedifferentiation, and this can markedly affect the relationship between biotransformation of a xenobiotic and its toxicity by altering the metabolite profile.

Organs and Cells in Culture

Concomitant with the development of successful epithelial cell culture techniques over the last few years, there has been a dramatic increase in the investigation of chemical metabolism, particularly of carcinogens, in extrahepatic organs and cells in culture. These preparations are also used to study the metabolic activation of compounds to mutagens by coculture with an appropriate bacterium (e.g., Ames test) or cell line. Organs and cells in culture overcome some of the deficiencies of freshly isolated, enriched populations of extrahepatic cells, including the labor-intensive nature of cell isolation, low cell yields, and the detrimental effects of proteolytic enzymes. However, there are limitations, at least in terms of extrapolation to the *in vivo* situation. These include the presence of mixed cell populations, rapid dedifferentiation of cells in culture, and the requirement for added growth factors and hormones, which can selectively affect cytochrome P-450 isozymes.

Advantages of the cultured preparations are that chemical metabolism can be studied in extrahepatic organs and cells of human origin and that metabolism can be investigated by *in vitro* test systems that undergo neoplastic transformation after exposure to carcinogens (e.g., 188). Furthermore, because metabolites and metabolite–DNA adducts formed during incubation of carcinogens with cultured organs or cells can be identified and quantified, and because selective removal of metabolite–DNA adducts and the repair of damaged DNA can be measured, these systems allow the elucidation of relationships between metabolism and at least two events thought to be critical to nitrosamine and PAH-mediated carcinogenesis.

Harris and his collaborators at NCI have been very active in this particular area of research. The diversity of organs and cells in culture that have been used to study carcinogen metabolism and, almost always, covalent interaction with DNA are illustrated in Tables 10 and 11, respectively. In general, these studies have shown that cultured extrahepatic cells and organs metabolize BP, that this metabolism is induced during culture with a PAH such as benz(a)anthracene, that the deoxyguanosine adduct of BPDEI is the major BP metabolite–DNA product formed, and that repair may be selective for certain adducts or nonexistent. The observations emphasize that DNA alkylation by BPDEI is, at most, a contributing factor to BP-mediated tumorigenesis. Other, more

TABLE 10. *Some organs in culture that have been used to study the metabolism of chemical carcinogens*

Organ in culture	Animal source	Chemical carcinogen	Ref.
Bladder	Human, rat	2-AAF, BP; 2-AAF, BP	133
Bronchus	Human	Aflatoxin, BP, 1,2-DMH, DMN	8,9,11,78
Colon	Human	Aflatoxin, BP, 1,2-DMH	8–10,12
Duodenum	Human	BP	9
Endometrium	Human	BP	122
Esophagus	Human	BP, DEN, DMN, acyclic and cyclic nitrosamines	9,13,79
	Rat	Acyclic and cyclic nitrosamines	79
Pancreatic duct	Human	BP, DMBA	80
Prostate	Human	BP	105
Skin	Mouse, rat	BP; BP	120,204
Trachea	Hamster, rat	BP; BP	36,121

TABLE 11. *Some cells in culture that have been used to study the metabolism of chemical carcinogens*

Cell in culture	Animal source	Chemical carcinogen	Ref.
Amnion	Human	BP	71
Bladder (epithelial)	Human; Rat	NMEA, NPD; 2-AAF, BP	133,137
Bronchial (mucosal)	Human; Rat	BP	14
	Bovine; Hamster; Mouse	BP	14
Dermal (fibroblasts)	Human; Mouse	BP; BP, DMBA	54,92,110
Embryo	Hamster	BP	15
Epidermal (keratinocytes)	Human	BP	110,111,148
	Hamster; Mouse	BP, DMBA; BP, DMBA	20,55,92,110
Lung (mixed)[a]	Rat	BP, DMN	113,193
Mammary (epithelial)	Human; Rat	BP; BP, DMBA, NNMU	73,165,187
Mammary (fibroblast)	Human	BP	187
Prostate (epithelial)	Human	BP	105
Tracheal (epithelial)	Hamster; Rat	BP; BP	36,60

[a] 70% epithelial-like and 30% fibroblast-like cells.

critical factors determine whether extrahepatic cells will become neoplastic.

The fact that cells in culture undergo rapid dedifferentiation makes them an interesting potential model system for study of the modulation of individual cytochrome P-450 isozymes in cells of extrahepatic origin. Now that immunochemical assays for individual forms of cytochrome P-450 are available (discussed below), it is possible to determine selective increases or decreases of the various isozymes in cells cultured under varying conditions.

SUBCELLULAR FRACTIONS OF EXTRAHEPATIC TISSUES

The vast majority of information describing xenobiotic metabolism by extrahepatic tissues is derived from studies performed with subcellular fractions of homogenate. Many important xenobiotic-metabolizing enzymes, including the cytochrome P-450-dependent monooxygenase system, the flavin-dependent monooxygenase, epoxide hydrolase, prostaglandin synthetase, and UDP-glucuronosyltransferase, are localized in the endoplasmic reticulum. Consequently, much information is available that describes the problems and appropriate methodology for disruption of extrahepatic tissues and for isolation of microsomes from tissue homogenate. A comprehensive review of this subject, which includes an extensive literature survey of cytochrome P-450-dependent monooxygenase activities in extrahepatic tissues, is available (30). It is recommended reading for anyone planning experiments with subcellular fractions of extrahepatic organs. Because of this recent review, these topics are not discussed in detail here. Rather, the types of experiments that can best be accomplished in subcellular fractions are briefly mentioned with some examples.

Some advantages of subcellular fractions (nuclear membranes, mitochondria, microsomal fraction, cytosolic fraction, etc.) for the study of xenobiotic metabolism include optimization of reaction rates by addition of saturating amounts of substrate and cofactor, selection of a single enzymatic reaction or class of reactions by choice of cofactor, and enhancement of specific activity relative to whole homogenate. Disadvantages in comparing data generated *in vitro* to the *in vivo* situation are that some enzymes (e.g., the flavin-dependent monooxygenase) can be denatured during cell disruption, that cellular structure is destroyed, and that, at least for heterogeneous organs such as the lung and kidney, the relative contributions of different cell types localized in different anatomical regions of the organ to the isolated subcellular fraction are unknown. In spite of these limitations, subcellular fractions remain the method of choice for investigating certain aspects of the relationships between xenobiotic metabolism and target organ toxicity.

A frequent use of the microsomal fraction or the microsomal plus cytosolic fractions (the mitochondrial supernatant or S-9 fraction) of extrahepatic tissues is to test the ability of an organ to convert xenobiotics to mutagenic and/or chemically reactive metabolites. The microsomes are coupled with various strains of *Salmonella typhimurium* (the Ames test), with cells in culture, or sometimes even with single-stranded DNA. Recently, for example, Scarpelli et al. (171) used the postmitochondrial fraction of hamster pancreas, supplemented with NADPH, to convert various nitrosamines to bacterial mutagens. Andersson et al. (7) incubated ram seminal vesicle microsomes, arachidonic acid, and phenacetin (4-ethoxyacetanilide) or its metabolites along with cultured human skin fibroblasts; DNA strand breaks were induced in the fibroblasts by *p*-phenetidine and *p*-aminophenol but not by phenacetin. The implication of each of these experiments seems clear. Nitrosamines are metabolized to mutagens by cytochrome P-450-dependent monooxygenase activity in hamster pancreas, a toxication mechanism that is known to occur in many other tissues (153). *p*-Phenetidine and *p*-aminophenol are converted, presumably by prostaglandin synthetase, to products that damage fibroblast DNA. These *in vitro* experiments demonstrate conclusively that the reactions occur in a specific tissue; they indicate that a toxic metabolite will be formed *in vivo;* but they can not predict whether or not toxicity will be observed in the intact animal or in an experimental system with intact cellular structure.

More definitive information about xenobiotic metabolism by extrahepatic tissue results when the metabolites formed are identified chemically. If the metabolite happens to be unique to, or preferentially formed in, an extrahepatic organ, subcellular fractions can be used to biosynthesize enough of the product for detailed chemical analysis. Microsomal fractions are especially useful for compounds formed by reductive or oxidative pathways that ordinarily would be rapidly converted to secondary metabolites *in vivo* by perfused organs or intact cells.

Subcellular fractions also serve as an intermediate experimental system between *in vivo* xenobiotic biotransformation and the eventual characterization of biochemical reaction mechanisms with homogeneous enzyme preparations. Metabolic studies on the antiinflammatory drug sulindac, (*Z*)-5-fluoro - 2 - methyl - 1 - [*p* - (methylsulfinyl)benzylidene]indene-3-acetic acid, readily illustrate this point. Sulindac is metabolized *in vivo* to a pharmacologically active sulfide derivative via sulfoxide reduction; it is also oxidized to the pharmacologically inert sulfone analog (58,88). Because little was known about the enzyme(s) responsible for sulfoxide reduction in mammals, the reaction was studied *in vitro* with rat tissue preparations (163). Kidney cytosolic fraction has the highest activity (75.9 ± 23.8 pmole/min per mg protein, mean $\pm$ SD, $N = 3$) of the tissues sampled (liver, lung, brain, muscle, and kidney), although liver also has significant activity. Sulfoxide reduction by rat renal cytosol was investigated in more detail (5). NADPH is required for enzyme activity, and disulfides, such as GSH disulfide, that interact with thioredoxin-dependent enzymes inhibit sulindac reduction. If thioredoxin is removed from the renal cytosolic fraction, there is a dramatic loss of enzyme activity, which can be recovered by addition of bacterial thioredoxin. Thus, thioredoxin-dependent sulfoxide reduction occurs in mammalian kidney. This series of experiments illustrates how subcellular fractions can be used to investigate mechanistic aspects of xenobiotic metabolism and that investigations in such systems are a logical extension of *in vivo* observations detailing novel metabolic pathways.

Based on past experience, the most frequent use of subcellular fractions of extrahepatic tissues will likely be to investigate the effects of exogenous and endogenous chemicals on the induction, repression, or inhibition of xenobiotic metabolizing enzymes. Often a substrate, such as BP, that is oxidatively metabolized to many different products is used because its metabolite profile gives some information about the properties of the major form(s) of cytochrome P-450 catalyzing the reaction. Microsomal incubations are routinely conducted in the presence and absence of selective affectors of monooxygenase activity such as α-NF, metyrapone, and ellipticine. Montelius et al. (131) carried out such a study with rat adrenal gland. The BP metabolites obtained and inhibition of BP hydroxylase activity by α-NF demonstrate that the adrenal microsomal monooxygenase system resembles that of PAH-induced rat liver (i.e., cytochrome P-450_I and P-448 characteristics). The microsomal monooxygenase system metabolizing BP is distinct from the mitochondrial system responsible for the biosynthesis of mineralocorticoids and glucocorticoids from cholesterol. It is also known that rat microsomal adrenal BP hydroxylase activity is not induced by treatment with PAH (75).

One of the most interesting problems currently under investigation in extrahepatic tissues, one that is intimately involved with relationships between chemical metabolism and target organ toxicity, concerns the differential regulation of xenobiotic-metabolizing enzymes in different tissues and cells. For example, exogenous ACTH treatment restores adrenal microsomal cytochrome P-450-dependent AHH activity and an electrophoretic band of approximately 57,000 daltons to normal levels in hypophysectomized rats (75). Administration of LH to hypophysectomized rats significantly increases testicular microsomal cytochrome P-450 content, AHH, and epoxide hydrolase activities but does not affect GSH transferase activity (116). The increase in P-450 content occurs concomitantly with morphological recovery of the Leydig cell compartment in the testis.

There are also studies that demonstrate that the administration of steroid sex hormones to mice or rats selectively affects xenobiotic-metabolizing enzyme activities in different tissues. Testosterone administration increases flavin-containing monooxygenase-dependent *N,N*-dimethylaniline *N*-oxidase activity in renal microsomes, represses it in hepatic microsomes, and does not affect it in pulmonary microsomes of CF-1 mice (57). Chronic treatment of female rats with estradiol (1 mg/kg for 7 days) increases small intestinal microsomal AHH and 7-ethoxycoumarin *O*-deethylase activities but represses these enzyme activities in pulmonary microsomes (3). Pulmonary microsomal cytochrome P-450 content is higher in female rats than in male rats but is unaffected by treatment with estradiol or testosterone in either sex. However, estrogen administration to intact and castrated male rats selectively enhances pulmonary microsomal 7-ethoxyresorufin *O*-deethylase activity (relative to 7-ethoxycoumarin *O*-deethylase), implicating a selective change in the cytochrome P-450 isozyme content of lung (63).

It seems obvious that quantitation of individual cytochrome P-450 isozymes is requisite to understanding endogenous regulation of this monooxygenase system. Fortunately, sensitive immunochemical assays are available that can accomplish this task, at least for several cytochrome P-450 isozymes (discussed below). Thus, regulation of individual forms of cytochrome P-450 by endogenous (e.g., sex steroids, hormones, mineralocorticoids, glucocortoids) and exogenous (e.g., PAH, PB) factors can now be studied, at least with respect to tissue. In the future, this approach will undoubtedly be extended to individual cell types of extrahepatic tissues.

The ease of preparing subcellular fractions from tissue homogenate, relative to organ perfusion or cell isolation/enrichment procedures, guarantees that they will play an important role in xenobiotic metabolism studies of extrahepatic tissues. However, it is reemphasized that extrapolation of results of *in vitro* experiments investigating relationships between xenobiotic metabolism and toxicity to the *in vivo* situation requires caution at best and is impossible in certain situations.

PURIFIED COMPONENTS OF THE CYTOCHROME P-450-DEPENDENT MONOOXYGENASE SYSTEM

Homogeneous cytochrome P-450 isozymes and other xenobiotic-metabolizing enzymes purified from extrahepatic tissues are advantageous for certain types of experiments. First, the catalytic properties of individual forms of cytochrome P-450 can be investigated in reconstituted monooxygenase systems. This allows assessment of the position-specific or selective oxidation of diverse substrates of both exogenous and endogenous origin. Second, the preparation of specific inhibiting antibodies to individual forms of the hemoprotein allows immunochemical localization of cytochrome P-450 in extrahepatic tissues and cells, determination of the contribution of individual isozymes to total microsomal enzyme activity, and immunochemical quantitation of specific isozymes in microsomes from extrahepatic organs. These approaches are discussed in more detail below.

Rabbit Pulmonary Monooxygenase System

The cytochrome P-450-dependent monooxygenase system is very important in the oxidative metabolism and metabolic activation of many different xenobiotics. The potential for exposure to airborne pollutants and susceptibility to disease and chemical-mediated toxicity were significant factors in our laboratory's decision to select the lung for a long-term study of its cytochrome P-450-dependent monooxygenase system. However, the relatively low levels of these enzymes, cellular diversity, and the fibrous structure of this organ have been complicating factors in this endeavor. The number of forms of cytochrome P-450 isolated from liver continues to increase, and the most completely characterized cytochrome P-450 isozymes are those of the rat, rabbit, and mouse (138), which provide a good basis for comparison with the respective enzymes isolated from extrahepatic sources.

Of these species, the rabbit has the highest constitutive content of pulmonary cytochrome P-450 (155), which is advantageous for purification. However, as experimental strains of rabbits are not inbred, the characterization of isozymes may prove to be more complex because of polymorphisms, as has been observed for the hepatic isozyme form 3b (53). Nevertheless, of all the extrahepatic microsomal cytochrome P-450 systems studied, the rabbit pulmonary enzymes are currently the most fully characterized. Further, this has been accomplished with tissue from untreated rabbits.

Two isozymes have been purified to apparent homogeneity as determined by PAGE in the presence of SDS. A recent review (157) has summarized the purification, characterization, and cellular distribution of these isozymes; a brief overview of the work of Philpot and co-workers is presented here.

The nomenclature of the pulmonary isozymes, P-450_{I} and P-450_{II}, was changed to form 2 and form 5, respectively, to correspond to the nomenclature established to reflect the relative electrophoretic mobilities of rabbit hepatic isozymes. The necessity for this change was apparent once the properties of these isozymes were elucidated.

Pulmonary cytochrome P-450_{I} and the

major hepatic isozyme induced by PB, form 2, were indistinguishable by monomeric molecular weight (52,000), amino acid analysis, amino terminal sequence (MET-GLY-PHE-SER), monomeric molecular weights of peptides formed by partial proteolysis, UV–visible absorbance spectra, reconstituted catalytic activity, and immunoreactivity. These properties are distinct from those of cytochrome P-450, form 5, which is not similar to any previous identified rabbit isozyme and, in the presence of SDS, has an electrophoretic mobility (58,000 daltons) between those of hepatic forms 4 and 6.

In addition to the structural and immunochemical differences, forms 2 and 5, in purified reconstituted monooxygenase systems, exhibit distinct substrate specificity with the exception of activation of 4-ipomeanol, hydroxylation of benzo(a)pyrene, and formation of a metabolite–inhibitor complex from *N*-hydroxyamphetamine. The substrate specificity of the purified pulmonary isozymes correlates with pulmonary microsomal activities that are specifically inhibited by antibodies to the isozymes. Thus, isolation and characterization of these isozymes yielded biochemical and immunochemical means for monitoring them individually in tissue sections, isolated cells, or microsomes from untreated or treated rabbits.

The best example for induction of rabbit pulmonary cytochrome P-450 is that of TCDD-induced form 6. Although this isozyme has not been purified from lung, the structural, catalytic, and immunochemical evidence that it is significantly induced by TCDD is convincing; microsomal 7-ethoxyresorufin *O*-deethylation and cross reactivity with the antibody to form 6 are induced as well as a microsomal protein that, following extraction from polyacrylamide electrophoretic gels and partial proteolysis, yielded peptides with the same electrophoretic mobilities as those from purified hepatic form 6 (119). To a lesser degree, hydrocarbons such as 3-MC, BP (199), or PCBs (196) may also induce this isozyme. Pulmonary microsomes from untreated rabbits have variable low levels of 7-ethoxyresorufin *O*-deethylation activity that is not inhibited by antibodies to form 2 or 5, indicating the presence of form 6 (R. M. Philpot et al., *unpublished observation*).

Further evidence for form 6 in the lung and induction of this isozyme by TCDD has been obtained by the Western blotting technique. This procedure involves the separation of proteins on SDS polyacrylamide gels with subsequent electrophoretic transfer to nitrocellulose sheets followed by reaction with a specific antibody (194). The antibody binding can then be visualized by immunoperoxidase staining. The relative density of the stained band, which is proportional to the amount of antigen bound to the nitrocellulose sheet, is used to estimate the microsomal content of antigen (Fig. 3). Domin et al. (56) have used this method to determine that TCDD treatment induces form 6 by 10- to 20-fold in rabbit lung. This technique has also been used to demonstrate that the major P-450 isozymes induced by PB or β-NF in rat liver are present in rat pulmonary microsomes as well as to determine the cross reactivity among human pulmonary and hepatic microsomal samples to an antibody elicited against a purified human hepatic isozyme (74); as the monomeric molecular weight of the human pulmonary immunoreactive protein was found to be greater than that of the hepatic cytochrome, it is unlikely that these are identical isozymes.

The lack of induction of cytochrome P-450 by PB in rabbit lung (as well as in many other extrahepatic tissues) has been noted. Although the pulmonary content of forms 2 and 5 is not significantly altered by administration of PB, the content of form 6 is apparently decreased (B. A. Domin, and R. M. Philpot, *unpublished observation*). Polychlorinated biphenyl mixtures such as Aroclor 1260® contain TCDD-like components (coplanar congeners and tetrachlorodibenzofurans) capable of inducing form 6, as previ-

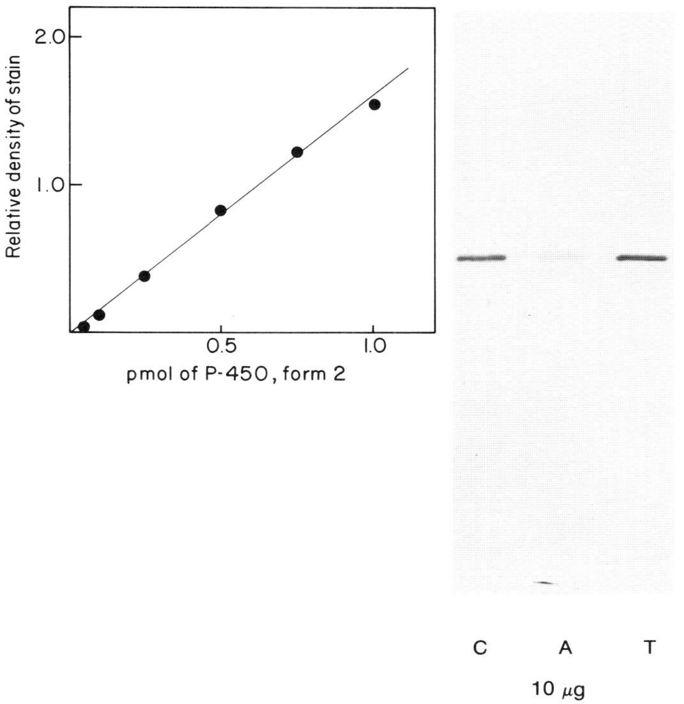

FIG. 3. Western blots of rabbit cytochrome P-450, form 2 in purified and pulmonary microsomal fractions. The samples were electrophoresed in 7.5% acrylamide gels in the presence of SDS (112) and subsequently electrophoretically transferred to a sheet of nitrocellulose, which was then incubated in saline containing 3% bovine serum albumin followed by the antibody to form 2 (194). The binding of the antibody was visualized by the bridged-immunoperoxidase diaminobenzidine stain (190). **Left:** densitometric measurements of stained bands (mm^2, area of absorbance peak from soft laser scan) were corrected for differences in band width and plotted versus the amount of form 2 per track applied to the acrylamide gel. **Right:** nitrocellulose blot of pulmonary microsomal samples (10 μg/track) from untreated (C), Aroclor 1260®-treated (A), and TCDD-treated (T) rabbits. The relative electrophoretic mobility of the stained bands is equal to that of purified form 2. (Data from B. A. Domin and R. M. Philpot, *unpublished*.)

ously mentioned, but perhaps of greater significance is the decrease in the pulmonary content of form 2 but not form 5 (195). It appears that the repressive effects of Aroclor 1260® are not caused by the components that induce form 6 and cannot be antagonized by administering PB (R. M. Philpot et al., *unpublished observation*).

Whether or not PB diminishes the hepatic content of form 6 has not been determined. However, it is clear that administration of Aroclor 1260® results in a loss of hepatic form 2 and that there is antagonism of induction by PB of this isozyme (174). The apparent repressive effects of these components on certain P-450 isozymes are more easily observed in the lung than in the liver because of the greater complexity and inducibility of the hepatic monooxygenase system.

The presence of form 5 in the liver and its induction by PB have been shown by immunoquantitation (immunodiffusion and Western blots), by inhibition by antibodies to form 5 of enzymatic activity, and by PAGE (156). The implications of these findings for the mechanism(s) of hepatic activation of aromatic amines to mutagens is currently under investigation. The efficiency of form 5 in the activation of 2-AAF to mutagens is the highest of any reported for rabbit P-450 isozymes (166).

Purification of form 5 from hepatic microsomes may be more arduous than from pulmonary microsomes, in which form 5 comprises a greater fraction of total P-450. Thus, as yet unidentified hepatic isozymes may in some instances be obtained in greater homogeneity from extrahepatic tissues.

The unique aspects of the rabbit lung in

its metabolism or susceptibility to xenobiotics can not be explained by the presence of tissue-specific isozymes, as all known pulmonary isozymes are also present in the liver. The relative proportions, concentrations, and control of synthesis of the isozymes are likely the pertinent parameters. In regard to the latter, hepatic but not pulmonary induction of the major pulmonary isozymes by PB represents a major biochemical difference between these organs. Whereas the importance of genetic differences in xenobiotic-metabolizing enzymes among species is recognized, the identification of factors that control the expression of the multiple genes (198) in various tissues of an animal will be no less significant to understanding activation and detoxication of xenobiotics.

As the activity of cytochrome P-450 isozymes is dependent on the supply of electrons, tissue differences in content and composition of reductive enzymes are obvious factors in the evaluation of monooxygenase activity of extrahepatic tissues. The pulmonary microsomal content of NADPH–cytochrome P-450 reductase is equivalent to that of untreated liver; the pulmonary and hepatic reductases are structurally, catalytically, and immunochemically indistinguishable. Thus, the ratio of reductase to cytochrome is three to five times greater in pulmonary microsomes. This difference perhaps results in the lower estimated specific activity of form 2 in the *N*-demethylation of benzphetamine in hepatic than in pulmonary microsomes (176).

Artificial though they are, purified enzymes have provided the means for studying this P-450-dependent monooxygenase in a more biologically realistic setting, whole cells. Although the cellular concentration of cytochrome P-450 monooxygenase components cannot be accurately determined, immunocytochemical methods employing specific antibodies to cytochrome P-450 isozymes or NADPH–cytochrome P-450 reductase allow qualitative comparisons of the cellular distribution of these enzymes. By means of the immunofluorescence assay, the relative fluorescent intensity caused by the binding of antibody to form 2 in nonciliated bronchiolar epithelial (Clara) cells is greater than that in hepatocytes of PB-treated rabbits (176). A high pulmonary intracellular concentration of enzymes that activate 4-ipomeanol (48,208) is consistent with the pulmonary specificity of this toxin. This interpretation of immunohistochemical data is also consistent with morphological evidence of high concentrations of agranular endoplasmic reticulum in Clara cells of mammals (161) that are susceptible to the pulmonary toxic effects of furans such as 4-ipomeanol, 3-methylfuran, or pirella ketone (25).

Admittedly, the comparison of immunofluorescence in different tissues is based on the assumption that the antigen, regardless of location, binds the same amount of antibody. However, in comparing immunofluorescence caused by the presence of various antigens, the assumption that each antigen binds the same amount of antibody has little validity unless the comparative immunoreactivity has been assessed. Such a difference in immunoreactivity of antibodies may explain the disagreement between the immunofluorescence data, which suggest that in hepatocytes the content of form 2 is greater than that of form 4 (43), and immunoquantitation of these isozymes in hepatic microsomes, which indicates the reverse (33). Also, form 4, determined immunohistochemically in rabbit lung, has not been identified in pulmonary microsomal samples by electrophoretic or immunochemical analysis (119).

Another restraint to this experimental approach is that the antibody may react with an inactive isozyme or even a functionally unrelated but antigenically similar protein (104). Thus, in determining the relative proportion of isozymes in extrahepatic tissues, cautious interpretation of immunofluorescence data is warranted. Nevertheless, immunohistochemical techniques are valuable for indicating anatomical regions that may contain xenobiotic-metabolizing enzymes, but the data must be confirmed by other means.

Isolated Clara and alveolar type II epithelial pneumocytes have permitted aspects of the cellular localization of cytochrome P-450 monooxygenases to be studied by several means: immunohistochemical distribution, enzymatic activity, and electrophoretic analysis (48,49). This is a valuable supplement to *in situ* studies, as it has established that the type II cell, which is difficult to identify by light microscopy, contains catalytically active, immunoreactive cytochrome P-450, forms 2 and 5. Electrophoretic analysis of microsomal fractions prepared from these cells indicates that the proportion of form 2 to form 5 as well as the total amount in each cell type may differ significantly, the Clara cell being the more enriched.

Other Extrahepatic Tissues

The cross reactivity of antibodies to rabbit cytochrome P-450 isozymes with endothelial cells determined by immunofluorescence as well as evidence of monooxygenase activity in aorta have been the basis for applying the Western blot technique to microsomal fractions from rabbit heart and aorta. Preliminary results in our laboratory demonstrate the presence of NADPH cytochrome *c* reductase, cytochrome P-450, form 2, form 5, and the induction of form 6 subsequent to treatment with TCDD in these tissues. The concentration of these proteins in heart and aorta fractions are less than 1 to 2% of that in pulmonary microsomes.

Two forms of cytochrome P-450 (P-450_{scc} and P-$450_{11\beta}$ purified from bovine renal mitochondria) have been quite well characterized by biochemical and immunochemical methods (127). In the rabbit renal proximal tubular epithelium, cross reactivity with antibodies against isozyme forms 2, 3, 4, and 6, purified from hepatic microsomes, has been histochemically demonstrated (43). Similar studies indicate that NADPH–cytochrome P-450 reductase and two inducible cytochrome P-450 isozymes are common to hepatocytes and renal epithelium of rats and miniature pigs (42).

The placenta, intestine, brain, skin, heart, eye, pancreas, and bladder contain cytochrome P-450 monooxygenase components, but the structural nature is unknown, and even with recent advances in purification, isolation of cytochrome P-450 from these sites would be an enormous undertaking. A possible exception is the ethmoturbinate, the cytochrome P-450 content of which is 60 to 70% of the hepatic content in the dog (40). Rats, mice, rabbits, guinea pigs, and Syrian hamsters also have significant amounts of cytochrome P-450 and monooxygenase activity in microsomal fractions from this nasal tissue.

The differences among species in the hepatic monooxygenase enzymes have precluded a common nomenclature or a generalized, yet comprehensive understanding of this system. Similarly, for other tissues, extrapolation of data obtained from one species to others would be erroneous.

It is clear that as the techniques for detection of cytochrome P-450 become more sensitive and specific, the effects of toxicants or therapeutic agents on these systems will be analyzed more explicitly. Reliable modulation by inducers/repressors of isozyme content in target organs will contribute to a clearer demonstration of the role of this ubiquitous and complex enzyme system in the biological fate of xenobiotics. However, the available data on cytochrome P-450-dependent monooxygenases in most extrahepatic tissues, adrenal and kidney being notable exceptions, are primarily observations of catalytic activities that may be induced or inhibited.

CONCLUSION

Over the last decade, we, along with our colleagues, have developed or adapted the necessary techniques to study relationships between xenobiotic metabolism and target organ toxicity in the rabbit lung at several levels of cellular organization, from *in vivo* to reconstituted monooxygenase systems containing the two homogeneous cytochrome P-450 isozymes that account for at least 70% of total P-450 in rabbit lung microsomes. Our experiments, which are performed with perfused lung, freshly isolated alveolar macrophages, Clara and alveolar type II cells, subcellular lung and cell fractions, and purified enzymes, allow us to elucidate both biochemical and chemical mechanisms involved in the metabolism of compounds that show selective acute and/or chronic toxicity to mammalian lung. We are currently developing the capability to isolate pulmonary cell populations enriched in endothelial and alveolar type I cells; we also wish to culture alveolar type II and Clara cells under conditions that retain both the amount of total cytochrome P-450 and the relative proportion of P-450 isozymes present in freshly isolated cells. Initial attempts to do this have been unsuccessful. Clara cells, for example, rapidly dedifferentiate in culture, losing almost 90% of their P-450-dependent monooxygenase activity over 24 hr (R. Wu and T. R. Devereux, *unpublished data*).

Several other laboratories are also using an integrated approach for the study of xenobiotic metabolism in extrahepatic tissues. Preparations available include rat lung, rat kidney, rat intestine, rat testis, and hamster pancreas. In our opinion, comprehensive, integrated approaches such as these are needed for unequivocal understanding of the role of extrahepatic tissues and cells in the metabolism of endogenous and exogenous chemicals, and such an understanding is required if we are ever to prevent chemical-mediated toxicity and disease.

ACKNOWLEDGMENTS

We are very grateful to our colleagues in the Laboratory of Pharmacology, N.I.E.H.S., who have shared unpublished data with us: Drs. M. W. Anderson, M. W. Coomes, T. R. Devereux, B. A. Domin, J. R. Fouts, and R. M. Philpot.

REFERENCES

1. Aitio, A. (1974): UDP-glucuronyltransferase activity in various rat tissues. *Int. J. Biochem.*, 5:325–330.
2. Aitio, A., and Marniemi, J. (1980): Extrahepatic glucuronide conjugation. In: *Extrahepatic Metabolism of Drugs and Other Foreign Compounds*, edited by T. E. Gram, pp. 365–387. S. P. Medical and Scientific Books, New York.
3. Al-Turk, A. W., Stohs, S. J., and Roche, E. B. (1980): Effect of acute and chronic estrone, estradiol, and estriol treatment on hepatic, pulmonary, and intestinal mixed-function mono-oxygenase activities in female rats. *Drug Metab. Dispos.*, 8:143–146.
4. Anders, M. W. (1980): Metabolism of drugs by the rat kidney. *Kidney Int.*, 18:636–647.
5. Anders, M. W., Ratnayake, J. H., Hanna, P. E., and Fuchs, J. A. (1981): Thioredoxin-dependent sulfoxide reduction by rat renal cytosol. *Drug Metab. Dispos.*, 9:307–310.
6. Anderson, M. W., Boroujerdi, M., and Wilson, A. G. E. (1981): Inhibition *in vivo* of the formation of adducts between metabolites of benzo(a)pyrene and DNA by butylated hydroxyanisole. *Cancer Res.*, 41:4309–4315.
7. Andersson, B., Nordenskjöld, M., Rahimtula, A., and Moldéus, P. (1982): Prostaglandin synthetase-catalyzed activation of phenacetin metabolites to genotoxic products. *Mol. Pharmacol.*, 22:479–485.
8. Autrup, H., Essigmann, J. M., Croy, R. G., Trump, B. F., Wogan, G. N., and Harris, C. C. (1979): Metabolism of aflatoxin B_1 and identification of the major aflatoxin B_1-DNA adducts formed in cultured human bronchus and colon. *Cancer Res.*, 39:694–698.
9. Autrup, H., Grafström, R. C., Brugh, M., Lechner, J. F., Haugen, A., Trump, B. F., and Harris, C. C. (1982): Comparison of benzo(a)pyrene metabolism in bronchus, esophagus, colon, and duodenum from the same individual. *Cancer Res.*, 42:934–938.
10. Autrup, H., Harris, C. C., Schwartz, R. D., Trump, B. F., and Smith, L. (1980): Metabolism of 1,2-dimethylhydrazine by cultured human colon. *Carcinogenesis*, 1:375–380.
11. Autrup, H., Harris, C. C., Stoner, G. D., Selkirk, J. K., Schafer, P. W., and Trump, B. F. (1978): Metabolism of [^{3}H]-benzo(a)pyrene by cultured human bronchus and cultured human pulmonary alveolar macrophages. *Lab. Invest.*, 38:217–224.
12. Autrup, H., Harris, C. C., Trump, B. F., and Jeffrey, A. M. (1978): Metabolism of benzo(a)pyrene and identification of the major benzo(a)pyrene–DNA adducts in cultured human colon. *Cancer Res.*, 38:3689–3696.
13. Autrup, H., and Stoner, G. D. (1982): Metabolism

of *N*-nitrosamines by cultured human and rat esophagus. *Cancer Res.*, 42:1307–1311.
14. Autrup, H., Wefald, F. C., Jeffrey, A. M., Tate, H., Schwartz, R. D., Trump, B. F., and Harris, C. C. (1980): Metabolism of benzo[a]pyrene by cultured tracheobronchial tissues from mice, rats, hamsters, bovines, and humans. *Int. J. Cancer*, 25:293–300.
15. Baird, W. M., Chern, C. J., and Diamond, L. (1977): Formation of benzo(a)pyrene–glucuronic acid conjugates in hamster embryo cell cultures. *Cancer Res.*, 37:3190–3197.
16. Bedell, M. A., Lewis, J. G., Billings, K. C., and Swenberg, J. A. (1982): Cell specificity in hepatocarcinogenesis: preferential accumulation of O^6-methylguanine in target cell DNA during continuous exposure of rats to 1,2-dimethylhydrazine. *Cancer Res.*, 42:3079–3083.
17. Bend, J. R., Holder, G. M., and Ryan, A. J. (1971): Metabolism of propham (isopropyl *N*-phenylcarbamate) in the rat. *Food Cosmetic Toxicol.*, 9:169–177.
18. Bend, J. R., Smith, B. R., Ball, L. M., Plummer, J. L., Wolf, C. R., Philpot, R. M., Devereux, T. R., and Fouts, J. R. (1982): Metabolism of benzo(a)pyrene and benzo(a)pyrene 4,5-oxide in rabbit lung. In: *Biological Reactive Intermediates II. Chemical Mechanisms and Biological Effects*, edited by R. Snyder, D. V. Parke, J. J. Kocsis, D. J. Jollow, C. G. Gibson, and C. C. Witmer, pp. 541–554. Plenum Press, New York.
19. Bickers, D. R., and Kappas, A. (1980): The skin as a site of chemical metabolism. In: *Extrahepatic Metabolism of Drugs and other Foreign Compounds*, edited by T. E. Gram, pp. 295–318. S. P. Medical and Scientific Books, New York.
20. Bickers, D. R., Marcelo, C. L., Dutta-Choudhury, T., and Mukhtar, H. (1982): Studies on microsomal cytochrome P-450, monooxygenases and epoxide hydrolase in cultured keratinocytes and intact epidermis from BALB/C mice. *J. Pharmacol. Exp. Ther.*, 223:163–168.
21. Bock, K. W., and Winne, D. (1975): Glucuronidation of 1-naphthol in the rat intestinal loop. *Biochem. Pharmacol.*, 24:859–862.
22. Boyd, M. R. (1977): Evidence for the Clara cell as a site of cytochrome P-450-dependent mixed-function oxidase activity in lung. *Nature*, 269:713–714.
23. Boyd, M. R. (1980): Effects of inducers and inhibitors on drug-metabolizing enzymes and on drug toxicity in extrahepatic tissues. *Ciba Found. Symp.*, 76:43–66.
24. Boyd, M. R. (1980): Biochemical mechanisms in chemical-induced lung injury: role of metabolic activation. *CRC Crit. Rev. Toxicol.*, 7:103–176.
25. Boyd, M. R. (1980): Biochemical mechanisms in pulmonary toxicity of furan derivatives. *Rev. Biochem. Toxicol.*, 2:71–102.
26. Boyd, M. R., and Burka, L. T. (1978): *In vivo* studies on the relationship between target organ alkylation and the pulmonary toxicity of a chemically reactive metabolite of 4-ipomeanol. *J. Pharmacol. Exp. Ther.*, 207:687–697.
27. Boyd, M. R., Burka, I. T., and Wilson, B. J. (1975): Distribution, excretion, and binding of radioactivity in the rat after intraperitoneal administration of the lung-toxic furan, 4-ipomeanol-^{14}C. *Toxicol. Appl. Pharmacol.*, 32:147–157.
28. Boyd, M. R., Statham, C. N., and Longo, N. S. (1980): The pulmonary Clara cell as a target for toxic chemicals requiring metabolic activation: studies with carbon tetrachloride. *J. Pharmacol. Exp. Ther.*, 212:109–114.
29. Breyer, U., and Winne, D. (1977): Absorption and metabolism of the phenothiazine drug perazine in the rat intestinal loop. *Biochem. Pharmacol.*, 26:1275–1280.
30. Burke, M. D., and Orrenius, S. (1979): Isolation and comparison of endoplasmic reticulum membranes and their mixed-function oxidase activities from mammalian extrahepatic tissues. *Pharmacol. Ther.*, 7:549–599.
31. Chasseaud, L. F. (1980): Extrahepatic conjugation with glutathione. In: *Extrahepatic Metabolism of Drugs and Other Foreign Compounds*, edited by T. E. Gram, pp. 427–452. S. P. Medical and Scientific Books, New York.
32. Chen, W. J., Chi, E. Y., and Smuckler, E. (1977): Carbon tetrachloride-induced changes in mixed-function oxidase and microsomal cytochromes in rat lung. *Lab. Invest.*, 36:388–394.
33. Chiang, J. Y. L., DiLella, A. G., and Steggles, A. W. (1982): Effect of inducers and aging on rabbit liver microsomal drug-metabolizing enzymes. *Mol. Pharmacol.*, 23:244–251.
34. Chuang, A. H. L., and Bresnick, E. (1976): Aryl hydrocarbon hydroxylase in mouse mammary gland. *Cancer Res.*, 36:4125–4129.
35. Ciaccio, E. I., and DeVera, H. (1976): Effect of benzo(a)pyrene and chlorpromazine on aryl hydrocarbon hydroxylase activity from rat tissues. *Biochem. Pharmacol.*, 25:985–987.
36. Cohen, G. M., Marchok, A. C., Nettesheim, P., Steele, V. E., Nelson, F., Huang, S., and Selkirk, J. K. (1979): Comparative metabolism of benzo(a)pyrene in organ and cell cultures derived from rat tracheas. *Cancer Res.*, 39:1980–1984.
37. Colby, H. D., and Rumbaugh, R. C. (1980): Adrenal drug metabolism. In: *Extrahepatic Metabolism of Drugs and Other Foreign Compounds*, edited by T. E. Gram, pp. 239–266. S. P. Medical and Scientific Books, New York.
38. Coomes, M. W., Norling, A. H., Pohl, R. J., Muller, D., and Fouts, J. R. (1983): Foreign compound metabolism by isolated skin cells from the hairless mouse. *J. Pharmacol. Exp. Ther.*, 225:770–777.
39. Coomes, M. W., Sparks, R. W., and Fouts, J. R. (1983): Oxidation of 7-ethoxycoumarin and conjugation of umbelliferone by intact, viable epidermal cells from the hairless mouse. (*submitted for publication*).
40. Dahl, A. R., Hadley, W. M., Hahn, F. F., Benson, J. M., and McCleellan, R. O. (1982): Cytochrome P-450-dependent monooxygenases in olfactory epithelium of dogs: possible role in tumorigenicity. *Science*, 216:57–59.
41. Davidson, D. G. D., and Eastham, W. M. (1966):

Acute liver necrosis following overdose of paracetamol. *Br. Med. J.*, 2:497–499.
41a. Dawson, J. R., and Bridges, J. W. (1979): Xenobiotic metabolism by isolated intestinal epithelial cells from guinea pigs. *Biochem. Pharmacol.*, 28:3299–3305.
42. Dees, J. H., Coe, L. D., Yasukochi, Y., and Masters, B. S. (1980): Immunofluorescence of NADPH–cytochrome *c* (P-450) reductase in rat and minipig tissues injected with phenobarbital. *Science*, 208:1473–1475.
43. Dees, J. H., Masters, B. S. S., Muller-Eberhard, U., and Johnson, E. F. (1982): Effect of 2,3,7,8-tetrachlorodibenzo-*p*-dioxin and phenobarbital on the occurrence and distribution of four cytochrome P-450 isozymes in rabbit kidney, lung and liver. *Cancer Res.*, 42:1423–1432.
44. Devereux, T. R., and Fouts, J. R. (1980): Isolation and identification of Clara cells from rabbit lung. *In Vitro*, 16:958–968.
45. Devereux, T. R., and Fouts, J. R. (1981): Xenobiotic metabolism in alveolar type II cells isolated from rabbit lung. *Biochem. Pharmacol.*, 30:1231–1237.
46. Devereux, T. R., and Fouts, J. R. (1981): Isolation of pulmonary cells and use in studies of xenobiotic metabolism. In: *Methods in Enzymology, Vol. 77*, edited by W. B. Jakoby, pp. 147–154. Academic Press, New York.
47. Devereux, T. R., Hook, G. E. R., and Fouts, J. R. (1979): Foreign compound metabolism by isolated cells from rabbit lung. *Drug. Metab. Disp.*, 7:70–75.
48. Devereux, T. R., Jones, K. G., Bend, J. R., Fouts, J. R., Boyd, M. R., and Statham, C. N. (1982): *In vitro* metabolic activation of the pulmonary toxin, 4-ipomeanol, in nonciliated bronchiolar epithelial (Clara) and alveolar type II cells isolated from rabbit lung. *J. Pharmacol. Exp. Ther.*, 220:223–227.
49. Devereux, T. R., Serabjit-Singh, C. J., Slaughter, S. R., Wolf, C. R., Philpot, R. M., and Fouts, J. R. (1981): Identification of cytochrome P-450 isozymes in nonciliated bronchiolar epithelial (Clara) and alveolar type II cells isolated from rabbit lung. *Exp. Lung Res.*, 2:221–230.
50. Diamond, G. L., Anders, M. W., Tremaine, L. M., and Quebbemann, A. J. (1982): Salicylate enhancement of renal glucuronide conjugation and tubular excretory transfer of phenols. *Drug Metab. Dispos.*, 10:573–578.
51. Diamond, G. L., and Quebbemann, A. J. (1981): *In vivo* quantification of renal sulfate and glucuronide conjugation in the kidney. *Drug Metab. Dispos.*, 9:402–409.
52. Diaz Gomez, M. I., Swann, P. F., and Magee, P. N. (1977): The absorption and metabolism in rats of small oral doses of dimethylnitrosamine. *Biochem. J.*, 164:497–500.
53. Dieter, H. H., and Johnson, E. F. (1982): Functional and structural polymorphism of rabbit microsomal cytochrome P-450 form 3b. *J. Biol. Chem.*, 257:9315–9323.
54. DiGiovanni, J., Miller, D. R., Singer, J. M., Viaje, A., and Slaga, T. J. (1982): Benzo(a)pyrene metabolism in primary cultures of mouse epidermal cells and untransformed and transformed epidermal cell lines. *Cancer Res.*, 42:2579–2586.
55. DiGiovanni, J., Sina, J. F., Ashurst, S. W., Singer, J. M., and Diamond, L. (1983): Benzo(a)pyrene and 7,12-dimethylbenz(a)anthracene metabolism and DNA adduct formation in primary cultures of hamster epidermal cells. *Cancer Res.*, 43:163–170.
56. Domin, B. A., Serabjit-Singh, C. J., and Philpot, R. M. (1983): A modified peroxidase-immunostaining procedure for rapid quantitation of cytochrome P-450, form 2, in microsomal preparations bound directly to nitrocellulose. *Fed. Proc.*, 42:806.
57. Duffel, M. W., Graham, J. M., and Ziegler, D. M. (1980): Changes in dimethylaniline *N*-oxidase activity of mouse liver and kidney induced by steroid sex hormones. *Mol. Pharmacol.*, 19:134–139.
58. Duggan, D. E., Hooke, K. F., Risley, E. A., Shen, T. Y., and Van Arman, C. G. (1977): Identification of the biologically active form of sulindac. *J. Pharmacol. Exp. Ther.*, 201:8–13.
59. Dutcher, J. S., and Boyd, M. (1979): Species and strain differences in target organ alkylation and toxicity by 4-ipomeanol. Predictive value of covalent binding in studies of target organ toxicities by reactive metabolites. *Biochem. Pharmacol.*, 28:3367–3372.
60. Eastman, A., Mossman, B. T., and Bresnick, E. (1981): Formation and removal of benzo(a)pyrene adducts of DNA in hamster tracheal epithelial cells. *Cancer Res.*, 41:2605–2610.
61. Emslie, K. R., Smail, K. C., Calder, I. C., Hart, S. J., and Tange, T. D. (1981): Paracetamol and the isolated perfused kidney: metabolism and functional effects. *Xenobiotica*, 11:43–50.
62. Fouts, J. R., and Devereux, T. R. (1972): Development aspects of hepatic and extrahepatic drug-metabolizing enzyme systems: microsomal enzymes and components in rabbit liver and lung during the first month of life. *J. Pharmacol. Exp. Ther.*, 183:458–468.
63. Franklin, R. B., and Vodicnik, M. J. (1981): Sex steroids and extrahepatic mixed-function oxidase activity. *J. Steroid Biochem.*, 14:367–375.
64. Fry, J. R. (1981): Preparation of mammalian hepatocytes. In: *Methods in Enzymology, Vol. 77*, edited by W. B. Jakoby, pp. 130–137. Academic Press, New York.
65. Fry, J. R., and Bridges, J. W. (1979): Use of primary hepatocyte cultures in biochemical toxicology. *Rev. Biochem. Toxicol.*, 1:201–247.
66. Fry, J. R., and Perry, N. K. (1981): The effect of Aroclor 1254 pretreatment on the phase I and phase II metabolism of 7-ethoxycoumarin in isolated viable rat kidney cells. *Biochem. Pharmacol.*, 30:1197–1201.
67. Fry, J. R., Wiebkin, P., Kao, J., Jones, C. A., Gwynn, J., and Bridges, J. W. (1978): A comparison of drug-metabolizing capability in isolated viable rat hepatocytes and renal tubule fragments. *Xenobiotica*, 8:113–120.
68. Gelboin, H. V., Wiebel, F., and Diamond, L. (1970): Dimethylbenzanthracene tumorigenesis and aryl hydrocarbon hydroxylase in mouse skin: in-

hibition by 7,8-benzoflavone. *Science,* 170:169–171.
69. Goldman, P. (1982): Role of the intestinal microflora. In: *Metabolic Basis of Detoxication: Metabolism of Functional Groups,* edited by W. B. Jakoby, J. R. Bend, and J. Caldwell, pp. 323–337. Academic Press, New York.
70. Goldman, W. E., and Baseman, J. B. (1980): Selective initiation and culture of a proliferating epithelial cell population from the hamster trachea. *In Vitro,* 16:313–319.
71. Goto, T., and Wiebel, F. J. (1980): Aryl hydrocarbon (benzo[a]pyrene) monooxygenase activity in human primary amnion cell cultures. *Eur. J. Cancer,* 16:751–761.
72. Gram, T. E. (1980): The metabolism of xenobiotics by mammalian lung. In: *Extrahepatic Metabolism of Drugs and Other Foreign Compounds,* edited by T. E. Gram, pp. 159–209. S. P. Medical and Scientific Books, New York.
73. Greiner, J. W., Malan-Shibley, L. B., and Janss, D. H. (1979): Characteristics of aryl hydrocarbon hydroxylase activity in rat mammary epithelial cells grown in primary culture. *Chem. Biol. Interact.,* 27:323–334.
74. Guengerich, F. P., Wang, P., and Davidson, N. K. (1982): Estimation of isozymes of microsomal cytochrome P-450 in rats, rabbits, and humans using immunochemical staining coupled with sodium dodecyl sulfate–polyacrylamide gel electrophoresis. *Biochemistry.,* 21:1698–1706.
75. Guenthner, T. M., Nebert, D. W., and Menard, R. H. (1979): Microsomal aryl hydrocarbon hydroxylase in rat adrenal: regulation by ACTH but not by polycyclic hydrocarbons. *Mol. Pharmacol.,* 15:719–728.
76. Habliston, D. L., Whitaker, C., Hart, M. A., Ryan, U. S., and Ryan, J. W. (1979): Isolation and culture of endothelial cells from the lungs of small animals. *Am. Rev. Respir. Dis.,* 179:853–868.
77. Hall, P. F., Irby, D. C., and DeKrester, D. M. (1969): Conversion of cholesterol to androgens by rat testes: comparison of interstitial cells and seminiferous tubules. *Endocrinology,* 84:488–496.
78. Harris, C. C., Autrup, H., Stoner, G. D., McDowell, E. M., Trump, B. F., and Schafer, P. (1977): Metabolism of dimethylnitrosamine and 1,2-dimethylhydrazine in cultured human bronchi. *Cancer Res.,* 37:2309–2311.
79. Harris, C. C., Autrup, H., Stoner, G. D., Trump, B. F., Hillman, E., Schafer, P. W., and Jeffrey, A. M. (1979): Metabolism of benzo(a)pyrene, *N*-nitrosodimethylamine, and *N*-nitrosopyrrolidine and identification of the major carcinogen–DNA adducts formed in cultured human esophagus. *Cancer Res.,* 39:4401–4406.
80. Harris, C. C., Autrup, H., Stoner, G., Yang, S. K., Leutz, J. C., Gelboin, H. V., Selkirk, J. K., Connor, R. J., Barrett, L. A., Jones, R. T., McDowell, E. M., and Trump, B. F. (1977): Metabolism of benzo[a]pyrene and 7,12-dimethylbenz[a]-anthracene in cultured human bronchus and pancreatic duct. *Cancer Res.,* 37:3349–3355.
81. Heinrichs, W. L., and Juchau, M. R. (1980): Extrahepatic metabolism: the gonads. In: *Extrahepatic Metabolism of Drugs and Other Foreign Compounds,* edited by T. E. Gram, pp. 319–332. S. P. Medical and Scientific Books, New York.
82. Hinson, J. A. (1980): Biochemical toxicology of acetaminophen. *Rev. Biochem. Toxicol.,* 2:103–129.
83. Hinson, J. A., Monks, T. J., Hong, M., Highet, R. J., and Pohl, L. R. (1982): 3-(Glutathione-S-yl)acetaminophen: a biliary metabolite of acetaminophen. *Drug Metab. Dispos.,* 10:47–50.
84. Hollinger, M. A. (1982): Biochemical evidence for pulmonary endothelial cell injury after carbon tetrachloride administration in mice. *J. Pharmacol. Exp. Ther.,* 222:641–644.
85. Hook, G. E. R., Bend, J. R., and Fouts, J. R. (1972): Mixed-function oxidases and the alveolar macrophage. *Biochem. Pharmacol.,* 21:3267–3277.
86. Hook, G. E. R., Bend, J. R., Hoel, D., Fouts, J. R., and Gram, T. E. (1972): Preparation of lung microsomes and a comparison of the distribution of enzymes between subcellular fractions of rabbit lung and liver. *J. Pharmacol. Exp. Ther.,* 182:474–490.
87. Hook, J. B., McCormack, K. M., and Kluwe, W. B. (1979): Biochemical mechanisms of nephrotoxicity. *Rev. Biochem. Toxicol.,* 1:53–78.
88. Hucker, H. B., Stauffer, S. C., White, S. D., Rhodes, R. E., Arison, B. H., Umbenhauer, E. R., Bower, R. J., and McMahon, R. G. (1973): Physiologic disposition and metabolic fate of a new antiinflammatory agent, *cis*-5-fluoro-2-methyl-1-[*p*-(methylsulfinyl)-benzylidenyl]-indene-3-acetic acid in the rat, dog, rhesus monkey, and man. *Drug Metab. Dispos.,* 1:721–726.
89. Ioannou, Y. M., Wilson, A. G. E., and Anderson, M. W. (1982): Effect of butylated hydroxyanisole, α-angelica lactone, and β-naphthoflavone on benzo(α)pyrene: DNA adduct formation *in vivo* in the forestomach, lung, and liver of mice. *Cancer Res.,* 42:1199–1204.
90. Ioannou, Y. M., Wilson, A. G. E., and Anderson, M. W. (1982): Effect of butylated hydroxyanisole on the metabolism of benzo[α]pyrene and the binding of metabolites to DNA, *in vitro* and *in vivo,* in the forestomach, lung, and liver of mice. *Carcinogenesis,* 3:739–745.
91. Iqbal, Z. M., Varnes, M. E., Yoshida, A., and Epstein, S. S. (1977): Metabolism of benzo(a)pyrene by guinea pig pancreatic microsomes. *Cancer Res.,* 37:1011–1015.
92. Irmscher, G., and Fusenig, N. E. (1980): Metabolism of 7,12-dimethylbenz(a)anthracene (DMBA) by mouse skin keratinocytes, fibroblasts, and carcinoma cells in culture. *Arch. Toxicol.,* 44:181–195.
93. Jakoby, W. B., and Habig, W. H. (1980): Glutathione transferases. In: *Enzymatic Basis of Detoxication, Vol. II,* edited by W. B. Jakoby, pp. 63–94. Academic Press, New York.
94. James, M. O., and Bend, J. R. (1978): A radiochemical assay for glycine *N*-acyltransferase activity: some properties of the enzyme in rat and rabbit. *Biochem. J.,* 172:285–291.
95. Jones, D. P., Moldéus, P., Stead, A. H., Ormstad, K., Jörnvall, H., and Orrenius, S. (1979): Metab-

olism of glutathione and a glutathione conjugate by isolated kidney cells. *J. Biol. Chem.*, 254:2787–2792.

96. Jones, D. P., Orrenius, S., and Jackobson, S. W. (1980): Cytochrome P-450-linked monooxygenase systems in the kidney. In: *Extrahepatic Metabolism of Drugs and Other Foreign Compounds*, edited by T. E. Gram, pp. 123–158. S. P. Medical and Scientific Books, New York.
97. Jones, D. P., Sundby, G.-B., Ormstad, K., and Orrenius, S. (1979): Use of isolated renal cells for study of drug metabolism. *Biochem. Pharmacol.*, 28:929–935.
98. Jones, K. G., Holland, J. F., Foureman, G. L., Bend, J. R., and Fouts, J. R. (1983): Induction of xenobiotic metabolism in Clara cells and alveolar type II cells isolated from rat lungs. *J. Pharmacol. Exp. Ther.*, 225:316–319.
99. Jones, K. G., Holland, J. F., and Fouts, J. R. (1982): Benzo(a)pyrene hydroxylase activity in enriched populations of Clara cells and alveolar type II cells from control and β-naphthoflavone-pretreated rats. *Cancer Res.*, 42:4658–4663.
100. Jostling, D., Winne, D., and Bock, K. W. (1976): Glucuronidation of paracetamol, morphine and 1-naphthol in the rat intestinal loop. *Biochem. Pharmacol.*, 25:613–616.
101. Juchau, M. R. (1972): Mechanisms of drug biotransformation reactions in the placenta. *Fed. Proc.*, 31:48–51.
102. Juchau, M. R. (1980): Extrahepatic drug metabolism in the placenta. In: *Extrahepatic Metabolism of Drugs and Other Foreign Compounds*, edited by T. E. Gram, pp. 211–238. S. P. Medical and Scientific Books, New York.
103. Juchau, M. R., Bond, J. A., and Benditt, E. P. (1976): Aryl 4-monooxygenase and cytochrome P-450 in the aorta: possible role in atherosclerosis. *Proc. Natl. Acad. Sci. U.S.A.*, 73:3723–3725.
104. Julliard, J. H., Shibasaki, T., Ling, N., and Guillemin, R. (1980): High-molecular-weight immunoreactive β-endorphin in extracts of human placenta is a fragment of immunoglobulin G. *Science*, 208:183–185.
105. Kahng, M. W., Liu, W., Sanefuji, H., Resau, J. H., Heatfield, B. M., and Trump, B. F. (1981): Aryl hydrocarbon hydroxylase in human prostate. *Chem. Biol. Interact.*, 34:249–256.
106. Kaubisch, N., Daly, J. W., and Jerina, D. M. (1972): Arene oxides as intermediates in the oxidative metabolism of aromatic compounds. Isomerization of methyl-substituted arene oxides. *Biochemistry*, 11:3080–3088.
106a. Kikkawa, Y., and Yoneda, K. (1974): The type II epithelial cell of the lung. I. Method of Isolation. *Lab. Invest.*, 30:76–84.
107. Kimmich, G. A. (1975): Preparation and characterization of isolated intestinal epithelial cells and their use in studying intestinal transport. *Methods Membr. Biol.*, 4:51–111.
108. Kluwe, W. M., and Hook, J. B. (1980): Effects of environmental chemicals on kidney metabolism and function. *Kidney Int.*, 18:648–655.
109. Kupfer, D., Bruggeman, L. L., and Munsell, T. (1969): Studies on the occurrence of *N*-demethylase activity in adrenal and hepatic preparations from guinea pigs and rats. The effect of various substances on the magnitude of this activity. *Arch. Biochem. Biophys.*, 129:189–195.
110. Kuroki, T., Hosomi, J., Munakata, K., Onizuka, T., Terauchi, M., and Nemoto, N. (1982): Metabolism of benzo(a)pyrene in epidermal keratinocytes and dermal fibroblasts of humans and mice with reference to variation among species, individuals, and cell types. *Cancer Res.*, 42:1859–1865.
111. Kuroki, T., Nemoto, N., and Kitano, Y. (1980): Metabolism of benzo[a]pyrene in human epidermal keratinocytes in culture. *Carcinogenesis*, 1:559–565.
112. Laemmli, U. K. (1970): Cleavage of structural proteins during the assembly of the head of bacteriophage T_4. *Nature*, 227:680–685.
113. Langenbach, R., Nesnow, S., Tompa, A., Gingell, R., and Kuszynski, C. (1981): Lung and liver cell-mediated mutagenesis systems: specificities in the activation of chemical carcinogens. *Carcinogenesis*, 2:851–858.
114. Lee, I. P., Mukhtar, H., Suzuki, K., and Bend, J. R. (1983): Metabolism of benzo(a)pyrene 4,5-oxide by the isolated perfused rat testis. *Biochem. Pharmacol.*, 32:159–163.
115. Lee, I. P., and Nagayama, J. (1980): Metabolism of benzo(a)pyrene by the isolated perfused rat testis. *Cancer Res.*, 40:3297–3303.
116. Lee, I. P., Suzuki, K., Mukhtar, H., and Bend, J. R. (1980): Hormonal regulation of cytochrome P-450-dependent monooxygenase activity and epoxide-metabolizing enzyme activities in testis of hypophysectomized rats. *Cancer Res.*, 40:2486–2492.
117. Levin, A. A., and Dent, J. G. (1982): Comparison of the metabolism of nitrobenzene by hepatic microsomes and cecal microflora from Fischer-344 rats *in vitro* and the relative importance of each *in vivo*. *Drug Metab. Dispos.*, 10:450–454.
118. Lewis, J. G., and Swenberg, J. A. (1980): Differential repair of O^6-methylguanine in DNA of rat hepatocytes and nonparenchymal cells. *Nature*, 288:185–187.
119. Liem, H. H., Muller-Eberhard, U., and Johnson, E. F. (1980): Differential induction by 2,3,7,8-tetrachlorodibenzo-*p*-dioxin of multiple forms of rabbit microsomal cytochrome P-450: evidence for tissue specificity. *Mol. Pharmacol.*, 18:565–570.
120. MacNicoll, A. D., Grover, P. L., and Sims, P. (1980): The metabolism of a series of polycyclic hydrocarbons by mouse skin maintained in short-term organ culture. *Chem. Biol. Interact.*, 29:169–188.
121. Mass, M. J., and Kaufmann, D. G. (1978): $[^3H]$-Benzo(a)pyrene metabolism in tracheal epithelial cell microsomes and tracheal organ cultures. *Cancer Res.*, 38:3861–3866.
122. Mass, M. J., Rodgers, N. T., and Kaufman, D. G. (1981): Benzo(a)pyrene metabolism in organ cultures of human endometrium. *Chem. Biol. Interact.*, 33:195–205.
123. Mattison, D. R., and Thorgeirsson, S. S. (1977):

Genetic differences in mouse ovarian metabolism of benzo(a)pyrene and oocyte toxicity. *Biochem. Pharmacol.,* 26:909–912.
124. McMurtry, R. J., Snodgrass, W. R., and Mitchell, J. R. (1978): Renal necrosis, glutathione depletion, and covalent binding after acetaminophen. *Toxicol. Appl. Pharmacol.,* 46:87–100.
125. Meister, A., and Tate, S. S. (1976): Glutathione and related γ-glutamyl compounds: biosynthesis and utilization. *Annu. Rev. Biochem.,* 45:559–604.
126. Menard, R. H., Stripp, B., and Gillette, J. R. (1974): Spironolactone and testicular cytochrome P-450: decreased testosterone formation in several species and changes in hepatic drug metabolism. *Endocrinology,* 94:1628–1636.
127. Mitani, F., Veno, R., Iizuka, T., Ishimura, Y., Kimura, T., Izumi, S., Komatsu, N., and Watanabe, K. (1982): Cytochrome P-450_{sec} and P-$450_{11\beta}$ in bovine adrenal cortex: localization and flash photolysis of CO-bound forms of cytochrome P-450 in both isolated and membrane-bound forms. In: *Microsomes, Drug Oxidations and Drug Toxicity,* edited by R. Sato and R. Kato, pp. 257–264. Wiley-Interscience, New York.
128. Moldéus, P., Andersson, B., Rahimtula, A., and Berggren, M. (1982): Prostaglandin synthetase catalyzed activation of paracetamol. *Biochem. Pharmacol.,* 31:1363–1368.
129. Moldéus, P., Högberg, J., and Orrenius, S. (1978): Isolation and use of liver cells. In: *Methods in Enzymology, Vol. 52,* edited by S. Fleischer and L. Packer, pp. 60–71. Academic Press, New York.
130. Moldéus, P., Jernström, B., and Dawson, J. (1983): The use of freshly isolated or cultured hepatocytes in studies of the metabolism of polycyclic hydrocarbons and other carcinogens. *Rev. Biochem. Toxicol.,* 5:239–265.
130a. Moldéus, P., Ormstad, K., and Reed, D. J. (1981): Turnover of cellular glutathione in isolated rat-kidney cells. Role of cystine and methionine. *Eur. J. Biochem.,* 116:13–16.
131. Montelius, J., Papadopoulos, D., Bengtsson, M., and Rydstrom, J. (1982): Metabolism of polycyclic aromatic hydrocarbons and covalent binding of metabolites to protein in rat adrenal gland. *Cancer Res.,* 42:1479–1486.
132. Montesano, R., and Bartsch, H. (1976): Mutagenic and carcinogenic *N*-nitroso compounds: possible environmental hazards. *Muta. Res.,* 32:179–228.
133. Moore, B. P., Hicks, R. M., Knowles, M. A., and Redgrave, S. (1982): Metabolism and binding of benzo(a)pyrene and 2-acetylaminofluorene by short-term organ cultures of human and rat bladder. *Cancer Res.,* 42:642–648.
134. Mudge, G. H., Gemborys, M. W., and Duggin, G. G. (1978): Covalent binding of metabolites of acetaminophen to kidney protein and depletion of renal glutathione. *J. Pharmacol. Exp. Ther.,* 206:218–226.
135. Mukhtar, H., Lee, I. P., and Bend, J. R. (1978): Glutathione *S*-transferase activities in rat and mouse sperm and human semen. *Biochem. Biophys. Res. Commun.,* 83:1093–1098.
136. Mukhtar, H., Lee, I. P., Foureman, G. L., and Bend, J. R. (1978): Epoxide metabolizing enzyme activities in rat testes: postnatal development and relative activity in interstitial and spermatogenic cell compartments. *Chem. Biol. Interact.,* 22:153–165.
137. Nebelin, E., Autrup, H., Christensen, B., and Blomkvist, B. (1982): Detection of metabolites of *N*-nitrosopyrrolidine and *N*-nitrosomethylethylamine in cultures of human bladder epithelial cells of normal origin. In: *Environmental N-Nitrosocompounds,* edited by H. Bartsch, pp. 473–482. International Agency for Research on Cancer, Lyon, France.
138. Nebert, D. W., Eisen, H. J., Negishi, M., Lang, M. A., Hjelmeland, L. M., and Okey, A. (1981): Genetic mechanisms controlling the induction of polysubstrate monooxygenase (P-450) activities. *Annu. Rev. Pharmacol. Toxicol.,* 21:431–462.
139. Newton, J. F., Braselton, W. E., Kuo, C.-H., Kluwe, W. M., Gemborys, M. W., Mudge, G. H., and Hook, J. B. (1982): Metabolism of acetaminophen by the isolated perfused rat kidney. *J. Pharmacol. Exp. Ther.,* 221:76–79.
140. Newton, J. F., and Hook, J. B. (1981): Isolated perfused rat kidney. In: *Methods in Enzymology, Vol. 77,* edited by W. B. Jakoby, pp. 94–105. Academic Press, New York.
141. Newton, J. F., Kuo, C.-H., Gemborys, M. W., Mudge, G. H., and Hook, J. B. (1982): Nephrotoxicity of *p*-aminophenol, a metabolite of acetaminophen, in the Fischer-344 rat. *Toxicol. Appl. Pharmacol.,* 65:336–344.
142. Oesch, F., Glatt, H. R., and Schmassman, H. (1977): The apparent ubiquity of epoxide hydratase in rat organs. *Biochem. Pharmacol.,* 26:603–607.
143. Oppelt, W. W., Zange, M., Ross, W. E., and Remmer, H. (1970): Comparison of microsomal drug hydroxylation in lung and liver of various species. *Res. Commun. Chem. Pathol. Pharmacol.,* 1:43–56.
144. Ormstad, K., Lastbom, T., and Orrenius, S. (1982): Evidence for different localization of glutathione oxidase and γ-glutamyltransferase activities during extracellular glutathione metabolism in isolated perfused rat kidney. *Biochim. Biophys. Acta,* 700:148–153.
145. Ormstad, K., and Orrenius, S. (1980): The localization of renal glutathione oxidase activity studied in the isolated, perfused rat kidney. *Biochem. Biophys. Res. Commun.,* 92:540–545.
146. Ormstad, K., Orrenius, S., and Jones, D. P. (1981): Preparation and characteristics of isolated kidney cells. In: *Methods in Enzymology, Vol. 77,* edited by W. B. Jakoby, pp. 137–146. Academic Press, New York.
147. Orrenius, S. A., Ellin, A., Jakobsson, S. V., Thor, H., Cinti, D. L., Schenkman, J. B., and Estabrook, R. W. (1973): The cytochrome P-450-containing monooxygenase system of rat kidney cortex microsomes. *Drug Metab. Dispos.,* 1:350–357.
148. Parkinson, E. K., and Newbold, R. F. (1980): Benzo[a]pyrene metabolism and DNA adduct formation in serial cultivated strains of human epidermal keratinocytes. *Int. J. Cancer,* 26:289–299.

149. Patel, J. M., Harper, C., and Drew, R. T. (1978): The biotransformation of *p*-xylene to a toxic aldehyde. *Drug Metab. Dispos.,* 6:368–374.
150. Patel, J. M., Wolf, C. R., and Philpot, R. M. (1979): Interaction of 4-methylbenzaldehyde with rabbit pulmonary cytochrome P-450 in the intact animal, microsomes, and purified systems. *Biochem. Pharmacol.,* 28:2031–2036.
151. Pegg, A. E. (1980): Formation and subsequent repair of alkylation lesions in tissues of rodents treated with nitrosamines. *Arch. Toxicol.* [*Suppl.*], 3:55–68.
152. Pegg, A. E. (1980): Metabolism of dimethylnitrosamine. In: *Molecular and Cellular Aspects of Carcinogen Screening Tests,* edited by R. Montesano, H. Bartsch, and L. Tomatis, pp. 3–22. International Agency for Cancer Research, Lyon.
153. Pegg, A. E. (1983): Alkylation and subsequent repair of DNA after exposure to dimethylnitrosamine and related carcinogens. *Rev. Biochem. Toxicol.,* 5:83–133.
154. Pegg, A. E., and Perry, W. (1981): Alkylation of nucleic acids and metabolism of small doses of dimethylnitrosamine in the rat. *Cancer Res.,* 41:3128–3132.
155. Philpot, R. M., Anderson, M. W., and Eling, T. E. (1977): Uptake, accumulation, and metabolism of chemicals in the lung. In: *Metabolic Functions of the Lung,* edited by Y. S. Bakhle and J. R. Vane, pp. 123–172. Marcel Dekker, New York.
156. Philpot, R. M., Robertson, I. G. C., and Serabjit-Singh, C. J. (1983): Increases in cytochrome P-450, form 5, and the metabolism of aromatic amines to mutagenic products following treatment of rabbits with phenobarbital. *Fed. Proc.,* 42:1324.
157. Philpot, R. M., and Wolf, C. R. (1981): The properties and distribution of the enzymes of pulmonary cytochrome P-450-dependent monooxygenase systems. *Rev. Biochem. Toxicol.,* 3:51–76.
158. Piciano, P. E., and Rosenbaum, R. M. (1978): The type I alveolar lining cells of the mammalian lung. *Am. J. Pathol.,* 90:99–122.
159. Pinkus, L. M. (1981): Separation and use of enterocytes. In: *Methods in Enzymology, Vol. 77,* edited by W. B. Jakoby, pp. 154–162. Academic Press, New York.
160. Plopper, C. G., Alley, J. L., Serabjit-Singh, C. J., and Philpot, R. M. (1983): Cytodifferentiation of the nonciliated bronchiolar epithelial (Clara) cell during rabbit lung maturation. Ultrastructural morphology. *Am. J. Anat.,* 167:329–357.
161. Plopper, C. G., Mariassy, A. T., and Hill, L. H. (1980): Ultrastructure of the nonciliated bronchiolar epithelial (Clara) cell of mammalian lung. *Exp. Lung Res.,* 1:139–180.
162. Pohl, R. J., Coomes, M. W., Sparks, R. W., and Fouts, J. R. (1983): 7-Ethoxycoumarin O-deethylation activity in viable basal and differentiated keratinocytes isolated from the skin of the hairless mouse (*submitted for publication*).
163. Ratnayake, J. H., Hanna, P. E., Anders, M. W., and Duggan, D. E. (1981): Sulfoxide reduction. *In vitro* reduction of sulindac by rat hepatic cytosolic enzymes. *Drug Metab. Dispos.,* 9:85–87.
164. Remel, R. P., Pohl, L. R., and Elmer, G. W. (1981): Influence of the intestinal microflora on the elimination of warfarin in the rat. *Drug Metab. Dispos.,* 9:410–414.
165. Richards, J., and Nandi, S. (1978): Primary culture of rat mammary epithelial cells. II. Cytotoxic effect and metabolism of 7,12-dimethylbenz[a]anthracene and *N*-nitroso-*N*-methylurea. *J. Natl. Cancer Inst.,* 61:772–777.
166. Robertson, I. G. C., Philpot, R. M., Zeiger, E., and Wolf, C. R. (1981): Specificity of rabbit pulmonary cytochrome P-450 isozymes in the activation of several aromatic amines and aflatoxin B_1. *Mol. Pharmacol.,* 20:662–668.
167. Ross, B., Tange, J., Emslie, K., Hart, S., Smail, M., and Calder, I. (1980): Paracetamol metabolism by the isolated perfused kidney. *Kidney Int.,* 18:562–570.
168. Roth, J. A. (1979): Use of the isolated perfused lung in biochemical toxicology. *Rev. Biochem. Toxicol.,* 1:287–309.
169. Rouet, P., Alexandrov, K., Markovits, P., Frayssinet, C., and Dansette, P. M. (1981): Metabolism of benzo(a)pyrene by brain microsomes of fetal and adult rats and mice. Induction by 5,6-benzoflavone, comparison with liver and lung activities. *Carcinogenesis,* 2:919–926.
170. Scarpelli, D. G., Kokkinakis, D. M., Rao, M. S., Subbarao, V., Luetteke, N., and Hollenberg, P. F. (1982): Metabolism of the pancreatic carcinogen *N*-nitroso-2,6-dimethylmorpholine by hamster liver and component cells of pancreas. *Cancer Res.,* 42:5089–5095.
171. Scarpelli, D. G., Rao, M. S., Subbarao, V., Beversluis, M., Gurka, D. P., and Hollenberg, P. F. (1980): Activation of nitrosamines to mutagens by postmitochondrial fraction of hamster pancreas. *Cancer Res.,* 40:67–74.
172. Scheline, R. R. (1980): Drug metabolism by the gastrointestinal microflora. In: *Extrahepatic Metabolism of Drugs and Other Foreign Compounds,* edited by T. E. Gram, pp. 551–580. S. P. Medical and Scientific Books, New York.
173. Schiller, C. M., and Lucier, G. W. (1978): The differential response of isolated intestinal crypt and tip cells to the inductive effects of 2,3,7,8-tetrachlorodibenzo-*p*-dioxin. *Chem. Biol. Interact.,* 22:199–209.
174. Serabjit-Singh, C. J., and Philpot, R. M. (1983): Modulation of the rabbit hepatic cytochrome P-450 isozyme, form 2, by Aroclor 1260. *Fed. Proc.,* 42:806.
175. Serabjit-Singh, C. J., Wolf, C. R., and Philpot, R. M. (1979): The rabbit pulmonary monooxygenase system: immunochemical and biochemical characterization of enzyme components. *J. Biol. Chem.,* 254:9901–9907.
176. Serabjit-Singh, C. J., Wolf, C. R., Philpot, R. M., and Plopper, C. G. (1980): Cytochrome P-450: localization in rabbit lung. *Science,* 207:1469–1470.
177. Shichi, H., Atlas, S. A., and Nebert, D. W. (1975):

Genetically regulated aryl hydrocarbon hydroxylase induction in the eye. Possible significance of the drug-metabolizing enzyme system for the retinal pigmented epithelial-choroid. *Exp. Eye Res.*, 21:557–567.
178. Shichi, H., and Nebert, D. W. (1980): Drug metabolism in ocular tissues. In: *Extrahepatic Metabolism of Drugs and Other Foreign Compounds*, edited by T. E. Gram, pp. 333–363. S. P. Medical and Scientific Books, New York.
179. Shirkey, R. J., Kao, J., Fry, J. R., and Bridges, J. W. (1979): A comparison of xenobiotic metabolism in cells isolated from rat liver and small intestinal mucosa. *Biochem. Pharmacol.*, 28:1461–1466.
180. Sirica, A. E., and Pitot, H. C. (1980): Drug metabolism and effects of carcinogens in cultured hepatic cells. *Pharmacol. Rev.*, 31:205–228.
181. Smith, B. R., and Bend, J. R. (1979): Metabolism and excretion of benzo(a)pyrene 4,5-oxide by the isolated perfused rat liver. *Cancer Res.*, 39:2051–2056.
182. Smith, B. R., and Bend, J. R. (1980): Prediction of pulmonary benzo(a)pyrene 4,5-oxide extraction ratio from kinetic parameters of epoxide metabolizing enzymes. *J. Pharmacol. Exp. Ther.*, 214:478–482.
183. Smith, B. R., and Bend, J. R. (1981): Metabolic interactions of hydrocarbons with mammalian lung. *Rev. Biochem. Toxicol.*, 3:77–122.
184. Smith, B. R., and Bend, J. R. (1981): Lung perfusion techniques for xenobiotic metabolism and toxicity studies. In: *Methods in Enzymology, Vol. 77*, edited by W. B. Jakoby, pp. 105–120. Academic Press, New York.
185. Smith, B. R., Plummer, J. L., Ball, L. M., and Bend, J. R. (1980): Characterization of pulmonary arene oxide biotransformation using the perfused rabbit lung. *Cancer Res.*, 40:101–106.
186. Smith, B. R., Plummer, J. L., Wolf, C. R., Philpot, R. M., and Bend, J. R. (1982): *p*-Xylene metabolism by rabbit lung and liver and its relationship to the selective destruction of pulmonary cytochrome P-450. *J. Pharmacol. Exp. Ther.*, 223:736–742.
187. Stampfer, M. R., Bartholomew, J. C., Smith, H. S., and Bartley, J. C. (1981): Metabolism of benzo[a]pyrene by human mammary epithelial cells: toxicity and DNA adduct formation. *Proc. Natl. Acad. Sci. U.S.A.*, 78:6251–6255.
188. Steele, V. E., Marchok, A. C., and Nettesheim, P. (1979): Oncogenic transformation in epithelial cell lines derived from tracheal explants exposed *in vitro* to *N*-methyl-*N*′-nitro-*N*-nitrosoguanidine. *Cancer Res.*, 39:3805–3811.
189. Steele, J. W., Yagen, B., Hernandez, O., Cox, R. H., Smith, B. R., and Bend, J. R. (1981): The metabolism and excretion of styrene oxide–glutathione conjugates in the rat and by isolated perfused liver, lung and kidney preparations. *J. Pharmacol. Exp. Ther.*, 219:35–41.
190. Sternberger, L. A. (1979): In: *Immunocytochemistry*, pp. 122–129. John Wiley & Sons, New York.
191. Stohs, S. J., Grafström, R. C., Burke, M. D., and Orrenius, S. (1977): Benzo(α)pyrene metabolism by isolated rat intestinal epithelial cells. *Arch. Biochem. Biophys.*, 179:71–80.
192. Strobel, H. W., Fang, W. F., and Oshinsky, R. J. (1980): Role of colonic cytochrome P-450 in large bowel carcinogenesis. *Cancer*, 45:1060–1065.
193. Tompa, A., and Langenbach, R. (1979): Culture of adult rat lung cells: benzo(a)pyrene metabolism and mutagenesis. *In Vitro*, 15:569–578.
194. Towbin, H., Staehalin, T., and Gordon, J. (1979): Electrophoretic transfer of proteins from acrylamide gels to nitrocellulose sheets: procedure and some applications. *Proc. Natl. Acad. Sci. U.S.A.*, 76:4350–4354.
195. Ueng, T.-H., and Alvares, A. P. (1981): Selective loss of pulmonary cytochrome P-450_I in rabbits pretreated with polychlorinated biphenyls. *J. Biol. Chem.*, 256:7536–7542.
196. Ueng, T.-H., and Alvares, A. P. (1982): Pulmonary cytochromes P-450 from rabbits treated with 3-methylcholanthrene. *Mol. Pharmacol.*, 22:221–228.
197. VanDemark, N. L., and Ewing, L. L. (1963): Factors affecting testicular metabolism and function. I. A simplified perfusion technique for short term maintenance of rabbit testis. *J. Reprod. Fertil.*, 6:1–8.
198. Walz, F. G., Vlasuk, G. P., Omiecinski, C. J., Bresnick, E., Thomas, P. E., Ryan, D. E., and Levin, W. (1982): Multiple, immunochemical forms of phenobarbital-induced rat liver cytochromes P-450 are encoded by different mRNAs. *J. Biol. Chem.*, 257:4023–4026.
199. Warren, B. L., Domin, B. A., and Philpot, R. M. (1983): Changes in the hepatic and pulmonary concentrations of cytochrome P-450 isozymes and rate of *O*-deethylation of 7-ethoxyresorufin following treatment of rabbit with benzo(a)pyrene. *Fed. Proc.*, 42:546.
200. Wattenberg, L. W. (1972): Inhibition of carcinogenic and toxic effects of polycyclic hydrocarbons by phenolic antioxidants and ethoxyquin. *J. Natl. Cancer Inst.*, 48:1425–1430.
201. Wattenberg, L. W., and Leong, J. L. (1971): Tissue distribution studies of polycyclic hydrocarbon hydroxylase activity. In: *Handbook of Experimental Pharmacology, Vol. 27*, edited by B. B. Brodie and J. R. Gillette, pp. 422–430. Springer-Verlag, Berlin.
202. Wattenberg, L. W., Leong, J. L., and Strand, P. J. (1962): Benzpyrene hydroxylase activity in the gastrointestinal tract. *Cancer Res.*, 22:1120–1125.
203. Weber, W. W., Radtke, H. E., and Tannen, R. H. (1980): Extrahepatic *N*-acetyltransferases and *N*-deacetylases. In: *Extrahepatic Metabolism of Drugs and Other Foreign Compounds*, edited by T. E. Gram, pp. 493–531. S. P. Medical and Scientific Books, New York.
204. Weston, A., Grover, P. L., and Sims, P. (1982): Metabolism and activation of benzo[a]pyrene by mouse and rat skin in short-term organ culture and *in vivo*. *Chem. Biol. Interact.*, 42:233–250.

205. Windmueller, H. G., and Spaeth, A. E. (1975): Intestinal metabolism of glutamine and glutamate from the lumen as compared to glutamine from blood. *Arch. Biochem. Biophys.*, 171:662–672.

206. Windmueller, H. G., and Spaeth, A. E. (1980): Respiratory fuels and nitrogen metabolism *in vivo* in small intestine of fed rats: quantitative importance of glutamine, glutamate, and aspartate. *J. Biol. Chem.*, 255:107–112.

207. Windmueller, H. G., and Spaeth, A. E. (1981): Vascular autoperfusion of rat small intestine *in situ*. In: *Methods in Enzymology, Vol. 77,* edited by W. B. Jakoby, pp. 120–129. Academic Press, New York.

208. Wolf, C. R., Statham, C. N., McMenamin, M. G., Bend, J. R., Boyd, M. R., and Philpot, R. M. (1982): The relationship between the catalytic activities of pulmonary cytochrome P-450 isozymes and the lung specific toxicity of the furan derivative, 4-ipomeanol. *Mol. Pharmacol.*, 22:738–744.

209. Wollenberg, P., and Ullrich, V. (1980): The drug monooxygenase system in the small intestine. In: *Extrahepatic Metabolism of Drugs and Other Foreign Compounds,* edited by T. E. Gram, pp. 267–276. S. P. Medical and Scientific Books, New York.

210. Zenser, T. V., Mattamal, M. B., Brown, W. W., and Davis, B. B. (1979): Cooxygenation by prostaglandin cyclooxygenase from rabbit inner medulla. *Kidney Int.*, 16:688–694.

Drug Metabolism and Drug Toxicity, edited by J. R. Mitchell and M. G. Horning. Raven Press, New York © 1984.

Environmental and Genetic Factors Influencing Drug Metabolism and Toxicity

Daniel W. Nebert and Masahiko Negishi

Laboratory of Developmental Pharmacology, National Institute of Child Health and Human Development, National Institutes of Health, Bethesda, Maryland 20205

The study of the genetic control of drug metabolism is often called pharmacogenetics. Simply, a pharmacogeneticist attempts to understand the hereditary reasons why two individuals (with the possible exception of monozygotic twins) respond differently to drugs or other foreign chemicals. These responses include therapeutic effects of a drug, e.g., anticoagulation or control of seizures, and also unwanted deleterious effects such as cancer or drug toxicity. The experimental system to be examined in detail in this chapter represents, principally, a genetic difference in receptor concentration; because of this defect, there are large genetic differences in the biotransformation and pharmacokinetics of certain drugs and other environmental pollutants, resulting in important differences in risk toward cancer, drug toxicity, mutation, and birth defects.

In this chapter, the general characteristics of the P-450-mediated monooxygenases and their coordinated enzymes are first described. Secondly, the genetic differences in a particular model system in mice, the *Ah* locus, are examined. Methods for determining phenotypic expression and linkage are described. Numerous other conditions in mice associated with this genetic system are also listed. Current evidence for this genetic difference in man is briefly assessed. Finally, the use of recombinant DNA technology is suggested as a new technique to study pharmacogenetics in the near future.

P-450-MEDIATED MONOOXYGENASES AND COORDINATED ENZYMES

Many environmental pollutants and other foreign compounds are chemicals that are so hydrophobic they would remain in the body indefinitely were it not for metabolism resulting in more polar derivatives. These drug-metabolizing enzyme systems, which are localized principally in the liver, are usually divided into two groups: phase I and phase II. During phase I metabolism, one or more polar groups (such as hydroxyl) are introduced into the hydrophobic parent molecule, thus creating a handle, or position, for the phase II conjugating enzymes (such as UDP-glucuronosyltransferase) to attack. The conjugated products are sufficiently polar that these detoxified chemicals are now excreted from the cell and from the body (95).

One of the most interesting of the phase I enzyme systems is a group of enzymes known collectively as the cytochrome P-450-mediated monooxygenases. These membrane-bound enzyme systems are known to metabolize polycyclic aromatic hydrocarbons such as benzo(a)pyrene (ubiquitous in city smog, cigarette smoke, and charcoal-cooked foods) and biphenyl; halogenated hydrocarbons such as polychlorinated and polybrominated biphenyls, insecticides, and ingredients in soaps and deodorants; strong mutagens such as *N*-methyl-*N'*-nitro-*N*-nitrosoguanidine and nitrosamines; aminoazo dyes and diazo compounds; *N*-acetylarylamines and nitrofurans; numerous aromatic amines, such as those found in hair dyes; nitro aromatics and heterocyclics; wood terpenes; epoxides; carbamates; alkyl halides; safrole derivatives; certain fungal toxins and antibiotics; many of the chemotherapeutic agents used to treat human cancer; most drugs; small chemicals such as benzene, thiocyanate, or ethanol; both endogenous and synthetic steroids; and other endogenous compounds such as biogenic amines, indoles, thyroxine, and fatty acids.

Evidence is growing that metabolism to reactive intermediates by the P-450-mediated monooxygenases is a prerequisite for mutagenesis, carcinogenesis, and toxicity by numerous drugs, polycyclic hydrocarbons, and other environmental pollutants. These reactive intermediates probably bind covalently to numerous cellular macromolecules. Most of this binding is probably random, but some may be nonrandom, i.e., specific binding dependent on the chemical structures of the reactive intermediate and the cellular macromolecule. Among these various types of covalent binding, there probably exists a very small amount of important binding of the ultimate carcinogen to its critical subcellular target, thereby initiating tumorigenesis. Two examples of apparent specific binding include the binding of benzo(a)pyrene 7,8-diol-9,10-epoxide to the ^{2}N-amino of guanine (94) and of aflatoxin B_1 2,3-oxide to the ^{7}N of guanine (15).

Although it is not yet clear what "signal" leading to carcinogenesis is evoked by the ultimate carcinogen metabolite, transmission of the signal clearly appears to involve DNA rather than RNA or protein (77). Transfection of DNA from certain chemically transformed cell lines into NIH 3T3 mouse cells can induce the appearance of transformation foci (76). NIH 3T3 cells that

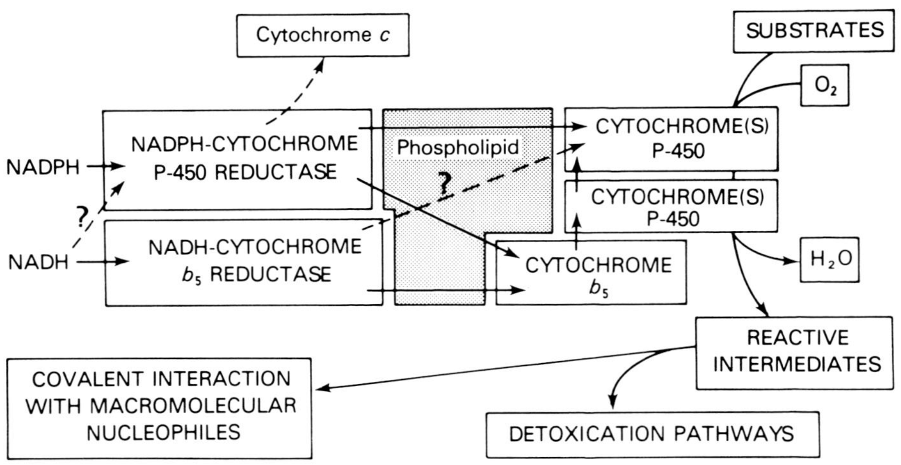

FIG. 1. Scheme for the membrane-bound multicomponent monooxygenase system(s) and the various possibly important pathways for hydrophobic substrates (53a). For any given substrate, the relative balance between toxification and detoxication likely would differ among different tissues, strains, and species. Age, genetic expression, nutrition, hormone concentration, diurnal rhythm, pH, saturating versus nonsaturating conditions of the substrate, K_m and V_{max} for each enzyme, subcellular compartmentalization of each enzyme, efficiency of DNA repair, and the immunological competence of the animal may all be important factors affecting this balance. (Reproduced with permission from Environmental Health Perspectives Press.)

have been transformed by transfected DNA from human, rabbit, and mouse tumors and tumor cell lines were shown in certain cases to be tumorigenic in mice and to contain human DNA sequences when the original transfected DNA had been human in origin (38,75).

The steady-state levels of these reactive electrophilic intermediates and, consequently, the rates at which they interact with the critical nucleophilic target are dependent on a delicate balance between their generation and detoxication (Fig. 1). Changes in the balance between toxification and detoxication in any particular tissue of an individual may therefore affect his risk of tumorigenesis or toxicity.

AHH ASSAY

The assay for AHH activity (Fig. 2) with the use of benzo(a)pyrene as the substrate and 3-hydroxybenzo(a)pyrene as the product formed has remained for years a reliable index of benzo(a)pyrene metabolism, although it was known long ago (79) that numerous oxygen-containing metabolites other than the 3-hydroxy derivative are formed. It was believed until recently that the formation of 3-hydroxybenzo(a)pyrene may occur by a direct hydroxylation. It has now been shown that 3-hydroxybenzo(a)pyrene arises from a very reactive 2,3-oxide (96). An additional point of interest is that an impure preparation of "recrystallized 3-hydroxybenzo(a)-pyrene" contains several different phenolic metabolites of benzo(a)pyrene, each of which is activated, and these fluoresce at similar wavelengths. In fact, the relatively major product 9-hydroxybenzo(a)pyrene is similar to 3-hydroxybenzo(a)pyrene in its degree of fluorescence at similar wavelengths of activation and emission (19).

Therefore, the well-known "AHH assay" probably takes into account the formation of several phenolic products (the 1-, 3-, 6-, 7-, and 9-hydroxy derivatives). Diols and quinones do not contribute significantly to fluorescence in this assay (reviewed in 19,61). If minor changes in benzo(a)pyrene metabolite profile are important in one's research, high-pressure liquid chromatographic techniques (26) are preferable. If very low levels of AHH activity are present (e.g., lympho-

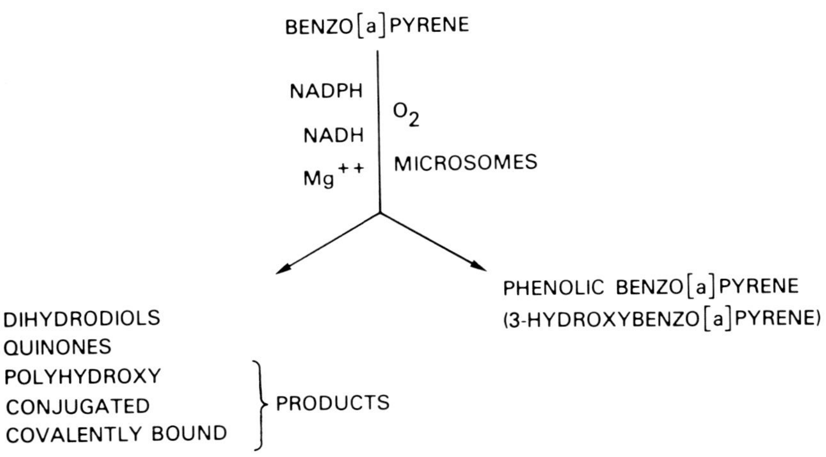

FIG. 2. Illustration of the aryl hydrocarbon [benzo(a)pyrene] hydroxylase (E.C. 1.14.14.1) (AHH) "activity" (57). The substrate benzo(a)pyrene is oxygenated to an arene oxide, which rearranges nonenzymatically to various phenols or is oxygenated by direct oxygen insertion to phenolic derivatives. The 3- and 9-phenols have the strongest fluorescence in alkali. Other oxygenated derivatives of benzo(a)pyrene, including dihydrodiols and quinones, are not measured by this assay. (From Nebert and Felton, ref. 57, with permission of *Federation Proceedings*.)

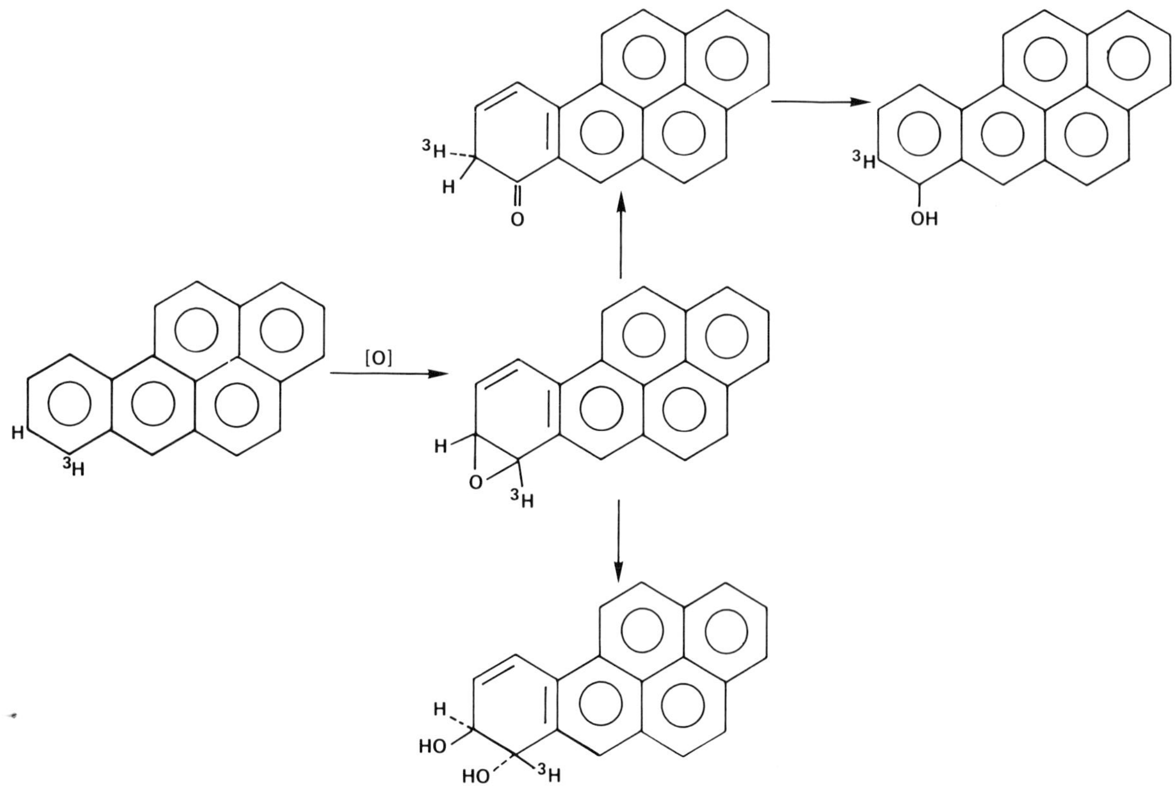

FIG. 3. Hypothetical example of tritiated benzo(a)pyrene, illustrating why the AHH assay using generally tritiated benzo(a)pyrene is less sensitive than the fluorescent AHH assay because of tritium retention. (From Nebert and Jensen, ref. 61, with permission of CRC Press.)

cytes in culture), the fluorometric microassay is preferable; this assay is described later in this chapter.

When we compared quantitatively the fluorescent AHH assay (58) with a more recently described radiometric assay (25), more "benzo(a)pyrene metabolized" was found in the former than in the latter. An apparent discrepancy exists. The "total" tritium exchange should include all quinone and other nonphenolic derivatives and therefore should theoretically reach a higher value than that found by a method in which only the phenolic products are measured. This apparent discrepancy can be explained by the fact that generally labeled [^{3}H]benzo(a)pyrene is used. As shown in Fig. 3, a benzo(a)pyrene molecule not having tritium on the two adjacent carbon positions involved in the epoxidative process will not be included in the assay (25) for "total" tritium exchange. When the oxygen becomes more strongly associated with carbon-7 than carbon-8 of benzo(a)pyrene, the tritium atom at position 7, by means of the "NIH shift" (11), will migrate to position 8. Because the carbon–tritium bond is thermodynamically stronger than the carbon–hydrogen bond, the hydrogen atom rather than the tritium atom will leave to become incorporated into water.

Thus, the only metabolites measured by the "total" tritium exchange assay are those benzo(a)pyrene molecules having tritium on the two adjacent carbons at which the oxygen attack occurs (or those phenols that are formed directly at a particular carbon–tritium bond by an oxygen "insertion" reaction, if this ever happens). In fact, the rate of tritium exchange, relative to that of phenolic product formation, could be used as an index for measuring the uniformity of tritium labeling for any radioactive preparation of [^{3}H]benzo(a)pyrene.

Preparation of Biological Samples

Our mice are usually permitted free access to food (Purina NIH Open Formula Rat and Mouse Ration 5018) and tap water. The animals are typically sacrificed between 8:00 and 10:00 a.m. by exsanguination. Livers are quickly removed, dissected free of the gallbladder and adhering tissues, and minced and rinsed several times in ice-cold 0.15 M KCl–0.25 M potassium phosphate buffer, pH 7.25. Nonhepatic tissues are treated similarly except that the pH of the buffer is 7.55. Each tissue of each species should, of course, be tested first for optimal pH of any monooxygenase activity. The tissues are typically homogenized in 10 volumes of the buffer with a Polytron® tissue homogenizer (Kinematica, Switzerland; distributed by Brinkmann) for 30 sec at setting no. 5 or with a motor-driven Potter–Elvehjem Teflon®–glass homogenizer. Liver homogenates are centrifuged at 15,000 *g* for 15 min; nonhepatic tissue homogenates are spun at 5,000 *g* for 10 min. The carefully decanted supernatant fraction is further centrifuged at 78,000 *g* for 90 min or 105,000 *g* for 60 min to obtain a pellet rich in microsomes. This pellet can be stored at −80° with negligible loss of AHH activity. Freezing at 0° to −10° in a "frost-free" refrigerator results in enough thawing and refreezing to slowly destroy AHH activity; the basal AHH activity is more easily destroyed than the polycyclic hydrocarbon-induced (i.e., P_1-450-associated) AHH activity, thereby causing artificially larger "induction ratios" (induced AHH:control AHH) than those seen when fresh tissues are assayed. The microsomal pellet is resuspended in 30% glycerol–0.25 M potassium phosphate buffer (pH 7.25 for liver, pH 7.55 for nonhepatic tissues) by gentle homogenization to give a final protein concentration of 8 to 12 mg/ml (determined by the method of Lowry with crystalline bovine serum albumin as the standard).

Enzyme Assay

The 1-ml reaction volume includes 50 μmole of potassium phosphate buffer (pH 7.25 for liver, usually pH 7.55 for nonhepatic tissues), 0.36 μmole of NADH, 0.010 to 0.10 ml of microsomal (or other tissue) homogenate, and 80 nmole of benzo(a)pyrene (in 40 μl of methanol). An NADPH-generating system can be substituted reasonably well for the NADPH and is less expensive. NADH is synergistic when used in combination with NADPH (59). The reaction is linear with 50 μg to 2.0 mg of protein. The mixture is shaken at 37° (for 10 min in the case of liver and 20 min or longer in the case of nonhepatic tissues), and the reaction is stopped with 4.25 ml of cold hexane–acetone (3.25:1.00). Ten more minutes of shaking at 37° insures the best extraction of benzo(a)pyrene and metabolites into the organic layer (3.33 ml by volume); covering the flasks prevents any evaporation. The assay at this point can be interrupted, even for several days, without appreciable change in products measured.

Aliquots (1 ml) of the organic phase are added to 3-ml volumes of 1.0 N NaOH, thereby extracting phenolic metabolites into the alkali phase. The phenolic benzo(a)pyrene metabolites are immediately determined spectrophotofluorometrically and equated with AHH activity. This determination can be accomplished by means of a recording spectrophotofluorometer with a slit width of 5 mm and with an activation wavelength of about 396 nm and emission wavelength of about 522 nm (58) or with an inexpensive fluorocolorimeter with a slit width of 1/32 inch and a Corning no. 7-51 filter and a no. W-58 filter. The limit of sensitivity of this macroassay is about 0.1 pmole of 3-hydroxybenzo(a)pyrene detected per minute per milligram of protein. The limit of sensitivity can easily be enhanced 10-fold by the microassay.

AHH "Microassay"

For certain nonhepatic tissues (e.g., skin, lymph nodes) and cells in culture (e.g., some tumor-derived continuous lines, lymphocytes activated with mitogens, monocytes, etc.), maximal sensitivity is desirable. In the 1-ml reaction mixture, if protein content is less than 300 μg, 3 μmole of $MgCl_2$ and 600 μg of bovine serum albumin (to aid solubility of benzo(a)pyrene) are routinely included (59). The optimal pH for lymphocyte AHH activity is 8.5 (3), thereby necessitating the use of Tris chloride instead of potassium phosphate buffer. Of course, the pH optimum should be established for every new tissue and species to be studied.

Cultured lymphocytes are typically centrifuged, washed free of growth medium, and resuspended directly in 2.4 ml of the reaction mixture (3). The reaction is started at 37° by adding 80 nmole of benzo(a)pyrene (in 40 μl of methanol) to duplicate 0.96-ml aliquots of whole-cell suspension (containing 1 to 3 mg of cellular protein per milliliter). There is no need for homogenization or sonication of the cells. The reaction at 37° is terminated after 45 or 60 min by adding 4.25 ml of cold hexane–acetone (3.25:1.00), and phenolic metabolites from 3.0 ml of the organic phase are extracted for 1 min with 0.50 ml of 1.0 N NaOH. After centrifugation (100 rpm for 2 min), the alkali extract is transferred to a quartz microcuvette (0.7 ml capacity), and fluorescence is immediately determined in a spectrophotofluorometer at maximal sensitivity (396 nm activation; 522 nm emission). In control flasks, either the benzo(a)pyrene or the microsomal or cell protein is added after the termination of the 37° incubation with cold hexane–acetone, or the usual assay is performed in the presence of boiled microsomes or bovine serum albumin alone in order to determine background fluorescence.

Maximal AHH activity induced by 3-methylcholanthrene per unit of NADH–cytochrome *c* reductase activity appears to be the best assessment for human AHH phenotype in cultured mitogen-activated lymphocytes (36). The "inducibility ratio" to study human AHH phenotype is a more difficult assay with greater intraindividual variability (3).

A careful recrystallization of the substrate benzo(a)pyrene will result in a lower background fluorescence and therefore a more sensitive assay. Recrystallization is performed as follows. The crude benzo(a)pyrene is dissolved (0.5 g in 5 ml) in benzene. This solution is washed three times in a separatory funnel with 10 ml of 1.0 N NaOH and then with 10 ml of water three times. Methanol (6 ml) and water (20 ml) are added to the benzene, and the mixture is thoroughly shaken. The mixture is heated 60° to 70° for 10 min and then cooled on ice for 60 min. The formed crystals are filtered with a Büchner funnel and Whatman no. 1 filter paper. The crystals are washed once with methanol–water (1:3, vol/vol). The entire recrystallization procedure may be repeated a second time. The purified benzo(a)pyrene is now dissolved in a minimal volume of benzene, and the solution for use in the AHH assay is made 2.0 mM with methanol.

The rate of formation of 3-hydroxybenzo(a)pyrene and therefore the apparent K_m value are dependent on the microsomal protein concentration; i.e., AHH activity does not strictly follow Michaelis–Menten kinetics. Presumably this also is true for monooxygenase activities other than AHH activity if the substrate is very hydrophobic and its solubility is aided by protein in the reaction mixture. These data are consistent with those of "mutual depletion systems," in which the substrate is apparently reversibly bound to nonspecific enzyme sites on the microsomes. The velocity of the AHH reaction depends on the concentration of free benzo(a)pyrene. Therefore, either a high relative enzyme concentration or a low dissociation constant favors a mutual depletion in free concentrations (discussed in 58).

Benzo(a)pyrene (or other polycyclic hydrocarbon) metabolism in cell culture can also be assessed with the use of radioactive substrate and extraction of the growth medium with hexane–acetone or with 1% SDS followed by extraction with chloroform–methanol (2:1); these procedures detect metabolites in the "organic phase" and "water-soluble phase" (discussed further in 49). Again, recrystallization of the radioactive polycyclic hydrocarbon substrate will improve the sensitivity of the assay.

Standardization Curves

The standard curve is most accurately obtained by adding known amounts of purified 3-hydroxybenzo(a)pyrene to the reaction mixture cofactors and the cell or microsomal protein, after which the usual incubation and extraction procedures are performed. The resultant standard curve (Fig. 4A) indicates a lack of linearity at low 3-hydroxybenzo(a)pyrene concentrations. This lack of linearity is not inherent in the fluorometer itself, because the direct addition of 3-hydroxybenzo(a)pyrene to 1.0 N NaOH results in a linear calibration curve. Similar standard curves are obtained when no microsomes or cells are present in the reaction mixture or when the samples are not incubated (3). The nonlinearity is thus apparently a result of inefficient extraction at low 3-hydroxybenzo(a)pyrene concentrations. This lack of linearity becomes important principally in tissues or cultured cells in which AHH activity is low (<750 pmole of total 3-hydroxybenzo(a)pyrene formed).

Because of the difficulties in obtaining, using, and storing authentic 3-hydroxybenzo(a)pyrene as a standard, it is desirable to have on hand a readily available stable standard that can be used routinely to calibrate the instrument each day. Quinine sulfate, stable in water, fluoresces strongly in 0.1 N H_2SO_4 at the peak excitation and emission wavelengths of 3-hydroxybenzo(a)pyrene. Figure 4B shows the concentrations of quinine sulfate and 3-hydroxybenzo(a)pyrene at which fluorescence is the same.

Ah LOCUS: GENETIC EXPRESSION OF INDUCED AHH ACTIVITY AND CYTOCHROME P_1-450 INDUCTION

The *Ah* locus represents an experimental model system that has provided several good examples of a delicate balance between genetic and environmental factors in the etiol-

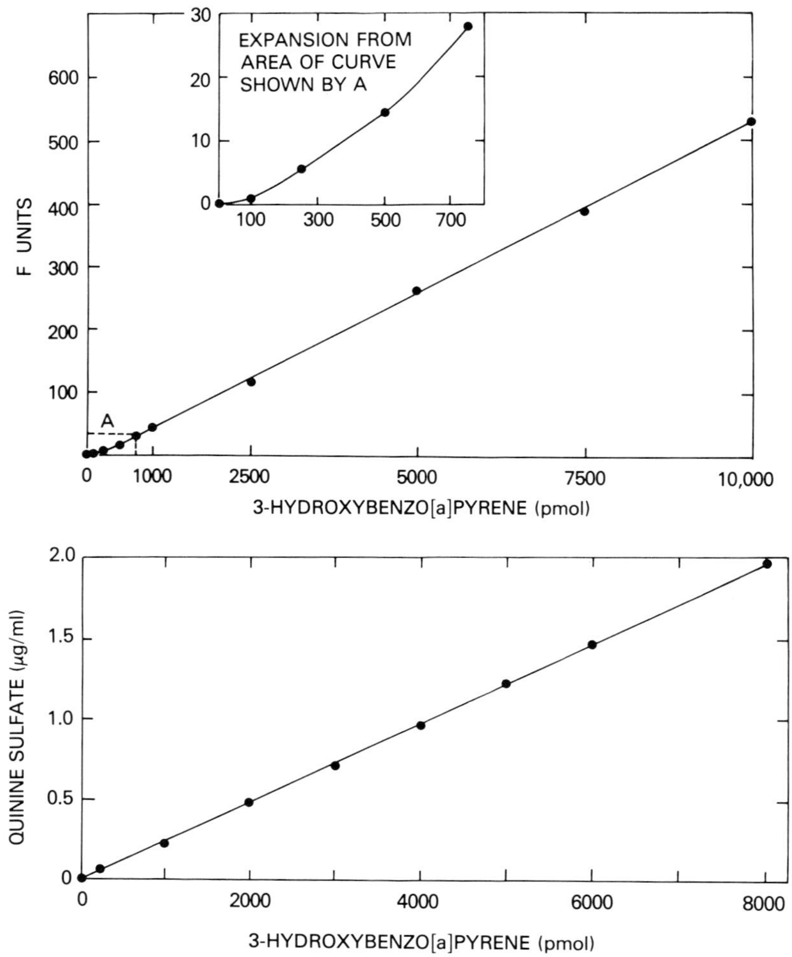

FIG. 4. A: Relative fluorescence as a function of 3-hydroxybenzo(a)pyrene concentrations added to the reaction mixture and incubated for the usual 10-min time period. **B:** Correlation of concentrations of quinine sulfate having the same relative fluorescence as solutions of 3-hydroxybenzo(a)pyrene. The fluorescence of quinine sulfate solutions is determined in 0.1 N H_2SO_4. (From Nebert, ref. 49, with permission of Academic Press.)

ogy of cancer, drug toxicity, and birth defects (61). The *Ah* gene of the mouse regulates the induction (by polycyclic aromatic compounds such as 3-methylcholanthrene, benzo(a)pyrene, or 2,3,7,8-tetrachlorodibenzo-*p*-dioxin) of numerous drug-metabolizing enzyme "activities" associated with several new induced forms of cytochrome P_1-450. At any given dose of inducer, the induction of AHH activity and at least two dozen other monooxygenase activities and associated forms of P_1-450 occurs in 3-methylcholanthrene-treated C57BL/6N and other genetically "responsive" inbred strains and is always much lower in 3-methylcholanthrene-treated DBA/2N and other genetically "nonresponsive" strains. In addition to the liver, this genetic expression is seen in such tissues as lung, kidney, intestine, lymph nodes, skin, bone marrow, pigmented epithelium of the retina, brain, mammary gland, uterus, ovary, and testis. The genetic re-

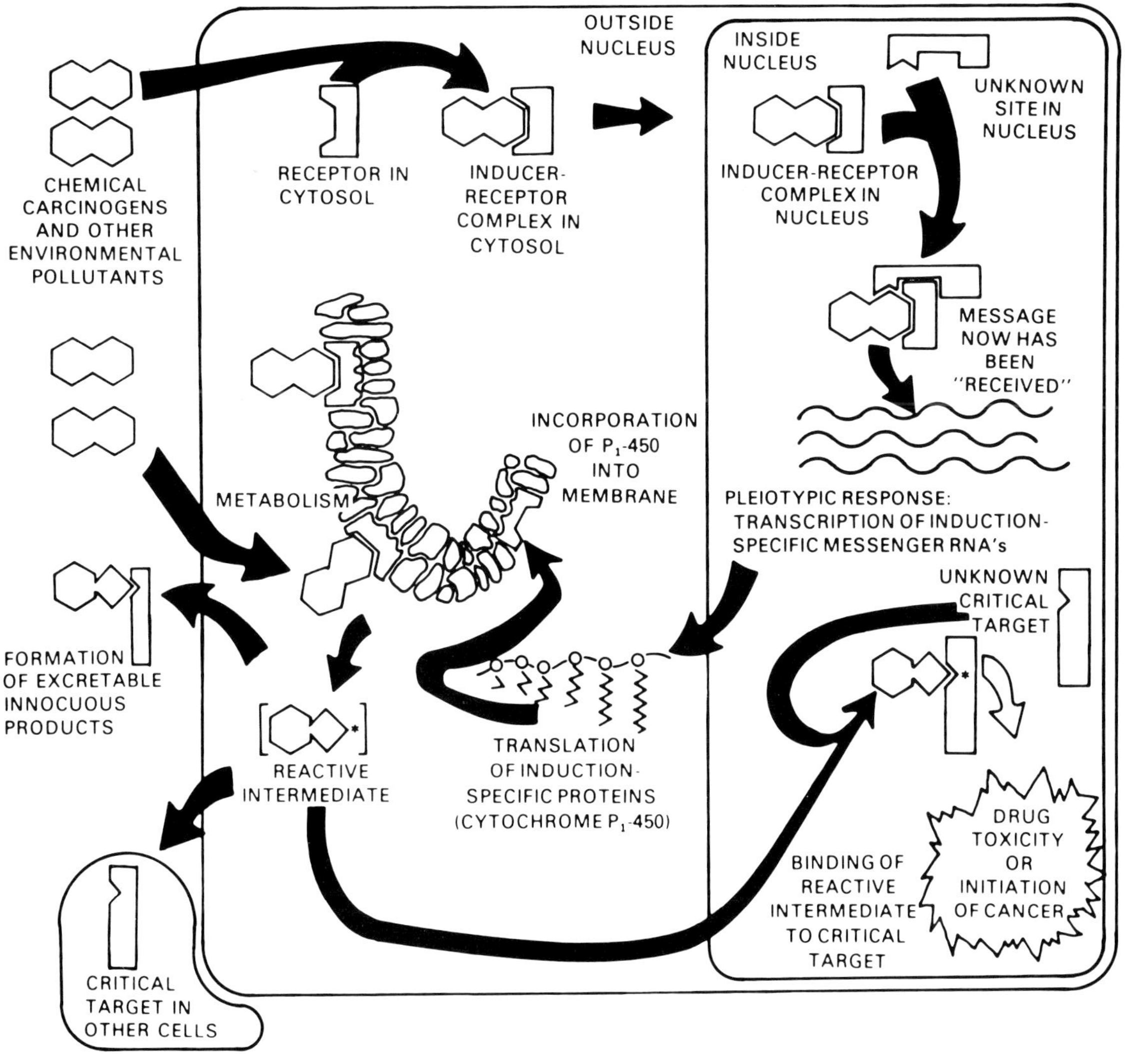

FIG. 5. Diagram of a cell and the hypothetical scheme by which a cytosolic receptor, product of the regulatory *Ah* gene, binds to inducer (51). Depending on the half-life of the reactive intermediate, the rate of formation of the intermediate, and the rate of conjugation and other means of detoxifying the intermediate, important covalent binding may occur in the same cell in which metabolism took place or in some distant cell. Although the "unknown critical target" is illustrated here in the nucleus, there is presently no experimental evidence demonstrating unequivocally the subcellular location of the "critical target(s)" required for the initiation of drug toxicity or cancer. (From Nebert, ref. 51, with permission.)

sponse is therefore called "systemic," or occurring throughout virtually all tissues of the animal. Responsiveness to aromatic hydrocarbons has been designated the *Ah* locus: Ah^b is the dominant allele; Ah^d is the recessive allele; the Ah^b/Ah^d heterozygote is phenotypically similar to the Ah^b/Ah^b mouse in terms of degree of responsiveness.

Several studies indicate that the fundamental genetic difference resides in the *Ah* cytosolic receptor (Fig. 5) which is capable of binding to inducers such as 3-methylcholanthrene, benzo(a)pyrene, and 2,3,7,8-tetrachlorodibenzo-*p*-dioxin. To our knowledge, only certain foreign chemicals bind to this receptor with saturability and high affinity (less than 1 nM). The C57BL/6N receptor appears to have at least 50 times better affinity toward inducers of P_1-450 than the Ah^d/Ah^d mouse (66). Translocation of the inducer–receptor complex into the nucleus has been demonstrated in the *Ah*-responsive heterozygote and homozygote (66) and requires a temperature-dependent step (67). Discrepancies between the dextran–charcoal adsorption assay and the sucrose density-gradient assay have recently been understood through chromatographic studies of the *Ah* receptor (24).

What happens in the nucleus is not yet known, but somehow the "information" (that these inducers of P_1-450 exist in the cell's microenvironment) is received; the response is transcription of specific mRNAs, translation of these mRNAs into specific enzymes such as P_1-450, and incorporation of P_1-450 into cellular membranes. These induced enzymes may aid in detoxication, or they may generate increased amounts of reactive intermediates.

TYPES OF GENETIC INHERITANCE SEEN AT THE *Ah* LOCUS

Induction of AHH activity and cytochrome P_1-450 by 3-methylcholanthrene is expressed almost exclusively as an autosomal dominant trait among offspring of the appropriate crosses between C57BL/6 and DBA/2 inbred strains of mice and as an additive trait among offspring of the appropriate crosses between the C3H/He and DBA/2 inbred strains (reviewed in 61). On the other hand, the lack of induction of AHH activity and P_1-450 by 3-methylcholanthrene is expressed as an autosomal dominant trait among offspring of the appropriate crosses between C57BL/6N and AKR/N parent strains.

The genetic interaction of AHH inducibility between C57BL/6 and DBA/2 may therefore be regarded as similar to the dominance of red over white garden pea blossoms (Fig. 6A), as described by Mendel more than 100 years ago. The expression of AHH inducibility between C3H/He and DBA/2 appears, on the other hand, to be similar to the additive inheritance found in crosses between red and white snapdragons (Fig. 6B); with this type of inheritance, the F_1 expresses the trait codominantly. If two or more genes are more or less equally involved, genetic inheritance would appear multifactorial, or polygenic, as is the case for the ear length in corn (Fig. 6C). It is perhaps surprising for us to have found the expression of aromatic hydrocarbon responsiveness so "simple" in crosses between C57BL/6 and DBA/2 mice given the apparent complexities of the P-450 monooxygenase system illustrated in Fig. 1.

A minimum of two loci and six alleles is needed so far to explain most of the genetic experiments (61). And, although the (C57BL/6)(DBA/2)F_1 heterozygote can in fact be distinguished (61) from the inbred dominant C57BL/6 parent, the autosomal dominant expression shown in Fig. 7 closely approximates our data. When a responsive C57BL/6 is crossed with a nonresponsive DBA/2 (upper left), the F_1 animal is essentially as responsive as the dominant C57BL/6. When the F_1 is back crossed with the C57BL/6 (upper right), all offspring are essentially as responsive as the C57BL/6 parent. When the F_1 is back crossed with the DBA/2 parent (lower right), one-half of the offspring are

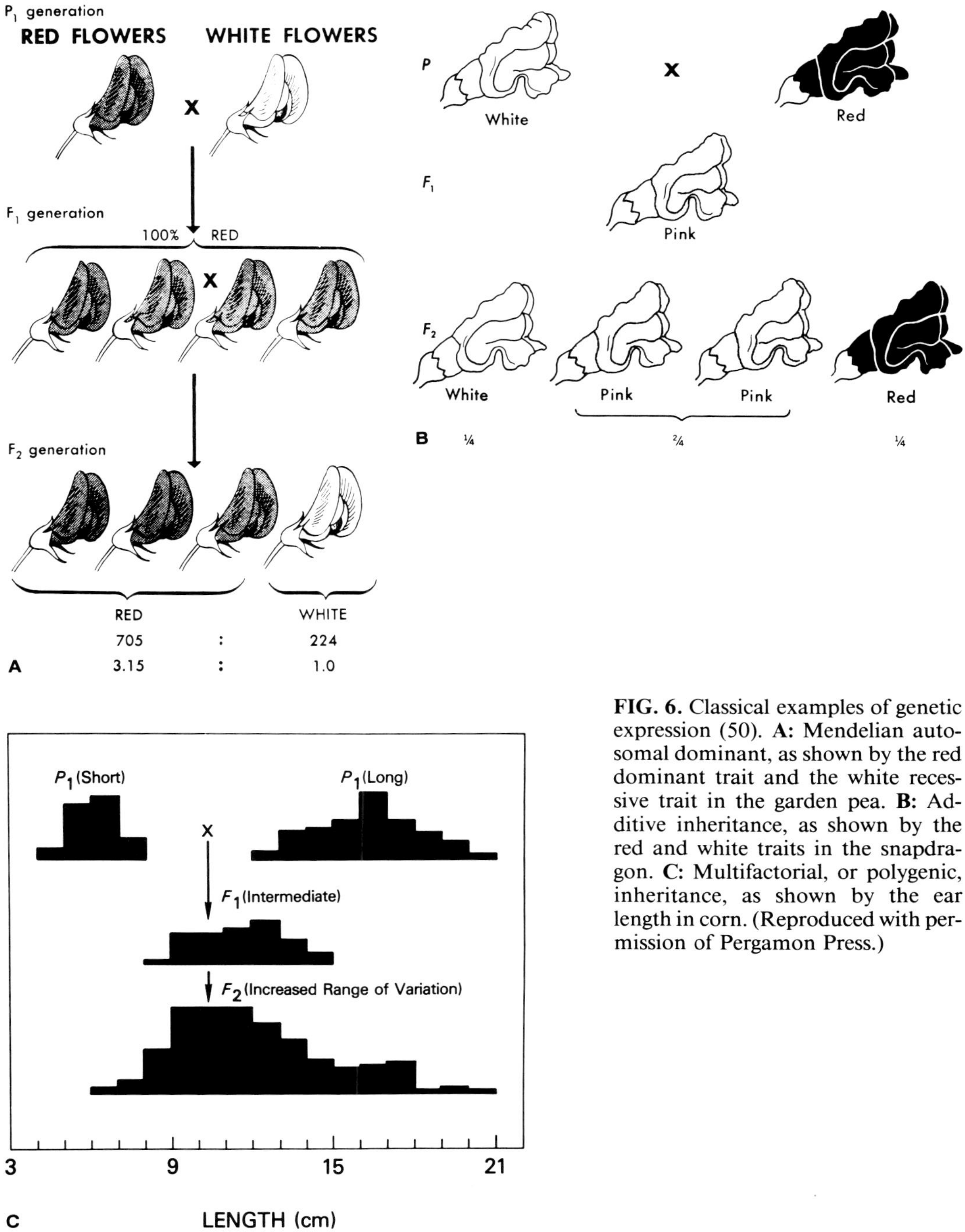

FIG. 6. Classical examples of genetic expression (50). **A:** Mendelian autosomal dominant, as shown by the red dominant trait and the white recessive trait in the garden pea. **B:** Additive inheritance, as shown by the red and white traits in the snapdragon. **C:** Multifactorial, or polygenic, inheritance, as shown by the ear length in corn. (Reproduced with permission of Pergamon Press.)

essentially as responsive as the C57BL/6 parent, and the other half are similar to the nonresponsive DBA/2 parent. When F_1 mice are intercrossed (lower left), three-fourths of the offspring are similar to the C57BL/6 parent, and one-fourth are similar to the DBA/2 par-

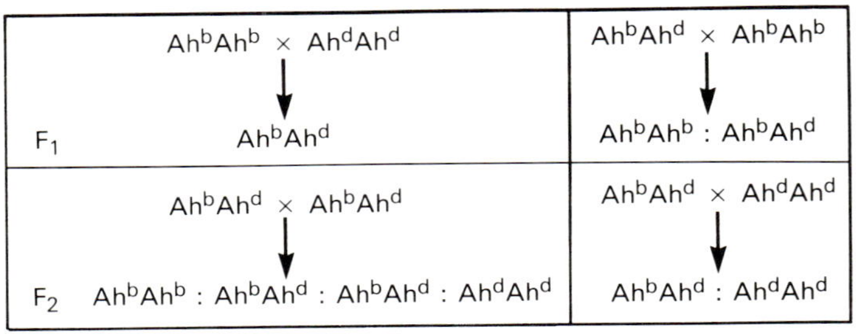

FIG. 7. Simplified genetic scheme for aromatic hydrocarbon "responsiveness" in the mouse (56). Ah^b/Ah^b are responsive (C57BL/6) mice; Ah^d/Ah^d are nonresponsive (DBA/2) mice. (From Nebert and Felton, ref. 56, with permission.)

ent. The offspring from the $F_1 \times$ DBA/2 back cross and the $F_1 \times F_1$ intercross are therefore valuable for use as a genetic probe in studies of chemical carcinogenesis, pharmacology, toxicology, and teratology, because specific events related to the phenotype of the *Ah* locus can be divorced from nonspecific pathophysiologic events (e.g., malnutrition, sedation, hormonal imbalance) associated with the test compound given during the experiment.

GENETIC EXPRESSION IN OTHER TISSUES BESIDES LIVER

The genetic regulation of an induced enzyme in one tissue need not be the same in other tissues. However, the induction of AHH, and several other monooxygenase activities as well, appears to have similar genetic expression in all tissues examined (61). There are difficulties in a very careful genetic analysis of this point, because most "control" responsive animals have, in fact, slightly induced AHH activity in many of their tissues, which can be lowered by changing the diet (41).

A responsive polycyclic hydrocarbon-treated mouse is subject to both quantitative and qualitative increases in the steady-state levels of certain reactive intermediates because of both an increase in cytochrome(s) P_1-450 content and an increased P_1-450/P-450 ratio in numerous tissues. The relative content of P_1-450, compared with other forms of P-450, may be especially large (e.g., ratios of 10:1 or 500:1) in tissues such as skin and lung but never reaches even a 1:1 ratio in liver. This relatively large change in the profile of cytochrome(s) P-450, compared with much smaller increments of change in epoxide hydrase, UDP-glucuronosyltransferase, and glutathione *S*-transferase activities with benzo(a)pyrene as substrate, might be a factor in explaining why polycyclic hydrocarbons cause tumors in skin and lung but rarely in liver (reviewed in 55).

WHAT IS AN "INBRED MOUSE?"

The Jackson Laboratory (Bar Harbor, Maine) sells dozens of inbred strains of mice that are readily available. Most of the standard inbred strains were developed between 1909 and 1924, and more than 240 strains have been well described (80). This expanding list does not include hundreds of fostered and otherwise manipulated lines (e.g., congenic and recombinant inbred sublines). The nomenclature may be confusing to a novice. DBA/2N, for example, is derived from the original DBA stock; the N denotes NIH. DBA/1J is also derived from the original DBA stock; the J denotes Jackson Laboratory. An "inbred strain" denotes 20 or more generations of exclusive brother–sister matings; after 20 generations of inbreeding, the probability of heterozygosity is less than 1% in the absence of mutation or of selection favoring heterozygotes.

For breeding mice, one male is typically placed with three to six females. This male:female ratio for mice thus may be considered similar to that found to be optimal for human populations. For pharmacologic or toxicologic studies, a constant day:night light cycle (14:10 hr) and absence of insecticides, cigarette smoke, and aromatic wood bedding are recommended. Five DBA/2N females crossed with one C57BL/6N male constitutes a DBA/2N × C57BL/6N cross, and the offspring are termed (DBA/2N)(C57BL/6N)F_1; i.e., the female progenitor is listed first. Five C57BL/6N females crossed with one DBA/2N male constitutes a C57BL/6N × DBA/2N cross, and the offspring are called (C57BL/6N)(DBA/2N)F_1. Early in any genetic study, it should be determined whether there exists any maternal factor—transmitted, for example, in the breast milk. In other words, is transmission of the genetic trait you are studying the same in (DBA/2N)(C57BL/6N)F_1 and (C57BL/6N)(DBA/2N)F_1 individuals? Pregnant females and newborn mice are generally safe within this "family unit" of three to six females and one male per cage, but this will vary from strain to strain. Particular individuals within a strain may be "fighters" or "fur eaters." Breeding frequencies and the size of the litter clearly vary with the time of the year, and there are inbred strain differences as well.

STRUCTURAL GENES ASSOCIATED WITH THE *Ah* LOCUS

Recent studies have shown (Table 1) that the induction of at least two dozen monooxygenase "activities" is closely associated with the Ah^b allele. Cytochrome P-450-mediated monooxygenases not associated with the *Ah* locus include the induction of aminopyrine *N*-demethylase, *d*-benzphetamine *N*-demethylase, diphenylhydantoin hydroxylase, hexobarbital hydroxylase, aniline hydroxylase, benzenesulfonanilide hydroxylase, chlorocyclizine *N*-demethylase, ethylmorphine *N*-demethylase, pentobarbital hydroxylase, aflatoxin B_1 2,3-oxide formation, and testosterone 7α-, 16α-, and 6β-hydroxylases. Also not associated with the *Ah* receptor is the induction of NADPH–cytochrome *c* reductase, NADPH–cytochrome P-450 reductase, epoxide hydrolase, and glutathione *S*-transferase (61).

TABLE 1. *All induced monooxygenase "activities" known to be associated with the* Ah^b *allele*[a]

Aryl hydrocarbon (benzo(a)pyrene) hydroxylase (AHH)
7-Ethoxycoumarin *O*-deethylase
p-Nitroanisole *O*-demethylase
Dimethylaminoazobenzene *N*-demethylase
Zoxazolamine 6-hydroxylase
Acetylarylamine (2-acetylaminofluorene) *N*-hydroxylase
Biphenyl 2-hydroxylase
Biphenyl 4-hydroxylase
Acetanilide 4-hydroxylase
Naphthalene monooxygenase
Acetaminophen *N*-hydroxylase
p-Chloroacetanilide *N*-hydroxylase
Phenacetin *O*-deethylase
Ethoxyresorufin *O*-deethylase
Aflatoxin B_1 4-hydroxylase (21)
Amaranth azoreductase (17)
β-Naphthoflavone metabolism to unidentified products[b]
α-Naphthoflavone metabolism to unidentified products[b]
Ellipticine metabolism to unidentified products[b]
Lindane metabolism to unidentified products[b]
Niridazole metabolism to unidentified products[b]
Caffeine metabolism to unidentified products[b]
Theophylline metabolism to unidentified products[b]
Theobromine metabolism to unidentified products[b]

[a] This list is taken from Nebert (50). All basal enzyme activities so far tested, with the exception of biphenyl 2-hydroxylase, are preferentially inhibited by metyrapone *in vitro,* indicating an association of these catalytic activities with one or more forms of control P-450 other than P_1-450. All polycyclic aromatic compound-induced enzyme activities so far tested, plus basal biphenyl 2-hydroxylase activity, are preferentially inhibited by α-naphthoflavone, indicating an association of these catalytic activities with cytochrome P_1-450 or P-448 (or other inducible form of P-450) (see 61 for further discussion).

[b] Unpublished data.

Reproduced with permission from Pergamon Press, Ltd.

Other inducible enzymes that are not monooxygenases but that appear to be associated with the Ah^b allele (and therefore probably require the cytosolic receptor protein) include microsomal UDP-glucuronosyltransferase, cytosolic reduced NAD(P): menadione oxidoreductase, and cytosolic ornithine decarboxylase (61). Also, an architectural difference in the microsomal electron transport system may exist between control untreated Ah^d/Ah^d mice and control untreated Ah^b/Ah^b or Ah^b/Ah^d mice (6). Just because an enzyme activity is much higher

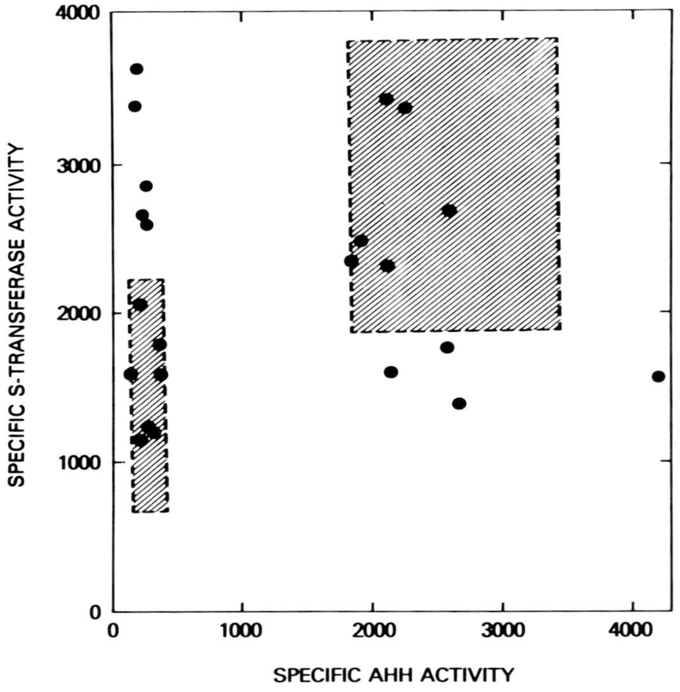

FIG. 8. Distribution of hepatic glutathione transferase and AHH activities among individual offspring from the (C57BL/6N)-(DBA/2N)F_1 × DBA/2N back cross (16). The substrate used in this experiment was 1-chloro-2,4-dinitrobenzene. *Each point* represents an individual mouse treated 6 days previously with a single dose of 3-methylcholanthrene. The *shaded regions* denote the means ± standard deviations for the transferase and AHH activities in eight C57BL/6N mice (**upper right**) and eight DBA/2N mice (**lower left**), each individually assayed for the two enzyme activities 6 days after a single dose of 3-methylcholanthrene. (Reproduced with permission of Academic Press.)

in 3-methylcholanthrene-treated C57BL/6 and (C57BL/6)(DBA/2)F_1 mice than in 3-methylcholanthrene-treated DBA/2 mice, one cannot conclude an association with the Ah^b allele until progeny from the DBA/2 × F_1 back cross are studied. An excellent example (16) is depicted in Fig. 8. The 10 offspring having 3-methylcholanthrene-inducible AHH activities of 1,900 or more are known (66) to have sufficient quantities of the *Ah* receptor, i.e., the *Ah* regulatory gene product. The 12 3-methylcholanthrene-treated offspring having AHH activities of 400 or less are known (66) to have undetectable cytosolic *Ah* receptor. Five of 12 *Ah*-nonresponsive back-cross individuals had transferase activities of greater than 2,500, and 4 of 10 *Ah*-responsive individuals had transferase activities of less than 1,800; these mice are regarded as "recombinants" (50). It can therefore be concluded that this 3-methylcholanthrene-induced glutathione transferase activity is not genetically linked to the *Ah* locus.

HOW TO DETERMINE THE Ah^b ALLELE PHENOTYPE

Among the inducible monooxygenase "activities" shown in Table 1 is zoxazolamine 6-hydroxylase. Hence, increased metabolism of the parent drug (which causes paralysis) will result in a shorter length of time during which the animal's muscles are paralyzed (Fig. 9). It has long been known that zoxazolamine paralysis is decreased in rats previously treated with polycyclic hydrocarbons. Such a noninvasive "paralysis time" test is a successful means for separating responsive (i.e., Ah^b/Ah^b and Ah^b/Ah^d) from nonresponsive (i.e., Ah^d/Ah^d) individuals. We routinely test in our laboratory on the same day 20 to 100 weanling mice from the (C57BL/6N)(DBA/2N)F_1 × DBA/2N back cross or the (C57BL/6N)(DBA/2N)F_1 × (C57BL/6N)(DBA/2N)F_1 intercross. First, the 3- to 4-week-old (weighing 10–14 g) weanlings are treated intraperitoneally with 200 mg of β-naphthoflavone per kilogram

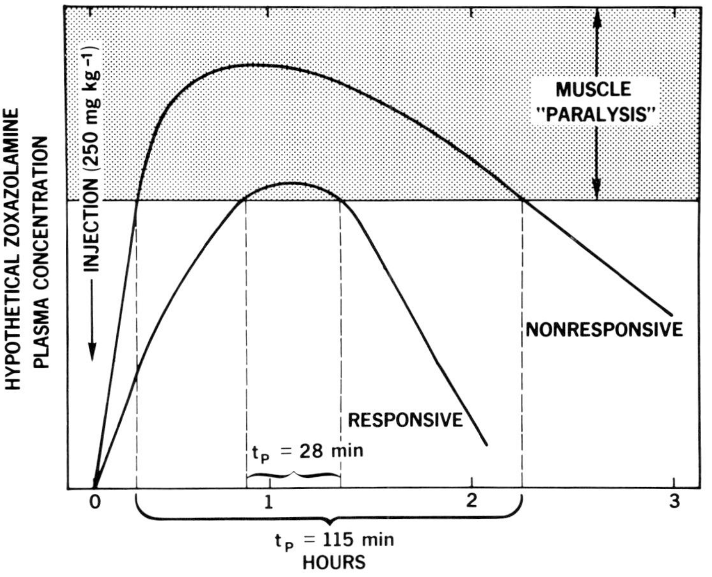

FIG. 9. Illustration of the principle for the zoxazolamine paralysis time, whereby the phenotype—with respect to the *Ah* locus—can be determined without killing the mouse (57). In β-naphthoflavone-treated responsive mice, because of considerably more hepatic cytochrome P_1-450, zoxazolamine is hydroxylated more rapidly than in β-naphthoflavone-treated nonresponsive mice. (From Nebert and Felton, ref. 57, with permission.)

body weight. β-Naphthoflavone (dissolved at 8 mg/ml corn oil) is not believed to be carcinogenic and is less toxic than polycyclic hydrocarbon inducers. About 40 hr later, zoxazolamine (McNeil Laboratories, Inc., Fort Washington, Pennsylvania) dissolved at 5 mg/ml of corn oil is given intraperitoneally at a dose of 250 mg/kg body weight. Responsive mice are usually paralyzed for 30 min or less; nonresponsive mice are usually paralyzed for more than 90 min. Any questionable individuals (paralyzed between 30 and 90 min) are discarded. These weanlings from the $F_1 \times$ DBA/2N back cross or the $F_1 \times F_1$ intercross can be regarded, for all intents and purposes, as siblings. After a week or more to allow full recovery from this phenotyping test, experimental protocols designed to test these two different phenotypes in response to carcinogenic, toxic, mutagenic, or teratogenic drugs or other chemicals is now possible.

IMPORTANCE OF THE ROUTE OF ADMINISTRATION

The results of numerous cancer and toxicity studies are categorized in Table 2. When the carcinogen (or other toxic drug) is placed in relatively direct contact with the tissue being studied, the genetically responsive Ah^b/Ah^b or Ah^b/Ah^d mouse is at increased risk for developing a tumor or toxicity in that tissue, compared with the nonresponsive Ah^d/Ah^d receiving the same dose of xenobiotic (Fig. 10). On the other hand, if the malignancy or toxicity is found at a site distant from the administered drug, the Ah^d/Ah^d mouse is at increased risk compared with the Ah^b/Ah^d or Ah^d/Ah^d individual receiving the same dose of xenobiotic. In this latter case, we believe that the data are explainable by the "first-pass effect," also termed "presystemic drug elimination" (reviewed in 74). Fundamentally, presystemic elimination reflects the metabolism and excretion of a drug before the drug reaches its site of action. How benzo(a)pyrene metabolism in the intestine can be induced 400- to 800-fold by oral benzo(a)pyrene and yet not exhibit any apparent toxicity (62) is not clear; an increase in conjugating enzymes or mechanism of efficient excretion of toxic metabolites must be involved. It will be of interest to see if the Ah^d/Ah^d mouse is more susceptible than the Ah^b/Ah^d mouse to *in utero* fetal toxicity or

TABLE 2. *Summary of toxicity and tumorigenesis in the mouse associated with the* Ah *locus*

Individual at increased risk	Tumor or toxicity	Route of administration	Chemical	Ref.
Ah^b/Ah^b and Ah^b/Ah^d	Skin inflammation	Topical	7,12-Dimethylbenzo(a)anthracene	81
	Fibrosarcomas	Subcutaneous	3-Methylcholanthrene or benzo(a)pyrene	37
	Pulmonary tumors	Intratracheal	3-Methylcholanthrene ≫ benzo(a)pyrene	35
	In utero fetal toxicity	Intraperitoneal	Benzo(a)pyrene, 3-methylcholanthrene, 7,12-dimethylbenzo(a)anthracene	78
	Primordial oocyte depletion	Intraperitoneal	7,12-Dimethylbenzo(a)anthracene, 3-methylcholanthrene, benzo(a)pyrene	46
	Epidermal carcinoma	Topical	Benzo(a)pyrene	40
	Cleft palate in fetus	Intraperitoneal	2,3,7,8-Tetrachlorodibenzo-*p*-dioxin	72
	Experimental porphyria	Intraperitoneal	Chlorinated aromatic compounds	30
Ah^d/Ah^d	Lymphoma, lymphosarcoma	Intraperitoneal	7,12-Dimethylbenzo(a)anthracene	4
	Bone marrow toxicity	Oral	Benzo(a)pyrene	73
	Leukemia	Subcutaneous	3-Methylcholanthrene	13
	Leukemia	Oral	Benzo(a)pyrene	60

Modified from Nebert (53), with permission from Academic Press, Inc.

primordial oocyte depletion when the polycyclic hydrocarbon is administered daily in the diet.

These data thus demonstrate that P_1-450 induction represents a "double-edged sword." Therefore, in all cancer and toxicity experiments, the size and timing of the dose(s), the route of administration, and the tissue in which the malignancy or toxicity develops (relative to the route of administration) are all very important factors in interpretation of the data.

EVIDENCE OF THE *Ah* LOCUS IN THE HUMAN

With the use of 20 to 40 cc of drawn blood, peripheral lymphocytes have been cultured in the presence of mitogens and an inducer of AHH activity such as 3-methylcholanthrene in order to assess the human *Ah* phenotype. In spite of the shortcomings of this assay method (reviewed in 2), a growing list of clinical disorders (Table 3) appears to be associated with the human *Ah* locus.

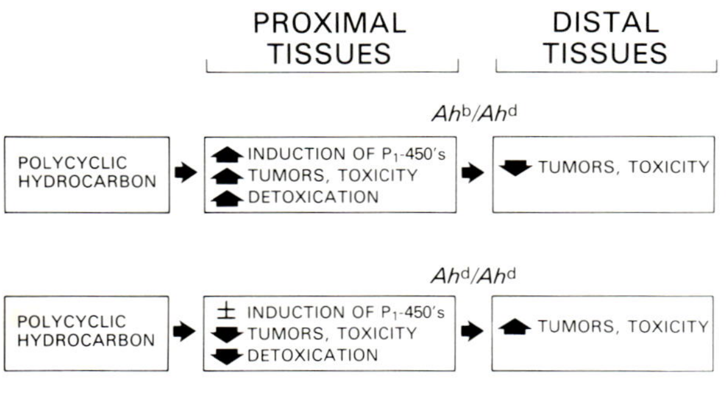

FIG. 10. Scheme indicating that the genetically responsive Ah^b/Ah^d individual (**top**) is at increased risk for tumors or toxicity at sites in direct contact with the xenobiotic (53). The nonresponsive Ah^d/Ah^d individual (**bottom**) is at increased risk for tumors or toxicity at distant sites because of decreased detoxication in many tissues of the body. (From Nebert, ref. 53, with permission.)

TABLE 3. *Human disorders that appear to be associated with the* Ah *locus*

Disorder	Association with high or low AHH inducibility	Ref.
Malignancy		
Bronchogenic carcinoma	High[a]	1,10,14,18,20,32–34,36,47
Bronchogenic carcinoma	No association found	22,28,42,69,70,93
Laryngeal carcinoma	High[b]	84
Cancer of oral cavity	High[b]	83,85
Cancer of renal pelvis or ureter	No association found	87
Cancer of urinary bladder	No association found	69,86
Acute leukemia of childhood	Low[a]	5
Toxicity		
Zoxazolamine-induced fetal hepatic necrosis	Unknown	44
Earlier onset of menopause among cigarette smokers	Unknown[c]	29
Infertility among cigarette smokers	Unknown[c]	23,71,82,92
Acetaminophen-induced diffuse bilateral cataracts	Unknown[c]	9

[a] Consistent with genetic data from inbred strains of mice (35, 61).

[b] Studies of these disorders in mice have not been specifically carried out, but the human data are consistent with what is known (53) about environmental carcinogens and their effect on local and distant tissue sites in genetically "*Ah*-responsive" and "*Ah*-nonresponsive" mice.

[c] Genetically responsive mice are at increased risk for these disorders (61). In retrospect (or in studies to be designed in the future), it would have been (or would be) of interest to know the *Ah* phenotype of afflicted clinical patients.

There clearly exists sufficient evidence that heritable variation of AHH inducibility occurs in man. Most likely, AHH induction is controlled by two or more loci (i.e., polygenic). Until one can increase the range of inducibility of AHH activity and/or decrease the magnitude of day-to-day variability of "control" AHH activity, however, AHH inducibility in cultured mitogen-activated lymphocytes or any other similar test system cannot be used as a promising biochemical marker for predicting who is at risk for aplastic anemia, leukemia, bronchogenic carcinoma, or other various types of environmentally caused toxicity or malignancy. We believe that a high ratio of P_1-450 to other forms of P-450 exists in many, if not all, extrahepatic tissues *in vivo,* just as appears to be the case in cultured lymphocytes, monocytes, pulmonary macrophages, and even skin fibroblasts. An alternative assay for assessing the human *Ah* phenotype (such as a receptor assay, a radioimmunoassay for induced P_1-450, or RNA–DNA hybridization to quantitate P_1-450 mRNA) might be more successful than the existing commonly performed AHH inducibility assay.

One major emphasis of this chapter has been to point out the importance of genetics in response to environmental stimuli. Such genetic heterogeneity in the human population undoubtedly reflects the large amount of "background noise," thereby making it difficult for the clinical investigator to discern distinct subgroups. If the genetic components can eventually be characterized among the clinical population, it should become easier to understand the etiology of environmentally caused malignancies and toxicity.

USE OF RECOMBINANT DNA TECHNOLOGY

It is anticipated that dozens of pharmacology laboratories will soon follow the example of this laboratory in studying genetic differences in drug-metabolizing enzymes by means of recombinant DNA technology (63). With the use of partially purified mouse liver 23 S mRNA (Fig. 11), known to be associated with the *Ah* locus and 3-methylcholanthrene-induced cytochrome P_1-450 (64), double-stranded complementary DNA (cDNA) was synthesized by the successive action of reverse transcriptase and the Klenow A fragment of *Escherichia coli* DNA polymerase I (Fig. 12). The double-stranded cDNA was inserted into pBR322 plasmid DNA by *Pst I* cleavage and homopolymeric "tailing" and cloned in *E. coli* LE392. One clone was shown to hybridize with ^{32}P-cDNA made from 23S mRNA from *Ah*-responsive C57BL/6N mice but not with similarly prepared ^{32}P-cDNA from *Ah*-nonresponsive DBA/2N mice (65).

By both genetic and immunologic criteria, the DNA from this clone (Fig. 13) was shown to be associated with anti-P_1-450 (65,90). With use of this clone, the mechanism of AHH (and associated P_1-450) induction is known to be under transcriptional control (90). Figure 14 summarizes the basic techniques for performing Southern or Northern blots. DNA fragments, or RNAs of different sizes, are electrophoresed on agarose gels. The migratory pattern of the nucleic acids in the gels then can be transferred directly (or "fixed" covalently) to hybridization paper. "Southern" refers to nitrocellulose paper; "Northern" refers to diazobenzyloxymethyl (or DBM) paper. The filter paper is then "probed" with radiolabeled single-stranded DNA or RNA. Following hybridization and posthybridization washes, the paper is exposed to X-ray film to produce the blot hybridization analysis. The radiolabeled probe is then added for possible hybridization with the DNA on the filter. If hybrid-

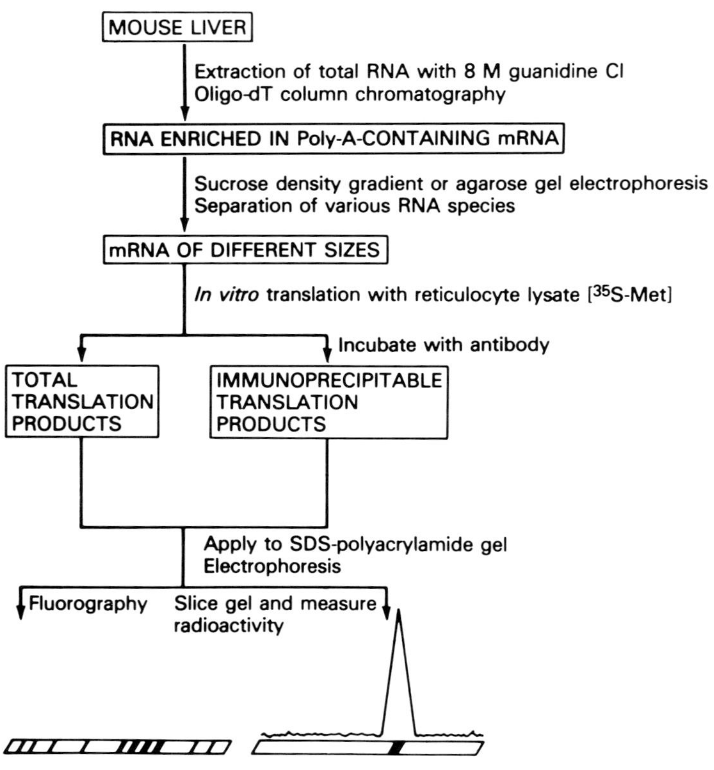

FIG. 11. Outline of methods by which mRNA for a particular protein can be sized (54). The method can only be as good as the antibody used for the immunoprecipitation of translation products. (From Nebert, ref. 54, with permission.)

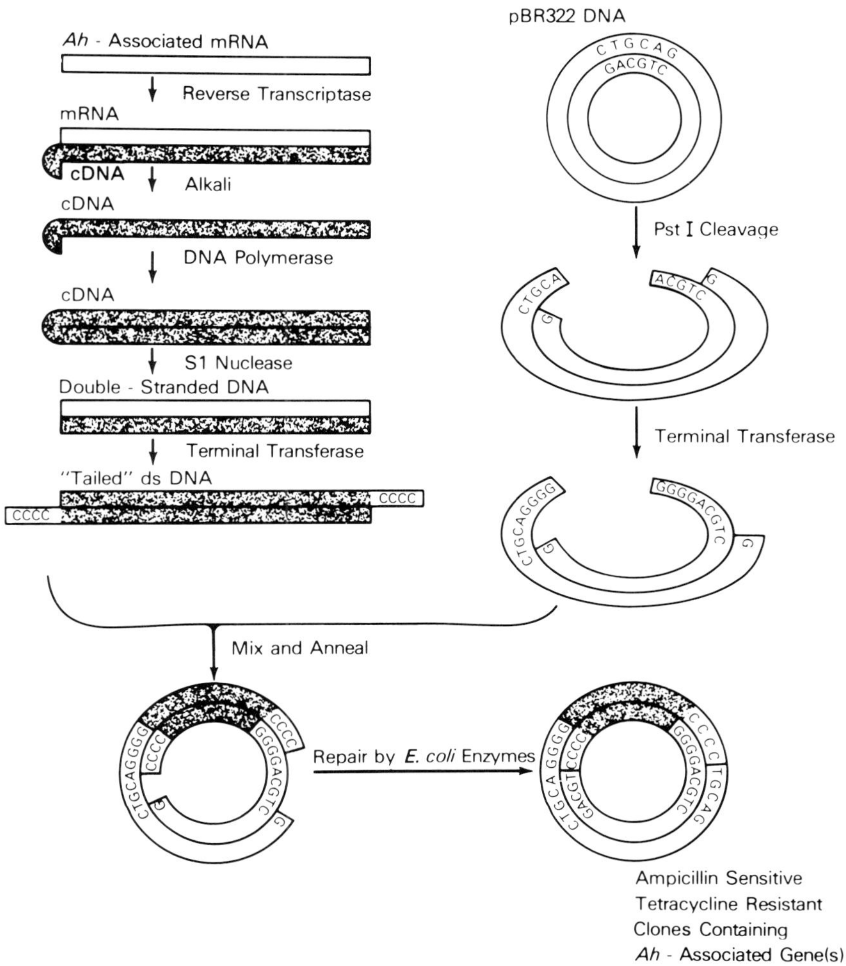

FIG. 12. Diagram of the cloning of double-stranded DNA derived from mouse liver 23 S mRNA. (From Lang et al., ref. 39, with permission.)

ization occurs, one can detect this colony or band as a "spot" on X-ray film that has been exposed to the paper filter for several hours or days.

Further characterization of the P_1-450 structural gene and the identification and characterization of other P-450 structural genes should provide valuable insight into understanding the genetic regulation of drug-metabolizing enzyme induction, the ultimate number of possible (constitutive and inducible) forms of P-450 (43,45), and the evolution of this multigene family (51). Moreover, such probes as the DNA of this clone may aid in the development of new potentially useful assays for determining genetic differences in individual risk of cancer, drug toxicity, and teratogenesis within the mouse (61) and human (52) populations.

ADDENDUM

This laboratory has recently uncovered several important points of information with

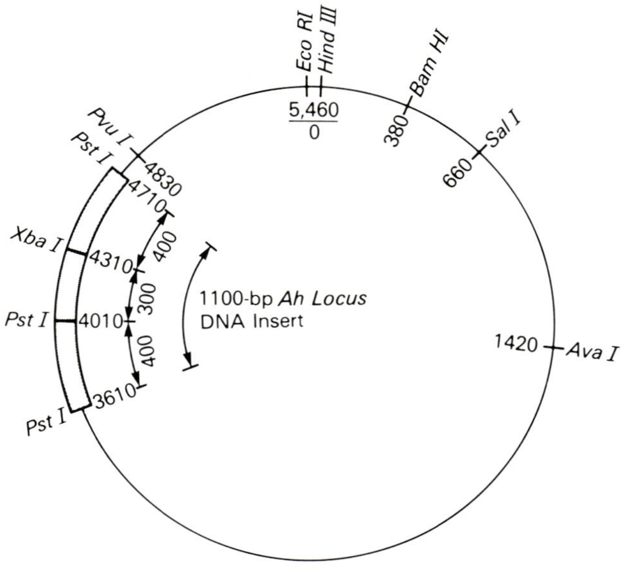

FIG. 13. Restriction map of pBR322-clone 46 (65). This cDNA clone has 1,100 base repairs, about one-third of the estimated total length of P_1-450 mRNA.

the use of the P_1-450 cDNA clone (Table 4). An association of clone 46 with the P_1-450 protein has been demonstrated by both immunologic and genetic criteria (65,90). We know that P_1-450 induction is under transcriptional control, because increased 23 S

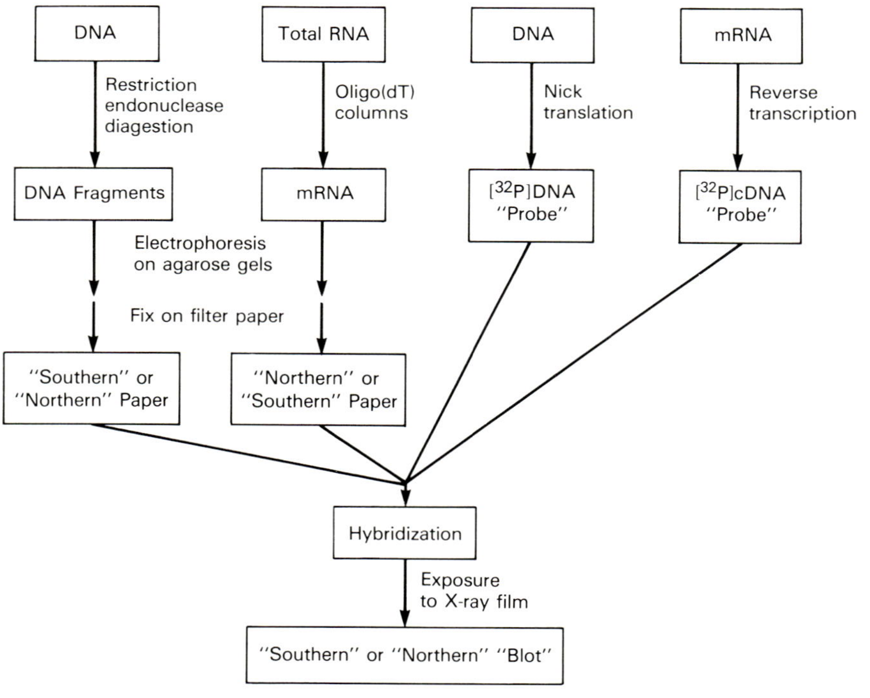

FIG. 14. General scheme of recombinant DNA techniques. (Reproduced from ref. 54, with permission.)

TABLE 4. *Our findings with clone 46 (cDNA clone; 1100 bp; 3'-unique sequence)*

Association with P_1-450 protein
a. Negative and positive translation arrest with anti-(P_1-450)
b. Correlation with Ah^b allele in offspring from B6D2F_1 × D2 back cross
P_1-450 induction under transcriptional control
a. Association with increased mRNA (23 S) levels
b. Correlation with intranuclear large-molecular-weight mRNA precursor
No evidence for gene amplification or gross form of genomic rearrangement
P_1-450 mRNA translation occurs on membrane-bound polysomes
Cross hybridization with rat and rabbit DNA, rat (23 S) mRNA
P_1-450 gene hypomethylated in adult B6 compared with that in adult D2 or sperm or embryonic B6
Other inducers (such as isosafrole) increase P_1-450 mRNA to small extent
P_1-450 genomic gene characterized by R-loop analysis (~5 kbp; at least five exons and four introns)
Evidence of genes for other polycyclic-aromatic-inducible forms of P-450
Excellent correlation ($r = 0.99$) between appearance of inducer–receptor complex in nucleus and P_1-450 mRNA induction

mRNA and an intranuclear large-molecular-weight mRNA precursor occur concomitantly during the induction process (90). No evidence for gene duplication or gross form of genomic rearrangement has been found, either during induction or during development (90).

The P_1-450 mRNA is translated probably exclusively on membrane-bound polysomes (7). Clone 46 hybridizes with rat and rabbit DNA and with rat but not rabbit mRNA; these data suggest that clone 46 hybridizes to a segment of the rabbit P_1-450 gene that is not transcribed into the messenger (8). We found that the P_1-450 gene in adult B6 is hypomethylated compared with the gene in B6 sperm, B6 embryo, or adult D2 mice; this hypomethylation pattern could be related to the increased expressivity of the P_1-450 gene in B6 compared with that in D2 mice (8). Other P-450 inducers, such as benzo(a)-anthracene and isosafrole, have been found to induce P_1-450 mRNA as measured by the clone 46 probe (91).

With the cDNA probe, we have isolated the chromosomal P_1-450 gene from a mouse genomic DNA library (27,48). By R-loop analysis, the gene spans about 4,600 base pairs and has at least five exons and four introns. We have cloned at least two genomic genes encoding different forms of polycyclic-aromatic-inducible P-450.

Polycyclic hydrocarbon metabolites appear to affect the replenishment of epidermal growth factor receptors on the cell surface; the mechanism for this is not understood (31). Finally, we have found an excellent correlation between the intranuclear appearance of the inducer–receptor complex and the induction of P_1-450 mRNA as measured by the clone 46 probe (88). With clone λAhP-1 and the surrounding regions of this mouse chromosome, we hope to understand a great deal about the regulation of P-450 induction, the evolution of the P-450 system, and perhaps the ultimate number of P-450 forms that an individual organism is genetically capable of expressing.

REFERENCES

1. Arnott, M. S., Yamauchi, T., and Johnston, D. A. (1979): Aryl hydrocarbon hydroxylase in normal and cancer populations. In: *Carcinogens: Identification and Mechanisms of Action,* edited by A. C. Griffin and C. R. Shaw, pp. 145–156. Raven Press, New York.
2. Atlas, S. A., and Nebert, D. W. (1978): Pharmacogenetics: A possible pragmatic perspective in neoplasm predictability. *Semin. Oncol.,* 5:89–106.
3. Atlas, S. A., Vesell, E. S., and Nebert, D. W. (1976): Genetic control of interindividual variations in the inducibility of aryl hydrocarbon hydroxylase in cultured human lymphocytes. *Cancer Res.,* 36:4619–4630.
4. Benedict, W. F., Considine, N., and Nebert, D. W. (1973): Genetic differences in aryl hydrocarbon hydroxylase induction and benzo(a)pyrene-produced tumorigenesis in the mouse. *Mol. Pharmacol.,* 9:266–277.
5. Blumer, J. L., Dunn, R., Esterhay, M. D., Yamashita, T. S., and Gross, S. (1981): Lymphocyte aromatic hydrocarbon responsiveness in acute leukemia of childhood. *Blood,* 58:1081–1088.
6. Blumer, J. L., and Mieyal, J. J. (1978): Genetic expression of microsomal electron transport in mice. Different patterns of dependence of constitutive cytochrome P-450 reductase activity on pyr-

idine nucleotide concentrations. *J. Biol. Chem.*, 253:1159–1166.
7. Chen, Y.-T., and Negishi, M. (1982): Expression and subcellular distribution of mouse cytochrome P_1-450 mRNA as determined by molecular hybridization with cloned P_1-450 DNA. *Biochem. Biophys. Res. Commun.*, 104:641–648.
8. Chen, Y.-T., Negishi, M., and Nebert, D. W. (1982): Cytochrome P_1-450 structural gene in mouse, rat and rabbit. Differences in DNA methylation and developmental expression of mRNA. *DNA*, 1:231–238.
9. Cohen, S. B., and Burk, R. F. (1978): Acetaminophen overdoses at a county hospital: A year's experience. *South. Med. J.*, 71:1359–1364.
10. Coomes, M. L., Mason, W. A., Muijsson, I. E., Cantrell, E. T., Anderson, D. E., and Busbee, D. L. (1976): Aryl hydrocarbon hydroxylase 16α-hydroxylase in cultured human lymphocytes. *Biochem. Genet.*, 14:671–685.
11. Daly, J. W., Jerina, D. M., and Witkop, B. (1972): Arene oxides and the NIH shift: the metabolism, toxicity and carcinogenicity of aromatic compounds. *Experientia*, 28:1129–1149.
12. Davidson, E. H., and Posakony, J. W. (1982): Repetitive sequence transcripts in development. *Nature*, 297:633–635.
13. Duran-Reynals, M. L., Lilly, F., Bosch, A., and Blank, K. J. (1978): The genetic basis of susceptibility to leukemia induction in mice by 3-methylcholanthrene applied percutaneously. *J. Exp. Med.*, 147:459–469.
14. Emery, A. E. H., Danford, N., Anand, R., Duncam, W., and Paton, L. (1978): Arylhydrocarbon-hydroxylase inducibility in patients with cancer. *Lancet*, 1:470–471.
15. Essigmann, J. M., Croy, R. G., Nadzan, A. M., Busby, W. F., Jr., Reinhold, V. N., Buchi, G., and Wogan, G. N. (1977): Structural identification of the major DNA adduct formed by aflatoxin B_1 *in vitro*. *Proc. Natl. Acad. Sci. U.S.A.*, 74:1870–1874.
16. Felton, J. S., Ketley, J. N., Jakoby, W. B., Aitio, A., Bend, J. R., and Nebert, D. W. (1980): Hepatic glutathione transferase activity induced by polycyclic aromatic compounds. Lack of correlation with the murine *Ah* locus. *Mol. Pharmacol.*, 18:559–564.
17. Fujita, S., and Peisach, J. (1978): Liver microsomal cytochromes P-450 and azoreductase activity. *J. Biol. Chem.*, 253:4512–4513.
18. Gahmberg, C. G., Sekki, A., Kosunen, T. U., Holsti, L. R., and Makela, O. (1979): Induction of aryl hydrocarbon hydroxylase activity and pulmonary carcinoma. *Int. J. Cancer*, 23:302–305.
19. Gelboin, H. V. (1980): Benzo(a)pyrene metabolism, activation, and carcinogenesis: Role and regulation of mixed-function oxidases and related enzymes. *Physiol. Rev.*, 60:1107–1166.
20. Guirgis, H. A., Lynch, H. T., Mate, T., Harris, R. E., Wells, I., Caha, L., Anderson, J., Maloney, K., and Rankin, L. (1976): Aryl hydrocarbon hydroxylase activity in lymphocytes from lung cancer patients and normal controls. *Oncology*, 33:105–109.
21. Gurtoo, H. L., Dahms, R. P., Kanter, P., and Vaught, J. B. (1978): Association and dissociation of the *Ah* locus with the metabolism of aflatoxin B_1 by mouse liver. Co-segregation of aflatoxin B_1 hydroxylase induction with aryl hydrocarbon (benzo[a]pyrene) hydroxylase induction. *J. Biol. Chem.*, 253:3952–3961.
22. Gurtoo, H. L., Minowada, J., Paigen, B., Parker, N. B., and Hayner, N. T. (1977): Factors influencing the measurement and the reproducibility of aryl hydrocarbon hydroxylase activity in cultured human lymphocytes. *J. Natl. Cancer Inst.*, 59:787–798.
23. Hammond, E. C. (1961): Smoking in relation to physical complaints. *Arch. Environ. Health*, 3:28–46.
24. Hannah, R. R., Nebert, D. W., and Eisen, H. J. (1981): Regulatory gene product of the *Ah* complex. Comparison of 2,3,7,8-tetrachlorodibenzo-*p*-dioxin and 3-methylcholanthrene binding to several moieties in mouse liver cytosol. *J. Biol. Chem.*, 256:4584–4590.
25. Hayakawa, T., and Udenfriend, S. (1973): A simple radioisotope assay for microsomal aryl hydroxylase. *Anal. Biochem.*, 51:501–509.
26. Holder, G., Yagi, H., Dansette, P., Jerina, D. M., Levin, W., Lu, A. Y. H., and Conney, A. H. (1974): Effects of inducers and epoxide hydrase on the metabolism of benzo(a)pyrene by liver microsomes and a reconditioned system: analysis by high pressure liquid chromatography. *Proc. Natl. Acad. Sci. U.S.A.*, 71:4356–4360.
27. Ikeda, T., Altieri, M., Nakamura, M., Tukey, R. H., Chen, Y.-T., Nebert, D. W., and Negishi, M. (1983): Characterization of P_2-450 (20 S) mRNA. Association with the P_1-450 genomic gene and differential response to the inducers 3-methylcholanthrene and isosafrole. *Eur. J. Biochem.* (*in press*).
28. Jett, J. R., Moses, H. L., Branum, E. L., Taylor, W. F., and Fontana, R. S. (1978): Benzo(a)pyrene metabolism and blast transformation in peripheral blood mononuclear cells from smoking and nonsmoking populations and lung cancer patients. *Cancer*, 41:192–200.
29. Jick, H., Porter, J., and Morrison, A. S. (1977): Relation between smoking and age of natural menopause. *Lancet*, 1:1354–1355.
30. Jones, K. G., and Sweeney, G. D. (1980): Dependence of the porphyrogenic effect of 2,3,7,8-tetrachlorodibenzo(*p*)dioxin upon inheritance of aryl hydrocarbon hydroxylase responsiveness. *Toxicol. Appl. Pharmacol.*, 53:42–49.
31. Kärenlampi, S. O., Eisen, H. J., Hankinson, O., and Nebert, D. W. (1983): Effects of cytochrome P_1-450 inducers on the cell-surface receptors for epidermal growth factor, phorbol 12,13-dibutyrate, or insulin of cultured mouse hepatoma cells. *J. Biol. Chem.* (*in press*).
32. Kärki, H. T., and Huhti, E. (1978): Aryl hydrocarbon hydroxylase activity in cultured lymphocytes from lung carcinoma patients and cigarette smokers. *Abstr. Int. Cong. Pharmacol.*, 19:254.
33. Kellermann, G., Shaw, C. R., and Luyten-Keller-

mann, M. (1973): Aryl hydrocarbon hydroxylase inducibility and bronchogenic carcinoma. *N. Engl. J. Med.*, 289:934–937.
34. Korsgaard, R., and Trell, E. (1978): Aryl hydrocarbon hydroxylase and bronchogenic carcinomas associated with smoking. *Lancet*, 1:1103–1104.
35. Kouri, R. E. (1976): Relationship between levels of aryl hydrocarbon hydroxylase activity and susceptibility to 3-methylcholanthrene and benzo(a)pyrene-induced cancers in inbred strains of mice. In: *Polynuclear Aromatic Hydrocarbons: Chemistry, Metabolism and Carcinogenesis*, edited by R. I. Freudenthal and P. W. Jones, pp. 139–151. Raven Press, New York.
36. Kouri, R. E., McKinney, C. E., Slomiany, D. J., Snodgrass, D. R., Wray, N. P., and McLemore, T. L. (1982): Positive correlation between high aryl hydrocarbon hydroxylase activity and primary lung cancer as analyzed in cryopreserved lymphocytes. *Cancer Res.*, 42:5030–5037.
37. Kouri, R. E., Ratrie, H., and Whitmire, C. E. (1974): Genetic control of susceptibility to 3-methylcholanthrene-induced subcutaneous sarcomas. *Int. J. Cancer*, 13:714–720.
38. Krontiris, T. G., and Cooper, G. M. (1981): Transforming activity of human tumor DNAs. *Proc. Natl. Acad. Sci. U.S.A.*, 78:1181–1184.
39. Lang, M. A., Nebert, D. W., and Negishi, M. (1980): Structural gene products of the *Ah* complex. Separation of multiple forms of liver microsomal cytochrome P-450 and characterization of mRNA associated with P_1-450 from 3-methylcholanthrene-treated mice. In: *Biochemistry, Biophysics and Regulation of Cytochrome P-450, Vol. 13*, edited by J.-Å. Gustafsson, J. Carlstedt-Duke, A. Mode, and J. Rafter, pp. 415–422. Elsevier/North-Holland Biomedical Press, Amsterdam, New York.
40. Legraverend, C., Mansour, B., Nebert, D. W., and Holland, J. M. (1980): Genetic differences in benzo(a)pyrene-initiated tumorigenesis in mouse skin. *Pharmacology*, 20:242–255.
41. Legraverend, C., Nebert, D. W., Boobis, A. R., and Pelkonen, O. (1980): DNA binding of benzo(a)pyrene metabolites: Effects on substrate and microsomal protein concentration *in vitro* and diet and tissue differences *in vivo*. *Pharmacology*, 20:137–148.
42. Lieberman, J. (1978): Aryl hydrocarbon hydroxylase in bronchogenic carcinoma. *N. Engl. J. Med.*, 298:686–687.
43. Lu, A. Y. H., and West, S. B. (1980): Multiplicity of mammalian microsomal cytochromes P-450. *Pharmacol. Rev.*, 31:277–295.
44. Lubell, D. L. (1962): Fatal hepatic necrosis associated with zoxazolamine therapy. *N.Y. State J. Med.*, 62:3807–3810.
45. Mannering, G. J. (1981): Hepatic cytochrome P-450-linked drug-metabolizing systems. In: *Concepts in Drug Metabolism, Vol. 2*, edited by B. Testa and P. Jenner, pp. 53–165. Marcel Dekker, New York.
46. Mattison, D. R., and Thorgeirsson, S. S. (1979): Ovarian aryl hydrocarbon hydroxylase activity and primordial oocyte toxicity of polycyclic aromatic hydrocarbons in mice. *Cancer Res.*, 39:3471–3475.
47. McLemore, T. L., Martin, R. R., Springer, R. R., Wray, N., Cantrell, E. T., and Busbee, D. L. (1979): Aryl hydrocarbon hydroxylase activity in pulmonary alveolar macrophages and lymphocytes from lung cancer and noncancer patients: A correlation with family histories of cancer. *Biochem. Genet.*, 17:795–806.
48. Nakamura, M., Negishi, M., Altieri, M., Chen, Y.-T., Ikeda, T., and Nebert, D. W. (1983): Structure of the mouse cytochrome P_1-450 genomic gene. *Eur. J. Biochem. (in press)*.
49. Nebert, D. W. (1978): Genetic differences affecting microsomal electron transport: The *Ah* locus. *Methods Enzymol.*, LII:226–240.
50. Nebert, D. W. (1979): Genetic differences in the induction of monooxygenase activities by polycyclic aromatic compounds. *Pharmacol. Ther.*, 6:395–417.
51. Nebert, D. W. (1979): Multiple forms of inducible drug-metabolizing enzymes. A reasonable mechanism by which any organism can cope with adversity. *Mol. Cell. Biochem.*, 27:27–46.
52. Nebert, D. W. (1980): The *Ah* locus. A gene with possible importance in cancer predictability. *Arch. Toxicol.* [*Suppl.*], 3:195–207.
53. Nebert, D. W. (1980): The *Ah* locus: Genetic differences in toxic and tumorigenic response to foreign compounds. In: *Microsomes, Drug Oxidations, and Chemical Carcinogenesis, Vol. II*, edited by M. J. Coon, A. H. Conney, R. W. Estabrook, H. V. Gelboin, J. R. Gillette, and P. J. O'Brien, pp. 801–812. Academic Press, New York.
53a. Nebert, D. W. (1981): Genetic differences in susceptibility to chemically induced myelotoxicity and leukemia. *Environ. Health Perspect.*, 39:11–22.
54. Nebert, D. W. (1982): Fundamental principles of cloning. In: *Cytochrome P-450, Biochemistry, Biophysics and Environmental Implications*, edited by E. Hietanen, M. Laitinen, and O. Hänninen, pp. 109–117. Elsevier/North-Holland Biomedical Press, Amsterdam.
55. Nebert, D. W., Atlas, S. A., Guenthner, T. M., and Kouri, R. E. (1978): The *Ah* locus: genetic regulation of the enzymes which metabolize polycyclic hydrocarbons and the risk for cancer. In: *Polycyclic Hydrocarbons and Cancer: Chemistry, Molecular Biology and Environment*, edited by P. O. P. Ts'o and H. V. Gelboin, pp. 345–390. Academic Press, New York.
56. Nebert, D. W., and Felton, J. S. (1975): Evidence for the activation of 3-methylcholanthrene as a carcinogen *in vivo* by cytochrome P_1450 from inbred strains of mice. In: *Cytochromes P-450 and* b_5, edited by D. Y. Cooper, O. Rosenthal, R. Snyder, and C. Witmer, pp. 127–149. Plenum Press, New York.
57. Nebert, D. W., and Felton, J. S. (1976): Importance of genetic factors influencing the metabolism of foreign compounds. *Fed. Proc.*, 35:1133–1141.
58. Nebert, D. W., and Gelboin, H. V. (1968): Substrate-inducible microsomal aryl hydroxylase in mammalian cell culture: I. Assay and properties of induced enzyme. *J. Biol. Chem.*, 243:6242–6249.
59. Nebert, D. W., and Gielen, J. E. (1972): Genetic

regulation of aryl hydrocarbon hydroxylase induction in the mouse. *Fed. Proc.,* 31:1315–1325.

60. Nebert, D. W., and Jensen, N. M. (1979): Benzo(a)pyrene-initiated leukemia in mice. Association with allelic differences at the *Ah* locus. *Biochem. Pharmacol.,* 27:149–151.
61. Nebert, D. W. and Jensen, N. M. (1979): The *Ah* locus: Genetic regulation of the metabolism of carcinogens, drugs, and other environmental chemicals by cytochrome P-450-mediated monooxygenases. *CRC Crit. Rev. Biochem.,* 6:401–437.
62. Nebert, D. W., Jensen, N. M., Levitt, R. C. and Felton, J. S. (1980): Toxic chemical depression of the bone marrow and possible aplastic anemia explainable on a genetic basis. *Clin. Toxicol.,* 16:99–122.
63. Nebert, D. W., and Negishi, M. (1982): Multiple forms of cytochrome P-450 and the importance of molecular biology and evolution. *Biochem. Pharmacol.,* 31:2311–2317.
64. Negishi, M., and Nebert, D. W. (1981): Structural gene products of the *Ah* complex. Increases in large mRNA from mouse liver associated with cytochrome P_1-450 induction by 3-methylcholanthrene. *J. Biol. Chem.,* 256:3085–3091.
65. Negishi, M., Swan, D. C., Enquist, L. W., and Nebert, D. W. (1981): Isolation and characterization of a cloned DNA sequence associated with the murine *Ah* locus and a 3-methylcholanthrene-induced form of cytochrome P-450. *Proc. Natl. Acad. Sci. U.S.A.,* 78:800–804.
66. Okey, A. B., Bondy, G. P., Mason, M. E., Kahl, G. F., Eisen, H. J., Guenthner, T. M., and Nebert, D. W. (1979): Regulatory gene product of the *Ah* locus. Characterization of the cytosolic inducer–receptor complex and evidence for its nuclear translocation. *J. Biol. Chem.,* 254:11636–11648.
67. Okey, A. B., Bondy, G. P., Mason, M. E., Nebert, D. W., Forster-Gibson, C., Muncan, J., and Dufresne, M. J. (1980): Temperature-dependent cytosol-to-nucleus translocation of the *Ah* receptor for 2,3,7,8-tetrachlorodibenzo-*p*-dioxin in continuous cell culture lines. *J. Biol. Chem.,* 255:11415–11422.
68. Paigen, B., Gurtoo, H. L., Minowada, J., Houten, L., Vincent, R., Paigen, K., Parker, N. B., Ward, E., and Hayner, N. T. (1977): Questionable relation of aryl hydrocarbon hydroxylase to lung-cancer risk. *N. Engl. J. Med.,* 297:346–350.
69. Paigen, B., Ward, E., Steenland, K., Havens, M., and Sartori, P. (1979): Aryl hydrocarbon hydroxylase inducibility is not altered in bladder cancer patients or their progeny. *Int. J. Cancer,* 23:312–315.
70. Paigen, B., Ward, E., Steenland, K., Houten, L., Gurtoo, H. L., and Minowada, J. (1978): Aryl hydrocarbon hydroxylase in cultured lymphocytes of twins. *Am. J. Hum. Genet.,* 30:561–571.
71. Pettersson, F., Fries, H., and Nillius, S. J. (1973): Epidemiology of secondary amenorrhea. I. Incidence and prevalence rates. *Am. J. Obstet. Gynecol.,* 117:80–86.
72. Poland, A., and Glover, E. (1980): 2,3,7,8-Tetrachlorodibenzo-*p*-dioxin: Segregation of toxicity with the *Ah* locus. *Mol. Pharmacol.,* 17:86–94.
73. Robinson, J. R., Felton, J. S., Levitt, R. C., Thorgeirsson, S. S., and Nebert, D. W. (1975): Relationship between "aromatic hydrocarbon responsiveness" and the survival times in mice treated with various drugs and environmental compounds. *Mol. Pharmacol.,* 11:850–865.
74. Routledge, P. A., and Shand, D. G. (1979): Presystemic drug elimination. *Annu. Rev. Pharmacol. Toxicol.,* 19:447–468.
75. Shih, C., Padhy, L. C., Murray, M., and Weinberg, R. A. (1981): Transforming genes of carcinomas and neuroblastomas introduced into mouse fibroblasts. *Nature,* 290:261–264.
76. Shih, C., Shilo, B., Goldfarb, M. P., Dannenberg, A., and Weinberg, R. A. (1979): Passage of phenotypes of chemically transformed cells via transfection of DNA and chromatin. *Proc. Natl. Acad. Sci. U.S.A.,* 76:5714–5718.
77. Shilo, B.-Z., and Weinberg, R. A. (1981): Unique transforming gene in carcinogen-transformed mouse cells. *Nature,* 289:607–609.
78. Shum, S., Jensen, N. M., and Nebert, D. W. (1979): The *Ah* locus: *In utero* toxicity and teratogenesis associated with genetic differences in benzo(a)pyrene metabolism. *Teratology,* 20:365–376.
79. Sims, P. (1967): The metabolism of benzo(a)pyrene by rat-liver homogenates. *Biochem. Pharmacol.,* 16:613–618.
80. Staats, J. (1980): Standardized nomenclature for inbred strains of mice: Seventh listing. *Cancer Res.,* 40:2083–2128.
81. Thomas, P. E., Hutton, J. J., and Taylor, B. A. (1973): Genetic relationship between aryl hydrocarbon hydroxylase inducibility and chemical carcinogen induced skin ulceration in mice. *Genetics,* 74:655–659.
82. Tokuhata, G. (1968): Smoking in relation to infertility and fetal loss. *Arch. Environ. Health,* 17:353–359.
83. Trell, E., and Korsgaard, R. (1978): Smoking and oral carcinoma. *Lancet,* 1:671.
84. Trell, E., Korsgaard, R., Hood, B., Kitzing, P., Nordén, G., and Simonsson, B. G. (1976): Aryl hydrocarbon hydroxylase inducibility and laryngeal carcinomas. *Lancet,* 2:140.
85. Trell, E., Korsgaard, R., Kitzing, P., Lundgren, K., and Mattiasson, I. (1978): Aryl hydrocarbon hydroxylase inducibility and carcinoma of oral cavity. *Lancet,* 1:109.
86. Trell, E., Oldbring, J., Korsgaard, R., Hellsten, S., Mattiasson, I., and Telhammar, E. (1978): Aryl hydrocarbon hydroxylase inducibility and carcinoma of the urinary bladder. *IRCS J. Med. Sci.,* 6:138.
87. Trell, E., Oldbring, J., Korsgaard, R., and Mattiasson, I. (1977): Aryl hydrocarbon hydroxylase inducibility in carcinoma of renal pelvis and ureter. *Lancet,* 2:612.
88. Tukey, R. H., Hannah, R. R., Negishi, M., Nebert, D. W., and Eisen, H. J. (1982): The *Ah* locus. Correlation of intranuclear appearance of inducer-receptor complex with induction of cytochrome P_1-450 mRNA. *Cell,* 31:275–284.
89. Tukey, R. H., Nakamura, M., Chen, Y.-T. Negishi, M., and Nebert, D. W. (1982): Genetic regulation of P-450 induction in the mouse. Studies with a cloned DNA sequence. In: *Microsomes, Drug Oxidations, and Drug Toxicity,* edited by R. Sato and

R. Kato, pp. 353–360. Japan Scientific Societies Press, Tokyo.

90. Tukey, R. H., Nebert, D. W., and Negishi, M. (1981): Structural gene product of the *Ah* complex. Evidence for transcriptional control of cytochrome P_1-450 induction by use of a cloned DNA sequence. *J. Biol. Chem.*, 256:6969–6974.
91. Tukey, R. H., Negishi, M., and Nebert, D. W. (1982): Quantitation of hepatic cytochrome P_1-450 mRNA with the use of a cloned DNA probe. Effects of various P-450 inducers in C57BL/6N and DBA/2N mice. *Mol. Pharmacol.*, 22:779–786.
92. Vessey, M. P., Wright, N. H., McPherson, K., and Wiggins, P. (1978): Fertility after stopping different methods of contraception. *Br. Med. J.*, 1:265–267.
93. Ward, E., Paigen, B., Steenland, K., Vincent, R., Minowada, J., Gurtoo, H. L., Sartori, P., and Havens, M. B. (1978): Aryl hydrocarbon hydroxylase in persons with lung or laryngeal cancer. *Int. J. Cancer,* 22:384–389.
94. Weinstein, I. B., Jeffrey, A. M., Jennette, K. W., Blobstein, S. H., Harvey, R. G., Harris, C., Autrup, H., Kasai, H., and Nakanishi, K. (1976): Benzo(a)pyrene diol epoxides as intermediates in nucleic acid binding *in vitro* and *in vivo*. *Science,* 193:592–595.
95. Williams, R. T. (1959): *Detoxication Mechanisms,* second edition. John Wiley & Sons, New York.
96. Yang, S. K., Roller, P. P., Fu, P. P., Harvey, R. G., and Gelboin, H. V. (1977): Evidence for a 2,3-epoxide as an intermediate in the microsomal metabolism of benzo(a)pyrene to 3-hydroxybenzo-(a)pyrene. *Biochem. Biophys. Res. Commun.,* 77:1176–1182.

Drug Metabolism and Drug Toxicity,
edited by J. R. Mitchell and M. G. Horning.
Raven Press, New York © 1984.

Role of DNA Excision Repair in Preventing Cytotoxic, Mutagenic, and Oncogenic Effects of Carcinogens in Human Cells

J. Justin McCormick and Veronica M. Maher

Carcinogenesis Laboratory and Department of Biochemistry, Michigan State University, East Lansing, Michigan 48824

Most chemical mutagens are now thought to exert their biological action as a result of their covalent linkage to DNA (adduct formation). The adducts are premutagenic in that a mutation, which can broadly be defined as any change in DNA sequence, ordinarily occurs as a result of a DNA polymerase attempting to replicate DNA containing such adducts or secondary lesions resulting from them, e.g., apurinic sites. During replication, the DNA polymerases may insert an incorrect nucleotide or set of nucleotides opposite the modified nucleotide. The former would result in a base substitution, leading to a transition or transversion mutation; the latter would result in a frame shift. Alternatively, the polymerases may fail to insert any nucleotide opposite the altered base, which would also result in a frame shift. Failure to replicate a larger section of the DNA could also occur, resulting in a large deletion. If such changes occur in a critical part of a structural gene coding for a cellular protein, the result could be synthesis of an inactive protein or no protein at all. Similarly, if the changes occur in a regulatory gene or control region, this could alter the amount of a protein or proteins produced.

Irradiation of cells with ultraviolet (UV) radiation of wavelengths between 254 and 310 nm causes photoproducts in DNA that can lead to mutations by the same processes as DNA adducts do (21). The best known of the UV photoproducts are pyrimidine dimers. However, there also are a number of less-well-studied photoproducts induced in DNA by UV radiation (9,23). From extensive work in bacterial and mammalian systems, it seems extremely likely that pyrimidine dimers are premutagenic lesions (25,46). Whether the other lesions are also premutagenic is not yet known.

The above sequence of events leaves unanswered several important questions. First, if DNA synthesis is required for the induction of mutations, is this semiconservative synthesis or the DNA synthesis that takes place during excision repair? In bacteria, mutations can be induced by both processes (46). Second, the doses of chemical mutagens or UV radiation that induce mutations in human cells also produce cytotoxicity. Is this cytotoxicity caused by DNA adducts or photoproducts or by some other lesions in the cells induced by these agents? Most importantly, since UV radiation and almost all chemical mutagens are carcinogenic, can one extrapolate from the results of studies on the induction of the mutations and/or transformation of human cells in culture to the mechanisms involved in carcinogenesis in humans?

To address the above questions, we have developed quantitative assays for measuring the cytotoxic, mutagenic, and oncogenic effect of carcinogens in diploid human skin fibroblasts derived from neonatal foreskin or skin biopsy material (25,27,28,30–32,41). The use of human cells offers a number of advantages. They grow well in culture and clone with 40 to 80% efficiency. They can be treated with direct-acting mutagens, and the cytotoxic effect quantitated from the decrease in their cloning ability. Compounds requiring activation can also be used if the cells are provided with a source of activation, such as metabolizing feeder cells (1,2). The dose-dependent induction of mutations by carcinogens can be quantitated by determining the frequency of cells able to grow in the presence of the base analogs 8-azaguanine or 6-thioguanine as a result of inactivation of a functional hypoxanthine (guanine) phosphoribosyltransferase (HPRT) (25,29). Another genetic marker we have used to quantitate mutation induction is resistance to diphtheria toxin, which results from inactivation of its receptor site on the elongation factor 2 used in protein synthesis (12). The frequency of transformation of normal human cells into tumorigenic cells can be measured by determining the frequency of cells able to exhibit anchorage-independent growth, i.e., colony formation in semisolid medium containing 0.33% agar (41). We and others have shown that human cells isolated from anchorage-independent colonies form tumors when injected into athymic mice, whereas cells that do not express this phenotype do not grow in these animals (30,34). We now routinely treat human fibroblasts with mutagens and measure the cytotoxicity and the induction of thioguanine and diphtheria toxin resistance as well as anchorage independence in the same cell population (30).

Although strains of human fibroblasts in culture do not have an infinite life-span (14), the number of cells one can obtain from a single fibroblast population is so large (11) that we routinely use a cell strain for several years, with many workers using the same strain of cells. The advantage of using human fibroblast cell strains over the commonly used rodent cell lines with infinite life-spans is that the former retain their diploid karotype throughout their life-span, whereas the latter usually are aneuploid (42) and therefore no longer faithfully represent the normal cells of the species from which they were obtained.

Another advantage of working with strains of diploid human fibroblasts is that they retain the excision repair capability present in the individual from which they were obtained, whereas cell lines, especially those of rodent origin, lose their characteristic excision repair capabilities with time in culture (36). Most importantly, human fibroblast cell strains that have low rates of excision repair synthesis are available from xeroderma pigmentosum (XP) patients (39). Although the molecular nature of the defect(s) in such cells is not known, they have little or no excision repair capability for pyrimidine dimers (10) or for lesions induced by the covalent linkage of bulky ring structures to DNA, such as those formed by reactive derivatives of aromatic amines (15,24,26) or polycyclic aromatic hydrocarbons (47,48). Since the principal difference between XP cells and normal cells is in their rate of excision repair, a comparison of the cytotoxic, mutagenic, and/or transforming effect of various agents on such cells allows one to determine the biological effect of the DNA excision repair process.

SURVIVAL AND FREQUENCY OF INDUCED MUTATIONS IS INVERSELY PROPORTIONAL TO A CELL'S EXCISION REPAIR CAPACITY

In our earlier studies, we found that after 254-nm irradiation, the survival of fibroblasts and induction of mutations paralleled their excision repair capability (24,25,27).

For example, when three strains of diploid human fibroblasts, each with a cell cycle of approximately the same length but with different rates of excision of UV-induced DNA damage, were irradiated and assayed for survival and induction of mutations, the results

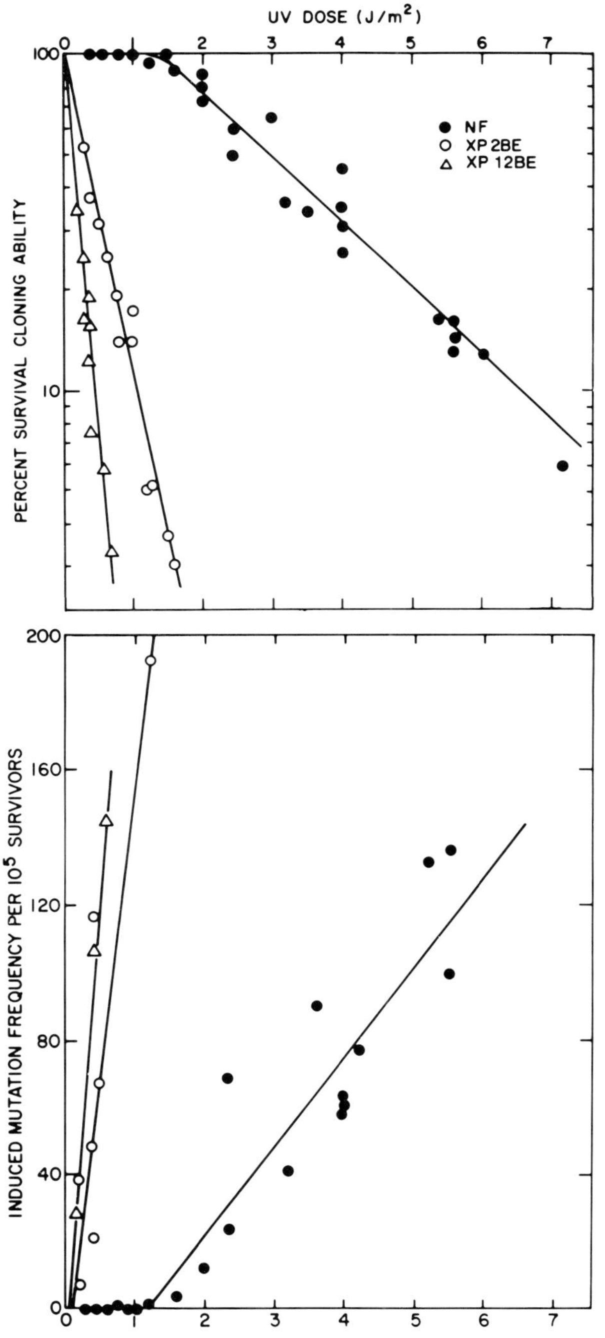

FIG. 1. Comparing the cytotoxic and mutagenic effect of UV radiation in human fibroblasts with different rates of excision repair. Cells from exponentially growing cultures were plated into culture dishes at appropriate densities, allowed 12 hr to attach, irradiated, and allowed to develop into colonies. Selection *in situ* with 20 μM AG was begun after 5 to 8 days of expression (>3 population doublings). (From Maher et al., ref. 25, with permission.)

(Fig. 1) indicated that the normal cells with rapid excision were much more resistant to the potentially lethal and mutagenic effect of UV than either XP strain. After exposure to 0.5 J/m^2, XP12BE cells with little or no excision repair capacity (37) exhibited ~5% survival; XP2BE cells, which excise damage slowly, exhibited a survival of ~25%; and normal cells exhibited 100% survival. The corresponding increase in mutant cells per 10^5 surviving cells assayed *in situ* was 140 for strain XP12BE, 75 for XP2BE, and no increase over background for the normal cells (25). This is the result one expects if the XP12BE cells exhibit the maximum potential cytotoxicity and mutagenicity of a given dose of UV whereas XP2BE cells reduce their load of DNA damage to a level approximately 40% of that initially received and the normal cells with rapid repair reduce their load to an insignificant number of photo lesions.

Such a result predicts that there is a finite amount of time for excision repair between the initial radiation and the onset of the critical events responsible for cell killing and/or mutation induction in these cells. A larger dose must be given to the normal cells to achieve the biological consequences observed in the repair-deficient XP cells. However, at equicytotoxic doses, the frequency of mutations induced in all three strains is approximately equal. Since an essential difference among these strains is their respective rates of excision repair of UV-induced damage, the data are consistent with the hypothesis that the loss of ability to form a clone and the frequency of mutations induced in these cells reflect the number of unexcised lesions remaining in DNA at the time of some "critical cellular event" that translates the DNA lesions into their biological manifestations. We suggested that within a specified time, the strains capable of excision (normal cells and XP2BE) removed many of the lesions initially introduced before these resulted in lethality or mutation induction and that this critical event could be semiconservative DNA synthesis on a damaged template (25).

LENGTHENING TIME BETWEEN EXPOSURE AND ONSET OF S PHASE REDUCES BIOLOGICAL EFFECTS OF THESE AGENTS

If mutations are introduced not by excision repair but by semiconservative DNA replication on a template containing unexcised lesions, then if one were to extend the time between the introduction of the lesions and the onset of DNA synthesis, it should be possible for a cell that has at least some capacity for excision repair to remove those lesions before they can cause mutations. Similarly, if cell killing reflects replication on a damaged template, then extending the time available for excision repair before allowing cells to replicate their DNA should result in increased survival. We tested this hypothesis by growing cells to confluence to achieve density inhibition of cell replication, treating them with a DNA-damaging agent, and then allowing them various lengths of time to remove potentially cytotoxic or mutagenic DNA lesions. After reaching confluence, cells were refed once and then held for 72 hr without refeeding. Autoradiography studies in cells maintained in the resting state under our conditions demonstrated that <0.5% of the cells incorporated tritiated thymidine during an 8-hr labeling period (25). However, such cells are capable of excision repair (15,22,47).

We irradiated confluent normal cells with a large enough dose of UV radiation to cause cell killing and to induce mutations in asynchronously growing populations, i.e., 5 to 10 J/m^2, and held them in the nonreplicating state for 7 days. They were then trypsinized and plated at lower densities to assay survival and induction of mutations, i.e., increase in frequency of thioguanine-resistant cells. The results are shown in Fig. 2. The normal cells, held for 7 days in the confluent state, showed

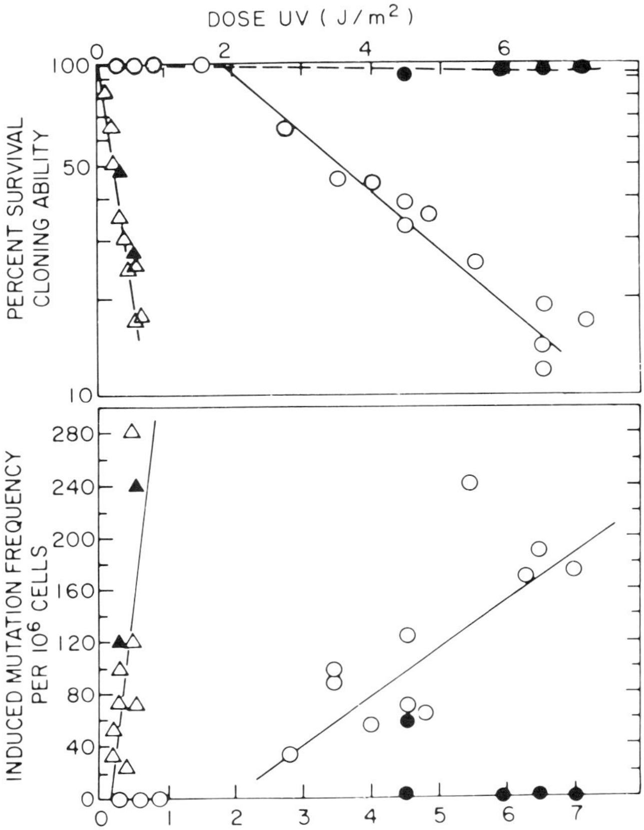

FIG. 2. Loss of potentially cytotoxic and mutagenic lesions induced by UV irradiation in NF in comparison to XP12BE cells. The XP12BE cells were grown to confluence and irradiated. One set was assayed immediately for survival and, after the appropriate expression period, for frequency of thioguanine-resistant cells by selection by replating (△). A second set was held confluent for 7 days and similarly assayed (▲). Alternatively, cells from exponentially growing cultures were plated, allowed 12 hr to attach, irradiated, and similarly assayed for survival and frequency of mutants (also shown as *open triangles*). Similar experiments were carried out in NF cells. *Closed circles* (●) indicate cultures irradiated and held in confluence for 7 days before assaying. *Open circles* (○) indicate cultures irradiated in confluence and immediately assayed for survival or cells from exponentially growing cultures plated, irradiated, and then assayed for survival and for frequency of UV-induced mutants. The frequency of mutants induced in normal cells irradiated at confluence was much lower than that of cells irradiated in exponential growth (see text for explanation). (From Maher et al., ref. 25, with permission.)

no cell killing and no mutation induction. In contrast, XP12BE cells irradiated at confluence exhibited the same degree of cell killing and mutation induction as we found in cycling cells (25).

To determine how much time it takes for the normal cells to remove potentially cytotoxic and/or mutagenic lesions, we irradiated a series of confluent cultures with 7 J/m^2 and released one immediately and the others at various times following radiation. There was a gradual decrease in the lethal and mutagenic effect of the radiation. After ~15 hr in the resting state, the cells that had exhibited an initial survival of 20% and an induced mutation frequency of 50×10^6 exhibited 100% survival and a frequency of mutations near background. A similar amount of time was required for XP5BE cells from complementation group D, with a slow rate of excision repair, to exhibit 100% survival after exposure to a 20%-survival dose of UV (i.e., 1 J/m^2). The XP5BE cells exposed to a sevenfold lower dose of UV light than normal cells had a lower number of lesions to excise, but since they can excise, although at a rate slower than normal cells, it is not surprising that they exhibited a gradual increase in survival and that their rate of recovery was similar to the rate of biologic recovery of normal cells given a much higher dose of UV. Twenty-four hours in the resting state was sufficient time for both sets of cells to remove a sufficient number of lesions so that when they were released, they exhibited 100% survival (25).

EVIDENCE OF BIOLOGICAL EFFECTS OF EXCISION REPAIR OF DNA LESIONS INDUCED BY CHEMICAL CARCINOGENS

Although one may measure the rate of excision of UV-induced pyrimidine dimers in human cells with reasonable accuracy at doses greater than 10 J/m^2, it is not possible to measure the cells' rate of removal of the low number of photoproducts induced by the low doses of UV that we used in these experiments. However, we demonstrated a high correlation between the rate of excision of DNA adducts induced by a series of radioactive labeled chemical carcinogens and the recovery of normal cells from potentially cytotoxic damage. The chemicals we selected were those we showed caused greater cell killing and much greater frequencies of mutations in XP cells than in normal cells, i.e., *N*-acetoxy-4-acetylaminobiphenyl (N-AcO-AABP), *N*-acetoxy-2-acetylaminofluorene (N-AcO-AAF), *N*-acetoxy-2-acetylaminophenanthrene (N-AcO-AAP), and *N*-acetoxy-4-acetylaminostilbene (N-AcO-AAS) (15,24,26).

Normal and repair-deficient cells grown to confluence were exposed to concentrations adjusted to result in ~20% survival. One set of cells was released immediately and assayed for survival and for the number of residues bound to the DNA. The other sets were held for 18, 36, 72, or 144 hr before being released and assayed for the number of residues remaining in the DNA and for survival. The results (Fig. 3) showed that the rate of recovery was directly related to the rate of removal of the bound carcinogen residues from DNA. In the XP12BE cells, there was little or no removal of the bound material and no evidence of recovery from the potentially le-

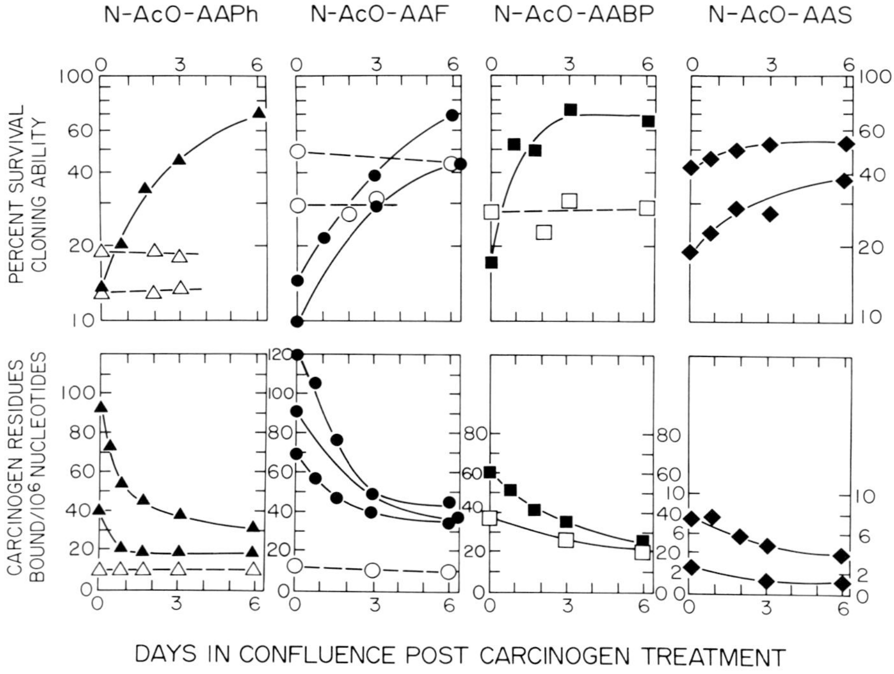

FIG. 3. Comparison of the rate of recovery from the potentially cytotoxic effects of four aromatic amine derivatives with the rate of removal of radioactively labeled residues from the DNA of NF cells (*closed symbols*) or XP12BE cells (*open symbols*). Cells were treated at confluence and assayed after the designated period of time at confluence. (From Maher et al., ref. 26, with permission.)

thal effects of the initial exposure, even over a period of 6 days (15).

We used the same approach to investigate the kinetics of removal of DNA adducts formed by radioactive 7β,8α-dihydroxy-9α,10α-epoxy-7,8,9,10-tetrahydrobenzo(a)-pyrene (anti-BPDE) and the rate of recovery of human cells from its potentially cytotoxic and mutagenic effects. Large populations of density-inhibited cells were treated, and a fraction of them were harvested immediately and assayed for DNA adducts, survival, and mutation induction. The rest were assayed after 2, 4, or 8 days in confluence (47). The results (Fig. 4) showed that residues were initially removed rapidly by the normal cells but that after 4 days excision repair slowed considerably. Similarly, the survival of the population increased during that same period, and the frequency of mutants decreased almost to background. These data indicate that the potentially cytotoxic and mutagenic lesions were removed with about the same kinetics as were the total number of DNA adducts.

The HPLC characterization of the DNA adducts indicated that the major adduct was the N^2-guanyl derivative (45). The kinetics of decrease of tritium label in the specific HPLC peak corresponded to the kinetics of decrease of radioactivity in the total DNA with time and also with the kinetics of recovery from the mutations and the cytotoxicity. There may be unstable adducts whose existence could not be noted or minor adduct(s) that escaped notice because the specific activity of the carcinogen did not permit their detection. Nevertheless, if such adducts are responsible for the mutagenic and/or cytotoxic effects of the anti-BPDE, they must be excised with the same kinetics as the N^2-guanyl derivative to account for these results.

A point of particular importance, which can be seen from the data in Fig. 4, is that the survival and mutagenic response manifested by the population of normal cells on release from confluence are directly related to the number of lesions in the DNA at the

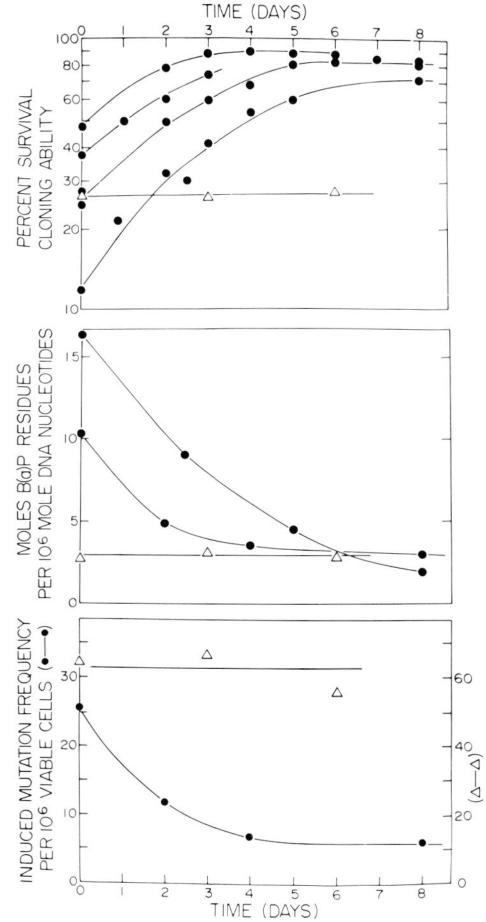

FIG. 4. Kinetics of removal of covalently bound adducts (**B**) and recovery of normal cells (*circles*) from the potentially cytotoxic (**A**) or mutagenic (**C**) effects of anti-BPDE. The cells were treated in confluence, released on the designated days, and assayed for survival of colony-forming ability, for the number of residues bound to DNA, and, after a suitable expression period, for the frequency of induced mutations. The *triangles* represent data from XP12BE cells. (From Yang et al., ref. 47, with permission.)

time the cells are plated to lower densities, regardless of whether the DNA contained this number of lesions because the cells had just been treated with the appropriate dose of anti-BPDE to give this frequency or because they had received a much higher dose originally and had removed some of the original adducts during the time they were held at confluence. These results indicate that RNA and protein lesions contribute only indirectly to the cytotoxic effects of such agents. Further evidence for this is shown in Fig. 5. Here, the cells were exposed to 0.15, 0.2, 0.25, or 0.3 μM tritiated anti-BPDE and assayed immediately for survival and number of adducts per 10^6 DNA nucleotides. The results, identified in Fig. 5 with the numeral 0, show that initial binding levels of 6.5, 10.2, 14.7, and 16.3 residues per 10^6 nucleotides result in survivals of 40%, 27%, 16%, and 12%, respectively.

When the data from Fig. 4, derived from cells treated and then held in confluence, were analyzed in the same manner and replotted with these data, the points fell on the identical line. Cells initially exposed to 0.3 μM tritiated anti-BPDE diol epoxide bound 16.3 residues per 10^6 DNA nucleotides and exhibited an initial survival of 12%. After 2.5 days in the nonreplicating state, when they had reduced the number of such residues per 10^6 nucleotides from 16 to 10, the survival they exhibited when released from confluence was the same as that obtained with cells exposed initially to a concentration giving 10 residues per 10^6 nucleotides and assayed immediately. Thus, the protein binding and RNA binding that presumably occurred as a result of the original treatment did not contribute significantly to the ultimate level of cell killing.

Additional evidence that cell killing does not reflect initial protein binding is the abnormal sensitivity of the XP cells. We suggest that cell killing and mutation induction seen when cells are plated at lower densities reflect DNA lesions remaining unexcised in the cells

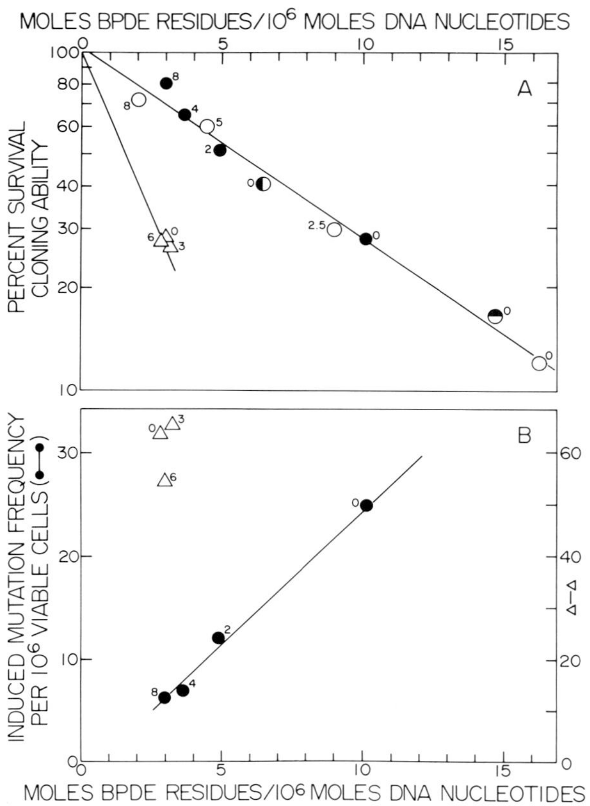

FIG. 5. Cytotoxicity (**A**) and induced mutation frequency (**B**) as functions of the number of BPDE-induced adducts present in DNA of normal fibroblasts (*circles*) and XP12BE cells (*triangles*) at the time they were released from confluence and plated for survival or for the beginning of expression of thioguanine resistance. The number of days cells were held in confluence before being analyzed is indicated next to each data point. The data represented by ○, ●, and △ have been replotted from the data given in Fig. 4. (From Yang et al., ref. 47, with permission.)

at the time of some critical event in the replicating state. This conclusion is supported by the lack of alteration in cytotoxicity or mutagenicity in the XP cells, which are unable to remove these DNA adducts.

SHORTENING TIME BETWEEN EXPOSURE TO DNA-DAMAGING AGENTS AND ONSET OF S PHASE INCREASES MUTAGENIC EFFECT

If the cellular event responsible for killing and mutation induction is semiconservative DNA replication on a damaged template, it should be possible to shorten the time available for excision by synchronizing cells and irradiating them or treating them with chemical carcinogens just before the onset of S. These cells should show significantly greater cell killing and mutagenesis than cells exposed many hours prior to the onset of S. XP12BE cells (with essentially no excision repair ability) should show no difference in sensitivity when treated at various times before the onset of S. We tested these predictions using UV (21) and the diol epoxide of BP (48) as the DNA-damaging agents in cells synchronized by density inhibition. Autoradiography indicated that cells released from the G_0 state after 72 hr in confluence and replated at lower densities (3 to 8 $\times$ 10^3 cells/cm^2) in fresh medium containing 15% fetal bovine serum begin semiconservative DNA synthesis (S phase) ~24 hr after the replating (Fig. 6). Normal cells and XP12BE cells were irradiated under conditions that would allow 24, 18, or 1 hr to occur between irradiation and the beginning of S phase. The cells that were to have 24 hr before S were irradiated in confluence and replated at lower densities. The cells that were to be irradiated 18 hr before S or just before S were released from confluence so as to have the appropriate number of hours prior to irradiation *in situ* at the lower densities. For greater accuracy of comparison, the cells were irradiated at a single time using the same lamp and incident dose of UV. The frequencies of mutants induced are shown in the bottom panel of Fig. 7. Normal cells irradiated shortly before S exhibited the highest frequency of thioguanine-resistant cells, and those irradiated 18 hr prior to S a sevenfold lower frequency. The cells irradiated in confluence and immediately replated exhibited the lowest frequency of mutations. The results of a similar study with XP12BE cells are also shown in Fig. 7. As expected, the frequency of mutations induced in these cells irradiated at the designated times before S did not vary significantly (21).

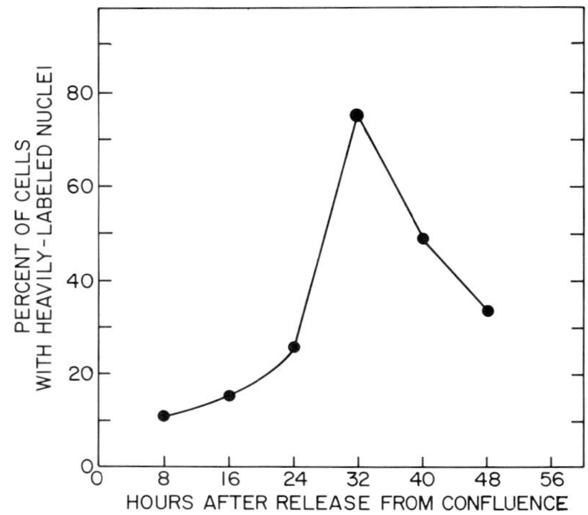

FIG. 6. Autoradiographic study of the time of onset and length of S phase. Normal human cells were replated from confluence at a density of ~9 $\times$ $10^3/cm^2$ into dishes containing coverslips and exposed to tritiated thymidine for 8-hr intervals. (From Konze-Thomas et al., ref. 21, with permission.)

The corresponding cytotoxic effect of UV in normal and XP12BE cells is compared in the top panel of Fig. 7. As expected, the survival of XP12BE cells did not depend on the number of hours available for excision repair between irradiation and the beginning of S. However, in contrast to the results for mutation induction, the survival curves for NF cells irradiated at 24, 18, or 1 hr prior to the onset of S showed only slight differences in sensitivity. The slope of the survival curve of cells irradiated just before S was only 1.1-fold

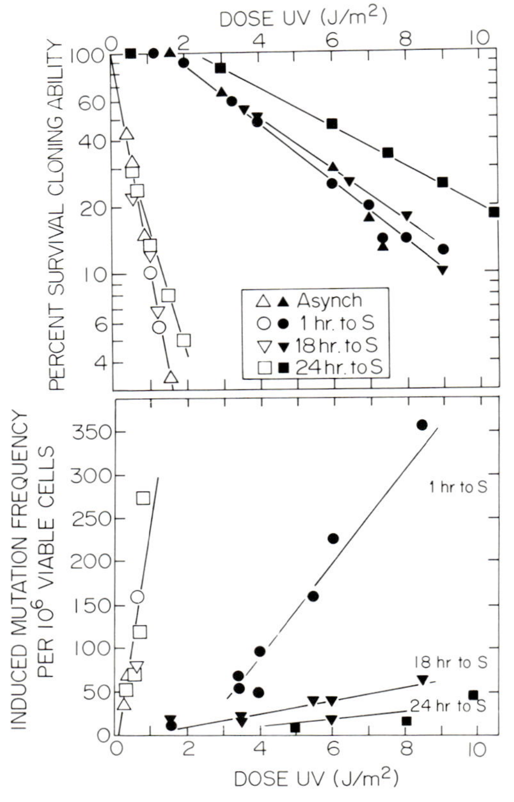

FIG. 7. Cytotoxicity and mutagenicity of UV in NF cells (*closed symbols*) or XP12BE cells (*open symbols*) irradiated under conditions designed to allow various lengths of time for excision repair to take place prior to the onset of S phase. Cells irradiated in confluence (G_0) and then released and plated at lower densities (■, □); cells released from G_0 and irradiated 6 hr later (▼, ▽); cells released and irradiated 24 hr later (●, ○); cells replated from asynchronously growing cultures and irradiated ~16 hr later (▲, △). (From Konze-Thomas et al., ref. 21, with permission.)

steeper than that of the cells irradiated 18 hr before S and only 1.3-fold steeper than that of cells irradiated in the confluent G_0 state and then released (24 hr to S).

These results indicate that in cells capable of removing lesions, the time available for excision repair between irradiation and S is, indeed, the determining factor for mutagenicity. Normal foreskin fibroblasts (NF cells) allowed 18 to 24 hr before onset of S significantly reduced their load of potentially mutagenic lesions, e.g., from the mutagenic equivalent of 8.5 J/m^2 to that of ~3 (18 hr) or 2 J/m^2 (24 hr). The fact that the XP12BE cells showed no significant difference in mutation frequency whether irradiated in G_0 and released or in early G_1 or just prior to S is consistent with their virtual lack of excision repair (37). If the increased mutation frequency exhibited by cells irradiated just prior to S reflects differences in the physical state of the DNA in these cells compared with that of cells in early G_1 so that a larger number of lesions were induced or lesions located in more critical sites, this could account for about a twofold increase in the mutation frequency (as seen in the XP population) but not for the sevenfold increase seen in the repair-proficient cells. Our data suggest that normal cells irradiated in G_1 have time to excise the potentially mutagenic damage before onset of S and support the hypothesis that the cellular event critical for mutation induction is semiconservative DNA synthesis on a template containing unexcised lesions.

In contrast to the mutation results, the cytotoxicity data indicate that no single-cell cycle-related event, such as DNA synthesis, is critical in translating DNA damage into cell death. Normal cells irradiated with 7 J/m^2 in G_1, S, or asynchronous growth showed approximately the same survival as XP12BE cells given 0.7 J/m^2, suggesting that each set of NF cells including those irradiated with 7 J/m^2 just at the onset of S had sufficient time to reduce the damage to the equivalent of 0.7 J/m^2. We suggest that the amount of time available for excision before cell death is regulated by the cells' need for critical cellular proteins and their respective mRNAs, so that if the DNA template for transcription of these mRNAs is still blocked by lesions at the time the cell has need of them, reproductive death (i.e., inability to form a colony) is the result (21). Although the kinds of proteins being synthesized by cells in early G_1 undoubtedly differ from those being synthesized by cells just prior to S, the overall average need for transcription and translation by the two populations may well be comparable. If so, this could explain why the lethal effect of low doses of UV was comparable in the two populations.

The hypothesis that the cells' need for some critical proteins at some point subsequent to irradiation is responsible for cell death can also explain why cells irradiated in confluence (G_0) and then held for 8 or 16 hr before being allowed to cycle showed a higher survival than cells released immediately (25): G_0 cells have a lower metabolic state than do cells in exponential growth, and, therefore, following irradiation, fewer critical proteins are needed immediately than are needed by cells released and allowed to begin the cell cycle. Therefore, these cells have time to remove the blocking DNA damage. This conclusion is consistent with the fact that XP12BE cells, which do not remove such lesions, show no dose-modifying effect when held in the G_0 state (25).

Recent biochemical evidence supports this hypothesis. Hildebrand and Strniste (16) measured the level of an inducible enzyme in NF and XP12BE cells after UV irradiation. Synthesis was initially blocked in both cell strains equally, but with time held in confluence, the NF cells recovered their ability to synthesize the enzyme, whereas the XP cells did not. Significantly, the kinetics of recovery of protein synthesis correlated with our data on the kinetics of recovery of NF cells from potentially lethal damage, dimer excision, and repair replication (22). Similarly, Ben-Hur et al. (6) showed in irradiated Chinese hamster cells a gradual recovery of synthesis of an inducible enzyme with time held in the plateau phase. Kantor et al. (20) came to a similar conclusion, that the lethal effect of UV results from faulty RNA transcription caused by photoproducts in DNA leading to inhibition of required protein synthesis, because they found that even in the absence of DNA synthesis and mitosis, it took a much higher dose of UV to cause NF cells to detach from the surface of the dishes after several days than was needed for XP12BE cells.

We carried out a similar study using anti-BPDE as the mutagenic agent (48). The results (Fig. 8) were essentially the same as those described here for UV radiation. The data support the hypothesis that the critical cellular event responsible for BPDE-induced

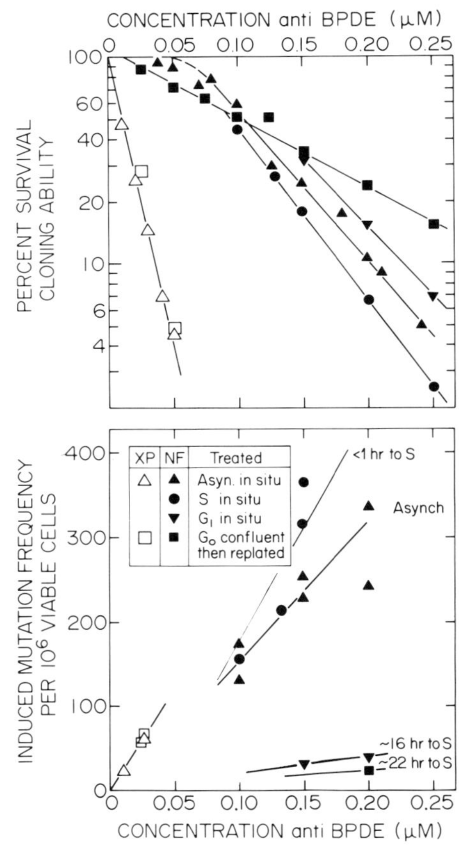

FIG. 8. Cytotoxicity (**upper panel**) and frequency of mutations to thioguanine resistance (**lower panel**) induced by low doses of anti BPDE in normal (**closed symbols**) and XP12BE (**open symbols**) cells treated under conditions designed to allow various lengths of time between treatment and the onset of S phase. (From Yang et al., ref. 48, with permission.)

mutagenesis is DNA synthesis on a template containing unexcised lesions but that this is not the major critical cellular event responsible for cell death. Instead, some cellular event occurring subsequent to carcinogen exposure and amenable to the dose-modifying effect of excision repair, yet not directly related to DNA synthesis, eventually brings about the lethality. We suggest that reproductive death results from inability to carry out required protein synthesis because of faulty or blocked transcription from DNA containing unexcised DNA–BPDE adducts (48).

QUANTITATIVE STUDIES OF TRANSFORMATION OF HUMAN CELLS BY CARCINOGENS

Carcinogen-induced transformation of mammalian cells has been carried out by a number of workers using cells obtained from various species (see 35 for review). Because cell lines that have unlimited life-spans are usually easier to handle in culture than primary or early-passage human or animal cells, they are often preferred. However, since cell lines already have some of the characteristics of transformed cells, transformation of such cells may not truly recapitulate the process by which a normal cell becomes a tumor cell. Therefore, for studies on the mechanisms of neoplastic transformation, it is preferable to utilize diploid cells with finite lifespans.

The most widely used system of this type is the cell transformation assay originally developed by Berwald and Sachs (7). Since then, a number of workers have developed this assay further (3–5,11a,38). In this assay, early-passage diploid cells derived from hamster embryos are treated with carcinogen and a portion plated at cloning density. Morphologically transformed colonies, characterized by abnormal growth patterns, develop in the treated populations at a high frequency (0.1–1%). The cells in these morphologically transformed colonies are not tumorigenic per se (3). However, cells able to cause tumors arise randomly in progeny of the carcinogen-treated cultures 35 to 70 population doublings after treatment. This delay makes it difficult to associate the ultimate tumorigenicity with the carcinogen treatment.

Since our purpose in carrying out transformation studies was to determine the mechanisms by which carcinogens induce cancer in human beings, diploid human fibroblasts in culture seemed to be the ideal cells. However, for many years, workers had tried without success to induce the transformation of human fibroblasts with carcinogens. Finally, in 1977, Kakunaga (17) demonstrated that human fibroblasts treated with a carcinogen could give rise to cells that formed foci (small areas, apparently clonal in origin, where cells grow in a three-dimensional array) on top of confluent monolayers. The progeny of these cells proved to be tumorigenic in athymic mice. Further work by Kakunaga (18), Milo and DiPaulo (33), Borek (8), Sutherland et al. (43,44), and ourselves (30,32,41) has extended this research to additional chemical carcinogens and radiation.

In the past, most workers who were developing transformation assays have assumed either explicitly or implicitly that the transformation events are not the result of mutations. This may seem surprising, since it is now a well-demonstrated fact that most carcinogens are mutagens. However, at the time, this view was not yet so widely accepted. Consequently, most transformation assays were not designed to simultaneously yield information on transformation frequencies and mutation frequencies using the same treated cell populations. Furthermore, the protocols used often prevented one from recognizing whether mutations were involved in transformation.

Since we had had extensive experience developing mutation assays for diploid human fibroblasts before we began development of a transformation assay, and since we believed that the transformation process was likely to involve one or more mutagenic events, we deliberately designed a human cell transformation assay modeled after our human cell mutagenesis assay (32). For example, we expected the process of transformation of human fibroblasts to have in common with the process of mutagenesis (a) an expression period, i.e., a period of time between carcinogen damage to cells and their ability to express the new (i.e., transformed) phenotype; (b) a linear increase in the frequency of transformants with increase in carcinogen dose; (c) a concentration dependence for the carcinogenic agent that resembled that required for induction of mutations, so that strong mutagens would usually be strong transforming agents; (d) a low but measurable frequency of transformed cells in non-carcinogen-treated cell populations just as one finds a low but measurable frequency of mutant cells in such populations; (e) a higher frequency of transformation per dose in DNA repair-deficient cells than in normal cells, as we had shown for the induction of mutants in XP cells; (f) a cell cycle dependence similar to that which occurs for mutation induction, so that populations of cells treated just before S phase would show a higher frequency of transformation than cell populations treated with the same dose of the agent far from S phase. As discussed below, our studies indicate that the human cell transformation process has each of these characteristics.

The protocol that we have developed to assay the transformation of human fibroblasts is based on the induction of ability to grow in an anchorage-independent manner following carcinogen treatment. The basic procedure is to treat human fibroblasts with reactive derivatives of chemical carcinogens or radiation (UV or ionizing), using doses that lower the survival as judged by cloning to between 40 and 10% of the control population. The surviving cells are kept in exponential growth for 8 to 10 population doublings to allow full expression of the anchorage-independent phenotype and are then plated as single cells into medium containing 0.33% agar. Colonies of anchorage-independent cells develop to a size that can be counted (>0.1 mm) after about 3 to 4 weeks. These anchorage-independent cells are tested for tumorigenicity by isolating colonies, propagating them into large populations, and injecting them s.c. into sublethally X-irradiated athymic mice. (In these animals, nontransformed human cells cannot grow, whereas malignant cells derived from human tumors are able to multiply.) We found that injection of 10^7 anchorage-independent cells yield fibrosarcomas at the site of injection. No tumors form when $>2 \times 10^7$ nontransformed cells are injected. When cells from the tumors are isolated and returned to culture, they are found to have a human karyotype and to produce new tumors on reinjection into athymic mice.

TRANSFORMATION AND MUTATION OF HUMAN CELLS BY PROPANE SULTONE

Our first large scale studies on human cell transformation were undertaken using the carcinogen propane sultone (41) because it was reported to give high frequencies of transformation (G. Milo, *personal communication*). We determined its cytotoxic effect on the cells using survival of colony-forming ability as our method because of the superiority of this method over other means of assessing cell toxicity (40). As can be seen in Fig. 9A, propane sultone produces dose-dependent killing. We next determined the optimal time for expression of anchorage-independent growth after propane sultone treatment by assaying the cells after various numbers of population doublings following treatment with a dose of propane sultone giving 22% survival. Figure 10 shows that the optimal expression period is 8 to 11 popu-

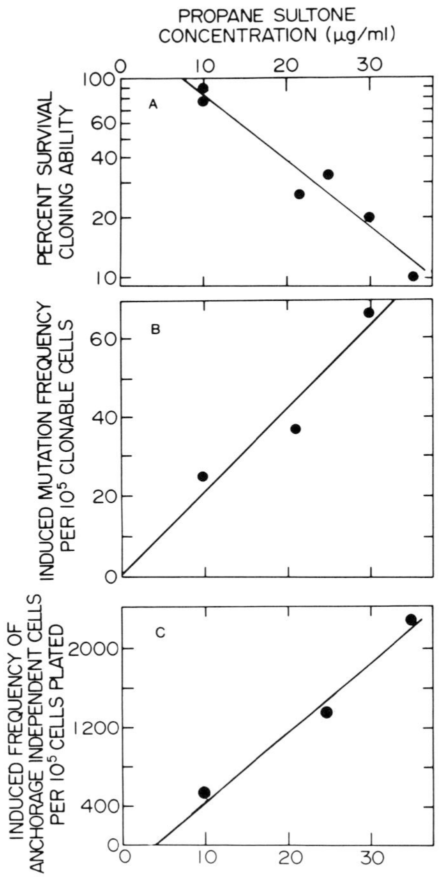

FIG. 9. The cytotoxicity, mutagenicity, and ability of various concentrations of propane sultone to induce anchorage-independent growth. Cells were synchronized and exposed to the carcinogen just after the onset of S phase. After 14 hr, an aliquot was assayed for initial cytotoxicity, and the rest was subcultured. The cells were assayed as described for resistance to thioguanine after five to six population doublings. They were assayed as described for anchorage independence after 10 to 11 doublings. (From Silinskas et al., ref. 41, with permission.)

lation doublings and that the frequency of anchorage-independent cells declines after 13 doublings. (Such a decline is expected if the anchorage-independent cells are at a slight selective growth disadvantage compared to anchorage-dependent cells when growing on plastic.)

Once we knew the optimal expression period, we carried out a study of the dose response for transformation using the agent. The results are shown in Fig. 9C. We then carried out mutagenicity studies to determine whether the concentrations of propane sultone required for the induction of thioguanine-resistant mutants were similar to those required for the induction of anchorage-independent growth in these cells. The results, shown in Fig. 9B, demonstrated this was indeed the case. When propane sultone-induced and spontaneously occurring anchorage-independent colonies were isolated from agar, grown to large cell populations, and injected into mice, they yielded fibrosarcomas in 2 to 3 weeks.

STUDIES OF THE ROLE OF DNA EXCISION REPAIR IN THE TRANSFORMATION PROCESS

Dose–response studies similar to those shown for propane sultone were also carried out with a number of other chemical carcinogens (J. J. McCormick, and V. M. Maher *unpublished data*). However, we wanted to determine whether DNA excision repair processes would protect human cells from the potentially transforming effect of exposure to carcinogens (30). In addition, we wanted to see if transformation to anchorage independence would exhibit the same cell cycle dependence we found for the induction of mutations to thioguanine resistance. Therefore, we chose UV radiation (254 nm) as our carcinogen and compared the frequency of transformation induced by UV in excision repair-proficient normal cells with that in repair-deficient xeroderma pigmentosum cells. For these particular studies, we chose XP cells from patient XP12BE of complementation group A (with little or no excision capability) and XP7BE of complementation group D (cells with ~25% the normal rate of DNA excision repair) (39) because they form colonies on plastic surfaces with ap-

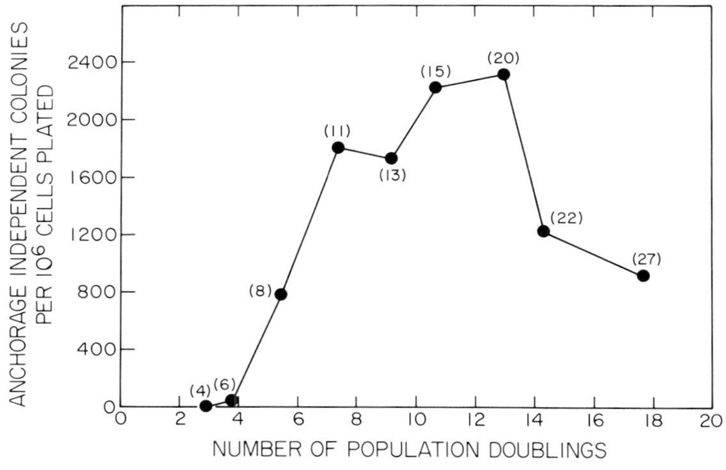

FIG. 10. Kinetics of expression of anchorage independence. Cells treated with 21.5 μg of propane sultone per ml for 14 hr after the cells entered S phase. The surviving population (28%) as well as the control population were trypsinized, diluted 1:2, replated, and kept in exponential growth by continuous subculturing as required. On each of the days indicated in parentheses, 2 to 5 × 10^6 cells were trypsinized, pooled, and counted to determine the number of population doublings which had occurred. For each determination, 10^6 cells were assayed for anchorage-independent growth (5 × 10^4 cells/dish), and the rest were replated for continued propagation and subsequent assay. (From Silinskas et al., ref. 41, with permission.)

proximately the same cloning efficiency as normal cells (i.e., 20–50%). Note that these XP cells are not malignant; the biopsies from which they are derived are always obtained from non-sunlight-exposed areas of the skin. This is confirmed by the fact that injection of >2 × 10^7 cells into athymic mice did not produce tumors (30).

The survival data (Fig. 11, top) show that the XP cells are significantly more sensitive than NF cells to the lethal effect of UV; e.g., a dose of 0.5 or 1.1 J/m^2 decreased their survival to 20%, whereas 7.5 J/m^2 was required to cause the same decrease in NF cells. The mutagenicity data (frequency of thioguanine-resistant cells in the population; Fig. 11, middle) show that the XP cells are significantly more sensitive than NF cells to the mutagenic action of UV radiation. Similar data were obtained earlier with XP12BE (cf. Figs. 2 and 7) and in XP7BE, using a different genetic marker (13). The mutant frequencies were corrected for the cloning efficiency of the cells because we showed that, under the selection conditions, their cloning efficiency is similar to that of cells plated at cloning density in the absence of selection.

The transformation frequency data (Fig. 11, bottom) indicate that the XP cells are also significantly more sensitive than the NF cells to UV-induced loss of anchorage dependence. These particular data were obtained by assaying the progeny of the irradiated cells after an expression period of about nine population doublings. However, in the majority of cases, the frequency of anchorage-independent cells was assayed twice, i.e., after 9 and 11 doublings, and yielded approximately the same frequencies both times. (Note that these data are the observed frequencies of agar colonies counted directly, without a correction factor.) The background frequencies have not been subtracted. The data indicate that to achieve a particular degree of cell killing, mutagenesis, and transformation, NF cells have to be exposed to 8- to 10-fold higher doses of UV radiation then XP cells. As discussed above,

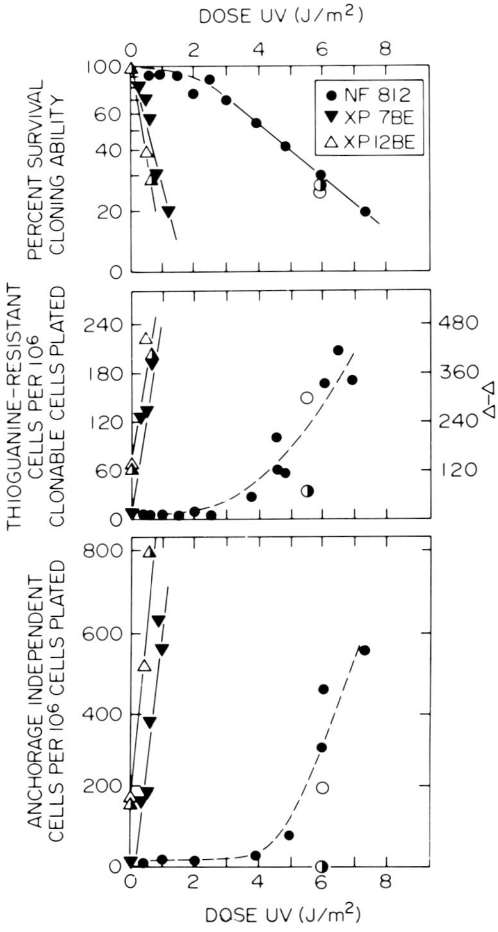

FIG. 11. Cytotoxicity, mutagenicity, and transforming ability of UV radiation in normal (*circles*) and XP cells (XP2BE, *triangle;* XP7BE, *inverted triangles*). The frequency of thioguanine resistant cells were assayed after six doublings; that of anchorage-independent cells, after 9 to 11 doublings. The former were corrected for cloning efficiency on plastic. *Solid symbols,* populations irradiated in exponential growth; *open symbols,* cells synchronized by release from confluence and irradiated shortly before onset of S phase; *half-solid symbols,* cells irradiated 18 to 20 hr prior to S. See text for details.

this is the result expected if induction of anchorage independence as well as thioguanine resistance results ultimately from DNA damage remaining unexcised in the cell at some critical time after irradiation and if, because of the difference in their respective rates of excision repair, the average number of lesions remaining at this critical time is approximately equal in the three populations.

EFFECT OF TIME FOR EXCISION REPAIR BEFORE S ON FREQUENCY OF ANCHORAGE INDEPENDENCE IN REPAIR-PROFICIENT NORMAL CELLS

We showed (Fig. 7) that if synchronous populations of NF cells are irradiated shortly before the onset of S phase, the frequency of induced thioguanine-resistant cells is sixfold higher than in the same cells treated 18 hr prior to S. No such difference was observed when the target cells were virtually incapable of excision repair. To determine if a similar cell cycle effect occurred for induction of transformation, we irradiated NF and XP12BE cells in early and late G_1 and assayed their progeny for frequency of anchorage independence. As shown in Fig. 11 as open and half-solid symbols, the survival of the two populations did not differ significantly and was similar to that of cells irradiated in exponential growth. In contrast, the transformation frequencies of the repair-proficient normal cells showed a strong cell cycle dependence; i.e., cells irradiated with 6 J/m^2 ~3 hr prior to onset of S phase yielded 200 anchorage-independent cells per 10^6 cells plated; cells irradiated ~20 hr prior to S gave no cells capable of soft agar growth out of 2×10^6 cells plated. The control cells in this experiment also gave no colonies out of 2×10^6. In contrast, the frequency of anchorage independence in XP12BE cells irradiated in early G_1 did not decrease; in fact, it was somewhat higher. In the corresponding mutation experiment, the frequencies were equal. In the mutagenesis experiments with normal cells from which the data in the middle panel were taken, the frequency of mutant cells did not decrease completely to the background level. However, in that experiment, the cells irradiated in G_1 had somewhat less time for excision repair before onset of S than was available in the transformation experiments.

An explanation for the fact that to obtain equal cell killing and equal frequencies of transformation (and mutagenesis) in the two cell strains, the normal cells had to be irradiated with 8- to 10-fold higher doses of UV is this: Low doses induced low numbers of DNA lesions in the XP cells, but they were unable to excise many of the potentially cytotoxic, mutagenic, and transforming lesions before these were permanently "fixed" in the cells, whereas high doses induced a high number of lesions in the normal cells but, before these could be permanently fixed, the repair-proficient cells were able to reduce the number to a level approximating that remaining in the XP7BE cells. The fact that allowing substantial time for excision before DNA synthesis eliminated the potentially mutagenic and transforming effect of UV radiation in normal cells but not in XP12BE cells suggests that DNA synthesis on a template still containing unexcised lesions is the cellular event responsible for fixing the mutations and transformation.

An experiment reported by Kakunaga (19) is consistent with this interpretation. He showed that when confluent cultures of a mouse cell line were exposed to 4-nitroquinoline-1-oxide and then allowed to carry out excision repair but not to replicate, the potential for focus formation was gradually eliminated. However, when the cells were allowed to undergo a single population doubling after treatment before attaining confluence, additional time in confluence did not decrease the transformation frequency.

In addition to the information that can be gained by analyzing the 8- to 10-fold differences between XP and NF cells in Fig. 11, it is useful to compare the frequencies of anchorage-independent cells with those of thioguanine-resistant cells. Resistant to thioguanine is a well-characterized mutation marker. As noted, the induction of anchorage independence in human fibroblasts has many characteristics in common with introduction of thioguanine resistance, including a similar expression curve. The similarity of the dose responses for the two phenotypes is obvious and supports the idea that acquisition of anchorage independence (transformation) in human cells occurs as the result of a single mutational event. The frequencies of mutations and transformation differ by a factor of ~2.5. In our earliest experiments, using propane sultone, the difference was ~22-fold (Fig. 9). However, a ratio of 2.5 is much closer to the ratios we now routinely observe with a number of agents. The higher value reported in the early experiments can be attributed in part to the use of a different lot of serum and a different type of agar. Small technical differences in the way the cells were handled may also have contributed to the difference. A third significant difference between our present experiments and those with propane sultone is that in the case of those early experiments, the agar colonies per dish were so numerous that only a representative fraction of them was counted, and the calculated numbers may have been systematically overestimated. In subsequent experiments with propane sultone, in which fewer cells per dish were assayed and every macroscopic colony was counted, the frequency was one-fourth of the early value (see Fig. 10).

If we assume that anchorage independence results from a mutation, we might speculate about the size of the DNA target involved. The observed number of thioguanine-resistant colonies (selected on plastic at a density equivalent to 10^4 cells per 60-mm dish) has been corrected for the cells' intrinsic cloning efficiency (i.e., 30–50%); the number of anchorage-independent cells (selected at a density of 10^5 cells per 3 ml of soft agar), on the other hand, was determined directly from the observed number of agar colonies without correction. There is no simple way to determine the "intrinsic cloning efficiency" under conditions in which 10^5 cells are plated per dish. If the cloning efficiency in agar were less than 100%, the frequencies would have to be increased accordingly. Nevertheless, the relationship between the frequencies observed for thioguanine resistance as well as anchorage independence in the three strains that differ in DNA repair capacity support the hypothesis that mutations are involved in transformation.

CONCLUSION

In summary, our studies indicate that excision repair in diploid human fibroblasts is essentially an error-free process and that the ability to excise potentially cytotoxic and potentially mutagenic or transforming lesions induced in DNA by UV radiation or by several classes of chemical carcinogens determines their ultimate biological consequences. Other classes of carcinogens that form "bulky" lesions in DNA can be expected to give similar results, whereas the results with carcinogens that methylate DNA and with ionizing radiation should be different, since the damage produced by these latter agents is repaired by pathways at least partially different from those studied here. Such studies are in progress. The data presented here suggest that there is a certain amount of time available between the initial exposure and the onset of the cellular events responsible for mutation induction, for cell transformation, and for cell killing and that the critical event for the mutation and transformation is DNA synthesis on a damaged template. In contrast, the cytotoxicity studies indicate that although a population's survival is determined by the extent of excision repair of potentially lethal damage from DNA before some critical cellular event(s), there is no single cell-cycle-related event such as DNA synthesis on a damaged template that determines cytotoxicity.

ACKNOWLEDGMENTS

We wish to express our indebtedness to our colleagues, A. E. Aust, J. C. Ball, N. R. Drinkwater, R. H. Heflich, B. Konze-Thomas, J. W. Levinson, K. C. Silinskas, and L. L. Yang for their invaluable contributions to the research summarized here. The excellent technical assistance of R. Corner, D. J. Dorney, R. M. Hazard, S. A. Kateley, T. E. Kinney, L. D. Milam, M. Moon, T. G. O'Callaghan, L. A. Rowan, D. Richmond, and T. VanNoord is gratefully acknowledged. The labeled anti-BPDE was provided by the Cancer Research Program of the National Cancer Institute, and the labeled aromatic amines by Dr. John Scribner of the Pacific Northwest Research Foundation. The research summarized in this report was supported in part by Contract ES-78-4659 from the Department of Energy and by Grants CA 21247, CA 21253, CA 21289, and ES 07076 from the Department of Health and Human Services, NIH. Additional financial assistance was provided by the Michigan Osteopathic College Foundation.

REFERENCES

1. Aust, A. E., Antczak, M. R., Maher, V. M., and McCormick, J. J. (1981): Identifying human cells capable of metabolizing various classes of carcinogens. *J. Supramol. Struct. Cell Biochem.,* 16:269–279.
2. Aust, A. E., Falahee, K. J., Maher, V. M., and McCormick, J. J. (1980): Human cell-mediated benzo(a)pyrene cytotoxicity and mutagenicity in human diploid fibroblasts. *Cancer Res.,* 40:4070–4075.
3. Barrett, J. C., Crawford, B. D., and Ts'o, P. O. P. (1980): The role of somatic mutation in a multistage model of carcinogenesis. In: *Mammalial Cell Transformation by Chemical Carcinogens,* edited by N. Mishra, V. Dunkel, and M. Mehlman, pp. 467–501. Senate Press, Princeton.
4. Barrett, J. C., and Ts'o, P. O. P. (1978): The relationship between somatic mutation and neoplastic transformation. *Proc. Natl. Acad. Sci. U.S.A.,* 75:3297–3301.
5. Barrett, J. C., and Ts'o, P. O. P. (1978): Evidence for the progressive nature of neoplastic transformation *in vitro. Proc. Natl. Acad. Sci. U.S.A.,* 75:3761–3765.
6. Ben-Hur, E., Heimer, Y. M., and Riklis, E. (1980): Recovery from inhibition by radiation of transcriptionally controlled enzyme induction. *FEBS Lett.,* 120:21–23.
7. Berwald, Y., and Sachs, L. (1965): *In vitro* transformation of normal cells to tumor cells by carcinogenic hydrocarbons. *J. Natl. Cancer Inst.,* 35:641–661.

8. Borek, C. (1980): X-ray-induced *in vitro* neoplastic transformation of human diploid cells. *Nature,* 283:776–778.
9. Cerutti, P. A., and Remsen, J. F. (1977): Formation and repair of DNA damage induced by oxygen radical species in human cells. In: *DNA Repair Processes,* edited by W. W. Nichols and D. G. Murphy, pp. 147–166. Symposium Specialists, Miami.
10. Cleaver, J. E., and Bootsma, B. (1975): Xeroderma pigmentosum: Biochemical and genetic characteristics. *Annu. Rev. Genet.,* 9:19–38.
11. Didinsky, J. B., and Rheinwald, J. G. (1981): Failure of hydrocortisone or growth factors to influence the senescence of fibroblasts in a new culture system for assessing replicative lifespan. *J. Cell. Physiol.,* 109:171–179.
11a. DiPaolo, J. A. (1980): Quantitative in vitro transformation of Syrian golden hamster embryo cells with the use of frozen stored cells. *J. Natl. Cancer Inst.,* 64:1485–1489.
12. Drinkwater, N. R., Corner, R. C., McCormick, J. J., and Maher, V. M. (1982): An *in situ* assay for induced diphtheria toxin resistant mutants of diploid human fibroblasts. *Mutat. Res.,* 106:277–289.
13. Glover, T. W., Chang, C.-C., Trosko, J. E., and Li, S. S.-L. (1979): Ultraviolet light induction of diphtheria toxin-resistant mutants in normal and xeroderma pigmentosum human fibroblasts. *Proc. Natl. Acad. Sci. U.S.A.,* 76:3982–3986.
14. Hayflick, L. (1965): The limited *in vitro* lifetime of human diploid cell strains. *Exp. Cell Res.,* 37:614–636.
15. Heflich, R. H., Hazard, R. M., Lommel, L., Scribner, J. D., Maher, V. M., and McCormick, J. J. (1980): A comparison of the DNA binding, cytotoxicity and repair synthesis induced in human fibroblasts by reactive derivatives of aromatic amide carcinogens. *Chem. Biol. Interact.,* 29:43–56.
16. Hildebrand, C. E., and Strniste, G. F. (1981): Differential reactivation of zinc-mediated metallothionein induction in ultraviolet-irradiated normal and repair-deficient human cells. *J. Supramol. Struct. Cell Biochem.,* 16:121–133.
17. Kakunaga, T. (1977): The transformation of human diploid cells by chemical carcinogens. In: *Origins of Human Cancer, Vol. C,* edited by H. H. Hiatt, J. D. Watson, J. A. Winsten, pp. 1537–1548. Cold Spring Harbor Laboratory Press, Cold Spring Harbor, New York.
18. Kakunaga, T. (1978): Neoplastic transformation of human diploid fibroblast cells by chemical carcinogens. *Proc. Natl. Acad. Sci., U.S.A.,* 75:1334–1338.
19. Kakunaga, T. (1974): Requirement for cell replication in the fixation and expression of the transformed state in mouse cells treated with 4-nitroquinoline-1-oxide. *Int. J. Cancer,* 14:736–742.
20. Kantor, G. J., Warner, C., and Hull, D. R. (1977): The effect of ultraviolet light on arrested human diploid cell populations. *Photochem. Photobiol.,* 25:483–489.
21. Konze-Thomas, B., Hazard, R. M., Maher, V. M., and McCormick, J. J. (1982): Extent of excision repair before DNA synthesis determines the mutagenic but not the lethal effect of UV radiation. *Mutat. Res.,* 94:421–434.
22. Konze-Thomas, B., Levinson, J. W., Maher, V. M., and McCormick, J. J. (1979): Correlation among the rates of dimer excision, DNA repair replication, and recovery of human cells from potentially lethal damage induced by ultraviolet radiation. *Biophys. J.,* 28:315–326.
23. Lippke, J. A., Gordon, L. K., Brash, D. E., and Haseltine, W. A. (1981): Distribution of ultraviolet light induced damage in a defined sequence of human DNA: Detection of alkaline sensitive lesions at pyrimidine-nucleoside-cytidine sequences. *Proc. Natl. Acad. Sci. U.S.A.,* 78:3388–3392.
24. Maher, V. M., Birch, N., Otto, J. R., and McCormick, J. J. (1975): Cytotoxicity of carcinogenic aromatic amides in normal and xeroderma pigmentosum fibroblasts with different DNA repair capabilities. *J. Natl. Cancer Inst.,* 54:1287–1294.
25. Maher, V. M., Dorney, D. J., Mendrala, A. L., Konze-Thomas, B., and McCormick, J. J. (1979): DNA excision repair processes in human cells can eliminate the cytotoxic and mutagenic consequences of ultraviolet irradiation. *Mutat. Res.,* 62:311–323.
26. Maher, V. M., Heflich, R. H., and McCormick, J. J. (1981): Repair of DNA damage induced in human fibroblasts by N-substituted aryl compounds. In: *Carcinogenic and Mutagenic N-Substituted Aryl Compounds,* edited by E. K. Weisberger et al., pp. 217–222. National Cancer Institute, Bethesda.
27. Maher, V. M., and McCormick, J. J. (1976): Effect of DNA repair on the cytotoxicity and mutagenicity of UV irradiation and of chemical carcinogens in normal and xeroderma pigmentosum cells. In: *Biology of Radiation Carcinogenesis,* edited by J. M. Yuhas, R. W. Tennant, and J. D. Regan, pp. 129–145. Raven Press, New York.
28. Maher, V. M., and McCormick, J. J. (1982): Excision repair by human cells of the potentially mutagenic, carcinogenic and lethal lesions formed in DNA by carcinogens. In: *Mechanisms of Chemical Carcinogenesis,* edited by C. Harris and P. A. Cerutti, pp. 429–439. Alan R. Liss, New York.
29. Maher, V. M., McCormick, J. J., Grover, P. L., and Sims, P. (1977): Effect of DNA repair on the cytotoxicity and mutagenicity of polycyclic hydrocarbon derivatives in normal and xeroderma pigmentosum human fibroblasts. *Mutat. Res.,* 43:117–138.
30. Maher, V. M., Rowan, L. A., Silinskas, K. C., Kateley, S. A., and McCormick, J. J. (1982): Frequency of UV-induced neoplastic transformation of diploid human fibroblasts is higher in xeroderma pigmentosum cells than in normal cells. *Proc. Natl. Acad. Sci. U.S.A.,* 79:2613–2617.
31. McCormick, J. J., and Maher, V. M. (1981): Measurement of colony-forming ability and mutagenesis in diploid human cells. In: *DNA Repair: A Laboratory Manual of Research Procedures, Vol. 1, Part B,* edited by E. C. Friedberg and P. C. Hanawalt, pp. 501–521. Marcel Dekker, New York.
32. McCormick, J. J., Silinskas, K. C., and Maher,

V. M. (1980): Transformation of diploid human fibroblasts by chemical carcinogens. In: *Carcinogenesis, Fundamental Mechanisms and Environmental Effects,* edited by B. Pullman, P. O. P. Ts'o, and H. Gelboin, pp. 491–498. D. Reidel, Dordrecht.

33. Milo, G. E., Jr., and DiPaolo, J. A. (1978): Neoplastic transformation of human diploid cells in vitro after chemical carcinogen treatment. *Nature,* 275:130–132.
34. Milo, G. E., Oldham, J. W., Zimmerman, R., Hatch, G. G., and Weisbrode, S. A. (1981): Characterization of human cells transformed by chemical and physical carcinogens *in vitro. In Vitro,* 17:719–729.
35. Mishra, N., Dunkel, V., and Mehlman, M. (1980): *Mammalian Cell Transformation by Chemical Carcinogens.* Senate Press, Princeton Junction, New Jersey.
36. Peleg, L., Raz, E., and Ben-Ishai, R. (1976): Changing capacity for DNA excision repair in mouse embryonic cells *in vitro. Exp. Cell Res.,* 104:301–307.
37. Petinga, R. A., Andrews, A. D., Tarone, R. E., and Robbins, J. H. (1977): Typical xeroderma pigmentosum complementation group A fibroblasts have detectable ultraviolet light-induced unscheduled DNA synthesis. *Biochim. Biophys. Acta,* 479:400–410.
38. Pienta, R. J., Poiley, J. A., and Lebherz, W. B. (1977): Morphological transformation by early passage golden Syrian hamster embryo cells derived from cryopreserved primary cultures as a reliable in vitro bioassay for identifying diverse carcinogens. *Int. J. Cancer,* 19:642–655.
39. Robbins, J. H., Kraemer, K. H., Lutzner, M. A., Festoff, B. W., and Coon, H. G. (1974): Xeroderma pigmentosum, an inherited disease with sun sensitivity, multiple cutaneous neoplasms, and abnormal DNA repair. *Ann. Intern. Med.,* 80:221–248.
40. Roper, P. R., and Drewinko, B. (1976): Comparison of *in vitro* methods to determine drug-induced cell lethality. *Cancer Res.,* 36:2182–2188.
41. Silinskas, K. C., Kateley, S. A., Tower, J. E., Maher, V. M., and McCormick, J. J. (1981): Induction of anchorage independent growth in human fibroblasts by propane sultone. *Cancer Res.,* 41:1620–1627.
42. Stanford, K. K., Parshad, R., and Gantt, R. (1978): Light and oxygen effects on chromosomes, DNA, and neoplastic transformation of cells in culture. In: *Nutritional Requirements of Cultured Cells,* edited by H. Katsuta, pp. 117–148. University Park Press, Baltimore.
43. Sutherland, B. M., Cemino, J. S., Delihas, N., Shih, A. G., and Oliver, R. P. (1980): Ultraviolet light induced transformation of human cells to anchorage independent growth. *Cancer Res.,* 40:1934–1939.
44. Sutherland, B. M., Delihas, N. C., Oliver, R. P., and Sutherland, J. C. (1981): Action spectra for ultraviolet light-induced transformation of human cells to anchorage-independent growth. *Cancer Res.,* 41:2211–2214.
45. Weinstein, I. B., Jeffrey, A. M., Jennette, K. W., Blobstein, S. H., Harvey, R. G., Harris, C., Autrup, H., Kasai, H., and Nakanishi, K. (1976): Benzo(a)pyrene diol epoxides as intermediates in nucleic acid binding *in vitro* and *in vivo. Science,* 193:592–595.
46. Witkin, E. M. (1976): Ultraviolet mutagenesis and inducible DNA repair in *Escherichia coli. Bacteriol. Rev.,* 40:869–907.
47. Yang, L. L., Maher, V. M., and McCormick, J. J. (1980): Error-free excision of the cytotoxic, mutagenic N^2-deoxyguanosine DNA adduct formed in human fibroblasts by $(\pm)$-7β,8α-dihydroxy-9α,10α-epoxy-7,8,9,10-tetrahydrobenzo(a)pyrene. *Proc. Natl. Acad. Sci. U.S.A.,* 77:5933–5937.
48. Yang, L. L., Maher, V. M., and McCormick, J. J. (1982): Relationship between excision repair and the cytotoxic and mutagenic effect of the "anti" 7,8-diol-9,10-epoxide of benzo(a)pyrene in human cells. *Mutat. Res.,* 94:435–447.

Drug Metabolism and Drug Toxicity,
edited by J. R. Mitchell and M. G. Horning.
Raven Press, New York © 1984.

Metabolic Processing of Aromatic Amides

Snorri S. Thorgeirsson, Michael E. McManus, and Irene B. Glowinski

Laboratory of Carcinogen Metabolism, Division of Cancer Cause and Prevention, National Cancer Institute, National Institutes of Health, Bethesda, Maryland 20205

It is now well established that most known chemical carcinogens require metabolism in the organism before their carcinogenic potential is expressed (24,26). This metabolic processing of foreign chemicals generally involves several enzyme-catalyzed pathways and results in less toxic and readily excretable derivatives (detoxification). An exception to this general rule occurs when unstable and highly toxic metabolites are formed (metabolic activation), and these metabolites have been implicated in the initiation process of chemical carcinogenesis. Therefore, definition of the factors that determine the balance between detoxification and metabolic activation is central to an understanding of the process of chemical carcinogenesis.

Aromatic amines and amides have been among the most studied chemical carcinogens since the initial demonstration of the formation of liver tumors in rats following the administration of *o*-aminoazotoluene [2,2′-dimethyl-(-4-aminoazobenzene)] (45). Studies with 2-acetylaminofluorene (AAF) and its derivatives have provided the most extensive data on the mechanism by which aromatic amides cause neoplasia (24,26,42). Our laboratory has been studying the mechanism of metabolic activation of *N*-acetylarylamides and how the metabolic processing of these compounds influences their capacity to cause genotoxic damage (33,34,39,40, 43,44). In this chapter we use AAF as a model compound to examine the metabolic processing of chemical carcinogens.

OXIDATIVE METABOLISM

Compounds such as AAF are highly lipophilic and are extensively metabolized before excretion from the body. The numerous metabolic pathways that are involved in the metabolism of *N*-acetylarylamines are illustrated in Fig. 1. The discovery of *N*-hydroxy-2-acetylaminofluorene (N-OH-AAF) in urine of rats fed AAF (4) led to the hypothesis that *N*-hydroxylation was both the first and obligatory step in the metabolic activation of these compounds (24,25). The importance of *N*-hydroxylation in the metabolic activation of aromatic amines and amides has now been thoroughly substantiated by numerous laboratories (21,24,39,42).

In contrast to the *N*-hydroxylation of AAF, oxidation of various carbon atoms in the fluorene ring system (Fig. 2) are considered detoxification pathways (42). Both *N*- and *C*-hydroxylations of AAF are mediated via the cytochrome P-450 system (37,42), which is composed of a family of isoenzymes that differ with respect to both genetic regulation and substrate specificity (13,39). Evidence derived primarily from the effects of inducing agents on the activity of AAF *N*-hydroxylation has implicated specific forms (isoenzymes) of the cytochrome in AAF activation. In the rabbit (2,3) and several other species (36,39), *N*-hydroxylation of AAF is induced by both 2,3,7,8-tetrachlorodibenzo-*p*-dioxin (TCDD) and 3-methylcholanthrene (MC). Several isoenzymes of cytochrome

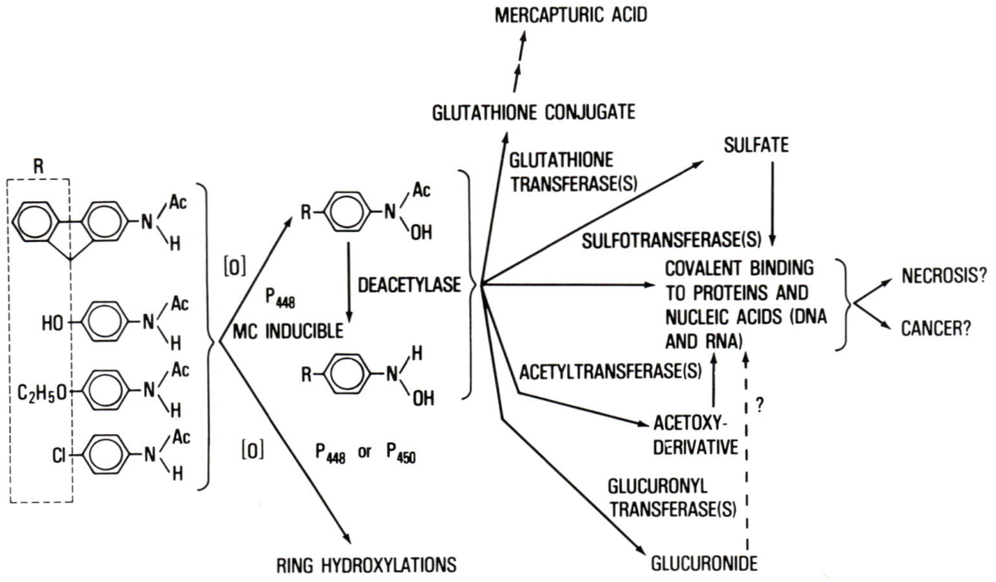

FIG. 1. Possible reaction pathways for *N*-acetylarylamides.

P-450 have been purified and their significance in the metabolism of AAF investigated. Johnson et al. (14) demonstrated that four highly purified forms of rabbit hepatic cytochrome P-450 differ with respect to both rate and site specificity of AAF oxidation (Table 1). Form 4, the major isoenzyme of cytochrome P-450 induced by TCDD in adult rabbits, was the only form that catalyzed *N*-hydroxylation. This accounted for approximately 75% of the metabolites produced by the action of this cytochrome (Table 1). In contrast, form 6, the major isoenzyme of cytochrome P-450 induced by TCDD in neonatal rabbit liver, and form 3, a constitutive form of the cytochrome, both catalyzed the hydroxylation of AAF exclusively in the 7-position. Form 2, the major phenobarbital-inducible cytochrome P-450 in rabbit liver, exhibited no catalytic activity with AAF as substrate. These *in vitro* data are in good agreement with earlier work on the urinary excretion of AAF metabolites by the rabbit, showing that 7-hydroxy-2-acetylaminofluorene (7-OH-AAF) and N-OH-AAF were the major metabolites (7).

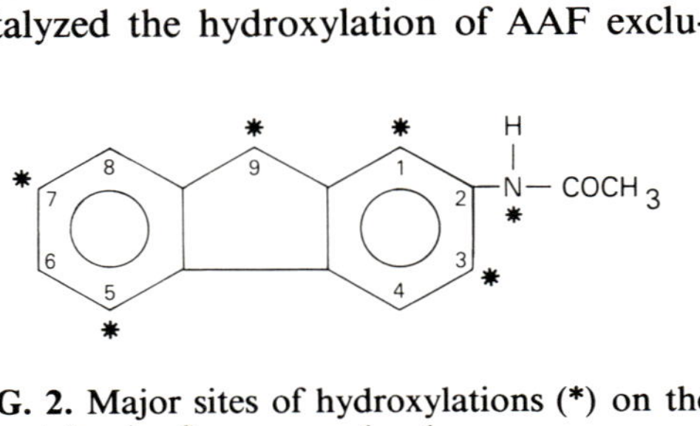

FIG. 2. Major sites of hydroxylations (*) on the 2-acetylaminofluorene molecule.

Cytochrome P-450 forms 3, 4, and 6 catalyze both the activation and detoxification of AAF to different extents (Table 1). This can be conveniently illustrated by representing the metabolism of AAF as a vector, which is the sum of a vector component *A*, giving the rate of *N*-hydroxylation or activation, and a vector component *D*, representing the rate of aromatic hydroxylation or detoxification (form 4 in Fig. 3). The vectors for forms 3 and 6 (not shown) are coincident with the abscissa, since these forms catalyze only the detoxification pathway.

The relationship between the microsomal metabolism of AAF and the activities of the purified cytochromes can be examined using microsomal preparations from PB-, TCDD-,

TABLE 1. *Metabolism of AAF by reconstituted forms of cytochrome P-450*

Metabolite formation	Moles of product formed/min/mole cytochrome P-450[b]		
	Form 3	Form 4	Form 6
7-OH-AAF	0.94 ± 0.07[a]	0.58 ± 0.13	1.13 ± 0.15
5-OH-AAF	0	0.13 ± 0.03	0
3-OH-AAF	0	0.04 ± 0.01	0
1-OH-AAF	0	0.14 ± 0.02	0
N-OH-AAF	0	2.09 ± 0.16	0

[a] Mean ± SD of triplicate experiments with two different preparations of each cytochrome.
[b] Form 2 exhibited no catalytic activity for AAF.
Reprinted with permission from Johnson et al. (14).

and nontreated newborn and adult rabbit livers (14). The relative occurrence of the four cytochromes are different in these preparations. The results of these experiments are shown in Table 2 and are in good agreement with the data obtained in the reconstituted system (Table 1), showing 7-OH-AAF and N-OH-AAF as the major metabolites in microsomes.

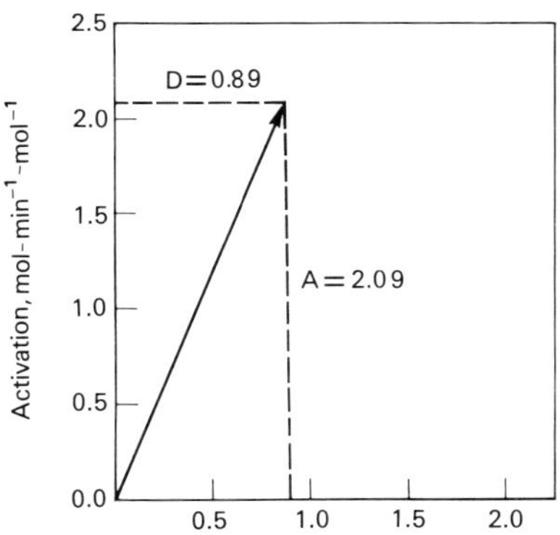

FIG. 3. Vectorial representation of AAF metabolism by rabbit microsomal P-450 form 4. The vector shown is the result of two vectors, *A* and *D*, representing the rates of *N*-hydroxylation and aromatic hydroxylation, respectively. Vectors for forms 3 and 6 (not shown) are coincident with the detoxification axis. The units along each axis are moles of product formed per minute per mole cytochrome P-450. (From Johnson et al., ref. 14, with permission.)

Microsomal metabolism can also be represented as a vector (Fig. 4). In this case, microsomal metabolism will reflect the vector sum of the catalytic contributions of all the cytochrome P-450 forms, including the three purified isoenzymes that are capable of metabolizing AAF. The direction of the metabolic vector for purified form 4 is indicated in Fig. 4 for comparison. In this representation, the correspondence between neonate microsomes (CN, PN, TN) and the detoxification cytochromes (forms 3 and 6) is clearly shown by the coincidence of these vectors with the abscissa (Figs. 3 and 4). The magnitude of neonatal metabolism is lower than the adult activity, reflecting the lower amounts (20%) of cytochrome P-450 in newborn rabbit liver microsomes. Pretreatment of the animal with TCDD increases the cytochrome P-450 content of neonate microsomes (fivefold) by induction of form 6 exclusively (30). As a result, the magnitude of AAF hydroxylation increases, but the direction is not altered. In contrast, the increase in *N*-hydroxylation following TCDD induction in adult animals, reflecting a selective increase in form 4, results in a change in both magnitude and direction of AAF metabolism (Fig. 4). Thus, microsomal metabolism reflects the behavior of the reconstituted cytochromes in a qualitative fashion.

Since form 2 exhibited no measurable AAF hydroxylase activity, its contribution to

TABLE 2. *Effect of age and inducing agents on the* in vitro *microsomal metabolism of AAF*

Sources of microsomes	AAF metabolite formation (nmole of product formed/min/mg protein)		
	7-OH	5-OH	N-OH
Control neonate	0.28 ± 0.02[a]	Trace[b]	Trace
	0.16 ± 0.01	Trace	Trace
TCDD neonate	0.80 ± 0.03	0.04 ± 0.01	Trace
	0.62 ± 0.03	0.03 ± 0.01	Trace
PB neonate	0.39 ± 0.01	Trace	Trace
	0.50 ± 0.01	Trace	Trace
Control adult	0.86 ± 0.04	0.12 ± 0.01	0.17 ± 0.02
	1.65 ± 0.09	0.10 ± 0.01	0.19 ± 0.07
TCDD adult	0.70 ± 0.09	Trace	0.69 ± 0.05
	2.10 ± 0.05	Trace	1.27 ± 0.03
PB adult	2.82 ± 0.01	0.07 ± 0.01	0.31 ± 0.03
	2.41 ± 0.06	0.17 ± 0.01	0.85 ± 0.03

[a] Mean ± SD of duplicate determinations.
[b] Trace, values not significantly greater than blank values ($p > 0.01$).
Reprinted with permission from Johnson et al. (14).

the direction of AAF metabolism is uncertain. Phenobarbital (PB) pretreatment increases AAF *N*-hydroxylase activity in several species (23). However, unlike TCDD, PB induces the cytochrome P-450 reductase in addition to specific cytochrome forms. This in turn could increase the enzymatic activities of cytochromes that are not specifically

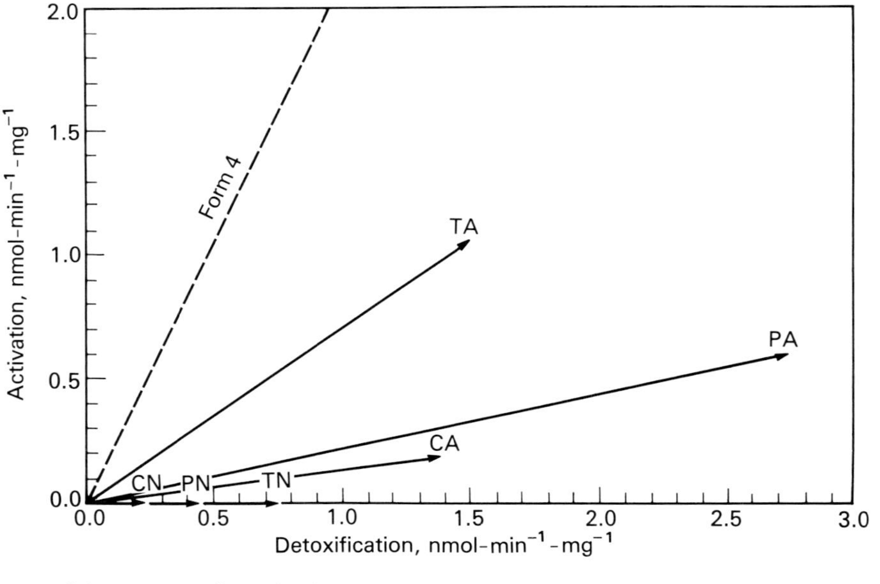

FIG. 4. Vectorial representation of microsomal AAF metabolism. Metabolic vectors are shown for reactions catalyzed by liver microsomes from TCDD-treated (T), PB-treated (P), control (C), and adult (A), and neonate (N) rabbits. *Dashed line,* direction of the vector corresponding to purified cytochrome P-450 form 4. Induction of cytochrome P-450 by TCDD in newborn rabbits increases the magnitude but not the direction of AAF metabolism. In contrast, both the magnitude and the direction of AAF metabolism are affected in the adult. The units along each axis are nmole of product formed per minute per milligram of protein.

induced by PB. Thus, liver microsomes isolated from neonates pretreated with PB were examined. Form 2 was induced in these microsomes against a background of low cytochrome P-450 content (35). In addition, form 4 was not detectable in neonatal microsomes (30). The results of these experiments are also presented in Table 2 and Fig. 4. Phenobarbital pretreatment does not alter the direction of AAF metabolism in the neonate (PN), although the rate of AAF metabolism is increased relative to untreated neonatal microsomes (CN). However, PB effects a change in both the direction and magnitude of AAF metabolism catalyzed by adult rabbit liver microsomes (PA). The observation that PB affects the direction of adult and neonatal metabolism differently, even though form 2 is induced in each case, suggests that the effect of PB on AAF metabolism is mediated primarily by factors other than the induction of form 2.

It is evident from the data presented above that the catalytic activity of the individual cytochromes towards AAF differs in both magnitude and direction. Of the four cytochromes isolated from rabbit liver, forms 3 and 6 catalyze the detoxification of AAF exclusively, whereas form 4 predominantly catalyzes its activation. Form 2, the major PB-inducible cytochrome, does not participate to a significant degree in the metabolism of AAF. Since numerous factors determine the expression of cytochrome P-450, and as carcinogenesis is a multistep process, it is difficult to predict with precision the impact of metabolic differences arising from isoenzyme variability on this carcinogenic process. However, the proportion of the dose of carcinogen that is processed via the initial activation step, as in the case of AAF, is clearly dependent on the relative composition of the different forms of cytochrome P-450 in the organism.

OTHER METABOLIC PATHWAYS

As illustrated in Fig. 5, N-OH-AAF is a substrate for several metabolic pathways that can convert this hydroxamic acid into reactive electrophiles capable of covalent interaction

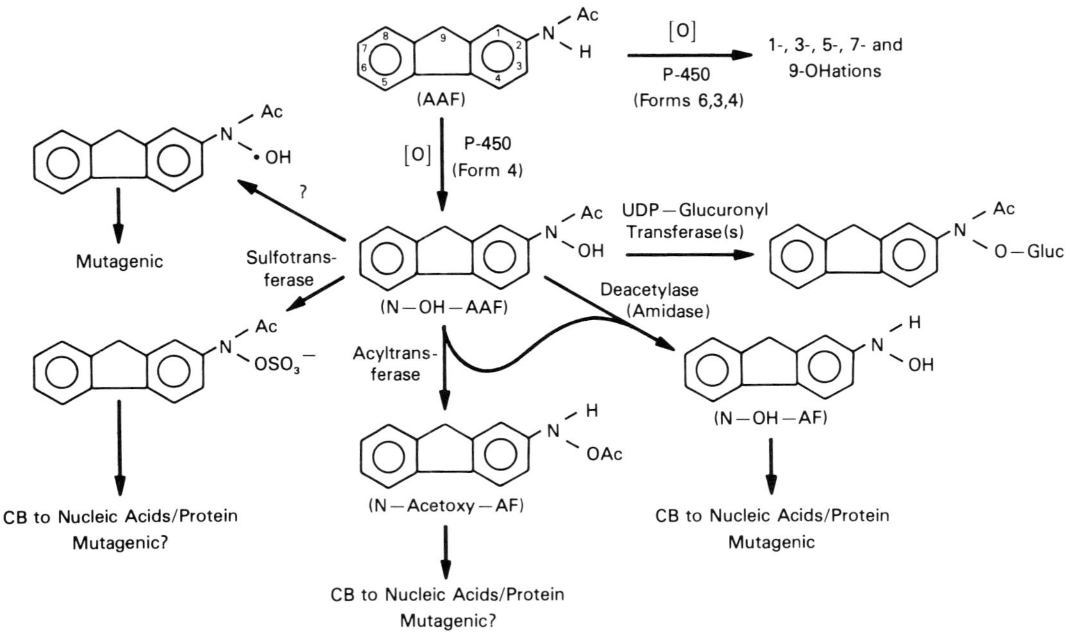

FIG. 5. Metabolic pathways for 2-acetylaminofluorene.

with cellular macromolecules. Although we do not know with certainty the role of each of these pathways in the toxicity and/or the carcinogenicity of N-OH-AAF, the available evidence indicates that sulfotransferase, *N-O*-acyltransferase, and deacetylase are the most important enzymes (44). We therefore devote the remainder of this chapter to the discussion of these three metabolic pathways.

N-Hydroxy-AAF Sulfotransferase

The first indication that sulfotransferase might play an important role in the metabolic activation of N-OH-AAF came from the laboratories of King and Philips (19) and the Millers (5,6). These data demonstrated that incubation of cytosolic (soluble) rat liver proteins with N-OH-AAF, 3′-phosphoadenosine 5′-phosphosulfate, Mg^{2+} or Mn^{2+}, and methionine or tRNA resulted in accumulation of 1- and 3-methylmercapto-AAF and tRNA adducts of AAF, respectively.

The possible importance of the sulfuric acid ester in the hepatic carcinogenicity of N-OH-AAF was assessed in the Millers' laboratory (5,26). It is evident from Table 3 that there is a positive association between hepatic sulfotransferase activity and the hepatocarcinogenicity of N-OH-AAF in the species that were tested. However, other target organs of AAF carcinogenesis such as the mammary gland and Zymbal's gland do not have measurable N-OH-AAF sulfotransferase activity (10). Moreover, analysis of DNA adducts in rat liver after administration of AAF or N-OH-AAF show that the major adduct is *N*-(deoxyguanosin-8-yl)-2-aminofluorene analog (11,20,32). This indicates that the acetyl group is lost from AAF and/or N-OH-AAF before or during arylation of DNA *in vivo*.

These observations led to a reexamination of the role of sulfotransferase in the hepatocarcinogenesis of AAF and/or N-OH-AAF. Experiments with the sulfate ester of N-OH-AAF formed *in situ* showed that no mutations were induced in the *Salmonella* mutagenesis test system (28,34; Fig. 6). Moreover, in experiments using purified rat liver sulfotransferase in the *Salmonella* system, it was clearly shown that this enzyme did not contribute to the mutagenic activation of N-OH-AAF (44; Fig. 7). However, Maher et al. (22) had shown that when the preformed DNA adduct of the sulfate ester of N-OH-AAF was added to the *Bacillus subtilis* system, both inactivation of transforming activity and induction of mutations occurred. It is therefore apparent that the sulfate ester of N-OH-AAF has the capacity to mutate the DNA if it is formed and/or placed in the immediate proximity of the nucleic acid. However, this situation does not

TABLE 3. *Comparison of hepatic* N-*hydroxy-AAF sulfotransferase activity and* in vivo *formation of hepatic protein-bound methionyl-AAF derivatives in species susceptible and resistant to* N-*hydroxy-AAF hepatocarcinogenesis*[a]

	O-methylmercapto-AAF from		
Species and sex	Liver sulfotransferase *in vitro* (μg/0.04 ml supernatant/30 min)	Liver protein *in vivo* (μg/5 g liver)	Hepatocarcinogenicity of N-OH-AAF
Rat (M)	23 ± 2 (13)	38 ± 9 (17)	+++++
Rat (F)	4 ± 0.5 (3)	4 ± 1 (5)	+
Mouse (M)	<0.5 (3)	<1.5 (3)	+
Hamster (M)	<0.5 (3)	<0.3 (3)	+
Rabbit (M)	2 ± 0.5 (3)	<0.5 (3)	−
Guinea pig (M)	<0.3 (3)	<0.5 (3)	−

[a] Data reprinted with permission from Miller (26).

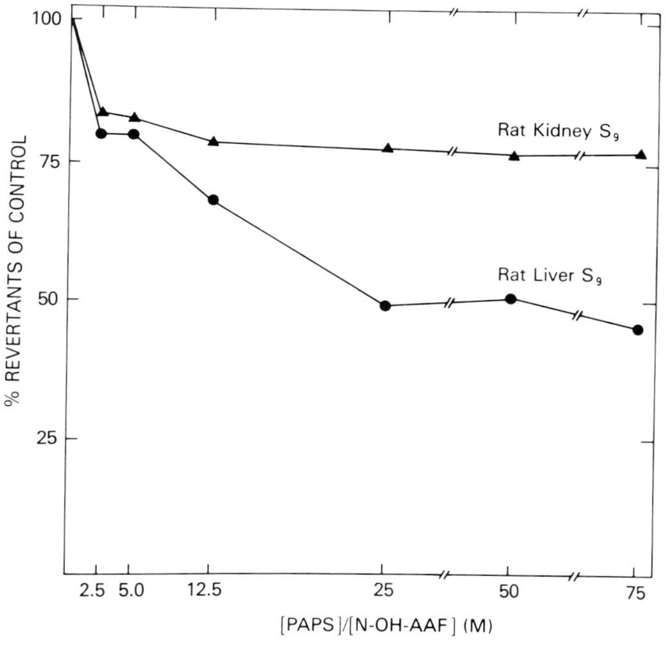

FIG. 6. Effect of PAPS on N-OH-AAF mutagenicity mediated by liver (●) and kidney (△) S-9 fractions from untreated rats. A concentration of 10 μg of N-OH-AAF per plate was used. Values are averages of two determinations on S-9 fractions prepared from pooled organs. The *abscissa* is the molar ratio of PAPS to the N-OH-AAF concentration on each plate. (From Schut et al., ref. 34, with permission.)

exist either *in vivo* or in the *Salmonella* system, indicating that the lack of interaction between the sulfate ester of N-OH-AAF and DNA results from the extreme instability of this compound in the aqueous environment of the cytosol.

In the context of the two-stage model of liver carcinogenesis (31), the role of N-OH-AAF sulfotransferase may not involve the initiation phase but rather contribute to the promotional aspects of carcinogenesis. Evidence for the possible promotional role of the sulfotransferase stems from both the lack of mutagenic effect in the *Salmonella* system and from the *in vivo* cytotoxic effect of N-OH-AAF (9,33,38,44). It has been proposed that the highly reactive and cytotoxic sulfate ester of N-OH-AAF causes cell death and induces subsequent cellular proliferation (38). This cellular proliferation may in turn promote the process of carcinogenesis of initiated cells that have been transformed by N-hydroxy-2-aminofluorene (N-OH-AF) or subsequent metabolites of N-OH-AF (44; Fig. 8).

N-O-Acyltransferase

Although the sulfate conjugation of N-OH-AAF and other arylhydroxamic acids appear to be confined to a single target organ in one species (i.e., the liver of the rat), activation of N-OH-AAF by *N-O*-acyltransferase has been demonstrated in the liver of a number of species and in several extrahepatic tissues of the rat in which arylamines are known to induce tumors (17,18). The activation of *N-O*-acyltransferase is believed to occur through enzyme-catalyzed generation of acyloxy intermediates via removal of the acyl group of the nitrogen and subsequent transfer to the oxygen. The unstable intermediates are then capable of covalent interaction with macromolecules. Because of the extreme reactivity of *N*-acetoxyarylamines, the synthesis of *N*-acetoxy-*N*-2-aminofluorene (derived from N-OH-AAF) has not been successful, and indirect measurements are used to assess this enzyme activity (17). Therefore, data from *in vitro* nucleic acid binding experiments and/or *in vitro* muta-

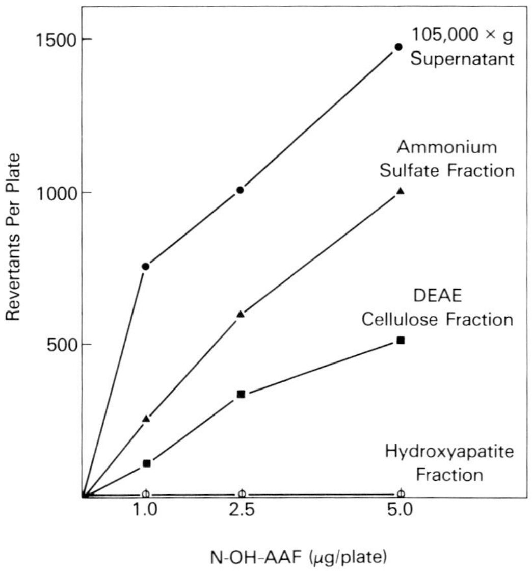

FIG. 7. Mutagenicity *in vitro* of N-OH-AAF in *Salmonella* TA 98 mediated by partially purified fractions of rat liver sulfotransferase. *Points* are the mean number of revertants per plate observed in two experiments and have been corrected for spontaneous (background) revertants observed with N-OH-AAF in the absence of partially purified sulfotransferase fractions. The protein concentration of each fraction was 1.0 mg/plate. ●, Experiments utilizing 105,000 × *g* supernatant; ▲, fraction obtained after ammonium sulfate precipitation; ■, fraction obtained after DEAE-cellulose chromatography; ○, experiments utilizing sulfotransferase activity following hydroxyapatite chromatography. (From Wirth and Thorgeirsson, ref. 44, with permission.)

genesis systems have been used to evaluate the role of *N-O*-acyltransferase in the metabolic activation of N-OH-AAF (Fig. 9) and its position in the two-stage hepatic carcinogenesis model (31).

Various investigators have shown that the mutagenic activation of N-OH-AAF by *N-O*-acyltransferase in the *Salmonella* mutagenesis system is independent of the metabolic activation resulting in nucleic acid binding (33,41,44; Figs. 10, 11). *N-O*-acyltransferase-catalyzed metabolic activation of N-OH-AAF, as measured by *in vitro* nucleic acid binding, can be inhibited by primary arylamines that compete with the initial product of deacetylation (N-OH-AF) for the acetyl group, thereby inhibiting the formation of *N*-acetoxy-2-aminofluorene (Fig. 9). Incubation of equimolar amounts of 2-aminofluorene (AF) with N-OH-AAF and partially purified *N-O*-acyltransferase decreased the incorporation of the fluorene nucleus into tRNA by more than 90% (Fig. 10A). In contrast, AF had no effect on the mutation frequency normally observed with *N-O*-acyltransferase when identical molar quantities of N-OH-AAF and AF were used in the mutagenesis assay system (Fig. 10B). Furthermore, guanosine monophosphoric acid [Guo-3′(2′)-P] competes with nucleic acids for the reactive electrophile generated from N-OH-AAF by *N-O*-acyltransferase activation, resulting in a reduction of adduct formation. However, the mutagenicity of N-OH-AAF was not decreased after addition of Guo-3′(2′)-P to the *Salmonella* test system (Fig. 11). Thus, the capacity of the reactive electrophile of *N*-acetoxy-2-aminofluorene to induce mutations and/or other genotoxic effects *in vivo* is questionable.

The mutagenic species derived from the metabolism of N-OH-AAF by *N-O*-acyltransferase has not been rigorously defined, but is most likely the highly mutagenic N-OH-AF (33,41,44). Whether N-OH-AF is formed by a deacetylase-type reaction by the *N-O*-acyltransferase that is independent of the acyltransfer or is a secondary "byproduct" of the *N-O*-acyltransfer itself (i.e., displacement of N-OH-AF from the enzyme and/or hydrolysis of the *N*-acetoxy-2-aminofluorene to N-OH-AF) remains to be clarified. However, it is important to note that *N-O*-acyltransferase is much more proficient in forming the *N*-acetoxy-2-aminofluorene (i.e., measured as formation of tRNA adducts) than it is in forming the mutagenic derivative(s) in the *Salmonella* system. It therefore appears that *N-O*-acyltransferase may play a dual role in the carcinogenic process of N-OH-AAF. *N-O*-acyltransferase catalyzes the formation of both *N*-acetoxy-2-

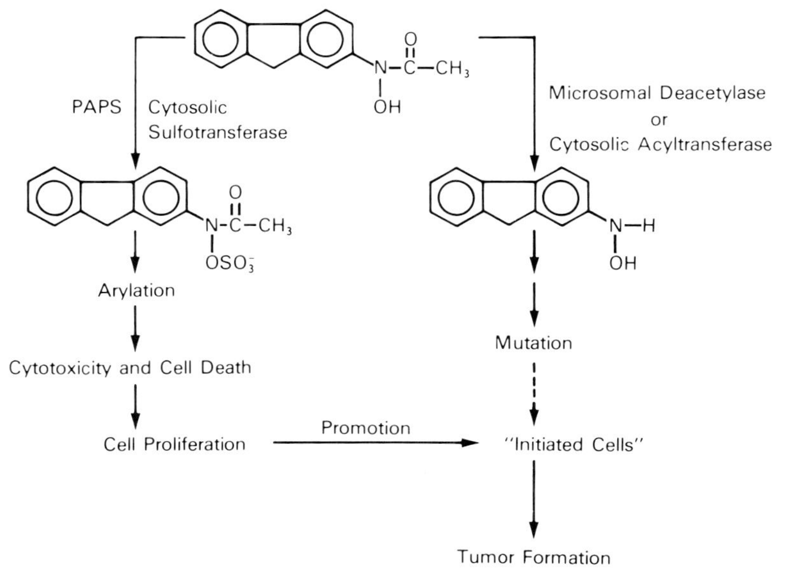

FIG. 8. Proposed role of sulfotransferase and deacetylase in N-OH-AAF-induced carcinogenesis.

aminofluorene and a mutagenic derivative, presumably N-OH-AF, from N-OH-AAF. The reactivity of *N*-acetoxy-AF is such that, like the sulfate ester of N-OH-AAF, it will probably react exclusively with nucleophilic sites on macromolecules in the cytoplasm and not interact with nuclear DNA. The consequence of this covalent interaction with cytosolic macromolecules may, as in the case of the sulfate ester, be primarily a cytotoxic effect and, as such, contribute to the promotional aspects of N-OH-AAF-induced car-

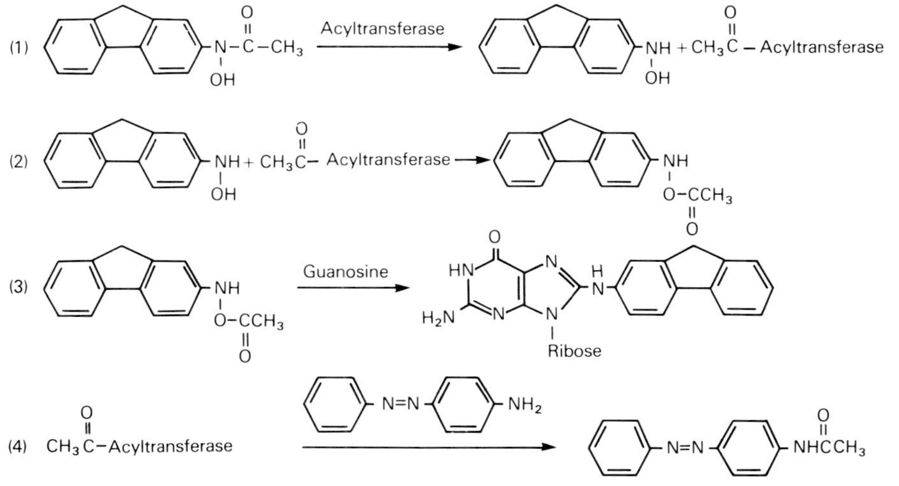

FIG. 9. Acetyltransferase-catalyzed formation of N-OH-AAF:guanosine adducts and acetylation of 4-aminoazobenzene.

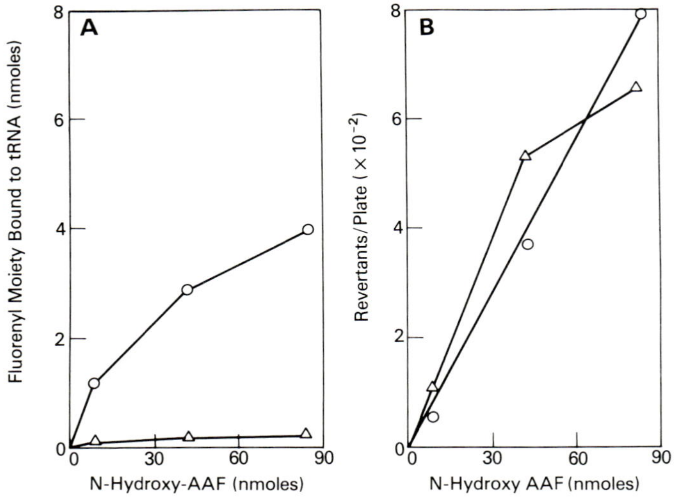

FIG. 10. Effect of AF on the acyltransferase-catalyzed formation of nucleic acid adducts (**A**) and mutations in *S. typhimurium* (**B**). Equimolar amounts of AF and *N*-hydroxy-AAF were incubated with acyltransferase preparations partially purified by fractional precipitation with ammonium sulfate in both *S. typhimurium* strain TA 1538 and the acyltransferase assay. △, with AF; ○, without AF. (From Weeks et al., ref. 41, with permission.)

cinogenesis. However, since *N-O*-acyltransferase catalyzes the formation of a mutagenic derivative(s) from N-OH-AAF, it is probable that metabolic activation by this enzyme also contributes to the initiation step in N-OH-AAF-induced carcinogenesis.

Deacetylation

Enzymatic deacetylation of both AAF and N-OH-AAF is catalyzed by two different deacetylases that are members of the carboxyesterase/amidase family (12,15). These enzymes are membrane bound and localized principally in the endoplasmic reticulum of the liver cell, but enzyme activity is also found in other tissues (8,15).

Early studies suggested the possible importance of acetylation and/or deacetylation of *N*-acetylarylamines and arylhydroxamic acids in the mechanism of their carcinogenicity (19,29). The low reactivity of N-OH-AF towards nucleic acids at neutral pH tended to negate the assumption that deacetylation of N-OH-AAF played a significant role in the metabolic activation of this com-

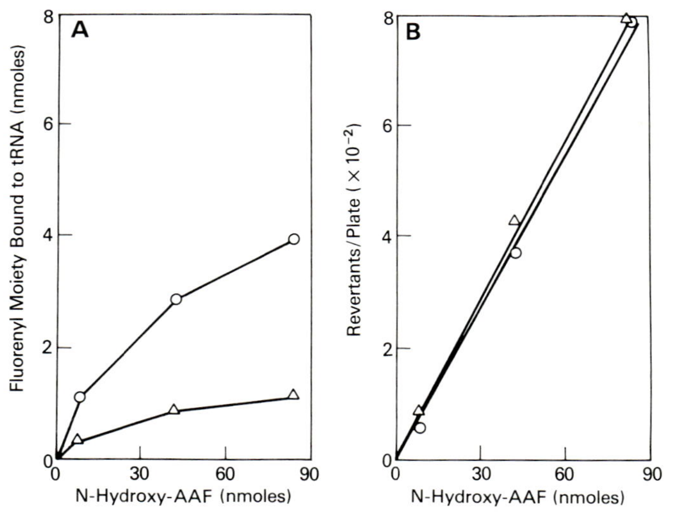

FIG. 11. Effect of Guo-3′(2′)-P on the acyltransferase-catalyzed formation of nucleic acid adducts (**A**) and mutations in *S. typhimurium* (**B**). Guo-3′(2′)-P (2.5 μmole) was incubated with *N*-hydroxy-AAF and acyltransferase preparations partially purified by fractional precipitation with ammonium sulfate in the acyltransferase assay system and *S. typhimurium* TA 1538. △, with Guo-3′(2′)-P; ○, without Guo-3′(2′)-P. (From Weeks et al., ref. 41, with permission.)

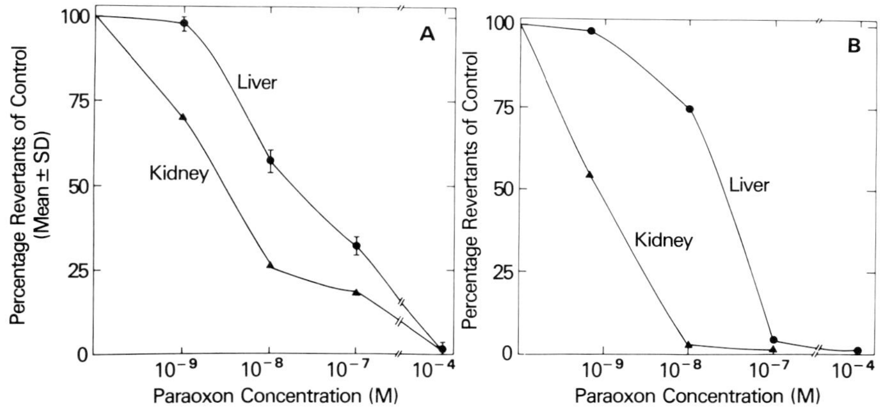

FIG. 12. Effect of paraoxon on N-OH-AAF mutagenicity mediated by liver and kidney microsomes from mice (**A**) and rats (**B**). A concentration of 5 μg of N-OH-AAF per plate was used. Values represent mean percentage revertants of control (uninhibited) ± standard deviations of four experiments in the case of mouse liver microsomes (●) and the means of two experiments in the case of microsomes of mouse kidney (▲), rat liver (●), and rat kidney (▲). (From Schut et al., ref. 34, with permission.)

pound (21). However, renewed interest in the possible role of N-OH-AF in the carcinogenicity of N-OH-AAF was generated when Ames et al. (1) demonstrated that it was a potent direct-acting frameshift mutagen in the *Salmonella* mutagenesis system.

The importance of microsomal deacetylation in the mutagenic activation of N-OH-AAF was clearly demonstrated by use of the carboxyesterase/amidase inhibitor diethyl-*p*-nitrophenylphosphate (paraoxon) (33,34; Figs. 12, 13). Complete inhibition of both mutagenesis (Fig. 12) and deacetylation (Fig. 13) of N-OH-AAF was observed in the *Salmonella* system containing liver and/or kidney microsomes in the presence of paraoxon (0.1 mM). Paraoxon is neither toxic nor mutagenic at the concentrations (0.1 μM to 0.1

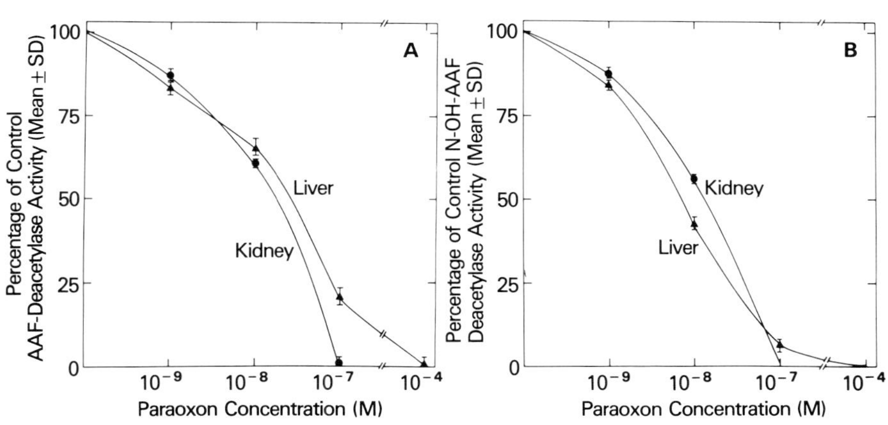

FIG. 13. Effect of paraoxon on microsomal AAF deacetylase (**A**) and N-OH-AAF deacetylase (**B**) of liver (▲) and kidney (●) from mice. Values (percentage of control) represent means ± standard deviations of four determinations on microsomes prepared from pooled organs. (From Schut et al., ref. 34, with permission.)

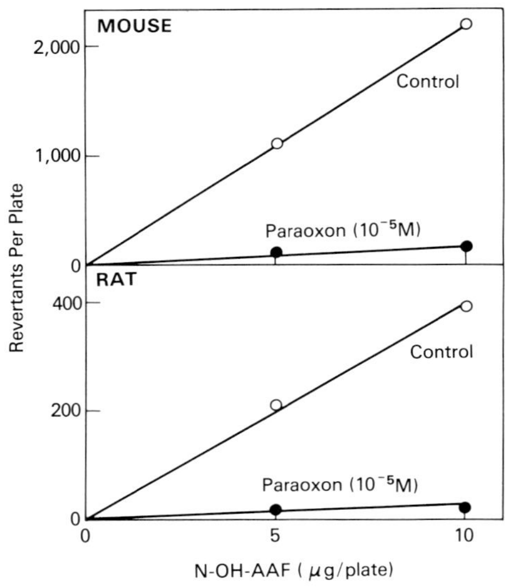

FIG. 14. Effect of paraoxon on mutagenic activation of N-OH-AAF by liver cell nuclei from mouse and rat. The nuclear protein concentration was 0.90 and 1.10 mg/plate for mouse and rat, respectively. ○, control; ●, paraoxon-treated (10^{-5} M) nuclei. *Points* represent the mean of two experiments done in triplicate. (From Sakai et al., ref. 33, with permission.)

mM) used in these experiments (34). These data indicate that the endoplasmic reticulum may be an important site for the metabolic activation not only of AAF but also of N-OH-AAF. Moreover, since the outer nuclear membrane of the hepatocyte is in a continuum with the endoplasmic reticulum and contains qualitatively the same enzymes (16), it may provide a critical location for the metabolic activation of N-OH-AAF. For example, liver cell nuclei from guinea pigs have been shown to deacetylate N-OH-AAF (8). The notion that the outer nuclear membrane may participate in the metabolic activation of N-OH-AAF was supported by results from experiments in the *Salmonella* system using isolated and purified rat and mouse liver cell nuclei (33). Both rat and mouse liver nuclei were capable of mutagenic activation of N-OH-AAF, which could be completely blocked by paraoxon (Fig. 14). Furthermore, the liver cell nuclei were capable of activating N-OH-AAF to a derivative(s) capable of covalent interaction with intranuclear macromolecules, and this activation was blocked by paraoxon (Table 4).

In light of data presented above, it seems reasonable to propose a role for N-OH-AAF deacetylase not only in the *in vitro* mutagenic activation of N-OH-AAF and other arylhydroxamic acids (Fig. 15) but also in the *in vivo* carcinogenic process of this compound.

TABLE 4. *Effect of paraoxon and PAPS on* in vitro *covalent binding of N-OH-AAF to nuclear nucleic acids and proteins and soluble proteins (100,000 × g supernatant fraction) from rat liver*

Subcellular fractions	Covalent binding of N-OH-AAF (pmole/mg/10 min) Soluble protein	Nuclear protein	RNA	DNA
Nuclei		4768 ± 134[a]	4860 ± 405	22.0 ± 3.0
Nuclei + paraoxon (10^{-4} M)		2235 ± 161[b]	1578 ± 170[b]	1.3 ± 0.3[b]
Nuclei + soluble fraction	1920 ± 212	3770 ± 450	3842 ± 296	28.0 ± 4.0
Nuclei + soluble fraction + PAPS	3125 ± 240[c]	3504 ± 312[b]	3540 ± 222[b]	26.0 ± 3.0
Nuclei + soluble fraction + paraoxon (10^{-4} M)	1862 ± 187	4020 ± 160	4440 ± 188	23.0 ± 4.0
Nuclei + DMSO (3.2×10^{-2} M)		4440 ± 83	4293 ± 275	20.0 ± 3.0

[a] Mean ± SE of three experiments.
[b] Significantly lower ($p < 0.05$, *t*-test) covalent binding of N-OH-AAF than in control nuclei.
[c] Significant increase ($p < 0.05$, *t*-test) in covalent binding of N-OH-AAF to the soluble proteins when PAPS was added.
Data reprinted with permission from Sakai et al. (33).

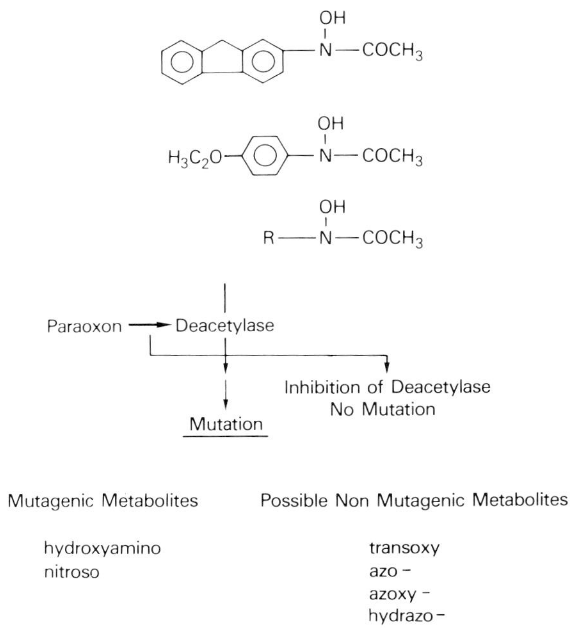

FIG. 15. Proposed mutagenic activation of *N*-acetylarylhydroxamic acids.

Consequently, we propose that the membrane-bound deacetylase catalyzes the major activation process for N-OH-AAF in the liver and perhaps in other target organs (Fig. 8).

REFERENCES

1. Ames, B. N., Gurney, E. G., Miller, J. A., and Bartsch, H. (1972): Carcinogens as frameshift mutagens: Metabolites and derivatives of 2-acetylaminofluorene and other aromatic amine carcinogens. *Proc. Natl. Acad. Sci. U.S.A.*, 69:3128–3132.
2. Atlas, S. A., Boobis, A. R., Felton, J. S., Thorgeirsson, S. S., and Nebert, D. W. (1977): Ontogenetic expression of polycyclic aromatic compound inducible monooxygenase activities and forms of cytochrome P-450 in rabbit. *J. Biol. Chem.*, 252:4712–4721.
3. Atlas, S. A., Thorgeirsson, S. S., Boobis, A. R., Kumaki, K., and Nebert, D. W. (1975): Differential induction of murine *Ah* locus-associated monooxygenase activities in rabbit liver and kidney. *Biochem. Pharmacol.*, 24:2111–2116.
4. Cramer, J. W., Miller, J. A., and Miller, E. C. (1960): *N*-Hydroxylation: A new metabolic reaction observed in the rat with the carcinogen 2-acetylaminofluorene. *J. Biol. Chem.*, 235:885–888.
5. De Baun, J. R., Miller, E. C., and Miller, J. A. (1970): *N*-Hydroxy-2-acetylaminofluorene sulfotransferase: Its probable role in carcinogenesis and in protein-(methion-*S*-yl) binding in rat liver. *Cancer Res.*, 30:577–595.
6. De Baun, J. R., Rowley, J. Y., Miller, E. C., and Miller, J. A. (1968): Sulfotransferase activation of *N*-hydroxy-2-acetylaminofluorene in rodent livers susceptible and resistant to this carcinogen. *Proc. Soc. Exp. Biol. Med.*, 129:268–273.
7. Irving, C. C. (1962): *N*-Hydroxylation of 2-acetylaminofluorene in the rabbit. *Cancer Res.*, 22:867–873.
8. Irving, C. C. (1966): Enzymatic deacetylation of *N*-hydroxy-2-acetylaminofluorene by liver microsomes. *Cancer Res.*, 26:1390–1396.
9. Irving, C. C. (1975): Comparative toxicity of *N*-hydroxy-2-acetylaminofluorene in several strains of rats. *Cancer Res.*, 35:2959–2961.
10. Irving, C. C., Janss, D. H., and Russell, L. T. (1971): Lack of *N*-hydroxy-2-acetylaminofluorene sulfotransferase activity in the mammary gland and Zymbal's gland of the rat. *Cancer Res.*, 31:387–391.
11. Irving, C. C., and Veazey, R. A. (1969): Persistent binding of 2-acetylaminofluorene to rat liver DNA *in vivo* and consideration of the mechanism of binding of *N*-hydroxy-2-acetylaminofluorene to rat liver nucleic acids. *Cancer Res.*, 29:1799–1804.
12. Järvinen, M., Santi, R. S. S., and Hopsu-Havu, V. K. (1971): Partial purification and characterization of two enzymes from guinea-pig liver microsomes that hydrolyze carcinogenic amides 2-acetylaminofluorene and *N*-hydroxy-2-acetylaminofluorene. *Biochem. Pharmacol.*, 20:2971–2982.

13. Johnson, E. F. (1979): Multiple forms of cytochrome P-450: Criteria and significance. *Rev. Biochem. Toxicol.,* 1:1–26.
14. Johnson, E. F., Levitt, D. S., Muller-Eberhard, U., and Thorgeirsson, S. S. (1980): Catalysis of divergent pathways of 2-acetylaminofluorene metabolism by multiple forms of cytochrome P_{450}. *Cancer Res.,* 40:4456–4459.
15. Junge, W., and Krisch, K. (1975): The carboxylesterases/amidases of mammalian liver and their possible significance. *CRC Crit. Rev. Food Sci. Nutr.,* 3:371–434.
16. Kashing, D. M., and Kasper, C. E. (1969): Isolation, morphology, and composition of the nuclear membrane from rat liver. *J. Biol. Chem.,* 244:3786–3792.
17. King, C. M. (1974): Mechanism of reaction, tissue distribution, and inhibition of arylhydroxamic acid acyltransferase. *Cancer Res.,* 34:1503–1515.
18. King, C. M., and Olive, C. W. (1975): Comparative effects of strain, species, and sex on the acyltransferase- and sulfotransferase-catalyzed activations of *N*-hydroxy-*N*-2-fluorenylacetamide. *Cancer Res.,* 35:906–912.
19. King, C. M., and Phillips, B. (1968): Enzyme-catalyzed reactions of the carcinogen *N*-hydroxy-2-fluorenylacetamide with nucleic acid. *Science,* 159:1351–1353.
20. Kriek, E. (1969/1970): On the mechanism of action of carcinogenic aromatic amines. 1. Binding of 2-acetylaminofluorene and *N*-hydroxy-2-acetylaminofluorene to rat-liver nucleic acids *in vivo. Chem. Biol. Interact.,* 1:3–17.
21. Kriek, E. (1974): Carcinogenesis by aromatic amines. *Biochim. Biophys. Acta,* 355:177–203.
22. Maher, V. M., Miller, E. C., Miller, J. A., and Szybalski, W. (1968): Mutations and decreases in density of transforming DNA produced by derivatives of the carcinogens 2-acetylaminofluorene and *N*-methyl-4-aminoazobenzene. *Mol. Pharmacol.,* 4:411–426.
23. Matsushima, T., Grantham, P. H., Weisburger, E. K., and Weisburger, J. H. (1972): Phenobarbital-mediated increase in ring- and *N*-hydroxylation of the carcinogen *N*-2-fluorenylacetamide and decrease in amounts bound to liver deoxyribonucleic acid. *Biochem. Pharmacol.,* 21:2043–2051.
24. Miller, E. C. (1978): Some current perspectives of chemical carcinogenesis in humans and experimental animals: Presidential address. *Cancer Res.,* 38:1479–1496.
25. Miller, E. C., Miller, J. A., and Hartmann, H. A. (1961): *N*-Hydroxy-2-acetylaminofluorene: A metabolite of 2-acetylaminofluorene with increased carcinogenic activity in the rat. *Cancer Res.,* 21:815–824.
26. Miller, J. A. (1970): Carcinogenesis by chemicals: An overview—G. H. A. Clowes Memorial Lecture. *Cancer Res.,* 30:559–576.
27. Miller, J. A., Wyatt, C. S., Miller, E. C., and Hartmann, H. A. (1961): The *N*-hydroxylation of 4-acetaminobiphenyl by the rat and dog and the strong carcinogenicity of *N*-hydroxy-4-acetylaminobiphenyl in the rat. *Cancer Res.,* 21:1465–1473.
28. Mulder, G. J., Hinson, J. A., Nelson, W. L., and Thorgeirsson, S. S. (1977): Role of sulfotransferase from rat liver in the mutagenicity of *N*-hydroxy-2-acetylaminofluorene in *Salmonella typhimurium. Biochem. Pharmacol.,* 26:1356–1358.
29. Nagasawa, H. T., and Gutmann, H. R. (1957): A note on the deacylation of the carcinogen 2-acetamidofluorene and related compounds by rat liver and intestine. *Biochim. Biophys. Acta,* 25:186–189.
30. Norman, R. L., Johnson, E. F., and Muller-Eberhard, U. (1978): Identification of the major cytochrome P-450 form transplacentally induced in neonatal rabbits by 2,3,7,8-tetrachlorodibenzo-*p*-dioxin. *J. Biol. Chem.,* 253:8640–8647.
31. Peraino, C., Fry, R. J. M., and Staffeldt, E. (1971): Reduction and enhancement by phenobarbital of hepatocarcinogenesis induced in the rat by 2-acetylaminofluorene. *Cancer Res.,* 31:1506–1512.
32. Poirier, M. C., Williams, G. M., and Yuspa, S. H. (1980): Effect of culture conditions, cell type, and species of origin on the distribution of acetylated and deacetylated deoxyguanosine C-8 adducts of *N*-acetoxy-2-acetylaminofluorene. *Mol. Pharmacol.,* 18:581–587.
33. Sakai, S., Reinhold, C. E., Wirth, P. J., and Thorgeirsson, S. S. (1978): Mechanism of *in vitro* mutagenic activation and covalent binding of *N*-hydroxy-2-acetylaminofluorene in isolated liver cell nuclei from rat and mouse. *Cancer Res.,* 38:2058–2067.
34. Schut, H. A. J., Wirth, P. J., and Thorgeirsson, S. S. (1978): Mutagenic activation of *N*-hydroxy-2-acetylaminofluorene in the *Salmonella* test system: The role of deacetylation by liver and kidney fractions from mouse and rat. *Mol. Pharmacol.,* 14:682–692.
35. Schwab, G. E., Norman, R. L., Muller-Eberhard, U., and Johnson, E. F. (1980): Identification of the form of cytochrome P-450 induced in neonatal rabbit liver microsomes by phenobarbital. *Mol. Pharmacol.,* 17:218–224.
36. Thorgeirsson, S. S., Atlas, S. A., Boobis, A. R., and Felton, J. S. (1979): Species differences in the substrate specificity of hepatic cytochrome P-448 from polycyclic hydrocarbon-treated animals. *Biochem. Pharmacol.,* 28:217–226.
37. Thorgeirsson, S. S., Jollow, D. J., Sasame, H. A., Green, I., and Mitchell, J. R. (1973): The role of cytochrome P_{450} in *N*-hydroxylation of 2-acetylaminofluorene. *Mol. Pharmacol.,* 9:398–404.
38. Thorgeirsson, S. S., Mitchell, J. R., Sasame, H. A., and Potter, W. Z. (1976): Biochemical changes after hepatic injury by allyl alcohol and *N*-hydroxy-2-acetylaminofluorene. *Chem. Biol. Interact.,* 15:139–147.
39. Thorgeirsson, S. S., and Nebert, D. W. (1977): The *Ah* locus and the metabolism of chemical carcino-

gens and other foreign compounds. *Adv. Cancer Res.,* 25:149–193.

40. Thorgeirsson, S. S., Wirth, P. J., Nelson, W. L., and Lambert, G. H. (1977): Genetic regulation of metabolism and mutagenicity of 2-acetylaminofluorene and related compounds in mice. In: *Origins of Human Cancer,* edited by J. D. Watson and H. Hiatt, pp. 869–886. Cold Spring Harbor Laboratory, New York.
41. Weeks, C. E., Allaben, W. T., Louie, S. C., Lazear, E. J., and King, C. M. (1978): Role of arylhydroxamic acid acyltransferase in the mutagenicity of *N*-hydroxy-*N*-2-fluorenylacetamide in *Salmonella typhimurium. Cancer Res.,* 38:613–618.
42. Weisburger, J. H., and Weisburger, E. K. (1973): Biochemical formation and pharmacological, toxicological, and pathological properties of hydroxylamines and hydroxamic acids. *Pharmacol. Rev.,* 25:1–66.
43. Wirth, P. J., Dybing, E., von Bahr, C., and Thorgeirsson, S. S. (1980): Mechanism of *N*-hydroxyacetylarylamine mutagenicity in the *Salmonella* test system: Metabolic activation of *N*-hydroxyphenacetin by liver and kidney fractions from rat, mouse, hamster, and man. *Mol. Pharmacol.,* 18:117–127.
44. Wirth, P. J., and Thorgeirsson, S. S. (1981): Mechanism of *N*-hydroxy-2-acetylaminofluorene mutagenicity in the *Salmonella* test system. *Mol. Pharmacol.,* 19:337–344.
45. Yoshida, T. (1933): Uber die serienweise Verfolgung der Veranderungen der Leber der experimentellen Hepatomerzeugung durch *O*-Aminoazotoluol. *Trans. Jpn. Pathol. Soc.,* 23:636–638.

Drug Metabolism and Drug Toxicity,
edited by J. R. Mitchell and M. G. Horning.
Raven Press, New York © 1984.

Pharmacokinetics: Basic Principles and Its Use as a Tool in Drug Metabolism

Leslie Z. Benet

Department of Pharmacy, University of California, San Francisco, California 94143

Pharmacokinetics may be simply defined as what the body does to the drug, as opposed to pharmacodynamics, which may be defined as what the drug does to the body. The combination of pharmacokinetics and pharmacodynamics allows the clinician and the pharmacological scientist to define the appropriate drug dosage regimen in a particular patient. However, pharmacokinetics may also be useful as a tool in drug metabolism and drug toxicity. In this chapter, basic pharmacokinetic parameters and the calculation of these parameters are reviewed; we then illustrate the use of pharmacokinetics in the interpretation of a drug metabolism problem, specifically applied to the disposition of azathioprine and 6-mercaptopurine in the presence and absence of concomitant probenecid administration.

BASIC PHARMACOKINETIC PRINCIPLES

A large number of pharmacokinetic parameters may be determined in defining a drug substance as well as its metabolites. Table 1 lists those parameters that can be determined from initial studies in animal models as well as from studies in normal human volunteers. Each of these parameters is discussed with special emphasis on drug metabolism and toxicity in this chapter and/ or in the following chapter.

Clearance

Clearance is the most important pharmacokinetic term in defining the disposition of a drug or a metabolite. In most cases for drugs, the physician would like to maintain concentrations within a known therapeutic range, that is, at a given steady-state condition. Steady state will be achieved when the dosing rate of active drug into the systemic circulation equals the rate of active drug elimination. Therefore:

$$\text{Dosing rate} = CL \cdot C^{ss} \qquad (1)$$

Thus, if the desired steady-state concentration (C^{ss}) is known, the clearance value (CL) in that patient will dictate the dosing rate. For a metabolite, dosing rate becomes the rate of metabolite formation, and the steady-state concentration and clearance are defined for that metabolite. Knowledge of the clearance of a metabolite and measurement of its steady-state concentration allow the investigator to calculate the rate of metabolite formation. Conversely, one may know the fraction of drug clearance to a particular metabolite (f_{m_i}); then, measurement of drug and metabolite steady-state concentrations (C^{ss} and $C^{ss}_{M_i}$, respectively) allows the investigator to determine the clearance of the metabolite CL_{M_i} if the clearance of the parent drug (CL) is known.

TABLE 1. *Pharmacokinetic parameters that may be defined in animal models and in human volunteers*

Clearance
Fractional clearance by specific metabolic pathways
Fractional renal clearance
Rate of metabolite formation
Volume of distribution
Half-life
Protein binding
Blood to plasma ratio
Extent of systemic availability
Peak time and concentration
Rate of availability

$$\text{Rate of metabolite formation} = f_{m_i} CL\, C^{ss} = CL_{M_i}\, C^{ss}_{M_i} \quad (2)$$

At its simplest, clearance of a compound is the rate of elimination by all routes relative to the concentration of the compound in a biologic fluid:

$$CL = \text{rate of elimination}/C \quad (3)$$

where clearance is usually defined as either blood clearance (CL_B), plasma clearance (CL_P), or clearance based on unbound or free drug concentration (CL^u), depending on the concentration measured for the right-hand side of equation 3 (C_B, C_P, or C^u).

A drug or metabolite with an extremely low concentration because of a favorable partition into the red blood cells (e.g., mecamylamine) and a high rate of elimination can manifest a plasma clearance of tens of liters per minute, i.e., clearances that are not "physiologic." However, if blood concentration is used to define clearance, the maximum clearance possible is equal to the sum of the blood flows to the various organs of elimination. For a compound eliminated solely by the liver, blood clearance is therefore limited to liver blood flow, approximately 1,500 ml/min in man. Blood clearance may be determined from plasma clearance if the blood/plasma distribution ratio or the red blood cell-to-plasma concentration ratio is known, as shown in equation 4.

$$\frac{CL_P}{CL_B} = \frac{C_B}{C_P} = 1 + H\left(\frac{C_{RBC}}{C_P} - 1\right) \quad (4)$$

where H equals the hematocrit.

It is important to note the additive character of clearance. Elimination of a compound in the body may occur as a result of processes occurring in the kidney, the lung, the liver, and other sites of elimination. Dividing the rate of elimination at each organ by the concentration of the compound will yield the respective clearance at that organ. Added together, these separate clearances will equal total systemic clearance (CL with no subscript):

$$CL = CL_{\text{renal}} + CL_{\text{liver}} + CL_{\text{other}} \quad (5)$$

"Other" tissues of elimination could include lung, saliva, sweat, partition into the gut, and additional sites of metabolism, for example, hydrolysis in blood or muscle. The two major sites of drug elimination are the kidney and liver. Clearance of a compound detected in the urine is represented by renal clearance. Within the liver, drug elimination occurs via biotransformation of unchanged drug to one or more metabolites and/or excretion of unchanged drug into the bile.

Currently, most national regulatory agencies require the sponsor of a new drug candidate to define the biotransformation pathways for that drug and especially to determine whether any of the metabolic products are themselves active or toxic compounds. Most of the biotransformation processes occur in the liver. From a pharmacokinetic standpoint, the sum of the rates of elimination by all such pathways in the liver can be expressed in the classical pharmacologic terms of $V_{\max}$, K_m, and concentration (Michaelis–Menten kinetics):

$$\text{Rate of elimination} = \sum_{i=1}^{N} \frac{V_{\max,i} C}{K_{m,i} + C} \quad (6)$$

where there are N such different pathways. Since rate of elimination divided by concentration yields clearance (eq. 3), rearrangement of equation 6 gives:

$$CL = \sum_{i=1}^{N} \frac{V_{\max,i}}{K_{m,i} + C} \quad (7)$$

For compounds that exhibit linear kinetics, K_m values for all hepatic routes of elimination are substantially greater than C, and clearance is approximated by the ratio of $V_{\max}$ to K_m summed over all routes. For these compounds, clearance is constant over the plasma or blood concentration range encountered in the experimental setting. For compounds that exhibit nonlinear (concentration-dependent) pharmacokinetics, K_m for one or more routes of elimination may not be substantially greater than C, and clearance will vary depending on the concentration of drug in the blood or plasma. A more detailed consideration of concentration dependent elimination is given by G. R. Wilkinson (*this volume*).

A further definition of clearance is useful in understanding the effects of physiologic and pathologic variables on drug and metabolite elimination, particularly with respect to an individual organ. The rate of elimination of a compound by an individual body organ can be defined in terms of the blood flow entering and exiting from the organ and the concentration of the compound in the blood. The rate of presentation of compound to the organ is the product of blood flow and entering concentration ($Q \times C_{\text{in}}$), whereas the rate of exit of drug from the organ is the product of blood flow and exiting drug concentration ($Q \times C_{\text{out}}$). The difference between these rates at steady state is the rate of drug elimination:

$$\text{Rate of elimination} = QC_{\text{in}} - QC_{\text{out}} \quad (8)$$

Dividing equation 8 by concentration of drug entering the organ of elimination (C_{in}), we obtain an expression for organ clearance of drug:

$$CL_{\text{organ}} = \frac{QC_{\text{in}} - QC_{\text{out}}}{C_{\text{in}}} = Q\,\frac{C_{\text{in}} - C_{\text{out}}}{C_{\text{in}}} = QE \quad (9)$$

As shown in equation 9, the expression $(C_{\text{in}} - C_{\text{out}})/C_{\text{in}}$ is referred to as the extraction ratio of the drug (E).

The simple concepts developed in equation 9 have important implications for compounds that are eliminated by the liver. Consider a drug that is efficiently removed from the blood by hepatic processes. In this instance, the concentration of drug exiting from the liver will be small, the extraction ratio will approach unity, and organ blood clearance will become limited by flow. Highly hepatic-extracted drugs (e.g., desipramine, hydralazine, imipramine, lidocaine, meperidine, morphine, nortriptyline, propranolol) are restricted in their rate of elimination not by intrahepatic processes but by the rate at which they can be transported in the blood to hepatic sites of elimination. The concepts embodied in equations 3 and 9 can be derived from consideration of mass balance of a drug across an eliminating organ at steady state. No model is required to derive these equations. It is apparent, however, that the simple expressions for clearance, blood flow, and extraction cannot account for the complexity of hepatic or renal drug elimination. For example, these equations do not account for drug protein binding to blood and tissue components, nor do they permit an estimation of the intrinsic ability of the liver or kidney to eliminate a drug in the absence of limitations imposed by blood flow.

To extend the relationship of equation 9 to include expressions for protein binding and intrinsic clearance, it is necessary to formulate a model to describe organ elimination of drugs. The most straightforward and most commonly employed model relating the extraction ratio to physiological parameters is the so-called venous equilibrium or well-stirred model (16,19), which assumes that the unbound drug concentration leaving the organ is equal to the unbound concentration inside the organ and that the intrinsic ability to metabolize or clear unbound drug ($CL^{\text{u}}_{\text{int}}$) is equal to the rate of elimination divided by the unbound concentration in the organ. The clearance (with respect to blood concentration) for the eliminating organ then becomes:

$$CL = Q \frac{f_B CL^u_{int}}{Q + f_B CL^u_{int}} \quad (10)$$

where f_B is the unbound fraction of drug in blood.

This model indicates that when the capability of the eliminating organ to metabolize the drug is large in comparison to the rate of drug presentation to the organ ($f_B CL^u_{int} \gg Q$), the clearance will approximate the organ blood flow:

$$CL \simeq Q \quad (11)$$

i.e., drug elimination is blood-flow-rate limited, and the compound is called a high-extraction-ratio drug. On the other hand, when the metabolic capability is small in comparison to the rate of drug presentation ($Q \gg f_B CL^u_{int}$), the clearance will be proportional to the unbound fraction of drug in blood and to the intrinsic clearance; i.e.,

$$CL \simeq f_B CL^u_{int} \quad (12)$$

The drug is then called a low-extraction-ratio drug. When the capability of elimination is of the same order of magnitude as the blood flow, clearance would be dependent on the blood flow as well as the intrinsic clearance and plasma protein binding (eq. 10).

An appreciation of equation 10 allows the investigator to understand a number of heretofore unclear experimental results. For example, enzyme induction or hepatic disease may change the rate of desipramine metabolism in an isolated hepatic microsomal enzyme system, but no change in clearance is found in the whole animal. Since desipramine is a high-extraction-ratio drug, clearance is blood-flow-rate limited (eq. 11), and changes in CL^u_{int} as a result of enzyme induction or liver disease should have no effect on clearance. Also, although desipramine is highly protein bound ($f_P = 0.08$), changes in protein binding because of disease or competitive binding should have no effect on clearance.

The availability of drugs that are highly extracted by the liver is sensitive to small changes in the hepatic extraction ratio. For a drug that is completely absorbed from the gastrointestinal tract and enters the liver without biotransformation in the portal vein or gut wall, the systemic availability of the drug (F) is diminished by the extent of hepatic extraction:

$$F = 1 - E \quad (13)$$

Small changes in E for a highly extracted drug can result in dramatic changes in availability, as discussed in the chapter by G. R. Wilkinson, this volume.

Volume of Distribution

The second pharmacokinetic parameter that might be expected to vary as a function of physiologic or pathologic changes is the volume of distribution, the measure of the apparent space in the body available to contain the drug. Volume of distribution (V) relates the amount of drug in the body to the concentration of drug (C) in the blood or plasma, depending on the fluid measured:

$$V = \text{Amount of drug in body}/C \quad (14)$$

The plasma of a normal 70-kg man is 3 liters; blood volume is about 5.5 liters; extracellular fluid outside plasma is 12 liters; and total body water is approximately 42 liters; yet, many drugs and some metabolites will exhibit a distribution volume (according to eq. 14) far in excess of these known body fluid volumes. That is, the volume of distribution does not represent a real volume but rather must be considered as the size of a pool of body fluids assuming that the drug or metabolite was equally distributed throughout all portions of the body.

Øie and Tozer (11) have developed a model for V that takes into account the plasma volume, the extracellular fluid outside the plasma, and the fluids in the rest of the body. For a drug bound to albumin, the relationship can be simplified to:

$$V = 7.2 + 7.8\, f_P + 27\, f_P/f_T \quad (15)$$

where f_P and f_T are the fractions of the drug unbound in plasma and outside the extracellular fluids (or "tissues"), respectively. For a drug extensively bound to plasma proteins but not bound to tissue proteins (i.e., $f_P \simeq 0$, $f_T \simeq 1$), the volume of distribution has a lower limit of approximately 7 liters as exemplified by furosemide and warfarin. In contrast, drugs such as desipramine, nortriptyline, and propranolol have high volumes of distribution even though these compounds are more than 90% bound to plasma proteins. From equation 15, it would appear that these drugs are even more extensively bound to tissue proteins (i.e., $f_T \ll f_P$). Further discussion of the effect of protein binding on volume of distribution as well as the consequence of nonlinear plasma and tissue binding may be found in the chapter by G. R. Wilkinson, this volume.

Half-Life

Half-life ($t_{1/2}$) is an expression of the relationship between volume and clearance. For the simplest case, the body may be considered as a single compartment of volume V. However, the organs of elimination can only clear drug from the blood or plasma in direct contact with those organs. Thus, the time course of a drug or metabolite in the body will depend on both of these physiologic parameters, volume of distribution and clearance.

$$t_{1/2} \simeq 0.693 V/CL \quad (16)$$

Half-life is a useful kinetic parameter in that it indicates the time required to attain and decay from steady-state conditions after institution of a particular rate of drug administration (i.e., the dosing regimen) or metabolite formation. As an indicator of whether disease changes either elimination or distribution, half-life has little value. Early studies of drug and metabolite pharmacokinetics in disease were compromised by the reliance on drug half-life as the sole measure of alteration in drug disposition. Disease can affect either or both of the physiologically related parameters of volume and clearance; thus, the derived parameter, $t_{1/2}$, will not necessarily reflect the expected change in drug elimination.

Up to now we have considered the parameters listed in Table 1 as general values without reference to a specific pharmacokinetic compartmental model. However, for most drugs and metabolites, the time course of plasma concentrations appears to follow a multiexponential pattern, which would indicate the presence of more than one half-life value. Therefore, equation 16 was written as an approximately equal relationship, where $t_{1/2}$ reflects an overall half-life for the compound in the body. The incorporation of the different half-lives in the calculation of clearance and volume of distribution is addressed below.

Bioavailability

Drug input efficiency is described as bioavailability, a term used to indicate a measure of both the relative amount of an administered dose that reaches the general circulation and the rate at which this occurs. In most clinical situations, the extent of drug availability (F) is considered to be a more important parameter than the rate of availability. The extent of bioavailability may be defined as the fraction of unchanged drug reaching the systemic circulation following administration by any route. For an intravenous dose of the drug, bioavailability is equal to unity. For a drug administered orally, bioavailability may be less than unity for several reasons. The drug may be incompletely absorbed. It may undergo enterohepatic cycling with incomplete reabsorption following elimination into the bile. It may be metabolized in the gut, the gut wall, the portal blood, or the liver prior to entry into the systemic circulation. This "first-pass" phenomenon (eq. 13) is extensively treated in the chapter by G. R. Wilkinson, this volume, with respect to drug availability and metabolite formation.

The final term listed in Table 1 is the rate of availability. Since pharmacokinetic concepts are most useful in the design of multiple-dose regimens, the extent (F) rather than the rate of availability is more critical in obtaining an appropriate concentration of drug in the body. Differences in rate of availability may become important for drugs given as a single dose, such as a hypnotic used to induce sleep. If a measure of the rate of availability is desired, it is necessary to fit the plasma concentration–time curve to a pharmacokinetic model to obtain a rate constant for absorption. However, in practice, comparisons of peak time and peak concentration yield relative measures of the rate of availability that suffice to define this parameter in most clinical situations. The rate of availability (or formation rate) of a metabolite is relevant when the metabolite elicits a pharmacologic response (either efficacious or toxic). Under steady-state conditions, this rate may be determined using equation 2.

NONCOMPARTMENTAL DETERMINATION OF PHARMACOKINETIC PARAMETERS

Except for the rate of availability and the fact that drugs often exhibit multiple half-lives, all of the parameters in Table 1 may be determined using so-called "noncompartmental methods." The treatment here considers only linear pharmacokinetic systems, i.e., situations in which there is a direct relationship between plasma concentration at a particular time and the intravenous dose administered.

Clearance

Under linear pharmacokinetic conditions, clearance may be determined as the ratio of the intravenous dose to the area under the plasma concentration–time curve measured from time zero to time infinity.

$$CL = \text{Dose}^{iv}/AUC = F\,\text{Dose}/AUC \qquad (17)$$

Or, with any dosing route, clearance will equal the available dose (F Dose) divided by the total area under the curve (AUC). This area may be measured directly using the trapezoidal rule or the log trapezoidal rule (20) or may be determined from the sum of the ratio of the coefficients and exponents for a multiexponential fit to the data (18). For example, if three exponential terms are required to fit the data (i.e., a three-compartment pharmacokinetic model), equation 18 describes the time course of the plasma concentration (C_P), and equation 19 defines the area under the curve for these data.

$$C_P = A_1e^{-\lambda_1 t} + A_2e^{-\lambda_2 t} + A_3e^{-\lambda_3 t} \qquad (18)$$

$$AUC = A_1/\lambda_1 + A_2/\lambda_2 + A_3/\lambda_3 \qquad (19)$$

Volume of Distribution

The volume of distribution may also be determined using both noncompartmental area methods as well as from the coefficients and exponents of the equation describing the plasma concentration–time curve. There are a number of volume terms reported in the literature that attempt to define the total space for distribution of a drug in the body. The volume of distribution at steady state (V_{ss}) represents the volume in which a drug would appear to be distributed during steady state if the drug existed throughout that volume at the same concentration as in the measured fluid (plasma or blood). This volume can be determined by the use of areas as described by Benet and Galeazzi (2):

$$V_{ss} = (\text{Dose}^{iv})(AUMC)/AUC^2 \qquad (20)$$

where $AUMC$ is the area under the first moment of the plasma concentration time curve, that is, the area under the curve of the product of time, t, and plasma concentration, C_P, over the time span zero to infinity. The volume of distribution at steady state may also be determined from coefficients and exponents in a manner similar to that for clearance since *AUMC* may also be defined in terms of these parameters, that is, the sum of the ratios of the coefficients to the exponents squared. For the three-exponential model given in equation 18:

$$AUMC = A_1/\lambda_1^2 + A_2/\lambda_2^2 + A_3/\lambda_3^2 \quad (21)$$

An alternative measure of the total volume of distribution is often used. This parameter, V_{area}, is calculated as the ratio of clearance and the terminal rate constant describing drug disposition (λ_z). For the three-compartmental model described by equation 18, λ_z equals λ_3.

$$V_{area} = CL/\lambda_z \quad (22)$$

Although V_{area} is a convenient and easily calculated parameter, this volume term varies when the rate constant for drug or metabolite elimination changes, even when there has been no change in the distribution space. As the rate constant for elimination decreases, V_{area} approaches V_{ss}. Since we may wish to know whether a particular disease state influences either clearance or the distribution of the drug within the body independently, it is preferable to define volume in terms of a parameter that is theoretically independent of changes in the rate of elimination. The difference between these two volume terms is illustrated in Table 2, where pharmacokinetic parameters for cefamandole in six normal volunteers (1) are compared to those obtained in three uremic patients (8). Since cefamandole is almost exclusively eliminated by the renal route, a marked difference in clearance (24-fold change) is noted between normals and uremics. However, the terminal half-life, $t_{1/2_z}$, and the terminal rate constant for elimination only change by a factor of 11. Note that a significant difference, more than a twofold change, is observed in V_{area}. This could be interpreted to mean that changes in renal function not only affect the elimination of cefamandole, as reflected by the clearance changes, but that there is also a decrease in the distribution volume of this drug. However, when V_{ss} is compared, it is obvious that no significant difference in the distribution volume between these two patient populations is noted.

Clearance to and of Metabolites—Sequential Metabolism

As noted in equation 2, the clearance of parent drug to a particular metabolite ($f_{m_i}\,CL$) and the clearance of that metabolite (CL_{M_i}) may be defined under steady-state conditions in terms of parent drug and metabolite concentrations in plasma or blood. Under nonsteady-state conditions, when an intravenous dose of drug is given, equation 2 may be integrated over time to yield the following relationship between area under the curve (*AUC*) measurements.

Amount of metabolite formed

$$= f_{m_i}\,CL\,AUC = CL_{M_i}\,AUC_{M_i} \quad (23)$$

where *AUC* is the area under the curve from time zero to infinity for unchanged drug con-

TABLE 2. *Cefamandole kinetics in normals and uremics*

Parameter	Normals[a]	Uremics[b]	Significance
CL (ml/min · kg)	2.81 ± 0.98[c]	0.115 ± 0.023	$p < 0.05$
$t_{1/2_z}$ (hr)	1.2 ± 0.2	13.0 ± 4.5	$p < 0.05$
λ_z (hr^{-1})	0.576 ± 0.096	0.0534 ± 0.0187	$p < 0.05$
V_{area} (liter/kg)	0.298 ± 0.104	0.138 ± 0.048	$p < 0.05$
V_{ss} (liter/kg)	0.161 ± 0.050	0.134 ± 0.045	n.s.

[a] Aziz et al. (1).
[b] Gambertoglio et al. (8).
[c] SD.

centrations, and AUC_{M_i} is the area for the metabolite concentrations following intravenous drug administration. When metabolite i is not further eliminated by the metabolizing organ, CL_{M_i} can be determined directly by administration of the metabolite and measurement of AUC_{M_i} (eq. 17). Then, f_{m_i} may be determined from equation 23. Note that for intravenous dosing of the drug, the product of CL and AUC equals dose. Equation 23 will not be valid for oral dosing, since some of the metabolite will be formed due to first-pass metabolism in the liver. In essence, both unchanged drug and metabolite are "dosed" into the systemic circulation. This complexity is discussed in the chapter by G. R. Wilkinson, this volume.

Further complexities arise when sequential metabolism of the drug occurs. Consider the situation where:

$$\begin{array}{ccccc} D & \rightarrow & M_1 & \rightarrow & M_2 \\ \downarrow & & \downarrow & & \downarrow \end{array}$$

That is, sequential metabolism occurs, and the drug and metabolite 1 may also be eliminated by alternate pathways. An equation analogous to equation 23 may be defined for the metabolic relationship between drug and metabolite 1.

$$\text{Amount of metabolite 1 formed} = f_{m_{D\to1}} CL\, AUC = CL_{M_1}\, AUC_{M_1} \tag{24}$$

where $f_{m_{D\to1}}$ is the fraction of the clearance of drug that results in the production of metabolite 1. Equation 24 might be valid for a drug for which metabolism to M_1 occurs in one organ of the body and further metabolism of M_1 to M_2 occurs in another organ. However, equation 24 will almost never be valid for a drug for which the sequential metabolic steps take place in the same organ of elimination. Under these conditions, metabolism of drug to M_1 and further to M_2 may occur within the hepatocyte, for example. That is, M_2 is formed and measured in the circulation without a corresponding measurement of M_1 in the circulation. This is analogous to the complexity resulting from first-pass metabolism following oral drug dosing. If M_2 is not further eliminated by the metabolizing organ, the fraction of the clearance of the drug that results in metabolite 2, f_{m_2}, can be determined following intravenous drug dosing as:

$$\text{Amount of metabolite 2 formed} = f_{m_2} CL\, AUC = CL_{M_2}\, AUC_{M_2} \tag{25}$$

Note that the restriction placed on equations 23 and 25 is that the metabolite not be further *eliminated* by the metabolizing organ rather than only further *metabolized.* Thus, if a hepatic metabolite is excreted in the bile, or if a compound metabolized in the kidney or lung is then excreted by that organ, AUC_{M_i} will be underestimated.

Pang, Gillette, and co-workers have attempted to solve the problems involved with sequential metabolism that make equation 24 invalid by the inclusion of an availability term to account for the "first-pass loss" of the metabolite (12–15).

$$f_{m_{D\to1}}\, F^{D}_{M_1} CL\, AUC = CL_{M_1}\, AUC_{M_1} \tag{26}$$

where $F^{D}_{M_1}$ is the availability of metabolite 1 when the parent drug is dosed. This term is included to account for the fraction of metabolite 1 formed that is then further metabolized or eliminated prior to leaving the metabolizing organ. As defined, equation 26 is correct. However, the products on the left- and right-hand sides of the equation are no longer equal to the amount of metabolite formed; rather, they are equal to the amount of metabolite measured in the circulation. Equation 26 can be redefined to calculate the fraction of the dose that appears in the circulation as metabolite 1 since $CL \cdot AUC$ equals the intravenous dose of parent drug:

$$f_{m_{D\to1}}\, F^{D}_{M_1}\, \text{Dose} = CL_{M_1}\, AUC_{M_1} \tag{27}$$

Equation 26 can also be rearranged to calculate, $CL^{\text{app}}_{D\to1}$, the apparent fractional clearance to metabolite 1 (i.e., as measured in the circulation):

$$CL^{\text{app}}_{D\to1} = f_{m_{D\to1}}\, F^{D}_{M_1}\, CL = CL_{M_1}\, AUC_{M_1}/AUC \tag{28}$$

The use of the noncompartmental methods defined above is demonstrated in the following section, where the influence of probenecid on the metabolism of azathioprine and 6-mercaptopurine is evaluated.

Although equation 26 is valid, it is often difficult to determine $F^{D}_{M_1}$ when sequential metabolism occurs. Pang and Gillette (13) have calculated $F^{D}_{M_1}$ following phenacetin dosing as the ratio of acetaminophen concentrations to the sum of acetaminophen plus conjugate concentrations in the blood flowing out of the liver, assuming no biliary excretion of acetaminophen in any form. Pang et al. (15) suggest that $F^{D}_{M_i}$ may be approximated by F_{M_i}, which is the ratio of areas under the metabolite curve after intraportal and intravenous doses of the metabolite (i.e., Eq. 13 for metabolite i). There is a major assumption in this treatment that has been addressed by Pang and Gillette (14); that is, the parent drug and metabolite 1 in equation 26 must have similar partition characteristics into the metabolic site (i.e., the hepatocyte in the case of liver metabolism). This is highly unlikely, since the usual effect of the metabolism of xenobiotics is to change the polarity of the compound to facilitate elimination by the body. Thus, it appears reasonable to assume that a metabolite formed within the hepatocyte would be more accessible to sequential metabolism than a metabolite infused into the liver. Therefore, $F^{D}_{M_1}$ in equation 26 is probably overestimated when it is determined from the extraction ratio of the dosed metabolite (i.e., when it is assumed that $F^{D}_{M_1} = F_{M_1}$).

APPLICATION OF PHARMACOKINETIC PRINCIPLES TO EVALUATE THE INTERACTION OF AZATHIOPRINE AND PROBENECID

Azathioprine (AZA) is widely used as a clinically effective immunosuppressive agent. The overall metabolic scheme of AZA is extremely complicated. One important metabolic step is cleavage to 6-mercaptopurine (6-MP), a step that is believed to be necessary for the pharmacologic action of the drug. 6-Mercaptopurine is anabolized to the biologically active thioinosinic acid, and this is transformed to other active nucleotides such as methylthioinosinic acid and thioguanylic acid (7). Azathioprine is readily split to 6-MP by sulfhydryl compounds. It has been demonstrated that glutathione plays an important role in mediating thiolysis of AZA to 6-MP *in vitro* and *in vivo* (3,4). Kaplowitz and Kuhlenkamp (9) reported the inhibition of hepatic AZA metabolism in the rat by probenecid and bilirubin. They concluded that the liver was the major site of the interaction of AZA with glutathione *in vivo* and that the inhibition of hepatic glutathione utilization by probenecid and bilirubin in the rat suggest that the conversion of AZA to 6-MP *in vivo* may be mediated enzymatically by the hepatic glutathione *S*-transferase. However, huge intraperitoneal doses (100 μmole/100 g) were employed in the above experiments in order to detect a measurable depletion of hepatic glutathione levels. Administering doses identical with the therapeutic dose for man (1 μmole/100 g) resulted in no significant change in glutathione levels.

Ling and Benet (10) attempted to identify a possible enzymatic thiolysis of AZA *in vivo* in the rhesus monkey. These workers determined the effect of probenecid on the metabolic clearance of AZA to 6-MP in the monkey using doses identical to those used clinically in man. The pharmacokinetics of AZA and 6-MP following oral and intravenous doses of both drugs has been described by Ding and Benet (5). The relevant metabolic scheme in terms of the probenecid interaction study is given below:

$$\text{AZA} \xrightarrow{\text{glutathione}} \text{6-MP} \xrightarrow{\text{xanthine oxidase}} \text{Thiouric acid}$$

AZA	6-MP	Thiouric acid
↓ other metabolic steps	↓ other metabolic and catabolic steps	↓

Note that this scheme is equivalent to that discussed previously. However, we investigate here not only the sequential metabolism of AZA but also the effect of probenecid on this metabolism.

Methods

Two male rhesus monkeys weighing 5.75 and 5.90 kg were studied. Azathioprine was administered to each monkey as a 10.83-μmole/kg intravenous bolus dose with and without concomitant probenecid. Probenecid was given as a 33-mg/kg bolus dose 15 min prior to the AZA dose. Blood was sampled for up to 3 hr after AZA administration. Plasma samples were frozen until analyzed for AZA, 6-MP, and probenecid. To determine the effect of probenecid on 6-MP kinetics, the above experiments were repeated with an equimolar i.v. dose of 6-MP (10.83 μmole/kg) given with and without probenecid. Plasma samples were then analyzed for 6-MP and probenecid.

Our previous method (6) for determining AZA and 6-MP levels in plasma by high-pressure liquid chromatography involves extraction of the drug with an organic solvent. The extremely polar nature of the thiopurines as well as their instability during the isolation procedure makes it difficult to achieve a high recovery of the thiopurines when extraction is attempted. A new direct injection method was developed (10), which does not involve any extraction steps and requires only small amounts of plasma (0.2 ml). Azathioprine was determined at 280 nm using a μBondapak® C-8 column, 10-μm particle size, and a solvent system consisting of 11% (v/v) acetonitrile in water, to which glacial acetic acid was added to give a final concentration of 0.02 M.

6-Mercaptopurine was analyzed at 325 nm using a Spherisorb® ODS column, 5-μm particle size, and a solvent system consisting of 14% (vol/vol) methanol in water, to which 0.5% of glacial acetic acid was added. 1-Heptane sulfonic acid sodium salt was added to give a concentration of 0.005 M in the HPLC buffer. Probenecid was measured using the HPLC method of Smith et al. (17).

Results

Figure 1 shows the effect of probenecid on AZA plasma levels in monkey I following i.v. AZA administration. The AZA levels were significantly higher when probenecid was given prior to AZA. The 6-MP levels following AZA dosing for this monkey were also significantly higher with concomitant probenecid (Fig. 2). Similar effects of probenecid on AZA and 6-MP were seen in monkey II following AZA dosing. Probenecid does not appear to have an effect on 6-MP levels when 6-MP is given i.v. to the monkey (Fig. 3).

Clearance of the drug dosed (AZA or 6-MP) may be calculated following intravenous administration as the ratio of Dose to *AUC* (equation 17). As seen in Table 3 and

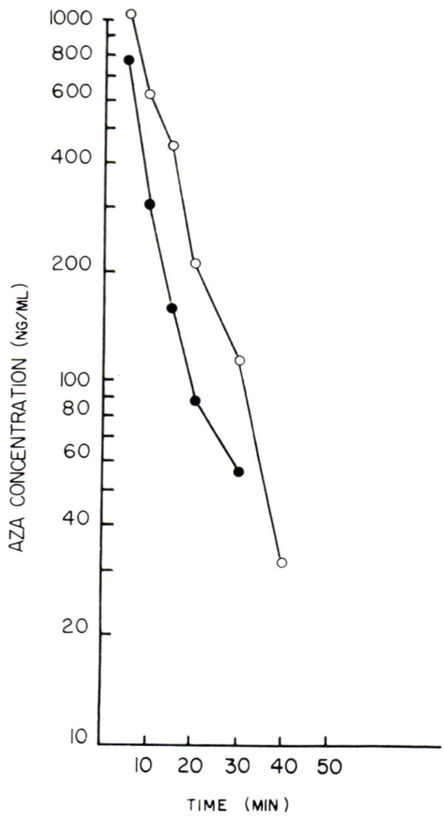

FIG. 1. Azathioprine plasma levels in monkey I following i.v. AZA administration (10.83 μmole/kg) with (○) and without (●) probenecid (33 mg/kg).

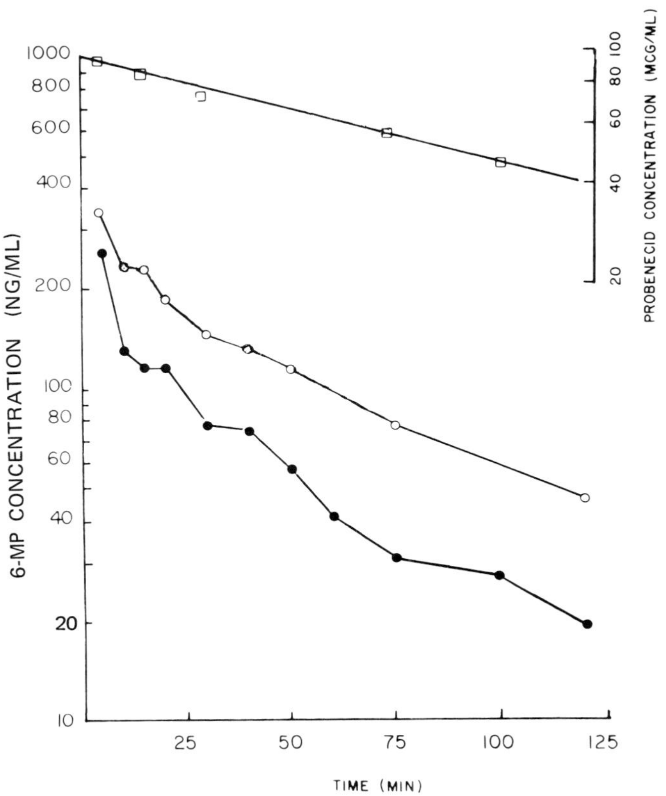

FIG. 2. 6-Mercaptopurine plasma levels in monkey I in the i.v. AZA studies with (○) and without (●) probenecid (33 mg/kg). Probenecid plasma levels (□) were measured in the experiment with probenecid.

Fig. 3, probenecid had little effect on the clearance of 6-MP when this drug was dosed to the monkeys. In contrast, probenecid had a marked effect on the clearance of AZA (>40% decrease), as shown in Table 4 and Fig. 1. The volume of distribution (equation 20) for AZA was also decreased when probenecid was present. Since the decrease in distribution space approximated the decrease in clearance when probenecid was dosed concomitantly, no change in $t_{1/2}$ (equation 16) was noted.

In the present study, it was not possible to separately determine $f_{m_{D \to 1}}$ and $F^{D}_{M_1}$ (see eq. 26), since studies of the metabolism of AZA were carried out in an intact animal. However, it was possible to calculate the apparent clearance of AZA to measured concentrations of 6-MP, i.e., $CL^{app}_{D \to 1}$, using equation 28. As noted in Table 4, probenecid had little effect on this apparent clearance of AZA to 6-MP. However, when this apparent clearance is subtracted from the total AZA clearance, probenecid has a marked effect. The apparent residual clearance ($CL - CL^{app}_{D \to 1}$) is more than halved when probenecid is administered concomitantly (Table 4).

Discussion

The higher AZA levels achieved with AZA and probenecid i.v. dosing (Fig. 1) might be expected if a glutathione-mediated thiolysis of AZA is inhibited by probenecid. The increased 6-MP levels following AZA and probenecid (Fig. 2) were not anticipated, since one would expect less 6-MP to be formed if the AZA interaction with glutathione is inhibited. In order to identify any changes in the pharmacokinetics of 6-MP with probenecid, experiments were conducted to see the effect of probenecid on 6-MP given i.v. Since there was no change in the plasma clearance of 6-MP with probenecid (Fig. 3 and Table

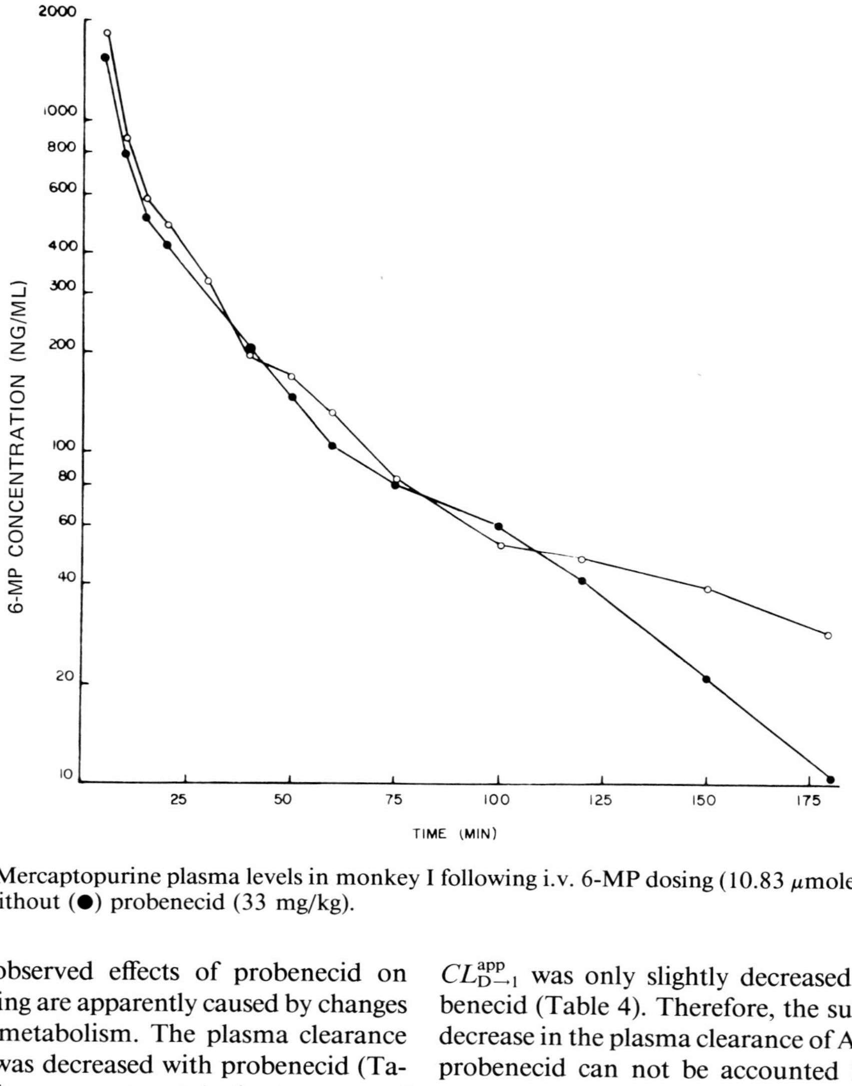

FIG. 3. 6-Mercaptopurine plasma levels in monkey I following i.v. 6-MP dosing (10.83 μmole/kg) with (○) and without (●) probenecid (33 mg/kg).

3), the observed effects of probenecid on AZA dosing are apparently caused by changes in AZA metabolism. The plasma clearance of AZA was decreased with probenecid (Table 4). The apparent metabolic clearance of AZA to 6-MP was subsequently calculated;

TABLE 3. *Effect of probenecid on the plasma clearance (ml/min · kg) of 6-MP following 10.8 µmole/kg intravenous bolus dosing*

	Monkey I	Monkey II
6-MP	44.7	30.6
6-MP + probenecid	44.3 (0.99)[a]	27.8 (0.91)

[a] Values in parentheses represent the clearance ratio with and without probenecid.

From Ling and Benet (10), with permission.

$CL^{\text{app}}_{\text{D}\rightarrow 1}$ was only slightly decreased by probenecid (Table 4). Therefore, the substantial decrease in the plasma clearance of AZA with probenecid can not be accounted for by a change in the apparent clearance of AZA to 6-MP and suggests that the probenecid effect may not result from alteration of the glutathione-mediated thiolysis of AZA to 6-MP (10). Rather, probenecid appears to markedly decrease the apparent residual clearance of AZA.

The metabolism of AZA is intricate and many faceted. The interaction study, briefly described here, is certainly not definitive, and the data may be interpreted in a number of ways (10). However, the example presented here does indicate how pharmacokinetics

TABLE 4. *Effect of probenecid on the pharmacokinetics of AZA following 10.8 μmole/kg intravenous bolus dosing*

	Monkey I		Monkey II	
	AZA	AZA + probenecid	AZA	AZA + probenecid
CL (ml/min · kg)	299	158 (0.53)[a]	160	87 (0.54)
V_{ss} (liter/kg)	2.87	1.59 (0.55)	1.84	1.08 (0.59)
$t_{1/2}$ (min)	9.6	10.1	11.5	12.4
$CL^{app}_{D\to 1}$ (ml/min · kg)	68	64 (0.94)	30	23 (0.77)
$CL - CL^{app}_{D\to 1}$ (ml/min · kg)	231	94 (0.41)	130	64 (0.49)

[a] Values in parentheses represent the parameter ratio with and without probenecid.
From Ling and Benet (10), with permission.

may serve as a tool in drug metabolism and how noncompartmental methods may be used.

REFERENCES

1. Aziz, N. S., Gambertoglio, J. G., Lin, E. T., Grausz, H., and Benet, L. Z. (1978): Pharmacokinetics of cefamandole using an HPLC assay. *J. Pharmacokinet. Biopharm.*, 6:153–164.
2. Benet, L. Z., and Galeazzi, R. L. (1979): Noncompartmental determination of the steady-state volume of distribution. *J. Pharm. Sci.*, 68:1071–1074.
3. Chalmers, A. H., Knight, P. R., and Atkinson, M. R. (1967): Conversion of azathioprine into mercaptopurine and mercaptoimidazole derivatives *in vitro* and during immunosuppressive therapy. *Aust. J. Exp. Biol. Med. Sci.*, 45:681–691.
4. DeMiranda, P., Beacham, L. M. III, Creagh, T. H., and Elion, G. B. (1973): The metabolic fate of the methylnitroimidazole moiety of azathioprine in the rat. *J. Pharmacol. Exp. Ther.*, 187:588–601.
5. Ding, T. L., and Benet, L. Z. (1979): Comparative bioavailability and pharmacokinetic studies of azathioprine and 6-mercaptopurine in the rhesus monkey. *Drug Metab. Dispos.*, 7:373–377.
6. Ding, T. L., and Benet, L. Z. (1979): Determination of 6-mercaptopurine and azathioprine in plasma by high-performance liquid chromatography. *J. Chromatogr.*, 163:281–288.
7. Elion, G. B., and Hitchings, G. H. (1975): Azathioprine. In: *Handbook of Experimental Pharmacology, Vol. 38, Part 2,* edited by A. C. Sartorelli and D. G. Johns, pp. 404–425. Springer-Verlag, Berlin.
8. Gambertoglio, J. G., Aziz, N. S., Lin, E. T., Grausz, H., Naughton, J. L., and Benet, L. Z. (1979): Cefamandole kinetics in uremic patients undergoing hemodialysis. *Clin. Pharmacol. Ther.*, 26:592–599.
9. Kaplowitz, N., and Kuhlenkamp, J. (1978): Inhibition of hepatic metabolism of azathioprine *in vivo*. *Gastroenterology,* 74:90–92.
10. Ling, T. L., and Benet, L. Z. (1984): Effect of probenecid on the metabolic clearance of azathioprine to 6-mercaptopurine in the rhesus monkey. *Pharmaceut. Res.* (*in press*).
11. Øie, S., and Tozer, T. N. (1979): Effect of altered plasma protein binding on apparent volume of distribution. *J. Pharm. Sci.,* 68:1203–1205.
12. Pang, K. S. (1981): Metabolite pharmacokinetics: The area under the curve of metabolite and the fractional rate of metabolism of a drug after different routes of administration for renally and hepatically cleared drugs and metabolites. *J. Pharmacokinet. Biopharm.*, 9:477–487.
13. Pang, K. S., and Gillette, J. R. (1978): Kinetics of metabolite formation and elimination in the perfused rat liver preparation: Differences between the elimination of preformed acetaminophen and acetaminophen formed from phenacetin. *J. Pharmacol. Exp. Ther.*, 207:178–194.
14. Pang, K. S., and Gillette, J. R. (1979): Sequential first-pass elimination of a metabolite derived from a precursor. *J. Pharmacokinet. Biopharm.*, 7:275–290.
15. Pang, K. S., Strobl, K., and Gillette, J. R. (1979): A method for the estimation of the fraction of a precursor that is converted to a metabolite in rat *in vivo* with phenacetin and acetaminophen. *Drug Metab. Dispos.*, 7:366–372.
16. Rowland, M., Benet, L. Z., and Graham, G. G. (1973): Clearance concepts in pharmacokinetics. *J. Pharmacokinet. Biopharm.*, 1:123–136.
17. Smith, D. E., Gee, W. L., Brater, D. C., Lin, E. T., and Benet, L. Z. (1980): Preliminary evaluation of furosemide-probenecid interaction in humans. *J. Pharm. Sci.*, 69:571–447.
18. Wagner, J. G. (1976): Linear pharmacokinetic equations allowing direct calculation of many needed pharmacokinetic parameters from the coefficients and exponents of polyexponential equations which have been fitted to data. *J. Pharmacokinet. Biopharm.*, 4:443–467.
19. Wilkinson, G. R., and Shand, D. G. (1975): A physiological approach to hepatic drug clearance. *Clin. Pharmacol. Ther.*, 18:377–390.
20. Yeh, K. C., and Kwan, K. C. (1978): A comparison of numerical integrating logarithms by trapezoidal, lagrange, and spline approximation. *J. Pharmacokinet. Biopharm.*, 6:79–98.

Drug Metabolism and Drug Toxicity,
edited by J. R. Mitchell and M. G. Horning.
Raven Press, New York © 1984.

Pharmacokinetic Considerations in Toxicology

Grant R. Wilkinson

Department of Pharmacology, Vanderbilt University, Nashville, Tennessee 37232

Toxicological studies in experimental animals form the basis of the safe use of drugs and chemicals in man and other species. The traditional approach to such extrapolations has been to establish a dosage or exposure level that produces no observable adverse effect in the test animal(s) and then to apply an arbitrary safety factor. However, the biological complexity and diversity of higher animals, particularly mammals, makes this approach difficult and uncertain even under the most optimal conditions. An alternative strategy that is receiving increasing attention is the identification of the causes and involved mechanisms responsible for interspecies differences in toxic responsiveness. The predictive reliability of the experimental data base is often considerably enhanced by the appropriate application of such information. An important component of this approach is an adequate understanding of the qualitative, quantitative, and temporal aspects of the absorption, distribution, metabolism, and excretion of the xenobiotic. Although the general principles of these processes are well recognized and have often been described, especially with respect to the usual dosage situation, their application to the special concerns of toxicity testing is not so well appreciated. Accordingly, a number of dispositional factors of particular relevance to toxicology are considered in this chapter.

ROUTE OF ADMINISTRATION

First-Pass Phenomenon

It has long been known that the effectiveness and toxicity of innumerable compounds are highly dependent on their route of administration. In general, delivery into the systemic circulation provides the most direct access to the ultimate site of action. However, when local effects are elicited in readily accessible tissues such as the skin, lung, and GI tract, other routes of administration than the intravascular may be more efficacious. Often the differences in toxicity, for example, among the intravenous, subcutaneous, intramuscular, oral, intraperitoneal, and inhalation routes are related to drug bioavailability, that is, the relative rate and extent at which the administered dose reaches the systemic circulation. This situation can be readily identified by well-established pharmacokinetic approaches based on the relative urinary excretion and/or plasma concentration/time profiles following drug administration by the various routes (31,60). Sometimes reduced bioavailability can be accounted for by an absorption problem; i.e., the drug has problems of dissolution from the dosage form, or it has difficulty in crossing the protective barriers of the body and being absorbed. However, in many instances, route-of-administration-dependent toxicity is caused by the presence of a first-pass effect.

Although the liver is frequently the major site of drug biotransformation within the body, many other organs have the capability to metabolize xenobiotics (see J. R. Bend and C. J. Serabjit-Singh, *this volume*). Whenever such an organ is interposed between the site of drug administration and the effector or sampling site, then drug elimination will occur during the overall "absorption" process, i.e., presystemic elimination. The extent of such a first-pass effect relative to a route of administration that bypasses the initial exposure, e.g., intravenous or intraarterial, is dependent on the efficiency of the removal process, as assessed by the organ's extraction ratio (E). Only that fraction (F) of the amount of drug entering the organ that is not metabolized and not excreted in the bile in the case of the liver, $(1 - E)$, escapes into the venous outflow of the organ and reaches the systemic circulation.

Quantitatively, organ bioavailability may be related to the three physiological determinants of organ elimination and measurable pharmacokinetic parameters by equation 1:

$$F = 1 - E = \frac{C_0}{C_{\text{in}}} = \frac{Q}{Q + f_B Cl^{\text{u}}_{\text{int}}} = \frac{AUC_2}{AUC_1} \times \frac{\text{Dose}_1}{\text{Dose}_2} \tag{1}$$

where Q is organ blood flow, f_B is the unbound fraction of drug in the blood, $Cl^{\text{u}}_{\text{int}}$ is the free intrinsic clearance of the drug from the organ's intracellular water, and C_{in} and C_o are the drug concentrations of the inflow and outflow blood of the organ; AUC is the total area under the blood concentration/time curve following administration of drug by the route involving first-pass elimination (Dose_2) compared to a reference route (Dose_1) in which presystemic elimination is absent, e.g., intravenous. In the case of the oral route, if the actual drug absorption step is incomplete, then equation 1 may be modified to reflect the absorbed fraction, F^*, that is available for first-pass elimination. Accordingly, the first-pass effect becomes increasingly significant as a drug's free intrinsic clearance increases and, to a lesser extent, as the binding in the blood decreases. From the practical standpoint, a drug with an extraction ratio above 60 to 70% is considered to exhibit an extensive first-pass effect.

Following oral, and to a lesser extent intraperitoneal, drug administration, several first-pass organs are arranged in series, e.g., GI tract, GI mucosa, liver, and lung. In this situation, the overall bioavailability as measured at a distal peripheral site is equal to the product of each sequential organ's bioavailability (34):

$$F_{\text{oral}} = F^*(1 - E_{\text{GI tract}})(1 - E_{\text{GI mucosa}}) \times (1 - E_{\text{liver}})(1 - E_{\text{lung}}) \tag{2}$$

The relative contribution of each organ to the net availability may be assessed by the relative areas under the blood or plasma concentration/time curves following drug administration at different sites. For example, Table 1 shows that only 3% of an orally administered dose of the extensively conjugated xenobiotic phenol reaches the systemic circulation intact (15). The similarities between the blood level/time profiles for the sum of the sulfate and glucuronide conjugates, however, indicates that this is not an absorption

TABLE 1. *Area under blood concentration/time curves (AUC) for phenol and phenyl conjugates following administration of phenol by different routes in the rat*

Route	AUC phenol (μg · ml^{-1} · min · kg^{-1})	AUC phenol conjugates (μg · ml^{-1} · min · kg^{-1})
Intraarterial	6.13 ± 1.83	39.74 ± 4.64
Intravenous	2.53 ± 0.94	49.48 ± 19.12
Hepatic portal venous	2.22 ± 0.72	41.66 ± 12.2
Oral	0.18 ± 0.12	46.25 ± 22.92

Modified from Cassidy and Houston (15), with permission.

problem. When phenol was given intraarterially, intravenously, orally, and also into the hepatic portal vein, the major contributor to this pronounced first-pass effect was shown to be the GI tract ($E = 92\%$), followed by the lung ($E = 62\%$), and the liver was, in fact, a minor site of metabolism ($E = 6\%$). In a similar fashion, it was shown that about 20 to 30% of an orally administered dose of acetylsalicylic acid is hydrolyzed in the GI mucosa of the dog during the absorptive process, and a further 25 to 50% is metabolized during the initial pass through the liver (36). Unfortunately, this type of approach is unable to separate the first-pass contribution of the microflora of the GI lumen from that of the various enzymes present in the GI mucosa. However, the use of germ-free and/or antibiotic-treated animals often provides insights into this matter (63).

Drug Metabolism and the First-Pass Effect

Conventional linear compartmental pharmacokinetics based on all of the drug clearance processes being within a single compartment indicates that the fraction of the absorbed dose excreted unchanged (f_e) and that metabolized, either totally ($f_m = 1 - f_e$) or to a specific metabolite (f_{m_i}), are independent of the route of administration (31,60). Moreover, the fractional contribution of any particular metabolic pathway is equal to the ratio of the clearance of parent drug to metabolite to the total systemic clearance of drug following intravenous administration (equation 5)

$$f_{m_i} = \frac{\text{Metabolic clearance by } i\text{th pathway}}{(\text{Renal} + \text{total metabolic} + \text{other}) \text{ clearance}} \quad (3)$$

Also, f_{m_i} may be estimated either from plasma (equation 4) or urinary excretion data (equation 5)

$$f_{m_i} = \frac{AUC^{D}_{M_i}/\text{Dose}^{D}}{AUC^{M_i,\text{iv}}_{M_i}/D^{M_i,\text{iv}}} \quad (4)$$

$$f_{m_i} = \frac{M_i^{D}/\text{Dose}^{D}}{M_i^{M_i,\text{iv}}/D^{M_i,\text{iv}}} \quad (5)$$

where AUC_{M_i} is the total area under the plasma level/time curve for metabolite following administration of parent drug by any route (Dose^D) and after intravenous administration of the metabolite itself ($D^{M_i,\text{iv}}$), and M_i is the ultimate amount of metabolite excreted in the urine following administration of parent M_i^D and metabolite M_i^M. Thus, not only is the metabolic/excretory pattern independent of the route of administration but so is the area under the metabolite's plasma level/time curve.

This conventional approach, however, fails to take into account the anatomical arrangement of the various organs capable of presystemic elimination. When this is considered, it readily becomes apparent that the ratio of the amount of drug excreted to that metabolized is route dependent except when all of the drug is eliminated by the first-pass organ (30). Regardless of whether drug is present in the systemic circulation by direct injection or reaches it following extravascular administration, there is an equal opportunity for all routes of elimination. In contrast, when a drug is administered by a route involving first-pass elimination, e.g., oral, then presystemic elimination occurs during this process, equivalent to the extraction ratio, and only a fraction $(1 - E)$ of the dose is available to the systemic circulation. Accordingly, the fraction of the absorbed dose metabolized (f_m^{po}) is given by equation 6.

$$f_m^{\text{po}} = E + Ff_m^{\text{iv}} \quad (6)$$

Substituting $(1 - F)$ for E and $(1 - f_e^{\text{iv}})$ for f_m^{iv} gives equation 7.

$$f_m^{\text{po}} = 1 - Ff_e^{\text{iv}} \quad (7)$$

Thus, the degree to which the ratio of metabolized to excreted drug changes according to the route of administration depends on the magnitude of the first-pass effect. Furthermore, a greater fraction of the absorbed dose is metabolized following oral and other first-pass-effect routes than when the drug is given intravenously. Conversely, more drug is excreted unchanged following intravascular injection. With salbutamol, for example, about 50% of an oral dose is eliminated in the urine as metabolites and 25% as unchanged drug, whereas only 22 to 25% of an intravenous injection is metabolized, and about 50% is excreted unchanged—a complete reversal of the elimination pattern (24).

If a metabolite immediately undergoes further elimination while it is still present within the organ responsible for its formation, then sequential elimination occurs. For example, in the liver, a compound may undergo phase-I-type metabolism, and the generated metabolite is then conjugated, or a glucuronidated metabolite is excreted into the bile. As a result, less metabolite escapes into the systemic circulation than is actually formed. Therefore, equation 4 gives an underestimation of the actual fractional conversion to metabolites, dependent on the extent of the metabolite's first-pass effect (50). By taking into account this factor, it is possible to estimate f_{m_i}. For example, if the liver is the only site of elimination for both parent drug and metabolite, then

$$f_{m_i} = \frac{AUC_{M_i}^{D,iv}/\text{Dose}^{D,iv}}{AUC_{M_i}^{M_i,po}/\text{Dose}^{M_i,po}} \quad (8)$$

That is, the parent drug must be administered intravenously and the metabolite given orally, and the plasma metabolite/time profile determined (50,51). Importantly, in this situation the area under the metabolite plasma concentration/time curve and the amount formed and excreted in the urine are the same for all routes of administration of parent drug.

When the metabolite undergoes sequential first-pass elimination in the organ in which it is formed and is also removed from the systemic circulation by another organ, e.g., kidney, then the situation becomes even more complex. The area under the metabolite plasma concentration/time curve and urinary excretion profile of metabolites then become dependent on the route of administration in the same way that first-pass elimination affects the disposition of parent drug. In the limited case in which the liver is only organ able to form the metabolite, the oral route of administration yields a higher area under the curve for metabolite than does intravenous administration by an additional term equal to the ratio of the renal clearance of parent drug to the hepatic perfusion rate (49). Accordingly, the smaller the renal clearance, the more comparable the areas. Also, consideration of the relative magnitudes of the determinants indicates that the maximal difference in the metabolite area between oral and intravenous is about 1.8. If this value is exceeded, then either incomplete gastrointestinal absorption and/or metabolism must be occurring.

The effect of different routes of administration on the metabolic fate of a xenobiotic is further complicated when the enzymes are compartmentalized; i.e., metabolism only occurs during the first pass, and systemically delivered drug is not available for biotransformation. Drug metabolism in the intestinal lumen by the microbial flora is an excellent example of this phenomenon, since the process is limited solely to the contents of the GI tract and is terminated immediately on drug absorption. The microflora of the GI lumen are capable of a multitude of reactions, with hydrolytic and reductive processes predominating over oxidation and conjugation (62,63). Furthermore, considerable qualitative and quantitative differences in the GI microflora may occur between various species, and this can account for differences in metabolic fate. An excellent example of this is the aromatization of quinic acid to benzoic acid, which is only found in man and Old-World monkeys and not in New-World primates or lower species (2).

Microbial biotransformation is often of toxicological significance, especially with regard to route-dependent metabolism and pharmacological effects. For example, amygdalin, a constituent of laetrile, is a glycoside that is practically nontoxic when given parenterally to mice ($LD_{50} > 5$ g/kg) but is toxic when given orally (LD_{50} 300 mg/kg). Hydrolysis by microbial enzymes to an unstable aglycone, mandelonitrile, which breaks down to yield cyanide is probably responsible for this difference in effects (23). The methemoglobinemia produced by nitrobenzene is associated with the formation of the reduction products, nitrosobenzene and phenylhydroxylamine. The nitroreductases of the microbial flora appear to be predominantly responsible for this toxicity, since germ-free or antibiotic-treated animals exhibit no measurable methemoglobin formation at doses producing 30 to 40% conversion in normal rats (56). A similar situation also occurs with the reduction of dinitrophenols to amino compounds, which cause methemoglobinemia (25).

Gastrointestinal metabolism may also play an important role in carcinogenesis. Various microorganisms have been isolated from the intestinal contents or feces of a variety of animals, including man, that are able to metabolize the artificial sweetening agent cyclamate to cyclohexylamine, and the latter compound has been postulated to be involved in the subsequent development of bladder cancer. Interestingly, hydrolysis of the sulfamate is only present in animals previously exposed to dietary cyclamate; naive animals do not metabolize the compound but acquire the ability on continued dietary intake and/or exposure via coprophagy to converted animals (57). It has also been suggested that the products of xenobiotic metabolism by the gastrointestinal flora are probably contributory in the etiology of colonic cancer, presumably by conversion of a potential carcinogen to an active carcinogen (22,57). Finally, there has been increasing recognition and concern over the carcinogenicity of *N*-nitroso compounds such as nitrosamines present in the diet and also formed in the GI tract. In the latter case, the microflora play a critical role in the reaction of dietary amines with endogenous nitrite and nitrate (39).

"True" first-pass metabolism may also occur with those metabolizing enzymes located in the epithelial lining of the GI tract. For example, about 70% of isoproterenol is conjugated with sulfate when instilled into a loop of the isolated canine intestinal preparation (29). However, no conjugation occurs if the drug is infused into the arterial blood supply of the loop (38). Similarly, biotransformation occurring in the pulmonary system may be restricted to drug passing through the bronchial membranes and not to that present in the alveolar blood supply. Again, the ethereal sulfation of isoproterenol demonstrates this possibility; conjugation is apparent after intrabronchial administration (12) but not following intravenous injection (17).

It is clear, therefore, that the route of administration of a xenobiotic can significantly affect the amount and plasma concentration/time profiles of both the parent drug and its metabolites. Also, the pattern of metabolism may be considerably affected even though linear pharmacokinetics are operative (see below). Such differences may be extremely informative in determining the site(s) of elimination of drug and metabolite(s). From a toxicological standpoint, however, the significance of route-dependent elimination will depend on the magnitude of the first-pass effect(s) and also on the relative toxicities of the xenobiotic and its metabolite(s).

DOSE-DEPENDENT DISPOSITION AND PHARMACOKINETICS

The processes involved in translocating a xenobiotic from its site of administration to the various tissues of the body and also its removal by either excretion or biotransformation are multitudinous and complex. However, from a descriptive–operational standpoint, most behave in a linear fashion characteristic of pseudo-first-order kinetics. This arises even if a process is mechanistically controlled by the law of mass action, since the xenobiotic is present at a concentration far below (<10%) the level at which the process is half-saturated (K_m). For example, only a handful of drugs used in man have been shown to be metabolized by hepatic enzymes in a nonlinear fashion over the therapeutic range. However, in toxicological investigations that use large to massive doses of a compound, nonlinearity of the various dispositional processes is a distinct possibility, which may considerably affect the experimental findings and their interpretation. This is particularly so when extrapolation is made from results obtained under nonlinear conditions to those expected at lower, nonsaturating doses.

Dose-Dependent Drug Availability

Presystemic or first-pass elimination of xenobiotics was extensively discussed in the previous section; however, an additional factor associated with this phenomenon is dose dependency. Following systemic administration, a xenobiotic has the opportunity to distribute to the tissues before it is exposed to the various drug-metabolizing enzymes. Accordingly, the presented drug concentration is considerably attenuated compared to that at the site of administration. In contrast, first-pass-effect organs such as the GI tract, liver, and lungs are exposed to the total administered dose present at much higher concentrations than after systemic dosing.

Many examples in both animals and man exist, particularly if the xenobiotic has a large volume of distribution and the absorption rate is rapid, indicating that in this situation the metabolizing enzymes may become saturated. As a result, bioavailability is nonlinear such that an increase in administered dose produces a disproportionate increase in the systemic blood levels. For example, in man, after oral doses of less than 1 g of salicylamide, virtually all of the drug enters the systemic circulation as inactive glucuronide and sulfate conjugates formed in the gastrointestinal epithelium and liver. Bioavailability is only a fractional percentage compared to an equal intravenous dose. However, above a 1-g oral dose, the area under the salicylamide plasma level/time curve increases enormously (Fig. 1); doubling the dose to 2 g increases the plasma levels several hundred-fold with a concomitant unexpected rise in therapeutic and toxic effects (7). Such "hockey-stick"-shaped bioavailability/dose curves, especially when comparable systemic doses yield a linear relationship, are indicative of saturation of a nonlinear process in the first-pass effect. Clearly, studies performed above the "breakthrough" dosage will bear little resemblance to those at lower doses, which in all probability may be the ultimately applicable range.

A further consequence of dose-dependent bioavailability, especially when the liver is involved, is that subsequent elimination of xenobiotic from the systemic circulation is affected so long as the involved enzymes remain "saturated." Thus, the rate of elimination following oral or pulmonary admin-

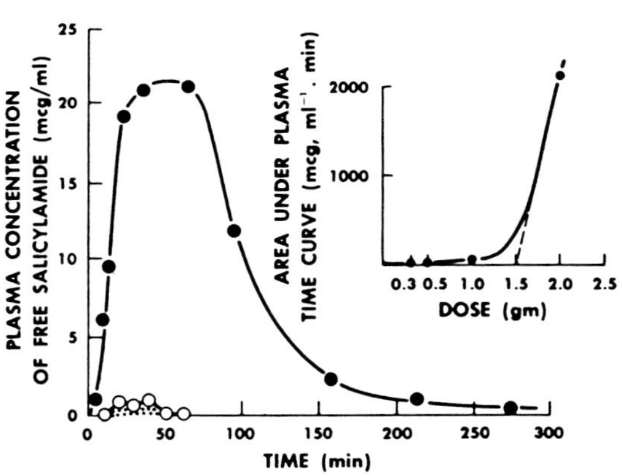

FIG. 1. Comparison of the plasma concentration/time profiles of unchanged (free) salicylamide following oral administration of a solution; 2 g dose (●), 1 g dose (○), *dotted lines* indicate the plasma concentrations after 0.5 and 0.3 g doses. The insert shows the corresponding areas under the plasma concentration/time curves (From Barr, ref. 7, with permission.)

istration may be slower and more complex than after intravenous administration (see below).

It is also possible that the saturation of one or more routes of metabolism in an involved first-pass organ may alter the pattern of metabolites formed and available to the systemic circulation. As a result, effects and toxicity may be considerably different from those observed following other routes of administration, especially when active and reactive metabolites are involved. For example, propranolol plasma concentrations following oral administration exhibit classical hockey-stick dose dependency in both animals (67) and man (65). In addition, the pharmacologically active 4-hydroxy metabolite is readily detectable in the plasma following an oral dose of propranolol but not after intravenous administration (52,70). Also, the pattern of excretion of the other oxidative metabolites of this β-adrenergic blocking agent is dependent on the administered dose (64). A similar situation has been shown to occur with the related β blocker, alprenolol (1). It has also been suggested that the increased incidence of side effects following oral lidocaine administration compared to the more conventional intravenous route is a reflection of increased production of a toxic metabolite during first-pass elimination (14).

A final consequence of a nonlinear first-pass effect is that the dose dependency is a function of the delivery rate of the xenobiotic. The slower the rate of presentation, the greater is the fraction of the administered dose removed by the presystemic elimination process. Accordingly, at any given dosage level, the more rapid the absorption, the larger is the bioavailability, and the greater the degree of enzyme saturation, the more pronounced is this effect (59).

It is also possible for oral bioavailability to decrease as the dosage is increased. In limited situations, this may arise because a saturable active transport process is involved in the absorption of the compound. Carrier-mediated intestinal absorption of physiologically important amino acids, sugars, and vitamins as well as a number of xenobiotics is well established. Moreover, only limited sections of the gastrointestinal tract are capable of such absorption; thus, GI transit time becomes an important addition factor in bioavailability. For example, with riboflavin, either increasing the dose or reducing gastric emptying, which leads to a prolongation of the residence time in the upper intestine, causes an increase in the extent of absorption (41). Gastric emptying has also been shown to be an important factor in the nearly 200-fold increase in the LD_{50} of chloroquine in the rat following oral dosing compared to the intravenous route. In this unusual case, the decreased bioavailability is a result of the dose-dependent inhibition of gastric emptying by the administered drug, which slows down its own rate of absorption from the intestine (41).

Problems of dose-dependent bioavailability may also arise because of dissolution considerations, especially if the compound of interest is only sparingly water soluble. Above the solubility limit, dissolution essentially becomes a zero-order process, and, therefore, with large doses, the time required for complete dissolution will exceed the intestinal transit time. As a consequence, a smaller fraction of the administered xenobiotic is absorbed as the dose is increased. Chronic oral toxicity studies involving large doses in small animals with short GI transit times are particularly prone to this type of problem.

Nonlinear Plasma and Tissue Binding

Many compounds are present in the circulating blood as reversible complexes with various macromolecules such as albumin, α_1-acid glycoprotein, lipoproteins, and certain specialized carrier globulins. In a similar fashion, intracellular tissue binding also occurs. In general, the binding macromolecules involved have a limited number of sites at which drugs and other compounds may bind, and the interaction follows the law of mass action. Accordingly, saturable binding is possible depending on the total number of available binding sites, the dissociation constant for the interaction(s), and the concentration of the xenobiotic. For example, the plasma albumin concentration in most common animal species is in the order of 0.75×10^{-3} M, which means for a compound with a molecular weight of about 300, plasma concentrations of approximately 200 μg/ml or greater lead to saturation of the binding to this protein. However, significant concentration-dependent binding is only present at these levels if the dissociation constant is less than about 10^{-4} to 10^{-5} M. With macromolecules present at lower concentrations, e.g., α_1-acid glycoprotein and the various carrier globulins, saturable binding occurs at significantly lower concentrations.

The major significance of nonlinear binding in the plasma is that the unbound moiety is generally considered to be the biologically active form of the compound. Thus, as the dose/concentration is increased, there is a disproportionate increase in the unbound fraction of xenobiotic at any particular concentration of total drug and, therefore, an augmented pharmacologic/toxicologic response. Moreover, the disposition of the compound with regard to its clearance from the body and also its distribution to the tissues may be significantly dependent on the fraction of xenobiotic present in the unbound form. This may readily be appreciated with respect to elimination by equation 9, which indicates the quantitative relationships between binding and clearance (73).

$$Cl = \frac{Q f_B Cl^u_{int}}{Q + f_B Cl^u_{int}} \qquad (9)$$

Cl is the irreversible clearance of compound by any given eliminating process/organ, Q is the organ's blood flow, Cl^u_{int} is the free intrinsic clearance of drug from tissue water, and f_B is the fraction of drug unbound in the blood. The latter is related to the more conventionally determined unbound fraction in the plasma (f_p) by the blood/plasma concentration ratio, which itself may be dependent on plasma binding ($f_B = f_P/(1 - H + HK_P f_P)$), where H is the hematocrit and K_p is the partition ratio of drug concentration in the formed elements in the blood to the unbound level in the plasma).

Accordingly, the effect of plasma binding on clearance depends on the relative magnitude of the free intrinsic clearance to the organ's blood flow. When Cl^u_{int}/Q is small, binding is the limiting factor in clearance of total drug, and there is an almost linear relationship between the two parameters. Such "restrictive" elimination is well established for excretion via glomerular filtration and also for poorly extracted compounds metabolized by the liver. Thus, if binding is dose/concentration dependent, clearance of total drug will not be a constant, but there will be an almost proportional change with the unbound fraction. Importantly, however, the nonlinear binding should not affect the clearance of the pharmacologically active, unbound moiety. In contrast, when an organ is very efficient at elimination, i.e., $Q \ll Cl^u_{int}$ then clearance is predominantly controlled by, and dependent on, organ blood flow. The clearance of total drug is then less sensitive to any changes in binding; however, the clearance of unbound drug is affected, an increase in the free fraction producing a reduction in this clearance. Accordingly, in a chronic toxicity study during which steady state is achieved, nonlinear plasma binding of a "nonrestrictively" cleared drug would result in disproportionately higher circulating levels of unbound drug as the administered dose is increased. This type of behavior would be expected for extensively bound drugs that are excreted by active secretion in the proximal renal tubule or are efficiently metabolized by the liver.

Only unbound drug is able to penetrate biological membranes; thus, the extent of distribution at equilibrium is dependent on binding in both the plasma and tissues. The simplest quantitative expression of the involved relationships in the volume of distribution (V_d) is shown in equation 10.

$$V_d = V_P + V_T f_P / f_T \qquad (10)$$

V_P is the plasma volume, V_T is the volume of other body tissue water and f_P and f_T are the fractions of unbound drug in the plasma and tissue, respectively (32,73). It is, therefore, apparent that the volume of distribution of a compound will increase as the unbound fraction in the plasma increases. Moreover, the change is almost directly proportional to the alteration in the unbound fraction except for extensively bound drugs that are distributed in a small volume, i.e., a large f_T. Drug distribution may also be expressed in terms of unbound drug (V_d/f_P). Although this term is essentially independent of the degree of binding for compounds that have large volumes of distribution, i.e., a small f_T, an increase in the unbound fraction in the plasma leads to a reduction in the value for drugs that are less extensively distributed, especially when binding is high.

Equation 10 also indicates that drug distribution is affected by changes in tissue binding (f_T). Unfortunately, the measurement of a xenobiotic in various tissues of the body as a function of time and dose has not been extensively investigated. However, there is considerable circumstantial and direct evidence to indicate that tissue binding in one or more organs can be saturated (69). As a result, the volume of distribution of both unbound and total drug will be reduced as the dose/concentration is increased.

When the effects of nonlinear binding in the plasma and/or tissues are considered together in terms of their predicted consequences on the time profile of drug elimination, the net result is dependent on the xenobiotic's particular pharmacokinetic characteristics, and it may be quite complex (47). For example, with a drug having a small volume of distribution in man (0.25 liter/kg) and a small free intrinsic clearance, saturable plasma binding in the presence of linear tissue binding produces biphasic, semilogarithmic, concave-decreasing elimination profiles for the amount of drug in the body and its total and unbound concentrations in the plasma. In contrast, if the distribution volume is large (14 liter/kg), then the total plasma concentration/time curve is convex-decreasing, whereas the amount in the body and the unbound plasma concentration decline almost monoexponentially. For a drug with a high free intrinsic clearance, nonlinear plasma binding tends to manifest itself by convex-decreasing profiles in all three variables regardless of the magnitude of the distribution volume.

The effects of saturable tissue binding alone are somewhat less complex since clearance is unaffected. Concave-decreasing curves are produced irrespective of the magnitude of free intrinsic clearance. When both plasma and tissue binding change concurrently, however, then even more complexity is predicted, including sigmoid-shaped elimination profiles. Unfortunately, experimental support for these predictions is not too extensive. However, they are based on a number of sound principles that have been independently validated. Therefore, it would appear essential to determine both total and unbound plasma concentrations when undertaking studies involving potentially saturating doses of xenobiotics as might occur in toxicity testing.

Concentration-Dependent Elimination by Michaelis–Menten Kinetics

The biotransformation of xenobiotics is usually controlled by enzymatic processes that are described by Michaelis–Menten kinetics. At low substrate concentrations relative to the K_m of the metabolic pathway(s), the rate of the process essentially becomes first order; i.e., metabolism is directly proportional to the substrate concentration. Similar considerations also apply to elimination routes involving active transport, such as biliary excretion and renal tubular secretion. Accordingly, levels in the body and in the plasma decline monoexponentially following completion of absorption and attainment of distribution equilibrium. As a result, the time to eliminate one-half of the xenobiotic present in the body or plasma is independent of the dose administered and the magnitude of the amount/concentration present. This is characterized by the first-order elimination half-life. Also, the area under the blood/plasma concentration/time curve is proportional to the dose. A further characteristic of a linear pharmacokinetic system is that drug levels at any specified time are directly proportional to the administered dose, the so-called principle of superimposition. Additionally, the proportions of drug excreted unchanged or metabolized along various pathways are unaffected by the dose given; i.e., the metabolic urinary excretion profile is dose independent.

The elimination from the body of most drugs and other xenobiotics typically may be described by such linear or first-order kinetics, especially within the therapeutic range. However, when a wider range of doses is administered, as often occurs in toxicity evaluation, then elimination processes may become saturated, and nonlinear pharmacokinetics result. The consequences of such elimination may be profound both in terms of disposition and biological effects (Table 2). The most characteristic indication of saturable elimination is that the postabsorption/distribution plasma concentration/time curve is not log-linear. Instead, as the dose is increased, the disappearance curve becomes convex-decreasing (Fig. 2). This is a result of desaturation of the metabolic process from a limiting situation in which elimination approaches a constant rate, equivalent to the V_{max} of the pathway, towards the first-order situation. As a result, the time taken to eliminate half of the administered dose increases with dose from the limiting and constant value under first-order conditions. It should be noted that the initial portions of the disappearance curves above the "saturation threshold" may appear log-linear, especially if only a few data points are available and the experimental "noise" is high. This could be incorrectly interpreted to indicate that an elimination half-life was present that increased with dose. Accordingly, the characterization of saturable elimination requires that plasma levels be followed after high doses until they pass through the same concentration range at which first-order elimination is exhibited.

TABLE 2. *Characteristics of nonlinear Michaelis–Menten elimination kinetics*

Disappearance of xenobiotic in the body/plasma is not exponential
Time required to eliminate 50% of an administered dose increases with increasing dose
Area under the blood/plasma concentration profile is curvilinearly related to dose in a concave-increasing fashion, and apparent total body clearance decreases in a convex-decreasing form
Composition of urinary excretion profile for unchanged xenobiotic and metabolites is altered by dose, rate, and route of delivery
Dose–response relationships may exhibit unusually large increases in pharmacological and/or toxicological effects with increasing dose, beginning at the dose level at which "saturation" effects become apparent

The elimination of ethanol in man has long been known to follow such kinetics (45), and more recent studies have shown that salicylate (40,43), phenytoin (5,58), theophylline (72), and certain anticancer agents (54) have similar characteristics over the therapeutic range. In animals, the phenomenon is much more common and, in fact, may be the rule rather than the exception provided that the xenobiotic's toxicity is not sufficiently high as to produce toxic effects or death at dosages below the threshold of saturation of the elimination processes. Thus, a wide variety of xenobiotics have been reported to exhibit saturable renal excretion, for example, the herbicide 2,4,5-trichlorophenoxyacetic acid (61), or capacity-limited metabolism such as styrene, ethylene glycol,

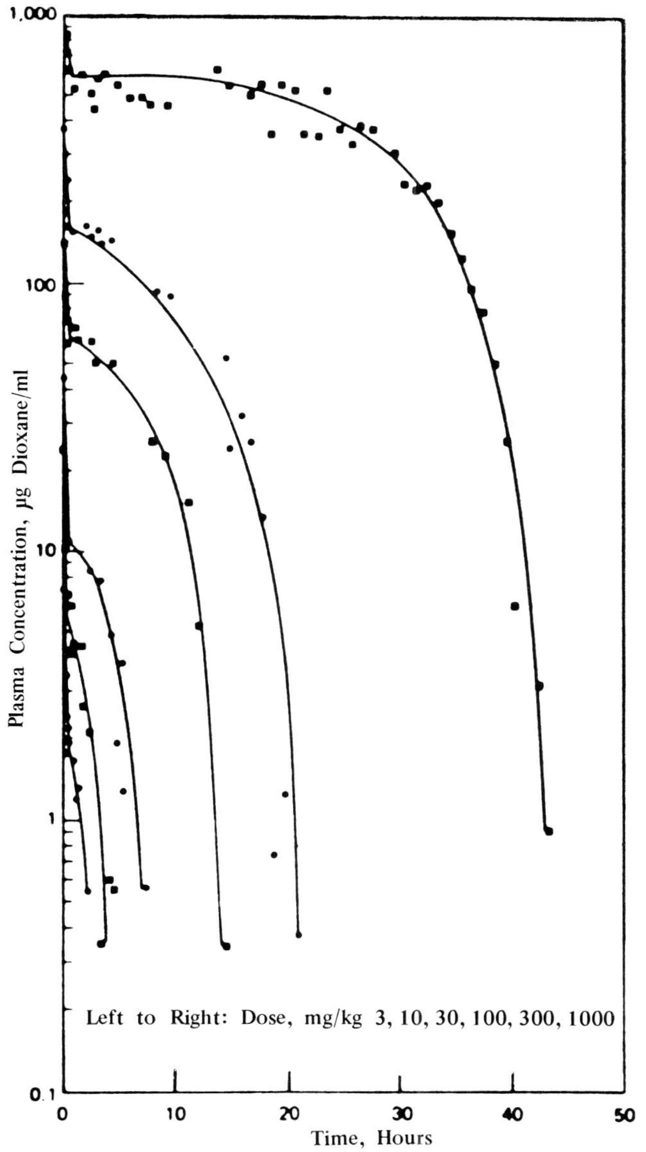

FIG. 2. Plasma concentration/time profiles of dioxane in rats given various intravenous doses, illustrating the shape of the convex-decreasing curves at higher doses that is characteristic of saturable elimination following Michaelis–Menten kinetics. (From Watanabe et al., ref. 71, with permission.)

aniline, carbon disulfide, 2-naphthylamine, benzopyrene, *bis*-hydroxycoumarin, bromobenzene, acetaminophen, isonicotinic acid hydrazide, vinyl chloride (27), acetone (35), and acetanilide (66).

Saturable elimination not only leads to a change in shape of the blood–plasma concentration/time profile but also affects the area under the curve, a quantitative measure of the time-integrated dose. As the dose increases, the area increases disproportionately. Studies with styrene in rats provide an excellent example of this effect (Table 3). At inhalation exposure levels below 200 ppm, the system appears to be linear, but as the concentration is increased to 600 and 1,200 ppm, the increase in the area under the curve is much greater than would be expected

TABLE 3. *Areas under curves (AUC) (0–24 hr) for the styrene blood concentration in rats exposed to 80, 200, 600, or 1,200 ppm for 6 hr*

Exposure concentration (ppm)	AUC ($\mu g \cdot hr \cdot ml^{-1}$)	Normalized exposure concentration	Normalized AUC
80	4.87	1.0	1.0
200	8.97	2.5	1.8
600	152	7.5	31
1,200	546	15	112

based on the increase in exposure level alone (55). Additional evidence for saturable pharmacokinetics is also provided by the different shape and nonsuperimposition of the blood concentration/time curves (Fig. 3).

Capacity-limited metabolism also results in disproportionate increases in the steady-state plateau level when the xenobiotic is administered continuously or chronically. With styrene, for example, a 15-fold increase in exposure produces a greater than 80-fold increase in the maximum blood concentration following continuous exposure (Fig. 3). The extent of an unanticipated increase is largely dependent on the relative contribution of the saturable pathway to the overall fate of the compound (Fig. 4). If the pathway is a major route of elimination, then the dose dependency may be extreme, and pronounced differences in the magnitude of pharmacological and toxicological effects may occur with very small dose increments. Most compounds, however, have competitive parallel first-order and Michaelis–Menten kinetics. The presence of such competitive routes of elimination tends to dampen the nonlinearity so that proportionality is approximately attained in the low dose range prior to saturation and also in the very high dose range, where the contribution of the saturated process to overall elimination is negligible (68).

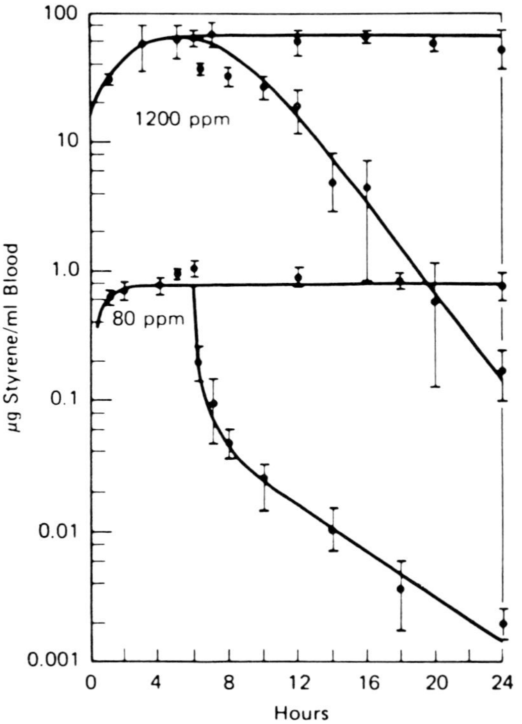

FIG. 3. Blood styrene concentrations in rats continuously exposed to either 80 or 1,200 ppm. (From Ramsey and Young, ref. 55, with permission.)

The existence of several competitive elimination processes also has repercussions on the effects of saturation of one pathway on the overall elimination pattern. Since the kinetic characteristics of each involved enzyme are different, the saturation of one route results in a greater contribution of the remaining linear pathways to the overall fate of the xenobiotic. For example, the percentage of salicylic acid recovered in the urine as the glycine conjugate, salicyluric acid, decreases with increasing dose in man (40), whereas the excretion of unchanged drug increases proportionally more than the dose (Table 4). The recovery of glucuronidated metabolites also increases, but only slightly, since phenolic glucuronide formation is also saturable at somewhat higher concentrations than glycine conjugation (43).

An important aspect of nonlinear elimination with regard to toxicology is the formation of reactive electrophilic metabolites that may covalently combine with important tissue nucleophiles such as nucleic acids, pro-

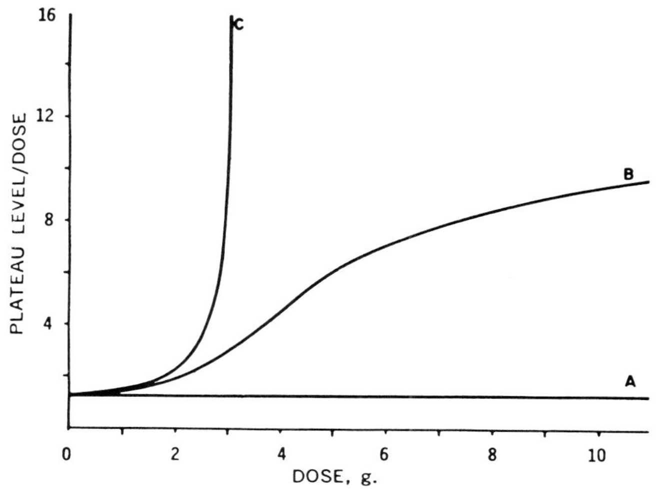

FIG. 4. Relationship between the maximum amount of xenobiotic in the body normalized to the dose administered as a function of dose, assuming that elimination proceeds by first-order (**A**), parallel first-order and Michaelis–Menten (**B**), and Michaelis–Menten kinetics (**C**). (From Tsuchiya and Levy, ref. 68, with permission.)

teins, etc. The net result of such irreversible binding is a toxic response that is a function of the total amount of reactive metabolite formed (cf. the more usual reversible pharmacokinetic response relationship, which is dependent on amount/concentration/time profile). Figure 5 illustrates a simple model of such a system involving interaction of the reactive metabolite with genetic material, which may lead to carcinogenesis. The total amount of reactive metabolite formed and covalently bound depends on the proportion of the xenobiotic that is converted to the reactive species and the proportion of this that becomes bound to the genetic material plus that covalently linked to other macromolecules. When the involved metabolic processes are all first order, then the various proportions may be obtained from the ratios of the involved clearances (equation 3), and the amount of irreversible binding is directly proportional to the dose (33). However, when saturable elimination is present, covalent binding may increase dramatically above a critical threshold dose (Fig. 6). If the events subsequent to covalent binding are also considered, including repair of genetic material by a saturable mechanism, then a very complex dose–response relationship exists even with the simplest of assumptions (28). Obviously, extrapolation of toxicity data obtained at high doses under these circumstances to the situation present at nonsaturating doses for risk assessment is fraught with difficulties (4).

TABLE 4. *Effect of dose on the metabolic fate of salicylate in a human volunteer*

	Dose (mg)		
Salicylate form	250	1,000	2,000
Salicylic acid (%)	2.5	7.3	23.7
Salicyluric acid (%)	79.6	67.5	59.2
Salicyl glucuronides (%)	17.9	25.2	23.7
Total	92.8	92.8	97.9

Consideration of the pharmacokinetics of covalent binding even under the assumption of linearity also provides insights into the effects of changing the activities of the involved metabolizing enzymes by induction and inhibition (33). When a large proportion of xenobiotic is converted to a reactive metabolite, increasing or decreasing the activity of the enzyme catalyzing its formation does not cause a marked change in the proportion of the dose converted to the reactive metabolite. Even when a relatively small fraction of the dose is biotransformed to reactive metabolite, changes in amount of covalent binding may not necessarily occur following enzyme induction or inhibition, since all par-

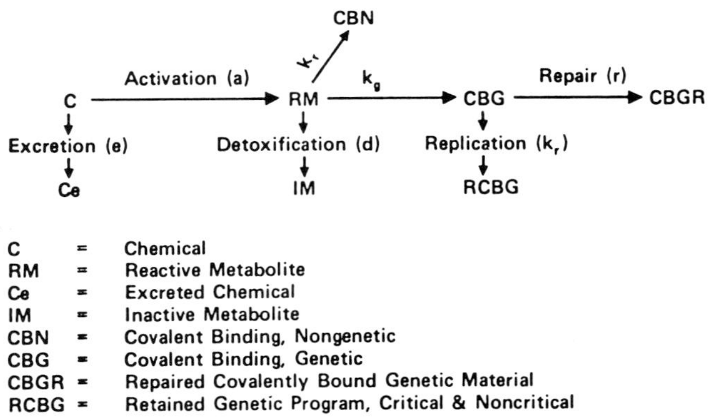

FIG. 5. Theoretical model for the fate of a chemical carcinogen in the body requiring, for expression of carcinogenicity, activation to a reactive metabolite and subsequent irreversible covalent reaction with a genetic receptor. Excretion (*e*), activation (*a*), detoxification (*d*), and repair (*r*) occur in accordance with dose-dependent (Michaelis–Menten) kinetics, whereas the remaining reactions follow first-order kinetics. (From Gehring et al., ref. 28, with permission.)

allel pathways of elimination may be equally affected. In fact, perturbing metabolism would be expected to have its greatest effect on covalent binding when the reactive metabolite pathway is minor but is selectively affected by pretreatment. Covalent binding may also be markedly changed if the rate of elimination of the reactive metabolite is altered. Considerations of this type indicate the difficulty of predicting the effects of enzyme induction and inhibition on covalent binding on the basis of simple measurements of xenobiotic disposition such as the elimination half-life (33).

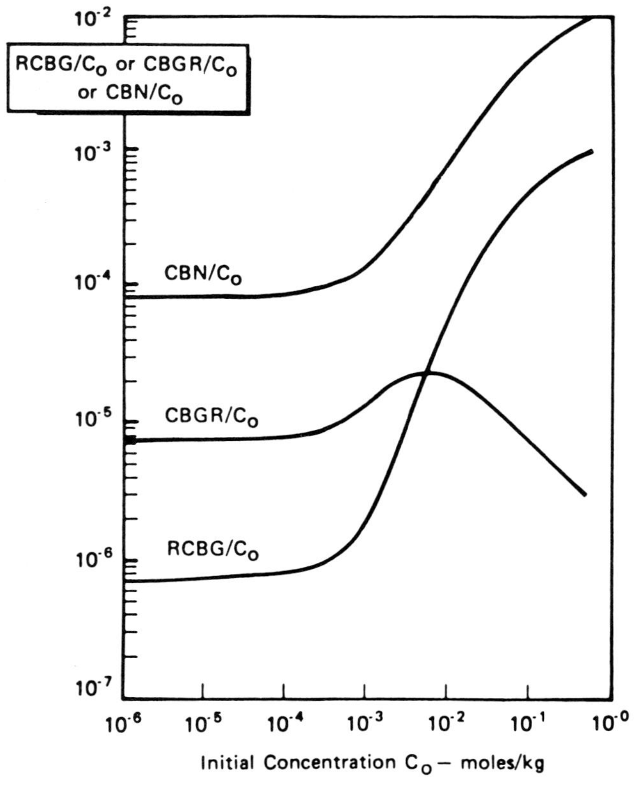

FIG. 6. Effect of increasing dose (C_0) on the fraction of chemical bound to nongenetic material (CBM/C_0), to genetic material that is subsequently repaired (CBGR/C_0), and to genetic material fixed by replication (RCBG/C_0) according to the model depicted in Fig. 5 using realistic parameter values. (From Gehring et al., ref. 28, with permission.)

Concentration-Dependent Elimination by Mechanisms Other than Saturation of Michaelis–Menten Kinetics

A characteristic of nonlinear elimination involving Michaelis–Menten kinetics is that at any substrate concentration the rate of elimination is the same regardless of how that level was attained. Also, the first-order half-life observed after a low dose is eventually attained even after the administration of saturating doses. However, certain xenobiotics have been shown to demonstrate dose/concentration-dependent elimination that does not fit these criteria. Instead, exponential elimination through several orders of magnitude is apparent at all dose levels, but with increasing dose the half-life increases. Also, different rates of elimination exist at a given plasma concentration dependent on the initial level that was present. The mechanism(s) responsible for this type of pharmacokinetic behavior are not always readily apparent.

In the case of acetaminophen (Fig. 7), not only does the half-life increase in a dose-dependent fashion, but the fractional amount of the dose excreted in the urine as the sulfate conjugate decreases significantly, as does the glucuronide but to a lesser extent, and unchanged acetaminophen excretion increases (26). Treatment with sodium sulfate or *N*-acetylcysteine significantly reduces and/or reverses these dose-dependent effects, strongly suggesting that the mechanism involves depletion of endogenous inorganic sulfate stores required for the formation of the sulfate conjugate (44). Cosubstrate depletion is also responsible for the dose-dependent increase in covalent binding and toxicity produced by many xenobiotics acting through a reactive intermediate. At low dose levels, endogenous glutathione in the liver and other organs is present in sufficiently high amounts to react with any electrophilic metabolites formed, and these are ultimately excreted as mercapturic acid conjugates. However, large doses of xenobiotic overwhelm the supply of glutathione, and the reactive metabolites then covalently bind to various tissue macromolecules, leading in some cases to toxicity. Since glutathione conjugation is only a minor pathway of metabolism, such depletion would not be expected to manifest itself as a significant change in the elimination kinetics of the parent xenobiotic.

Another putative mechanism whereby a dose-dependent increase in elimination half-life may occur is substrate–product inhibi-

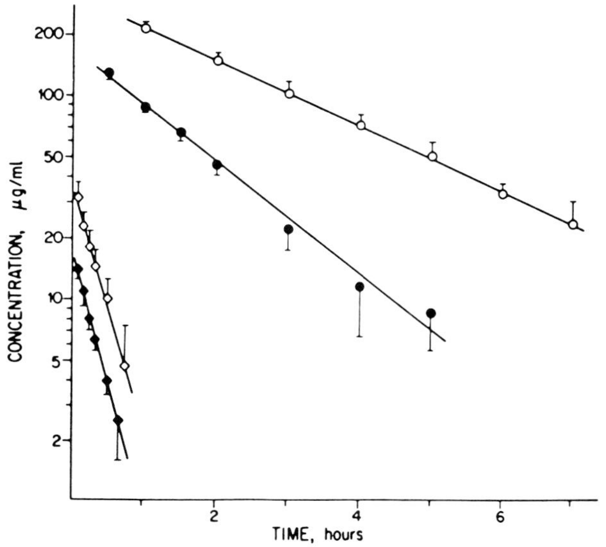

FIG. 7. Acetaminophen concentrations (mean ± SD) in the plasma of rats after intravenous administration of 15 (♦), 30 (◇), 150 (●), and 300 (○) mg/kg. (From Galinsky and Levy, ref. 26, with permission.)

tion; i.e., a metabolite impairs the biotransformation of the parent drug from which it is formed (53). For example, the hydroxy metabolite of phenytoin inhibits the metabolism of phenytoin, and this has been suggested to be a factor in the dose-dependent pharmacokinetics of phenytoin in the rat (6).

Several other examples exist for which the cause of the dose dependency is not so well understood, for example, dicumarol (48), biscoumacetate (18), and heparin (11). Similar behavior has been reported for probenicid and phenylbutazone and analogs (18); however, analytical artifacts were not ruled out (42), but, more importantly, the same concentration ranges were not examined following both low and high doses.

PHYSIOLOGICAL PHARMACOKINETICS

Classical pharmacokinetics is primarily a descriptive tool for events at the level of the total animal. The body is regarded as a "black box" with gross input and output functions, and little insight is provided regarding the biological aspects of the system. In recent years, significant progress has been made in understanding and relating the *in vivo* determinants of xenobiotic disposition. One approach has been to interpret the function of an eliminating organ, such clearance by the liver, in terms of the controlling physiological factors. An extension of this approach has been to model the whole body on the basis of actual anatomical, biochemical, and physiological considerations. Factors such as blood flow to tissues, tissue and organ size, metabolic and excretory clearances, membrane transport, and plasma and tissue binding may all be accounted for. As a result, factors that affect local tissue concentrations may be explored, providing insights into drug toxicity.

The fundamental unit of a physiological model is the "lumped compartment," which represents a region of the body at some uniform concentration (8). It may be equivalent to a single capillary with surrounding tissue, a discrete organ, or a widely distributed anatomical region such as fat or muscle. The body may then be represented as a number of such compartments interconnected according to the known anatomy of the system (Fig. 8). Mass balance considerations may be applied across each "tissue compartment" to

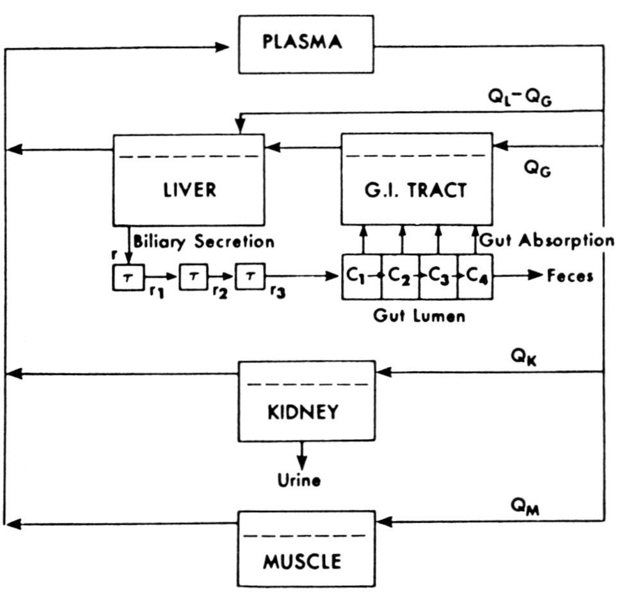

FIG. 8. A physiologically based model to describe the disposition of methotrexate. (From Bischoff et al., ref. 10, with permission.)

account for the delivery of drug in the blood, its uptake and binding in the tissue, clearance of the drug by either excretion or metabolism, and exit of the drug in the venous blood. Importantly, the parameters of the equations are actual anatomical or physiological values and empirically determined drug characteristics such as membrane permeability, plasma and tissue binding, renal clearance, apparent Michaelis–Menten kinetic parameters for metabolism, etc. The concentration/time profile of a typical "tissue compartment" is then given by an equation similar to equation 11.

$$V\frac{dC_T}{dt} = QC_B - Q\frac{C_T}{R} - K\frac{C_T}{R} - \frac{V_{max}C_T}{K_m + C_T} \qquad (11)$$

C_B and C_T are the total drug concentrations in the blood and compartment, respectively; V and Q are the actual volume and blood flow rate of the tissue; K is a first-order clearance rate; V_{max} and K_m are the Michaelis–Menten kinetic parameters for metabolism; and R is the distribution ratio of drug between blood and tissue. The latter often requires consideration of drug binding to the plasma and tissue proteins, involving either linear or non-linear kinetics. Thus, the rate of change of the amount of drug in the compartment is equal to the difference between the amount entering the compartment (QC_B) and the amount leaving by bulk flow (QC_T/R), excretion (KC_T/R), and metabolism $[V_{max}C_T/(K_m + C_T)]$. Solution of equation 11, and similar ones for other compartments, then provides a quantitative and temporal *a priori* description of drug concentrations in the various tissues (8,46). In the ideal case, only *in vitro* studies should be necessary to predict within reasonable limits the disposition *in vivo*.

The disposition and pharmacokinetics of a number of drugs such as barbiturates, polychlorinated biphenyls, salicylate, ethanol, digoxin, antibiotics, and a number of anticancer agents have been examined with considerable success using this approach (16,37,46). Investigation of the latter has been of particular value in the development of chemotherapeutic regimens in which the goal is to maintain drug levels in the target tumor sufficient to inhibit tumor growth while not producing unacceptable cytotoxicity in the normal tissues (8,46). For example, considerable success has been achieved in describing methotrexate's disposition at a gross organ level in experimental animals (Fig. 9) as well as examining its kinetics in the target tumor and also at the sites of toxicity, bone marrow and intestine (9,10,20). More recently, correlation of the cytotoxicity with the membrane transport parameters of the model has been successful (46).

The use of various animal species in the efficacy and toxicity evaluation of drugs is based on the belief that in general there are both qualitative and quantitative similarities between species. Most of the problems of interspecies extrapolation are related to the magnitude of any quantitative differences. Physiological pharmacokinetics has considerable potential to account for a large fraction of the species differences in disposition. This is because the mammalian system has remarkable constancy: the anatomical arrangement and vascular perfusion of organs are the same with few exceptions, most organs and tissues are similar fractions of body weight, and physiological processes are related to body weight according to the 0.7 to 0.8 power (3,13). Thus, physiological processes per unit body weight or organ size tend to decrease as body size increases; hemodynamically, 1 min in the life of a mouse is equivalent to about 2 min in the rat, 4 min in the dog, and 8 min in man. Accordingly, the same physiological model may be used for all species, the magnitude of the physiological and anatomical parameters being adjusted accordingly (20) along with modification of the drug's dispositional characteristics.

Tissue uptake and storage of xenobiotics is the least well understood and quantifiable

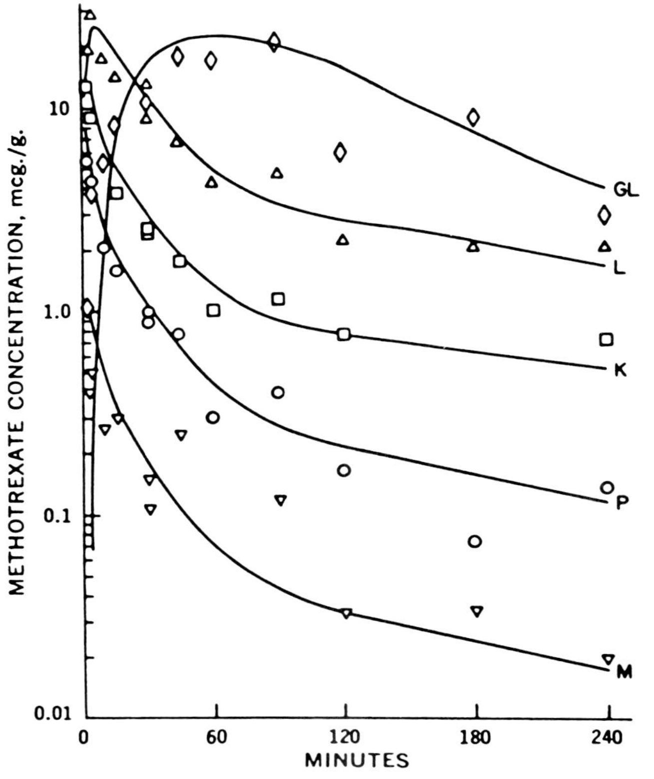

FIG. 9. Comparison of the methotrexate concentrations in various tissue of the rat following intraperitoneal dosing (6 mg/kg) as predicted by the physiologically based model shown in Fig. 8 (*solid line*) and the experimental data. (From Bischoff et al., ref. 10, with permission.)

area of drug disposition. However, the limited information that is presently available indicates that only minor interspecies variations occur in the equilibrium distribution ratios between blood and tissues (19). Therefore, for initial predictive purposes, the parameter values (the R term in equation 11) determined in one species may possibly be extrapolated to others. Renal clearance may also be extrapolated in a simple fashion, since in most instances it is proportional to glomerular filtration, which increases as a known function of body weight. The successful application of such a scaling approach may be appreciated by the findings with methotrexate (Fig. 10). Considerable variability (17,000-fold) exists among the mouse, rat, monkey, dog, and man with respect to the plasma levels attained with different doses of methotrexate and also the rate at which the drug is removed from the plasma. However, if the known physiological and kinetic differences are taken into account, a surprising degree of uniformity exists within all of the species (Fig. 10). This would indicate close similarities in the overall processes of distribution and drug elimination, which in this case is entirely by renal clearance (20).

The most problematic area in interspecies pharmacokinetic extrapolation is that of drug metabolism, since variability is the rule rather than the exception. Accordingly, the qualitative and quantitative metabolic characteristics must be defined for each xenobiotic. Such studies are routinely and inexpensively performed in *in vitro* systems such as crude and purified enzyme preparations and other systems such as microsomes, cell suspensions, tissue slices, and isolated perfused organs. The problem then is to correlate these

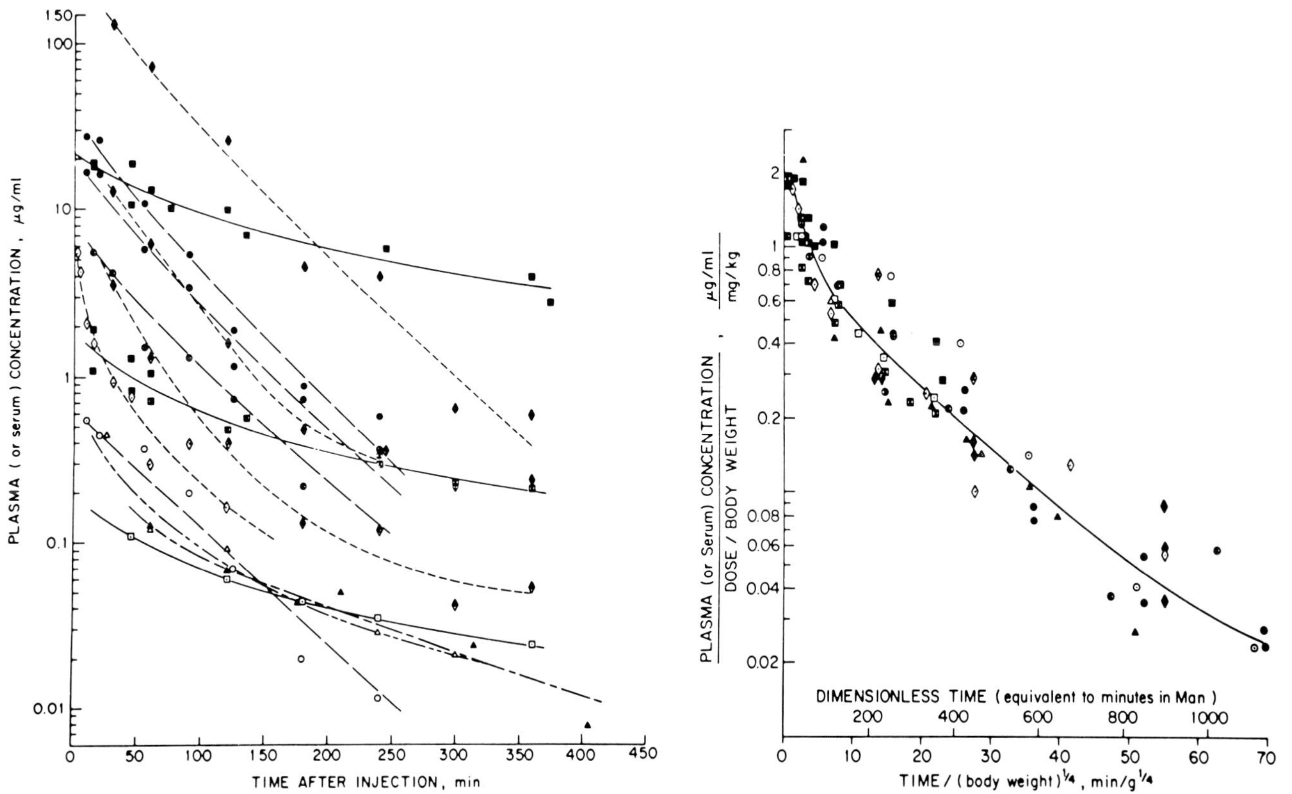

FIG. 10. Plasma or serum concentrations of methotrexate after intravenous or intraperitoneal injection of various doses indicated by different symbols. The **left panel** shows the raw data in the mouse - - -, rat — — —, monkey — - —, dog — - - —, and man ——, whereas the **right panel** shows the same data but scaled to take into account the dose, body size, and the "equivalent" time factor of the animals. (From Dedrick et al., ref. 20, with permission.)

in vitro findings with the *in vivo* situation. A modest and encouraging degree of success has been made in this regard, especially when intrinsic clearance has been the basis of the kinetic correlation (13,19). Figure 11 illustrates the relatively successful prediction of the plasma disposition of cytosine arabinoside is a human patient based on physiological modeling. Importantly, none of the parameters were individualized for this patient; the physiological and anatomical parameters were based on standard values, and the metabolic terms were obtained from *in vitro* data using human tissue homogenates (19). Obviously, not all situations will provide such satisfying predictions. However, the initial attempts of *in vitro/in vivo* correlation suggest that the appropriate kinetic data from a variety of simple preparations can provide estimates within an order-of-magnitude agreement. This is clearly an area that requires further investigation as a predictive tool for extrapolating animal data to man.

PERSPECTIVES

A basic objective of most toxicological studies, explicitly stated or otherwise, is the extrapolation of the experimental findings to the presumed situation that is likely to occur in man or any other exposed species. Such studies are based on the assumption that investigations performed at a variety of dosage levels bear some relationship to the level of concern, even though massive and often unrealistic dosages may be used in the evaluation procedure. As this chapter has indicated,

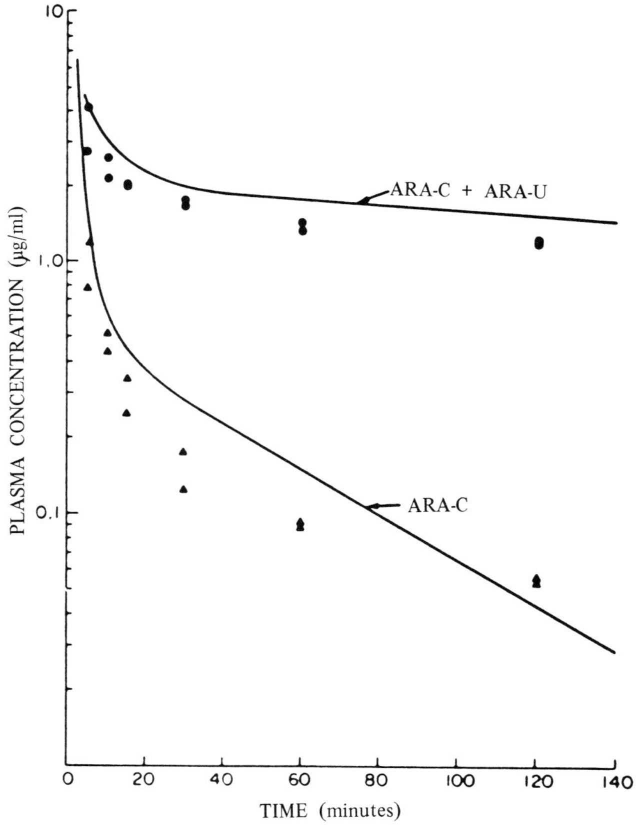

FIG. 11. Comparison of the plasma concentrations of cytosine arabinoside (Ara-C) and total radioactivity reflecting both Ara-C and its metabolite, Ara-U, in man as predicted *a priori* by a physiologically based model and actual data obtained from a patient. (From Dedrich and Bischoff, ref. 19, with permission.)

the relationship(s) may not be simple because of a variety of factors, especially nonlinear pharmacokinetics. However, the conceptual approaches and techniques for analyzing these situations are now well established and available for application to the often unique problems of toxicological evaluation.

There is frequently a further tacit assumption, or, more correctly, an intuitive belief that sufficient qualitative and quantitative similarities exist among species that reasonable limits of prediction are possible. Unfortunately, few studies have actually addressed this issue. In fact, there is considerable evidence that species differences tend to be the rule rather than the exception, at least with regard to disposition. Moreover, variability within a species, including the human, may be pronounced. Because of this, conventional drug metabolism studies designed to determine the metabolic fate of a compound in several species have become an integral part of toxicological evaluation. In the case in which toxicity is associated with the formation of a specific metabolite in only certain species, this type of information can be of great value. However, there is increasing recognition that consideration of the time course of the amount or concentration of the xenobiotic and its metabolites in various body fluids and tissue, i.e., pharmacokinetics, considerably enhances the utility of such metabolism studies.

The application of pharmacokinetics to the design and interpretation of toxicological studies will undoubtedly enhance the reliability of risk assessment both within and between animal species (27,28,71). It is increasingly becoming a conventional component of many toxicological studies. However, it must be recognized that pharmacokinetics is only a tool that is critically dependent on the quality of the experimental data and knowledge of the involved biological concepts. Its application will help but will not necessarily solve the challenging problems of toxicological predictions.

REFERENCES

1. Ablad, B., Ervik, M., Hallgren, J., Johnsson, G., and Sölvell, L. (1972): Pharmacological effects and serum levels of orally administered alprenolol in man. *Eur. J. Clin. Pharmacol.*, 5:44–52.
2. Adamson, R. H., Bridges, J. W., Evans, M. E., and Williams, R. T. (1970): Species differences in the aromatization of quinic acid *in vivo* and the role of gut bacteria. *Biochem. J.*, 116:437–443.
3. Adolph, E. F. (1949): Quantitative relations in the physiological constitutions of mammals. *Science*, 109:579–585.
4. Anderson, M. W., Hoel, D. G., and Kaplan, N. L. (1980): A general scheme for the incorporation of pharmacokinetics in low-dose risk estimation for chemical carcinogenesis: Example-vinyl chloride. *Toxicol. Appl. Pharmacol.*, 55:154–161.
5. Arnold, K., and Gerber, N. (1970): The rate of decline of diphenylhydantoin in human plasma. *Clin. Pharmacol. Ther.*, 11:121–134.
6. Ashley, J. J., and Levy, G. (1972): Inhibition of diphenylhydantoin elimination by its major metabolite. *Res. Commun. Chem. Pathol. Pharmacol.*, 4:297–306.
7. Barr, W. H. (1969): Factors involved in the assessment of systemic or biologic availability of drug products. *Drug Info. Bull.*, 3:27–45.
8. Bischoff, K. B. (1975): Some fundamental considerations of the applications of pharmacokinetics to cancer chemotherapy. *Cancer Chemother. Rep.*, 59:777–793.
9. Bischoff, K. B., Dedrick, R. L., and Zaharko, D. S. (1970): Preliminary model for methotrexate pharmacokinetics. *J. Pharm. Sci.*, 59:149–154.
10. Bischoff, K. B., Dedrick, R. L., Zaharko, D. S., and Longstreth, J. A. (1971): Methotrexate pharmacokinetics. *J. Pharm. Sci.*, 60:1128–1133.
11. Bjornsson, T. D., and Levy, G. (1979): Pharmacokinetics of heparin. I. Studies of dose dependence in rats. *J. Pharmacol. Exp. Ther.*, 210:237–242.
12. Blackwell, E. W., Briant, R. H., Conolly, M. E., Davies, D. S., and Dollery, C. T. (1974): Metabolism of isoprenaline after aerosol and direct intrabronchial administration in man and dog. *Br. J. Pharmacol.*, 50:587–591.
13. Boxenbaum, H. (1980): Interspecies variations in liver weight, hepatic blood flow, and antipyrine intrinsic clearance: Extrapolation of data to benzodiazepines and phenytoin. *J. Pharmacokinet. Biopharmacol.*, 8:165–176.
14. Boyes, R. N., Scott, D. B., Jebson, P. J., Godman, M. J., and Julian, D. G. (1971): Pharmacokinetics of lidocaine in man. *Clin. Pharmacol. Ther.*, 12:105–116.
15. Cassidy, M. K., and Houston, J. B. (1980): *In vivo* assessment of extrahepatic conjugative metabolism in first pass effects using the model compound phenol. *J. Pharm. Pharmacol.*, 32:57–59.
16. Chen, H.-S. G., and Gross, J. F. (1979): Physiologically based pharmacokinetic models for anticancer drugs. *Cancer Chemother. Pharmacol.*, 2:85–94.

17. Conolly, M. E., Davies, D. S., Dollery, C. T., Morgan, C. D., Paterson, J. W., and Sandler, M. (1972): Metabolism of isoprenaline in dog and man. *Br. J. Pharmacol.,* 46:458–472.
18. Dayton, P. G., Cucinell, S. A., Weiss, M., and Perel, J. M. (1967): Dose-dependence of drug plasma level decline in dogs. *J. Pharmacol. Exp. Ther.,* 158:305–316.
19. Dedrick, R. L., and Bischoff, K. B. (1980): Species similarities in pharmacokinetics. *Fed. Proc.,* 39:54–59.
20. Dedrick, R. L., Bischoff, K. B., and Zaharko, D. S. (1970): Interspecies correlation of plasma concentration history of methotrexate (NSC-740). *Cancer Chemother. Rep.,* 54:95–101.
21. Dedrick, R. L., Zaharko, D. S., and Lutz, R. J. (1973): Transport and binding of methotrexate *in vivo. J. Pharm. Sci.,* 62:882–890.
22. Drasar, B. S., and Hill, M. J. (1974): *Human Intestinal Flora.* Academic Press, New York.
23. Drasar, B. S., Hill, M. J., and Williams, R. E. O. (1970): In: *Metabolic Aspects of Food Safety,* edited by F. J. C. Roe, pp. 245–260. Blackwell, Oxford.
24. Evans, M. E., Walker, S. R., Brittain, R. T., and Paterson, J. W. (1973): The metabolism of salbutamol in man. *Xenobiotica,* 3:113–120.
25. Fraslie, A. (1973): Methaemoglobin formation by diamino metabolites of DNOC and DNBP. *Acta Pharmacol. Toxicol.,* 32:257–265.
26. Galinsky, R. E., and Levy, G. (1981): Dose and time-dependent elimination of acetaminophen in rats: Pharmacokinetic implications of cosubstrate depletion. *J. Pharmacol. Exp. Ther.,* 219:14–20.
27. Gehring, P. J., Watanabe, P. G., and Blau, G. E. (1976): In: *Advances in Modern Toxicology—Newer Concepts in Safety Evaluation,* edited by M. A. Mehlman, R. E. Shapiro, and H. Blumenthal, pp. 195–270. Hemisphere Publishing Co., Washington, D.C.
28. Gehring, P. J., Watanabe, P. G., and Blau, G. E. (1979): Risk assessment of environmental carcinogens utilizing pharmacokinetic parameters. *Ann. N.Y. Acad. Sci.,* 329:137–152.
29. George, C. F., Blackwell, E. W., and Davies, D. S. (1974): Metabolism of isoprenaline in the intestine. *J. Pharm. Pharmacol.,* 26:265–267.
30. Gibaldi, M., and Feldman, S. (1972): Route of administration and drug metabolism. *Eur. J. Pharmacol.,* 19:323–329.
31. Gibaldi, M., and Perrier, D. (1982): *Pharmacokinetics,* Marcel Dekker, New York.
32. Gillette, J. R. (1971): Factors affecting drug metabolism. *Ann. N.Y. Acad. Sci.,* 179:43–66.
33. Gillette, J. R. (1974): A perspective on the role of chemically reactive metabolites of foreign compounds in toxicity. II. Alteration in the kinetics of covalent binding. *Biochem. Pharmacol.,* 23:2927–2938.
34. Gillette, J. R., and Pang, K. S. (1977): Theoretic aspects of pharmacokinetic drug interactions. *Clin. Pharmacol. Ther.,* 22:623–639.
35. Hallier, E., Filser, J. G., and Bolt, H. M. (1981): Inhalation pharmacokinetics based on gas uptake studies. II. Pharmacokinetics of acetone in rats. *Arch. Toxicol.,* 47:293–304.
36. Harris, P. A., and Riegelman, S. (1969): Influence of the route of administration on the area under the plasma concentration–time curve. *J. Pharm. Sci.,* 58:71–75.
37. Himmelstein, K. J., and Lutz, R. J. (1979): A review of the applications of physiologically based pharmacokinetic modeling. *J. Pharmacokin. Biopharm.,* 7:127–145.
38. Ilett, K. F., Dollery, C. T., and Davies, D. S. (1980): Isoprenaline conjugation—a "true first-pass effect" in the dog intestine. *J. Pharm. Pharmacol.,* 32:362.
39. Lai, D. Y., and Arcos, J. C. (1980): Dialkylnitrosamine bioactivation and carcinogenesis. *Life Sci.,* 27:2149–2165.
40. Levy, G. (1965): Pharmacokinetics of salicylate elimination in man. *J. Pharm. Sci.,* 54:959–967.
41. Levy, G. (1968): In: *Importance of Fundamental Principles in Drug Evaluation,* edited by D. H. Tedeschi and R. E. Tedeschi, pp. 141–172. Raven Press, New York.
42. Levy, G. (1970): Apparent dose-dependent elimination kinetics as an experimental artifact. *J. Pharm. Sci.,* 59:1847–1848.
43. Levy, G., Tsuchiya, T., and Amsel, L. P. (1972): Limited capacity for salicyl phenolic glucuronide formation and its effect on the kinetics of salicylate elimination in man. *Clin. Pharmacol. Ther.,* 13:259–268.
44. Lin, J. H., and Levy, G. (1981): Sulfate depletion after acetaminophen administration and replenishment by infusion of sodium sulfate or *N*-acetylcysteine in rats. *Biochem. Pharmacol.,* 30:2723–2725.
45. Lundquist, F., and Wolthers, H. (1958): The kinetics of alcohol elimination in man. *Acta Pharmacol. Toxicol.,* 14:265–289.
46. Lutz, R. J., Dedrick, R. L., and Zaharko, D. S. (1980): Physiological pharmacokinetics: An *in vivo* approach to membrane transport. *Pharmacol. Ther.,* 11:559–592.
47. Øie, S., Guentert, T. W., and Tozer, T. N. (1980): Effect of saturable binding on the pharmacokinetics of drugs: a simulation. *J. Pharm. Pharmacol.,* 32:471–477.
48. O'Reilly, R. A., Aggeler, P. M., and Leong, L. S. (1964): Studies on the coumarin anticoagulant drugs: A comparison of the pharmacodynamics of dicumarol and warfarin in man. *Thromb. Diathes. Haemostas.,* 11:1–22.
49. Pang, K. S. (1981): Metabolite pharmacokinetics: The area under the curve of metabolite and the fractional rate of metabolism of a drug after different routes of administration for renally and hepatically cleared drugs and metabolites. *J. Pharmacokinet. Biopharmacol.,* 9:477–487.
50. Pang, K. S., and Gillette, J. R. (1979): Sequential first-pass elimination of a metabolite derived from a precursor. *J. Pharmacokinet. Biopharmacol.,* 7:275–290.

51. Pang, K. S., Strobl, K., and Gillette, J. R. (1979): A method for the estimation of the fraction of a precursor that is converted to a metabolite in rat *in vivo* with phenacetin and acetaminophen. *Drug. Metab. Dispos.*, 7:366–372.
52. Paterson, J. W., Conolly, M. E., Dollery, C. T., Hayes, A., and Cooper, R. G. (1970): Pharmacodynamics and metabolism of propranolol in man. *Pharmacol. Clin.*, 2:127–133.
53. Perrier, D., Ashley, J. J., and Levy, G. (1973): Effect of product inhibition on kinetics of drug elimination. *J. Pharmacokinet. Biopharmacol.*, 1:231–242.
54. Powis, G., Ames, M. M., and Kovach, J. S. (1981): Dose-dependent pharmacokinetics and cancer chemotherapy. *Cancer Chemother. Pharmacol.*, 6:1–9.
55. Ramsey, J. C., and Young, J. D. (1978): Pharmacokinetics of inhaled styrene in rats and humans. *Scand. J. Work Environ. Health*, 4(Suppl. 2):84–91.
56. Reddy, B. G., Pohl, L. H., and Krishna, G. (1976): The requirement of the gut flora in nitrobenzene-induced methemoglobinemia in rats. *Biochem. Pharmacol.*, 25:1119–1122.
57. Renwick, A. G. (1977): In: *Drug Metabolism—from Microbe to Man*, edited by D. V. Parke and R. L. Smith, pp. 169–189. Taylor and Francis, London.
58. Richens, A., and Dunlop, A. (1975): Serum phenytoin levels in the management of epilepsy. *Lancet*, 2:247–248.
59. Rowland, M. (1973): In: *Current Concepts in Pharmaceutical Sciences: Dosage Form Design and Bioavailability*, edited by J. Swarbrick, pp. 181–222. Lea & Febiger, Philadelphia.
60. Rowland, M., and Tozer, T. N. (1980): *Clinical Pharmacokinetics: Concepts and Applications.* Lea & Febiger, Philadelphia.
61. Sauerhoff, M. W., Braun, W. H., Glau, G. E., and Gehring, P. J. (1976): The dose-dependent pharmacokinetic profile of 2,4,5-trichloro-phenoxyacetic acid following intravenous administration to rats. *Toxicol. Appl. Pharmacol.*, 36:491–501.
62. Scheline, R. E. (1973): Metabolism of foreign compounds by gastrointestinal microorganisms. *Pharmacol. Rev.*, 25:451–523.
63. Scheline, R. R. (1980): In: *Extrahepatic Metabolism of Drugs and Other Foreign Compounds*, edited by T. E. Gram, pp. 551–580. S. P. Medical and Scientific Books, New York.
64. Schneck, D. W., Pritchard, J. F., Gibson, T. P., Vary, J. E., and Hayes, A. H. (1980): Effect of dose and uremia on plasma and urine profiles of propranolol metabolites. *Clin. Pharmacol. Ther.*, 27:744–755.
65. Shand, D. G., and Rangno, R. E. (1972): Disposition of propranolol. I. Elimination during oral absorption in man. *Pharmacology*, 7:159–168.
66. Shibasaki, J., Koizumi, T., and Tanaka, T. (1968): Drug absorption, metabolism and excretion. I. Some pharmacokinetic aspects of metabolism of acetanilide and 4-hydroxyacetanilide. *Chem. Pharm. Bull.*, 16:1661–1673.
67. Suzuki, T., Isozaki, S., Ishida, R., Saitoh, Y., and Nakagawa, F. (1974): Drug absorption and metabolism studies by use of portal vein infusion in the rat. II. Influence of dose and infusion rate on the bioavailability of propranolol. *Chem. Pharm. Bull.*, 22:1639–1645.
68. Tsuchiya, T., and Levy, G. (1972): Relationship between dose and plateau levels of drugs eliminated by parallel first-order and capacity-limited kinetics. *J. Pharm. Sci.*, 61:541–544.
69. Wagner, J. G. (1973): A modern view of pharmacokinetics. *J. Pharmacokinet. Biopharmacol.*, 1:363–401.
70. Walle, T., Conradi, E. C., Walle, U. K., Fagan, T. C., and Gaffney, T. E. (1980): 4-Hydroxy propranolol and its glucuronide after single and long-term doses of propranolol. *Clin. Pharmacol. Ther.*, 27:22–31.
71. Watanabe, P. G., Young, J. D., and Gehring, P. J. (1977): The importance of nonlinear (dose-dependent) pharmacokinetics in hazard assessment. *J. Environ. Pathol. Toxicol.*, 1:147–159.
72. Weinberger, M., and Ginchansky, E. (1977): Dose-dependent kinetics of theophylline disposition in asthmatic children. *J. Pediatr.*, 91:820–824.
73. Wilkinson, G. R., and Shand, D. G. (1975): A physiological approach to hepatic drug clearance. *Clin. Pharmacol. Ther.*, 18:377–390.

Drug Metabolism and Drug Toxicity,
edited by J. R. Mitchell and M. G. Horning.
Raven Press, New York © 1984.

Solvable and Unsolvable Problems in Extrapolating Toxicological Data Between Animal Species and Strains

James R. Gillette

Laboratory of Chemical Pharmacology, National Heart, Lung, and Blood Institute, National Institutes of Health, Bethesda, Maryland 20205

During the past several decades the variety and depth of toxicological studies have increased enormously. At the beginning of the present century, toxicological studies, if they were done at all, were usually restricted to observing whether an animal survived after the administration of a single dose of a substance. Now, studies are performed according to elaborate protocols in which different doses are administered for periods of time ranging from a day to several years, and even the most subtle changes in enzyme activities, cellular morphology, and animal behavior are assessed by sophisticated methods and instruments. The current toxicological studies in animals obviously reveal whether a substance can cause, either directly or indirectly, physiological or morphological changes in the test animals under the conditions of the experiment. But whether the substance would cause these changes in a given human being at the same doses used in the animal experiment is highly questionable.

The toxicologist is at a disadvantage for several reasons. He or she performs a toxicological study with a limited number of animals, usually no more than 100 to 1,000, and thus, the lowest incidence rate that can be detected would be within this range. With a compound that is to be widely distributed in the environment, however, an incidence rate of this order of magnitude may be deemed unacceptable in a human population. Hence, the doses of the substance used in toxicity studies frequently are larger than those expected to be present in the environment. The toxicologist is also at a disadvantage in that many toxicities are not evoked immediately but become manifest only after delays ranging from several hours to several weeks and, in the case of carcinogenesis, to several years. In the hope that the delays in onset may be shortened with increasing doses, the toxicologist also tends to administer higher doses of a compound in toxicity studies than the concentrations likely to be present in the environment. The toxicologist is at further disadvantage in that he or she never knows whether the population of the animals used in toxicity studies reasonably represents the populations of humans and of other organisms that are likely to be exposed to the compound in the environment.

Several mathematical models have been suggested as aids in making extrapolations from high doses to low doses and from experimental animals to the human population. Although these models still have their advocates, they are becoming increasingly in disrepute, largely because the validity of the assumptions made in their development is highly questionable. For example, in the derivation of the equation for the multistage model (9), it has been assumed that the relationship between the dose and the number of "hits" is always first order regardless of dose and that there are no individual differences among the animals in an experimental group. In other words, a group of 100 animals is visualized as a single animal 100 times the size of the individual animal. In the extrapolation of animals to humans, it is further assumed that all rats are like all humans. By contrast, in the development of the Mantel–Bryan approach (7), which is based on a probit response versus log-dose graph, it is recognized that there can be individual differences, but it is assumed that the probit response versus log-dose graph will be linear even when it is extrapolated far below the experimental range and that its slope is known without error. The slope of the graph is a measure of the variance of the incidence of the response within the group of the experimental animals. But since the toxicological tests become much more sensitive and meaningful when the slope of the probit response versus log-dose graph is large, the strain of animals selected for the test is as homogeneous as possible.

It is well known, however, that humans can be remarkably heterogeneous in their response to foreign compounds (5). Recognizing these differences, Mantel and Bryan (7) built into the models safety factors that they hoped would provide conservative estimates of the incidence rates. Such conservative safety factors, however, frequently provide estimates of acceptable doses that are below the capabilities of even the most sophisticated of the currently available analytical techniques. Indeed, some of them suggest the virtual elimination of the substance from the environment. Because the safety factors are arbitrary and have little or no sound scientific basis, their use is highly controversial.

It is evident that toxicological tests by themselves should not be expected to provide scientifically valid incidence rates in heterogeneous animal species or humans. What is needed is a better understanding of the mechanism of the toxicity and the ways that various parameters would be expected to alter the response of animals to chemicals. Some differences are caused by variations in the number and affinity of receptor sites or other sites with which the compound reacts. Some of the differences are caused by variations in the factors that govern the magnitude of the response after the compound reacts with the sites of action. But many of the differences are caused by variations in the time a compound is maintained at concentrations adequate to evoke the response. Moreover, in some instances, the response is caused by a metabolite of the substance rather than by the parent compound, and hence, the response is governed by the pharmacokinetics of the formation and elimination of the metabolite.

During the 1950s, considerable effort was expended in seeking an animal species that would be similar to man in the way it metabolized drugs and other foreign compounds in the hope that such an animal species would minimize the difficulties in extrapolating the results of toxicity studies to humans. At that time, it was believed that there were qualitative as well as quantitative differences in metabolism (2,10). For example, it was believed that cats did not form glucuronides, that dogs could not acetylate drugs, that guinea pigs could not form mercapturic acids, and that only primates could convert phenylacetic acid to phenacetyl glutamate. It was also thought that the intraspecies differences in the metabolism of foreign compounds would be negligible. Since that time, however, the quest has proved to be fruitless. Studies with drugs in humans revealed marked variability in the metabolism of foreign compounds. In some instances, there were genetic differences among humans in the metabolism of certain compounds; for example, the human population could be broadly separated into slow and fast acetylators of isoniazid and certain sulfanilamides (5). Moreover, the relative abundance of the fast and slow acetylators of isoniazid varied with racial origins; thus, nearly all orientals were fast acetylators, whereas only about 50% of the individuals in the white and black populations in the United States were fast acetylators. It also became evident that there were individual differences in the relative rates of metabolism of different drugs; thus, a given individual could metabolize one drug more rapidly than most of the human population but could metabolize another drug more slowly than the majority of the population.

It has also become evident that a drug may be metabolized at markedly different rates in different strains of the same animal species. Moreover, when the rates of metabolism of a drug in a set of strains of one animal species are compared with the rates of metabolism of the drug in a set of strains of another animal species, there can be considerable overlap. Thus, the distinctions implied by the term "species differences in drug metabolism" become blurred. It may well be that many apparent species differences in drug metabolism represent opposite extremes in the representative strains of the animal species rather than the average of all strains of the two animal species. Thus, it is difficult to establish the extent to which species differences in drug metabolism actually occur. One can only state that a given strain of one species differs from a given strain of another species used in the studies.

It has also become evident that the pattern and the rate constants of metabolism of a compound in an individual animal or human may not be constant. They may vary with age, diet, the time of day, the season, the presence of disease, or previous exposure to compounds that increase or decrease the activity of the enzymes that metabolize the compound (3). In certain instances, they may vary with the site of administration, the dose, or the rate of absorption of the compound. Moreover, the effect that age and these environmental factors may have on the metabolism of foreign compounds may differ with the animal strain or individual humans. The pattern and the rate constants of metabolism of a compound in a given strain of animals thus may be quantitatively different when the experiment is performed in different laboratories or when the experiment is repeated in the same laboratory at different times.

With these advances in our knowledge of drug metabolism, the question of "which animal species mimics humans in drug metabolism" began to be answered by a series of questions: "which human, which drug, which animal species under what conditions?" Moreover, since individuals having heritable differences in drug metabolism are heterogeneously distributed on earth, it thus became questionable whether a study of the metabolism of a drug in a small group of humans in a given location, as frequently occurs in clinical pharmacology studies, truly represents the metabolism of the drug in the human population as a whole.

Because of the interplay between genetic and environmental factors that affect the pattern and rate constants of metabolism, and because subpopulations resulting from the interplay are heterogeneously distributed, it seems unlikely that the variance in the metabolism of any given drug in the human population will ever be exactly known. Since there are now about 4 billion of us on earth, however, it seems likely that the range of values could be quite large. Indeed, it seems plausible that the range of values in humans may be so large that they include the ranges that occur in virtually every species or strain of laboratory animals used to test drugs. According to this view, any result obtained with virtually any strain or species of animal may mimic a subpopulation of humans. Even contradictory results obtained with two different strains or species of animals may both be relevant to humans. They simply would apply to two different subpopulations. It may thus be plausible that the administration of a given inducer may increase the toxicity of a metabolite of a compound in some humans and decrease it in others. Whether the subpopulation mimicked by a given strain of a given animal species represents a major or minor fraction of the total human population, however, may only be known after the metabolism of the compound is studied extensively in humans. Until that time, it is prudent to accept results obtained with any animal species as possibly relevant to some portion of the human population and to apply safety margins deemed appropriate by decision makers in regulatory agencies.

DO DRUG METABOLISM STUDIES PROVIDE USEFUL INFORMATION IN EVALUATING TOXICITY TESTS?

Although it is intuitively obvious that studies of the metabolism of a compound should aid in the extrapolation of toxicity data obtained with test animals to other animals and humans, attempts to use metabolic data for this purpose have frequently been disappointing. Occasionally, the responses used to assess the toxicity are too poorly defined to make any correlation possible. More often than not, however, neither the toxicity study nor the metabolic study is sufficiently well designed or coordinated to reach certain key objectives.

One of the key objectives of a coordinated study of toxicity and metabolism is to determine whether the response is caused by the parent compound or by one or more of the metabolites of the compound. If it can be established that the response is caused solely by the parent compound, the extrapolation of the results obtained in the toxicity study to other animals may be rather simple. Those factors that govern the concentration of the parent compound at the site of action would have to be compared, but species, strain, and individual differences in the relative abundance of the metabolites formed from the compound could be ignored. Moreover, nearly identical concentration–time curves of the parent compound may sometimes be simulated by appropriate changes in the dose and rate of administration, and thus, variations in the responsiveness of the action sites after the compound interacts with the sites may be assessed. If the action sites are nearly identical, the intensity and the time course of the response may be made to appear to be nearly identical even in animals in which the pharmacokinetics of the drug are quite different.

Because the rates of absorption, distribution, metabolism, and excretion of a compound can be altered by many different temporal and environmental factors, it is important that the studies of metabolism and toxicity of a compound be done with the same doses in the same strain of animals under the same environmental conditions. Indeed, whenever possible, both studies should be done with the same animals. All too often the studies of metabolism and toxicity of the compound are performed at different times with different doses of the compound under different conditions. Any hope of making meaningful correlations under those conditions is thus largely lost.

PHARMACOKINETICS AS A GUIDE TO THE INTEGRATION OF DATA FROM DIFFERENT KINDS OF EXPERIMENTS

Since the primary objective of studying the metabolism of a foreign compound as a part of an integrated toxicity–metabolism study is to determine the time courses of the unbound concentrations of the biologically active substances at sites of action, it is important to recognize how such information can be obtained from different kinds of drug metabolism studies.

Frequently, the drug is injected intravenously, and the concentration of the drug in the venous blood or plasma is measured at various times thereafter. But visualize the sequence of events that occur during the injection and subsequent distribution and elimination of the drug. Clearly, the highest concentration of the drug that is injected into the vein is the concentration of the drug within the syringe. But as the drug enters the vein and is carried to the heart, blood in the vein becomes mixed with the blood returning to the heart from other organs, and thus the drug is diluted. The maximal concentration of drug at extracellular receptor sites on the cellular membranes within the veins will be unmeasurable but will be between the concentration of the drug within the syringe and a value given by the rate of rapid injectior divided by volume of blood entering the heart during the injection of the drug. The concentration of the drug in blood leaving the right heart and entering the lungs will depend on the rate of injection. When the drug is injected instantaneously, the concentration will be no greater than the dose divided by the stroke volume, but when the compound is injected within a few seconds, the concentration will be the rate of injection divided by the cardiac output. As the compound in the blood leaves the right ventricle and enters the lung, some of the drug will diffuse out of the pulmonary capillaries and begin filling the lung extracellular and intracellular compartments. The drug then passes back to the heart and is distributed to other organs, where it diffuses out of the capillaries and enters the extracellular and intracellular spaces of the organs. The drug then returns to the heart via the venous system, but because the transit times of the blood infusing the various organs differ, the average concentration of the drug in the venous blood oscillates on recirculation until the drug in the blood and the other parts of the central compartment becomes completely mixed.

Although the drug in blood is completely mixed by the time the first blood sample is obtained, the concentration of the drug in the compartments of many organs of the body usually has not yet achieved a quasi-steady state with that in the blood. Consequently, the concentration of the drug in blood continues to fall, but the concentrations in many organs continue to increase. Ultimately, the concentration of the diffusible form of the compound in an organ reaches its concentration in blood. But the concentration in blood continues to decline as the compound is eliminated from the body. A concentration gradient for the diffusible form becomes established, and the concentration of the compound in the organ declines.

Complex though these processes may be, the decline in the concentration of the compound frequently may be simulated by the equation for two-compartment systems (Fig. 1).

$$C_b = \frac{\text{Dose}}{V_1}\left[\frac{(k_{21} - \alpha)\,e^{-\alpha t}}{\beta - \alpha} + \frac{(k_{21} - \beta)\,e^{-\beta t}}{\alpha - \beta}\right]$$

$$= \frac{\text{Dose}}{V_1}(A_0 e^{-\alpha t} + B_0 e^{-\beta t}) \qquad (1)$$

At $t = 0$, the equation degenerates to

$$C_b = \frac{\text{Dose}}{V_1} \qquad (1a)$$

In equation 1a, V_1 is a hypothetical volume of a central compartment into which the drug is initially distributed. Some investigators intuitively feel that the V_1 should be the volume of the blood, but this is almost never true. When the complex initial events described above are taken into account, it should be evident that the apparent volume of the central compartment will almost invariably include not only the volume of the blood but also at least a part of the extracellular space of all organs and a part of the intracellular space of many organs. Moreover, the sample of blood obtained for the assay of foreign

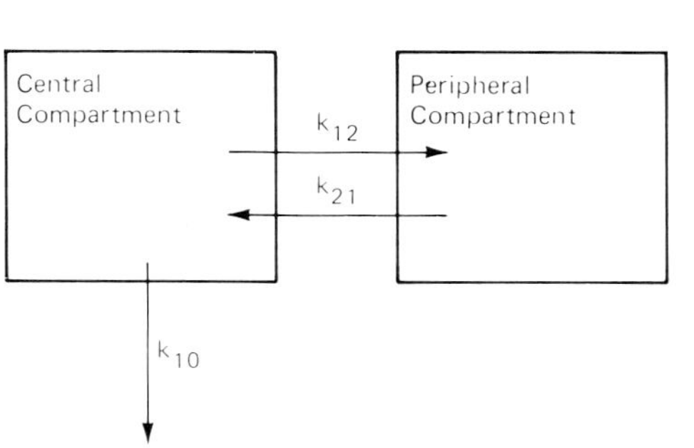

FIG. 1. Two-compartment model.

compounds frequently is venous blood that has passed through a capillary bed. Its measured concentration may therefore be smaller than the concentration in arterial blood, and the apparent value of V_1 would appear to be higher than its actual value.

Even if the premixing events of distribution of the drug were completely understood, the concept of V_1 would still be obscure. Because C_b is usually defined as the total concentration of drug in blood, it obviously represents not only the unbound drug but also the drug in erythrocytes and the drug that is bound to the various plasma proteins. But the volume of distribution of the unbound form of the drug will not be the same as the volumes of distribution of the bound forms of the drug. Moreover, the volumes of distribution of plasma proteins and therefore of the forms bound to plasma proteins are not the blood volume. Only about one-half of the albumin in the body, for example, is in the blood; the rest is in the lymph and the interstitial space (1). The investigator is thus left with the problem of deciding how much of the extracellular space in the body is incorporated into the central compartment and therefore how much of the total albumin was in the central compartment. If it were assumed that all of the albumin in the body were in the central compartment, the apparent volume of the central compartment would be

$$V_1 = \frac{\text{Dose}}{C_b}\left[\frac{C_{p(\text{free})}V_{\text{free}} + B_{\text{ev}} + C_{\text{rbc}}V_{\text{rbc}} + \Sigma C_{\text{bound to protein}(i)}A_{\text{protein}(i)}}{HC_{\text{rbc}} + [1-H][C_{p(\text{free})} + \Sigma C_{\text{bound to protein}(i)}C_{p(\text{protein}(i))}]}\right] \quad (2)$$

where B_{ev} is the amount of drug bound to components that are present in the central compartment but not present in the blood (for example, collagen), H is the hemocrit, C_{rbc} is the concentration of drug in the erythrocytes, V_{rbc} is the total volume of the erythrocytes in the central compartment, protein(i) is a protein or another binding component that is present in blood plasma and perhaps in other parts of the extracellular space in the body, $C_{\text{bound to protein}(i)}$ is the amount of drug bound to protein(i) per milligram of protein(i), $A_{\text{protein}(i)}$ is the total number of milligrams of protein(i) in the central compartment, $C_{p(\text{protein}(i))}$ is the number of milligrams of protein(i) in blood plasma per milliliter of plasma, $C_{p(\text{free})}$ is the concentration of unbound drug in blood plasma, and V_{free} is the volume into which the unbound drug is distributed, excluding that present in erythrocytes. Inspection of equation 2 reveals some of the reasons why pharmacokineticists consider it virtually impossible to assign any physiological significance to V_1.

Clearly, the maximum concentration of a drug at receptor sites achieved after an intravenous injection will depend on the localization of those receptor sites. If the receptor sites were located on the surface of the endothelium of the arteries, the maximum concentration of the receptor sites after intravenous administration of the drug would presumably occur during the first passage of the drug through the arteries in which they are located. Thus, the concentration of the drug at these receptor sites would exceed the initial concentration predicted by the compartmental model. If the receptor sites were located on surface of the endothelium of veins other than that into which the drug was injected, however, the time at which the maximum concentration would occur would depend on the extraction of the drug during the passage of the blood through capillary beds of the various organs. If very little of the drug were extracted by the organ, the maximum concentration in the veins might be achieved during the first passage of the drug. But if the drug were highly bound by the organ, the maximum concentration in the veins might occur considerably later. Thus, it is not always possible to assume that the blood in certain parts of the venous system is always a part of the central compartment.

Many receptors are located within cells, and, therefore, the concentration of unbound drug within target cells in an organ presumably would be more relevant to the pharmacological response than would the concentration of unbound drug in blood plasma.

If the cells were within the central compartment, the maximum concentration would have occurred during the mixing phase and before the first blood sample had been withdrawn. Thus, the maximum concentration at the receptor sites would be indeterminable and indeed may be somewhat higher than the initial concentration in blood predicted by equation 1a.

If the receptor sites were located in cells representing the deep compartment, the two-compartment model implies that the concentration at the receptor sites at any given time would be predicted from the equation.

$$C_{\text{deep compartment}} = \frac{\text{Dose}}{V_2} \frac{k_{12}}{\beta - \alpha} [(e^{-\alpha t} - e^{-\beta t})] \tag{3}$$

where V_2 is the hypothetical volume of distribution of the deep compartment, and k_{12} is the rate constant for the passage of the drug from the central compartment to the deep compartment.

In this model, the time at which the maximum concentration would occur may be estimated from the equation

$$t_{\max} = \frac{\ln (\alpha/\beta)}{\alpha - \beta} \tag{4}$$

On substitution of this equation into equation 3, the maximum concentration of the unbound drug may be estimated.

$$C_{\text{deep compartment,max}} = \left(\frac{\text{Dose}}{V_2}\right)\left(\frac{k_{12}}{\alpha}\right)\left(\frac{\alpha}{\beta}\right)^{[\beta/(\beta-\alpha)]} \tag{5}$$

However, the concentration of the unbound drug in the central compartment at $t_{\max}$ for the deep compartment may be expressed as

$$C_{\text{b(at deep compartment,max)}} = \left[\frac{\text{Dose}}{V_1}\right]\left[\frac{k_{21}}{\alpha}\right]\left[\frac{\alpha}{\beta}\right]^{[\beta/(\beta-\alpha)]} \tag{6}$$

The ratio of the maximum concentration of the drug in the deep compartment to the concentration of the drug in blood at $t_{\max}$ would be

$$\frac{C_{\text{deep compartment,max}}}{C_{\text{b(at deep compartment,max)}}} = \frac{V_1 k_{21}}{V_2 k_{21}} = \frac{Cl_{12}}{Cl_{21}} \tag{7}$$

Since there are ways of calculating the ratio of (Cl_{12}/Cl_{21}) (see below), it might seem possible to determine rather easily the maximum concentration in the peripheral compartment and thus the maximal concentration of the drug at receptor sites located in the peripheral compartment. Unfortunately, the two-compartment model is often inadequate for this purpose. The receptor sites frequently are in a group of cells that never contain a major fraction of the total amount of drug present in the body, and thus, the receptor compartment may not be represented by either the central or the peripheral compartments. Since the increase and subsequent decrease in the concentration of the drug in the receptor compartment would not be expected to affect markedly the concentration of the drug in blood, the equation for the concentration of the drug in blood would remain equation 1, but the equation for the amount of drug in the cells containing the receptors would be

$$V_{\text{cells}} C_{\text{cells in organ}} = \text{Dose} \frac{k_{13}(k_{21} - \alpha)e^{-\alpha t}}{(k_{31} - \alpha)(\beta - \alpha)} + \frac{k_{13}(k_{21} - \beta)e^{-\beta t}}{(k_{31} - \beta)(\alpha - \beta)} + \frac{k_{13}(k_{21} - k_{31})e^{-k_{31} t}}{(\alpha - k_{31})(\beta - k_{31})} \tag{8}$$

where k_{13} and k_{31} are the rate constants for the passage of the drug into and out of the receptor compartment, respectively. If the value of k_{31} were greater than β, the concentraion of the drug within the cells would continue to increase after the central compartment was established, reach a maximum, and then decrease biphasically (Fig. 2). Thus, after intravenous administration of the drug, the maximal concentration of the drug within the cells would occur at some time between the initial mixing phase and the time predicted by equation 6. If the value of k_{31} were

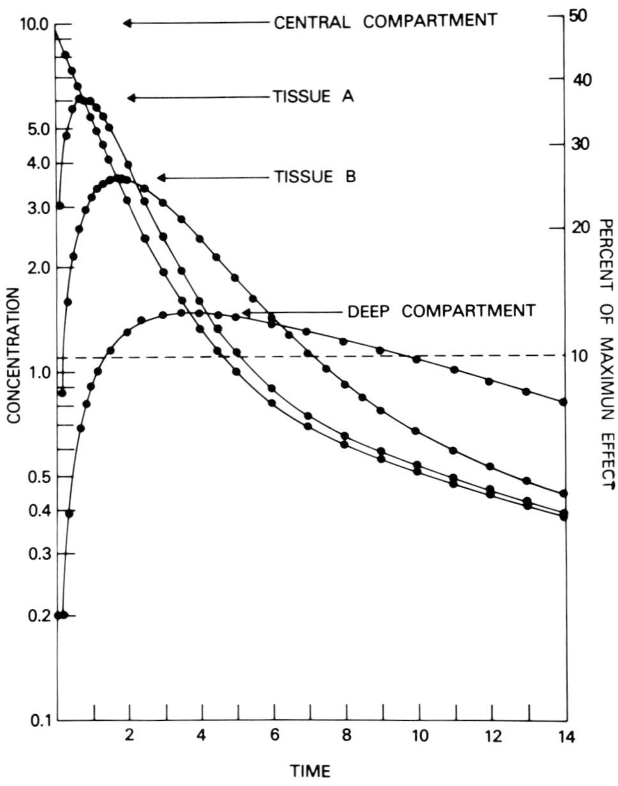

FIG. 2. Simulations of the time courses of the unbound concentrations of a hypothetical drug in blood, two small tissue compartments, and the deep compartment. The *right-hand scale* is the hypothetical concentration response relationship generated from [D]/([D] + EC_{50}), where EC_{50} equals 10 arbitrary units.

smaller than β, the two-compartment model would not be valid; instead, the kinetics of the concentration of the drug in blood would fit a system comprising three or more compartments, and thus the equations for these systems would be needed instead of equation 8.

Assays of the amounts of the drug in various organs at different times provide some idea of the kinetics of the passage of the drug into and out of organs. Unfortunately, the interpretation of such experiments is difficult because each organ frequently represents several compartments. The amount of drug present in an organ almost immediately after the intravenous administration of the drug reflects the contribution of the organ to the central compartment.

If the amount of drug in the organ has reached a maximum by this time and declines in parallel with the concentration of the drug in blood, the entire organ represents a part of the central compartment. If all processes were first order, the total amount of drug in the organ then would be described by multiplying both sides of equation 1 by the apparent volume of the organ [V_1 (organ)].

$$V_1 \text{ (organ) } C_b = \text{Dose } \frac{V_1 \text{ (organ)}}{V_1 \text{ (body)}} \left[\frac{(k_{21} - \alpha)e^{-\alpha t}}{\beta - \alpha} + \frac{(k_{21} - \beta)e^{-\beta t}}{\alpha - \beta} \right] \qquad (9)$$

In most organs, however, the amount of drug will continue to increase after completion of the initial mixing phase, reach a maximum, and then decline. The total amount of drug in the organ thus represents a composite of the amounts present in the various compartments within the organ. For example, if there were only one compartment other than the central compartment, the total amount of drug in the organ would be

$$A\text{ (organ)} = V_1\text{ (organ) } C_b + V_3\text{ (cells) } C_3\text{ (cells)} \tag{10}$$

where V_1 (organ) C_b is defined in equation 9 and V_3 (cells) C_3 (cells) is defined by equation 8. Thus, direct measurements of the amount of drug in an organ at any given time have only limited usefulness.

Area Under the Curve Measurement (Single Doses)

From the foregoing discussion, it should be clear that although rapid intravenous injection of drugs provides much valuable pharmacokinetic information, the relationship between the concentrations of the drug in blood and at the receptor sites at any given time is difficult to evaluate. When the drug is distributed to the various tissues and eliminated from the body solely by a first-order process, the relationship should theoretically be greatly clarified by measurements of the area under the curve of a plot of the concentrations of the drug in blood versus time and the areas under the curves of plots of the total amounts of drugs in the various organs versus time. The area under the curve of the blood concentration, which for a two-compartment system is obtained by integration of equation 1, will be

$$AUC_C\text{ (blood)} = \frac{\text{Dose } k_{21}}{V_1\alpha\beta} = \frac{\text{Dose}}{V_1 k_{10}} = \frac{\text{Dose}}{Cl_{10}} \tag{11}$$

If we visualized what the concentration of the drug would be in the deep compartment, however, and visualized what its area under the curve should be when the drug was not eliminated from the body by mechanisms in the deep compartment, we could calculate the area under the curve of the drug concentrations in the deep compartment by integrating equation 3. Thus,

$$AUC_C\text{ (deep compartment)} = \frac{\text{Dose}}{V_2}\frac{k_{12}}{\alpha\beta} = \frac{\text{Dose } k_{12}}{V_2 k_{21} k_{10}} \tag{12}$$

On dividing equation 12 by equation 11, we obtain

$$\frac{AUC_C\text{ (deep compartment)}}{AUC_C\text{ (blood)}} = \frac{V_1 k_{12}}{V_2 k_{21}} = \frac{Cl_{12}}{Cl_{21}} \tag{13}$$

Thus, the ratio of the areas under the curve of the concentrations of the drug in the deep compartment and the blood under these specified conditions would depend on the ratio of the clearances describing the passage of the drug into and out of the deep compartment.

As pointed out above, however, we are not always concerned solely with the average concentration of the drug in the hypothetical deep compartment, but we are concerned with the concentration of the drug in given organs containing the receptor sites. For cells that do not contain enzymes that metabolize the drug, we may obtain the equation for the area under the curve of the amount of drug within a given set of cells in an organ by integrating equation 8. That is

$$AUC_C\text{ (cells)} = \frac{\text{Dose } k_{13}k_{21}}{V_3 k_{31}\alpha\beta} = \frac{\text{Dose } k_{13}}{V_3 k_{31} k_{10}} = \frac{\text{Dose } Cl_{13}}{Cl_{31} Cl_{10}} \tag{14}$$

On dividing equation 14 by equation 11, we obtain

$$\frac{AUC_C\text{ (cells)}}{AUC_C\text{ (blood)}} = \frac{Cl_{13}}{Cl_{31}} \tag{15}$$

Thus, the ratio of the area under the curve of the concentration of the drug within any cell of any nonelimination organ to the area under the curve of the concentration of the drug in blood should equal the ratio of the clearance by which the drug enters and leaves the cell, provided that the drug is not eliminated from the organ by a fluid other than blood.

Because many animals would have to be killed in order to determine the amount of drug in the animal organs at various times, it is frequently not possible to obtain accurate measurements of the areas under the curves for the amount of drugs in the various organs of the body after rapid intravenous injection of the drug. Nevertheless, the ratios may be obtained after other methods of administration of drugs.

When the half-life of the β phase of a drug is short, the drug may be constantly infused intravenously until a steady state is attained, at which time the rate of elimination of the drug from the body would equal the rate of infusion of the drug. The time required to achieve 94% of the steady-state value should be four half-lives of the β phase. Under steady-state conditions, the rate of entrance of the drug into the cells of a nonelimination organ will equal the rate at which the drug leaves the cells. Thus, the ratio of the steady-state concentrations within the cells and in the blood plasma should be

$$\frac{C_{\text{cells,ss}}}{C_{\text{B,ss}}} = \frac{Cl_{13}}{Cl_{31}} \tag{16}$$

When the half-life of the β phase of a drug is long, the drug may be administered as several small doses until a steady state is reached. Again, the time required to reach 94% of the steady state should be four half-lives of the β phase. Under steady-state conditions, the ratio of the areas under the curves of the concentrations of the drug within cells of a nonelimination organ and in blood plasma during the dosage interval will be

$$\frac{AUC_C\,(\text{intracellular})_{ss}}{AUC_C\,(\text{blood})_{ss}} = \frac{Cl_{13}}{Cl_{31}} \tag{17}$$

Inspection of equations 15, 16, and 17 thus reveals that the following terms are theoretically equivalent:

$$\underset{\text{Single dose}}{\frac{AUC_C\,(\text{cells})}{AUC_C\,(\text{blood})}} = \underset{\text{Multiple doses}}{\frac{AUC_C\,(\text{cells})_{ss}}{AUC_C\,(\text{blood})_{ss}}} = \underset{\text{Infusion}}{\frac{C\,(\text{cells})_{ss}}{C\,(\text{blood})_{ss}}} = \frac{Cl_{13}}{Cl_{31}} \tag{18}$$

Ordinarily, clearance is defined as the rate of elimination of a substance from a compartment divided by the total concentration of the substance within the compartment under steady-state conditions. Thus, the values of Cl_{13} and Cl_{31} are

$$Cl_{13} = \frac{(\text{Rate of entrance into cells})_{ss}}{C\,(\text{blood})_{ss}} \tag{19}$$

$$Cl_{31} = \frac{(\text{Rate of exit from cells})_{ss}}{C\,(\text{cells})_{ss}} \tag{20}$$

Since the rate into and out of the cells under steady-state conditions must be equal, equations 19 and 20 may be combined.

$$Cl_{13}C\,(\text{blood})_{ss} = Cl_{31}C\,(\text{cells})_{ss} \tag{21}$$

When the clearances are calculated from the total concentrations of the drug in blood and the cells, the values of Cl_{13} and Cl_{31} for any given group of cells within an organ depend on the mechanisms by which the drug enters and leaves the cells and the extent of reversible binding of the drug to components in the blood and in the cells. Unfortunately, this is not the most useful form of the equation, because only the unbound forms of the drug pass into and out of the cells. We may define the unbound fraction of the drug in blood as ff (blood) and the unbound fraction in cells as ff (cells). By inserting the identities ff (blood)/ff (blood) and ff (cells)/ff (cells) into equation 21, we obtain

$$[Cl_{13}/ff\,(\text{blood})][ff\,(\text{blood})\,C\,(\text{blood})_{ss}] = [Cl_{31}/ff\,(\text{cells})][ff\,(\text{cells})\,C\,(\text{cells})_{ss}] \tag{22}$$

or

$$Cl_{13}\,(\text{free})\,C_{\text{free}}\,(\text{blood})_{ss} = Cl_{31}\,(\text{free})\,C_{\text{free}}\,(\text{cells})_{ss} \tag{22a}$$

If the unbound drug existed in only one form, and if it passed into and out of the cells solely by passive diffusion, then under steady-state conditions, C_{free} (blood)$_{ss}$ would equal C_{free} (cells)$_{ss}$, and thus, Cl_{13} (free) would equal Cl_{31} (free). The average concentration of such drugs at receptor sites in nonelimination tissues could therefore easily be calculated from the area under the curve of the concentration of unbound drug in blood during repeated-dose therapy.

Most drugs, however, are weak acids or weak bases. Ordinarily, such drugs pass through the lipoidal membranes of cells predominantly in their nonionized forms. In this situation, the concentration of the nonionized form of the drug in blood would be the same as the concentration of the nonionized form of the drug within cells of nonelimination organs under steady-state conditions (Fig. 3). The total concentration of unbound drug within the cells, however, would depend on the pK_a of the drug and the pH values of the blood plasma and the cells. For acids,

$$\frac{C_{free}\ (\text{cells})_{ss}}{C_{free}\ (\text{blood})_{ss}} = \frac{1 + 10^{(\text{pH}-\text{p}K_a)}\ (\text{blood})}{1 + 10^{(\text{pH}-\text{p}K_a)}\ (\text{cells})} = \frac{Cl_{13}\ (\text{free})}{Cl_{31}\ (\text{free})} \tag{23}$$

For bases,

$$\frac{C_{free}\ (\text{cells})_{ss}}{C_{free}\ (\text{blood})_{ss}} = \frac{1 + 10^{(\text{p}K_a-\text{pH})(\text{blood})}}{1 + 10^{(\text{p}K_a-\text{pH})(\text{cells})}} = \frac{Cl_{13}\ (\text{free})}{Cl_{31}\ (\text{free})} \tag{24}$$

Thus, if the pH values for the cells and blood were known, it should be possible to calculate the average concentration of unbound drug within cells of nonelimination organs from the pK_a of the drug and the steady-state concentration of unbound drug in blood plasma. Indeed, Waddell and Butler (8) have used these relationships with unbound drugs to calculate intracellular pH values.

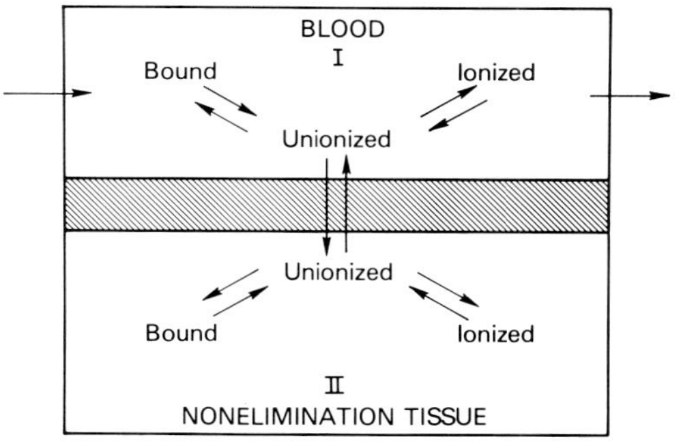

FIG. 3. Steady-state relationships in the concentrations of various forms of a drug between the blood and any nonelimination tissue in the body.

When a drug is eliminated from the cells either by metabolism or by active excretion, equation 22a should be modified to

$$Cl_{13}\ (\text{free})\ C_{free}\ (\text{blood})_{ss} = [Cl_{31}\ (\text{free}) + Cl_{30}\ (\text{free})]\ C_{free}\ (\text{cells})_{ss} \tag{25}$$

in which Cl_{30} (free) is the sum of the clearances of elimination of the drug from the cells. Equation 25 may be rearranged to

$$\frac{C_{free}\ (\text{cells})_{ss}}{C_{free}\ (\text{blood})_{ss}} = \frac{Cl_{13}\ (\text{free})}{Cl_{31}\ (\text{free}) + Cl_{30}\ (\text{free})} \tag{26}$$

Simple though equation 26 may be, it nevertheless illustrates one of the most important principles in pharmacokinetics. The degree to which enzymes in cells alter the concentration of the drug within the cells depends not only on the activity of the enzymes but also on the clearance of diffusion of the drug from the cells. Measurements of enzyme activity alone are not sufficient to determine the effects of enzyme on the intracellular concentration of the drug within cells. Knowledge of the clearance values for the passage of the drug into and out of the cells is also essential. It is nevertheless evident that a given activity of an enzyme will affect the intracellular concentration of a polar compound that does not pass membranes rapidly more than it will affect the intracellular concentration of a lipid-soluble compound.

The situation may be more complex than this. For example, in addition to passing into and out of cells by passive diffusion, a drug may be actively transported into cells and metabolized therein or otherwise eliminated from the cells. In this situation, the ratio of the intracellular and extracellular concentrations would be described by the following equation:

$$\frac{C_{\text{free}}\ (\text{cells})_{\text{ss}}}{C_{\text{free}}\ (\text{blood})_{\text{ss}}} = \frac{Cl_{13}\ (\text{free, active}) + Cl_{13}\ (\text{free, passive})}{Cl_{31}\ (\text{free}) + Cl_{30}\ (\text{free})} \quad (27)$$

where Cl_{30} is the sum of the clearance of elimination from the cells. In the brain, for example, Cl_{30} (free) would include not only the metabolic clearance but also the clearance by the flow of cerebrospinal fluid. Indeed, if the flow of cerebrospinal fluid did not serve as an effective way of removing from the brain polar compounds that are not metabolized in the brain, there would be no difference between the steady-state concentrations of the diffusible forms of compounds in brain and blood despite their poor diffusivity across the blood–brain barrier. The smallest value of Cl_{30} (free) for any foreign substance in the brain is thus the rate of flow of the cerebrospinal fluid. By the same reasoning, the smallest value of Cl_{30} (free) out of a fetus is either the fetal renal clearance or the clearance of the substance from the amniotic fluid into the mother's blood.

Because there may be species and strain differences in either the active transport or the metabolic mechanisms, the investigator should determine whether these mechanisms are present in cells containing the relevant receptor sites and, if they are present, whether their clearances are significantly larger than the clearance by diffusion. If the clearance by active transport or the clearance of metabolites in a small compartment containing the relevant receptor sites is significantly larger than the clearance of diffusion, studies based solely on the pharmacokinetics of the drug in blood will seldom provide sufficient information to account for the species or strain differences in the effects of the drug even though there may be no significant species differences in the affinity of the receptor sites for the drug.

Boundary Estimates of the Concentration of Drugs at Receptor Sites

Even without measurements of the concentrations of the drugs in organs, it is still possible to define the boundaries for the concentrations of the drug in the receptor compartment provided that (a) the drug enters and leaves the receptor compartment almost solely by passive diffusion and (b) the organ is not in the flow of blood from the site of administration to the arterial blood. After the intravenous administration, the concentration of drug in blood will decline, but the concentration in the receptor compartment will increase, reach a maximum, and then decline. At the maximum concentration of the drug in the receptor compartment, the rates at which the drug enters and leaves the receptor compartment must be equal. Unless there are other compartments between the receptor compartment and the blood, the concentrations of the diffusible form of the drug in the receptor compartment and the blood will also be equal (for example, compare equation 7 with equation 13). The ratio of the concentrations of unbound drug, however, would depend on the pK_a of the drug and the pH values of the receptor compartment and the blood plasma. But if these values were known, the concentration of unbound drug could be calculated from equation 23 or 24. If the time at which the concentration of the drug in the receptor compartment reached its maximum were known, the maximum concentration of the unbound drug in the receptor compartment could be calculated from the concentration of unbound drug in blood at that time. Thus, even without knowledge of the tissue distribution of the drug, the investigator may be reasonably confident that the concentration of the diffusible form of the drug at receptor sites will never be any higher than its maximum concentration in arterial blood.

When a drug is administered repeatedly until a steady state is attained, it is frequently possible to estimate minimum concentrations as well as maximum concentration. According to the two-compartment first-order model the concentration of unbound drug in blood under steady-state conditions may be expressed as follows:

$$C_b\ (\text{free})_{ss} = \frac{\text{Dose}}{V_1\ (\text{free})}\left[\frac{(k_{21}-\alpha)e^{-\alpha t}}{(\beta-\alpha)(1-e^{-\alpha\tau})} + \frac{(k_{21}-\beta)e^{-\beta t}}{(\alpha-\beta)(1-e^{-\beta\tau})}\right] \quad (28)$$

The concentration of unbound drug in a small compartment containing the receptors under steady-state conditions may be expressed as

$$C_{\text{cells}}\ (\text{free})_{ss} = \frac{\text{Dose}}{V_3\ (\text{free})}\left[\frac{k_{13}(k_{21}-\alpha)e^{-\alpha t}}{(k_{31}-\alpha)(\beta-\alpha)(1-e^{-\alpha\tau})} + \frac{k_{13}(k_{21}-\beta)e^{-\beta t}}{(k_{31}-\beta)(\alpha-\beta)(1-e^{-\beta\tau})} + \frac{k_{13}(k_{21}-k_{31})e^{-k_{31}t}}{(\alpha-k_{31})(\beta-k_{31})(1-e^{-k_{31}\tau})}\right] \quad (29)$$

In these equations, τ is the dosage interval. At the end of the dosage interval, t will be τ.

A solution of these equations would reveal that when the diffusional clearances of unbound drug into and out of the receptor compartment are equal, the concentration of unbound drug within the receptor compartment at the end of the dosage interval would be at least slightly higher than that in blood. Thus, unless there is reason to believe that the drug does not enter or leave the compartment solely by passive diffusion, the investigator can be reasonably confident that the concentration of the diffusible form of the drug in the receptor compartment is never higher than its highest concentration in blood (upper boundary) and never lower than its lowest concentration in blood (lower boundary) (Fig. 4).

Under the stated conditions, the areas under the curves of the concentrations of the diffusible form of the drug in blood and in the receptor compartment will be identical. The magnitude of fluctuation of the concentration within the receptor compartment depends on the value of the diffusional clearances: the smaller the clearance, the smaller the fluctuation during the dosage interval. Thus, if the investigator feels confident that the receptors are located in a deep compartment, measurements of the *AUC* of the unbound drug together with the use of equation 23 or 24 may provide a reasonable estimate of the concentration of unbound drug in the receptor compartment.

If the investigator is unsure of the "depth" of the receptor compartment but wishes to know more precisely the concentration of the drug in the receptor compartment, he or she may narrow the difference between the upper and lower boundaries by decreasing both the dose and the dosage interval. For example, halving both the dose and the dosage interval will not change the average concentration of the drug in either the blood or the receptor compartment but would decrease the maximum concentration and increase the minimum concentration in blood; indeed, the magnitude of the fluctuation in the concentration of the drug occurring during the dosage interval would now be one-half the magnitude of the fluctuation obtained with the other dosage schedule (Fig. 5). Decreasing both the dose and the dosage interval would decrease the difference between the upper and lower boundaries still further.

Thus, it should be possible in many instances to maintain the concentration of the drug at receptor sites between predefined limits in different animal strains or species even when the half-lives or clearances of the drug

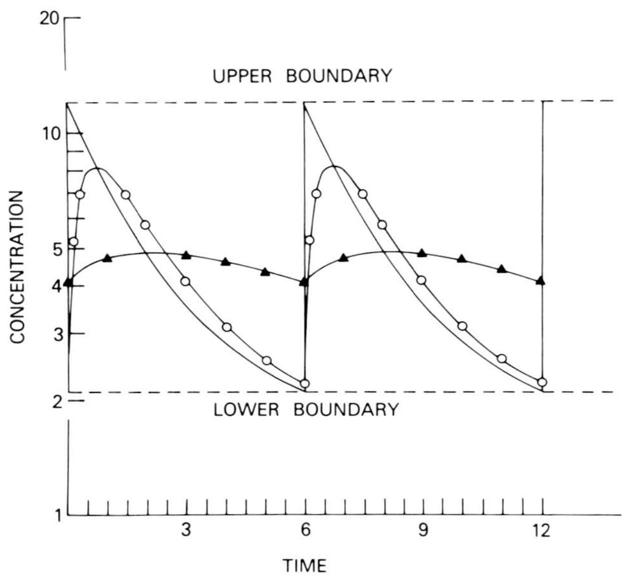

FIG. 4. Steady-state maximum and minimum blood concentrations of the diffusible form of a drug during its repeated intravenous administration. The concentrations represent the boundaries between which the concentrations of the diffusible form of the drug must lie in nonelimination tissues. When appropriate, equation 23 or equation 24 may be used to calculate the boundaries between which the total concentrations of unbound drug must be in any nonelimination organ in the body. (○) = Small shallow pool; (▲) = compartment.

differ markedly among the animals. Alternatively, it should be possible to estimate the boundaries that bracket the concentrations of the drug at receptor sites in different animals receiving the same dose per day of the drug.

Toxicologically Active Metabolites

Some toxicities are caused by metabolites of the drug rather than the drug itself. Thus, the concentration of an active metabolite at receptor sites in different organs may be more relevant than the concentration of the parent drug.

When the metabolite of interest is not formed or eliminated by the organ containing the receptor sites, the relationships between the areas under the curves of the concentrations of unbound metabolite in the receptor compartment and the blood would be exactly analogous to the relationships described by equations 15 to 24 for the parent compound. Moreover, under these conditions, the highest concentration of the diffusible form of the metabolite can never exceed its highest concentration in blood during either a single- or multiple-dosage schedule, nor can the lower concentration of the diffusible form ever be below its lowest concentration in blood. Thus, by use of equation 23 or 24, whichever is appropriate, the investigator should be able to calculate the boundaries that bracket the concentrations of the metabolite at receptors under steady-state conditions. Furthermore, decreasing both the dose and the dosage interval of the parent drug will decrease the difference between the upper and lower boundaries of the metabolite as well as that between the upper and lower boundaries of the parent drug.

At the other extreme, a short-lived metabolite generated within certain cells in the body may be converted to other substances so rapidly that it never leaves the cells in which it is formed. Thus, the rate constant of elimination of this kind of metabolite within the cells is considerably larger than the rate constant of diffusion of the metabolite out of the cells. The reactions within the cells rapidly achieve a quasisteady state in which the ratio of the concentration of the metabolite, C_M (cells), to that of the parent drug, C_D (cells), within the cells would be constant in a first-order system. Thus,

$$\frac{C_M\ (\text{cells})_{ss}}{C_D\ (\text{cells})_{ss}} = \frac{Cl_{(D \to M)}\ (\text{cells})}{Cl_{(M \to O)}\ (\text{cells})} \tag{30}$$

where $Cl_{(D \to M)}$ (cells) is the sum of the intrinsic clearances of the enzymes that cata-

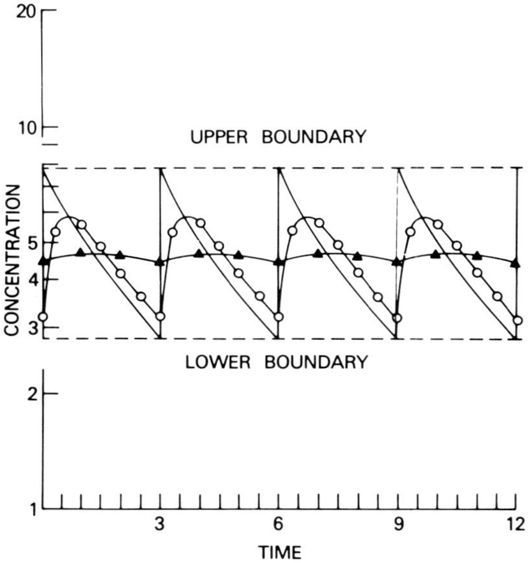

FIG. 5. Effect of halving both the dose and the dosage interval on the steady-state maximum and mininum blood concentrations of the diffusible form of a drug during its repeated intravenous administration. The difference between these concentrations will be one-half the difference shown in Fig. 4, but the average steady-state concentration of the diffusible form will not be changed. (○) = Small shallow pool; (▲) = compartment.

lyze the formation of the metabolite, and $Cl_{(M \rightarrow O)}$ (cells) is the sum of the intrinsic clearances of the enzymes and the clearances of the nonenzymatic reactions by which the metabolite is eliminated from the cells.

Thus, as long as neither $Cl_{(D \rightarrow M)}$ (cells) nor $C_{(M \rightarrow O)}$ (cells) is changed during the elimination of the parent compound, the concentration of the metabolite within the cells will be proportional to the concentration of the parent compound as predicted by equation 8. But there is no way that the actual concentration of the metabolite can be predicted at any given time. Even estimates of the total amount of the metabolite formed in the cells can be difficult. One might be able to determine the fraction of the dose that is converted to the metabolite by relating the total amount of the products formed from the metabolite in the body and excreted into urine. But this approach requires that the products be formed solely from the metabolite and that the metabolite be formed solely in the organ under investigation. Most estimates of the amount of short-lived metabolites require either direct measurements in tissue or *in vitro* experiments. One might measure a product of the metabolite that is retained in the cells—for example, the metabolite covalently bound to macromolecules including protein, RNA, DNA, and lipids. But this approach is limited because it depends on the fraction of the metabolite that becomes covalently bound and does not measure the products of the metabolite that leave the cells. Nevertheless, the approach is useful in relating changes in the area under the curve of the metabolite to changes in the incidence and severity of toxicities.

Most metabolites of drugs are sufficiently long-lived that they escape the cells in which they are formed and enter the systemic circulation, which serves other organs. Although the concentration of such a metabolite obviously will be higher in cells in which the metabolite is formed than in blood or the other cells in the body, the difference in the concentrations in the cells and blood is frequently trivial. Under steady-state conditions, the total rate at which the metabolite enters the cells by passive diffusion [$\text{Rate}_{M(in,dif)}$ (cells)] from the blood and metabolism [$\text{Rate}_{(D \rightarrow M)}$ (cells)] must equal the total rate at which the metabolite leaves the cells by diffusion [$\text{Rate}_{M(out,dif)}$ (cells)] and metabolism [$\text{Rate}_{M(met)}$ (cells)]. Thus,

$$\text{Rate}_{M(dif,out)}\ (\text{cells}) + \text{Rate}_{M(met)}\ (\text{cells}) = \text{Rate}_{M(dif,in)}\ (\text{cells}) + \text{Rate}_{(D \rightarrow M)}\ (\text{cells}) \quad (31)$$

These rates, however, can be expressed in terms of steady-state unbound concentrations of the drug and the metabolite and the clearances of the processes. Thus,

$$C_M\ (\text{cells})_{ss}\ [Cl_{M(dif,out)}\ (\text{cells}) + Cl_{(M \rightarrow O)}\ (\text{cells})] = C_M\ (\text{blood})_{ss}\ Cl_{M(dif,in)}\ (\text{cells}) + C_D\ (\text{cells})_{ss}\ Cl_{(D \rightarrow M)}\ (\text{cells}) \quad (32)$$

On rearrangement, equation 32 becomes

$$\frac{C_M\ (\text{cells})_{ss}}{C_M\ (\text{blood})_{ss}} = \frac{Cl_{M(\text{dif,in})}\ (\text{cells})}{Cl_{M(\text{dif,out})}\ (\text{cells}) + Cl_{(M\to O)}\ (\text{cells})} + \frac{C_D\ (\text{cells})_{ss}\ Cl_{(D\to M)}\ (\text{cells})}{C_M\ (\text{blood})_{ss}\ [Cl_{M(\text{dif,out})}\ (\text{cells}) + Cl_{(M\to O)}\ (\text{cells})]} \quad (33)$$

However, the steady-state concentration of the metabolite in blood depends on the total rates of formation and elimination of the metabolite from the body under steady-state conditions. Thus,

$$C_M\ (\text{blood})_{ss} = \frac{C_D\ (\text{blood})_{ss}\ Cl_{(D\to M)}\ (\text{body})}{Cl_{(M\to O)}\ (\text{body})} \quad (34)$$

Substitution of equation 34 into equation 33 gives

$$\frac{C_M\ (\text{cells})_{ss}}{C_M\ (\text{blood})_{ss}} = \frac{Cl_{M(\text{dif,in})}\ (\text{cells})}{Cl_{M(\text{dif,out})}\ (\text{cells}) + Cl_{(M\to O)}\ (\text{cells})} + \left[\frac{C_D\ (\text{cells})_{ss}}{C_D\ (\text{blood})_{ss}}\right]\left[\frac{Cl_{(D\to M)}\ (\text{cells})}{Cl_{(D\to M)}\ (\text{body})}\right] \times \left[\frac{Cl_{(M\to O)}\ (\text{body})}{Cl_{M(\text{dif,out})}\ (\text{cells}) + Cl_{(M\to O)}\ (\text{cells})}\right] \quad (35)$$

Inspection of equation 35 reveals that the steady-state concentration of an unbound metabolite within a given set of cells in the body is not governed solely by the activities of the enzymes that catalyze the formation and inactivation of the metabolite within the cells. It is also governed by the diffusional clearance of the metabolite into and out of the cells and the total body clearances of formation and elimination of the metabolite. In order to illustrate the relative effects of these factors on the steady-state concentration of the metabolite, visualize a situation in which $Cl_{(D\to M)}$ (cells) is zero. Thus,

$$\left[\frac{C_M\ (\text{cells})_{ss}}{C_M\ (\text{blood})_{ss}}\right]_{\text{absent}} = \frac{Cl_{M(\text{dif,in})}\ (\text{cells})}{Cl_{M(\text{dif,out})}\ (\text{cells}) + Cl_{(M\to O)}\ (\text{cells})} \quad (36)$$

The ratio of equation 35 to equation 36 can then be expressed as

$$\frac{[C_M\ (\text{cells})_{ss}/C_M\ (\text{blood})_{ss}]_{\text{present}}}{[C_M\ (\text{cells})_{ss}/C_M\ (\text{blood})_{ss}]_{\text{absent}}} = 1 + \left[\frac{C_D\ (\text{cells})_{ss}}{C_D\ (\text{blood})_{ss}}\right] \times \left[\frac{Cl_{(D\to M)}\ (\text{cells})}{Cl_{M(\text{dif,in})}\ (\text{cells})}\right] \times \left[\frac{Cl_{(M\to O)}\ (\text{body})}{Cl_{(D\to M)}\ (\text{body})}\right]_{\text{present}} \quad (37)$$

The factors that govern the relationship [C_D (cells)$_{ss}$/C_D (blood)$_{ss}$] are given by equation 26. Moreover, the relationship [$Cl_{(M\to O)}$ (body)/$Cl_{(D\to M)}$ (body)] may be estimated from the equation

$$\frac{[Cl_{(M\to O)}\ (\text{body})]}{[Cl_{(D\to M)}\ (\text{body})]} = \frac{C_{D(D)}\ (\text{blood})_{ss}}{C_{M(D)}\ (\text{blood})_{ss}} \quad (38)$$

where $C_{D(D)}$ (blood)$_{ss}$ is the steady-state concentration of the unbound drug in blood of animals receiving the parent drug, and $C_{M(D)}$ (blood)$_{ss}$ is the steady-state concentration of the unbound metabolite in blood of animals receiving the parent drug.

Equation 37 is an important pharmacokinetic relationship because it illustrates the interrelationship of the factors that govern whether the pharmacological and toxicological effects of a given dose of metabolite would be expected to be increased after the systemic administration of a prodrug that was converted to an equivalent amount of the metabolite in the body. The investigator might suspect that a prodrug would evoke a greater effect than the metabolite when one or more of the following events occur. (a) The prodrug but not the metabolite is actively transported into the receptor compartment. (The first ratio of equation 38 then would probably be greater than 1.0.) (b) The clearance of formation of the metabolite within the receptor compartment is greater than the diffusional clearance of the metabolite into the receptor compartment. (The second ratio of the equation would then be greater than 1.0.) (c) The total body clearance of the metabolite is greater than the total body clearance for the formation of the metabolite, i.e., the total body clearance of the prodrug times the fraction of the dose that is converted to the metabolite in the body.

It may be inferred from these principles that a prodrug usually will have a greater effect on the steady-state intracellular concentration of unbound metabolite when the metabolite is polar than when it is lipid soluble. The diffusional clearance of the metabolite will be smaller with polar metabolites than with lipid-soluble metabolites, and the urinary clearance of the metabolite will be larger with polar metabolites than with lipid-soluble metabolites. This rule of thumb should be used with caution, however, when both the prodrug and the metabolite are rapidly metabolized in the body.

Ordinarily, the investigator should be able to determine the amount of a metabolite formed from a given dose of drug administered to the animal and to compare the toxicological effects manifested by that amount of metabolite with the effects manifested by the dose of the parent drug. If the value obtained with equation 38 is substantially greater than 1, however, the same severity of the toxicity might not occur until the dose of the metabolite is increased. Since there may be species and strain differences in the activities of the enzymes that catalyze the formation of the metabolite within the receptor compartment, it is likely that there will be species and strain differences in the prodrug–metabolite relationships. Unfortunately, such differences would be impossible to detect solely from studies of the pharmacokinetics of the prodrug in blood.

RELATIONSHIPS BETWEEN DRUG CONCENTRATIONS IN BLOOD AND DRUG RESPONSES IN ORGANS

Ultimately, the toxicologist would like to be able to relate the concentration of the drug in blood with the intensity or duration of the response evoked by the drug in animals. However, such relationships will depend not only on the location of the sites of action of the drug but also on the mechanism and kinetics of the responses. Thus, researchers who fail to recognize differences in the mechanisms of drug action will frequently be disappointed in attempting to make such correlations. Some of these different mechanisms may be illustrated as follows.

Direct, Rapidly Acting Drugs

Many drugs exert their action by combining reversibly with receptor sites to form complexes that cause a physiological response almost instantaneously. The relationship between the responses (E) and the concentration of such drugs has been shown to be frequently predicted by the relationship

$$E = \frac{E_{\max} C^s}{C^s + (1/K)} \qquad (39)$$

where $(1/K)$ is the concentration of the drug that evokes 50% of the maximal response and is a constant. Although the simple occupancy theory predicts that s will be 1.0 as it is in Michaelis–Menten theory, s will differ from 1.0 when the receptor combines with more than one drug molecule before it evokes the response or when there are several populations of receptors having similar but not identical affinity constants. The value of s may also reflect the heterogeneity of a system in which a given number of drug–receptor complexes are required to evoke an all-or-none response such as the contraction of a muscle fiber. When the value of s is 1.0, a plot of effect against the concentration of the drug will be a hyperbola. But when the value of s is less than 1.0, the plot will be sigmoid.

However, a plot of the effect versus the logarithm of the concentration will always be sigmoid.

In the range of 20% to 80% of the maximal effect, the plot of the effect against the logarithm of the concentration of the drug will frequently be nearly linear regardless of the value of s. Indeed, the approximation to linearity of such plots forms the basis for reporting the results of most studies of the effects of drugs.

Levy and Nelson (6) combined the equation for drug response with the equation for the disappearance of drug from a one-compartment system in order to point out relationships between changes in concentration of the drug with changes in the intensity of the drug response. Within the range of 20 to 80% of the maximum effect, the rate of change of the intensity of the effect may be expressed as

$$\mathrm{d}E = -\frac{bk\,dt}{2.303} \tag{40}$$

where b is a constant, and k is the rate constant of elimination. Thus, within the range of 20 to 80% of the maximum effect, the decrease in the intensity of the effect should be linear with time.

For many drugs, there is a threshold concentration below which the effect is not manifested. The duration of action of such drugs (t_d), however, is not directly proportional to the dose of the drug but instead is related to the logarithm of the dose of the drug in a one-compartment system. The equation for threshold concentration, C_{thd}, would be as follows:

$$C_{thd} = C_0 e^{-kt_d} \tag{41}$$

and thus,

$$\log C_0 = \frac{kt_d}{2.303} + \log C_{thd} \tag{42}$$

In this form of the equation, estimates of the threshold concentration may be obtained.

Alternatively, the equation may be rearranged to

$$t_d = (2.303/k)\log (C_0/C_{thd}) \tag{43}$$

which illustrates the relationship between the duration of action of the drug and the initial concentration.

In multicompartment systems, the relationships between the intensity and duration of the effect of a drug and the blood concentration will depend on several interrelated factors including the dose of the drug, the relative sizes of the various compartments, and the location of the receptor sites. Although these relationships are difficult to illustrate mathematically, they can be easily illustrated graphically. For example, in a two-compartment system, the time course of the drug in blood after different doses would be similar to those shown in Fig. 6. If the log-concentration–response curve of drug were known, we could then construct a scale of the magnitude of the response that would be expected to occur in the central compartment at any given concentration of the drug (right hand scale, Fig. 6). By selecting a given intensity, we could easily determine the expected duration of action from the time required for the concentration to decrease to that required to evoke the given intensity. We then may plot these durations of action against the logarithm of the initial concentration (Fig. 7). These secondary plots would clearly reveal that when doses of the drug are selected so that the given effective concentration is crossed during the α phase, the duration of action will appear to be linearly related to the logarithm of the dose. But when the effective concentration is crossed during the α phase of low doses and the β phase of high doses, the relationship will not be linear (Fig. 7).

By converting the logarithms of the concentrations into corresponding fractions of the maximal intensities of the effects, we may also evaluate theoretical relationships between the intensity and duration of the effects of the drugs in deep compartments (Fig. 2) or after multidose therapy.

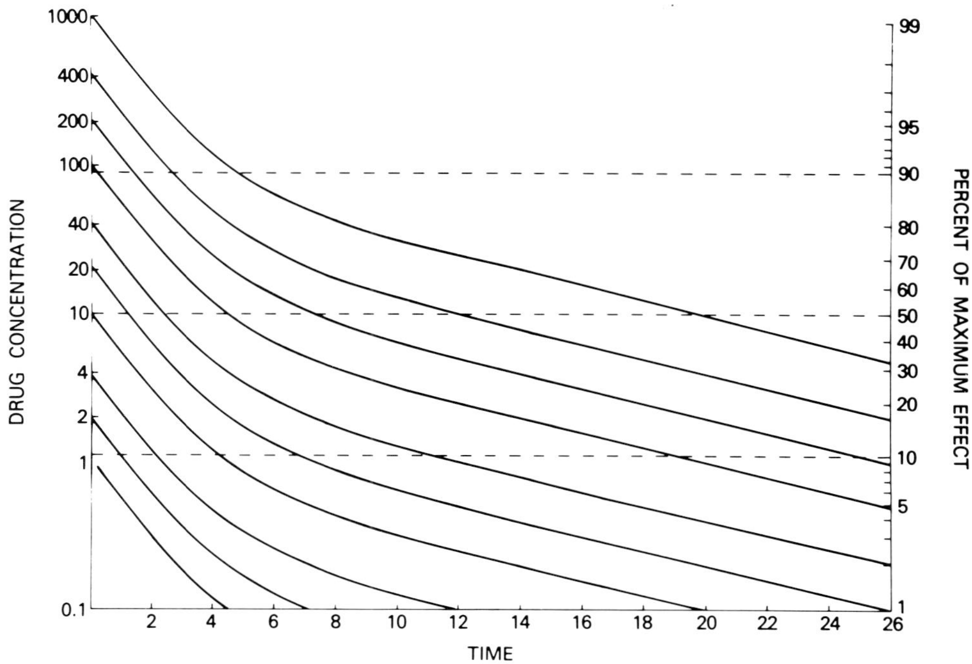

FIG. 6. A graphical method for estimating relationships among dose, the time course of the concentration of unbound drug in blood, and the magnitude of a pharmacologic effect at any given time in an organ in the central compartment. The *left-hand scale* is the concentration of the unbound drug. The *right-hand scale* is the percent of maximum effect. For the purpose of illustration, it was assumed that $E/E_{max} = [D]/([D] + EC_{50})$ and that the value of EC_{50} was 10 concentration units, where [D] is the concentration of unbound drug and EC_{50} is the concentration that causes 50% of the maximal effect. The *lines* are the concentrations that cause 10, 50, and 90% of the maximum effect of the drug.

Indirectly Acting Drugs

Many drugs evoke their effects indirectly by affecting the synthesis or catabolism of endogenous substances and thus their concentration in the body. In such mechanisms, the relationships between the drug concentration and the therapeutic or toxic effect may be frequently obscure and seemingly paradoxical.

To illustrate some of the difficulties in making these relationships, let us consider the effects of a hypothetical drug (I) that noncompetitively inhibits the synthesis of an endogenous substance (P). Let us further assume that the formation of the endogenous substance does not represent a major pathway of elimination of its precursor (S), and therefore, inhibition of the formation of P does not affect the concentration of the precursor (S). According to Michaelis–Menten theory, the rate of synthesis of the endogenous substance P in the absence of drug would be

$$\text{Rate}_{\text{syn(u)}} = V_m/[1 + (K_m/\text{S})] \tag{44}$$

Let us also assume that the rate of degradation of P in the body is first order and can be described as k_dP. The rate of change in the amount of P is the difference between the rates of synthesis and degradation of P; i.e.,

$$\frac{dP}{dt} = R_{syn} - k_dP \tag{45}$$

However, in the absence of drug, the amount of P does not change, and therefore, $R_{syn(u)} =$

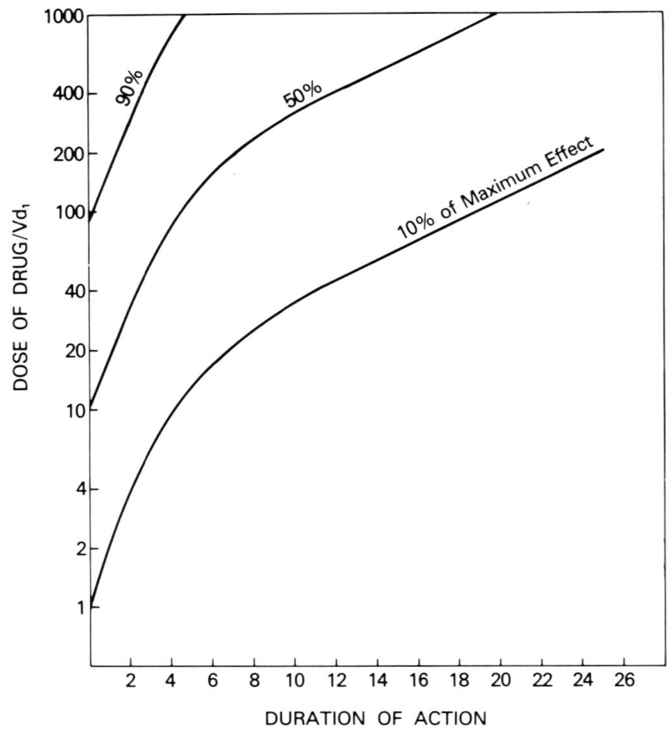

FIG. 7. The relationship between various Dose/V_1 (free) ratios and the duration of a pharmacologic effect of a hypothetical drug administered intravenously. The *lines* were constructed from the intersections of the lines shown in Fig. 6.

k_d P_0. In the presence of drug, the rate of synthesis of P would be

$$R_{syn(i)} = \frac{V_{max}}{\left[1 + \frac{K_s}{[S]}\right]\left[1 + \frac{[I]}{K_I}\right]} = \frac{R_{syn(u)}}{1 + \frac{[I]}{K_I}} = \frac{k_d P_0}{1 + \frac{[I]}{K_I}} \qquad (46)$$

On substitution of equation 46 into equation 45, we obtain

$$\frac{dP}{dt} = \frac{k_d P_0}{1 + [I]/K_I} - k_d P \qquad (47)$$

Although this equation is valid for multicompartment systems, we can illustrate many of the problems with a single-compartment system in which

$$I = I_0 e^{-k_e t}.$$

$$\frac{dP}{dt} = \frac{k_d P_0}{1 + (I_0/K_I)e^{-k_e t}} - k_d P \qquad (48)$$

Integration of this equation is difficult. Nevertheless, one can calculate the time course of the changes in P by iteration of the equation with small increments of time. Gibaldi and Perrier (4) have integrated an equation that gives reasonable answers for a system in which I_0 is never greater than $4K_I$ and I is never less than $0.25K_I$.

Inspection of curves generated by equation 48 reveals that the shape of the curves depends markedly on the turnover rate of the endogenous substance (Fig. 8). When the turnover rate is high (that is, k_d is very large), the maximum decrease in the amount of the endogenous substance will occur shortly after the intravenous administration of the inhibitor. The amount of the endogenous substance will then return to normal as the inhibitor is eliminated from the body. Moreover, if the volume of distribution of the inhibitor were decreased, thereby increasing the initial concentration but shortening the half-life of the inhibitor, the initial decrease

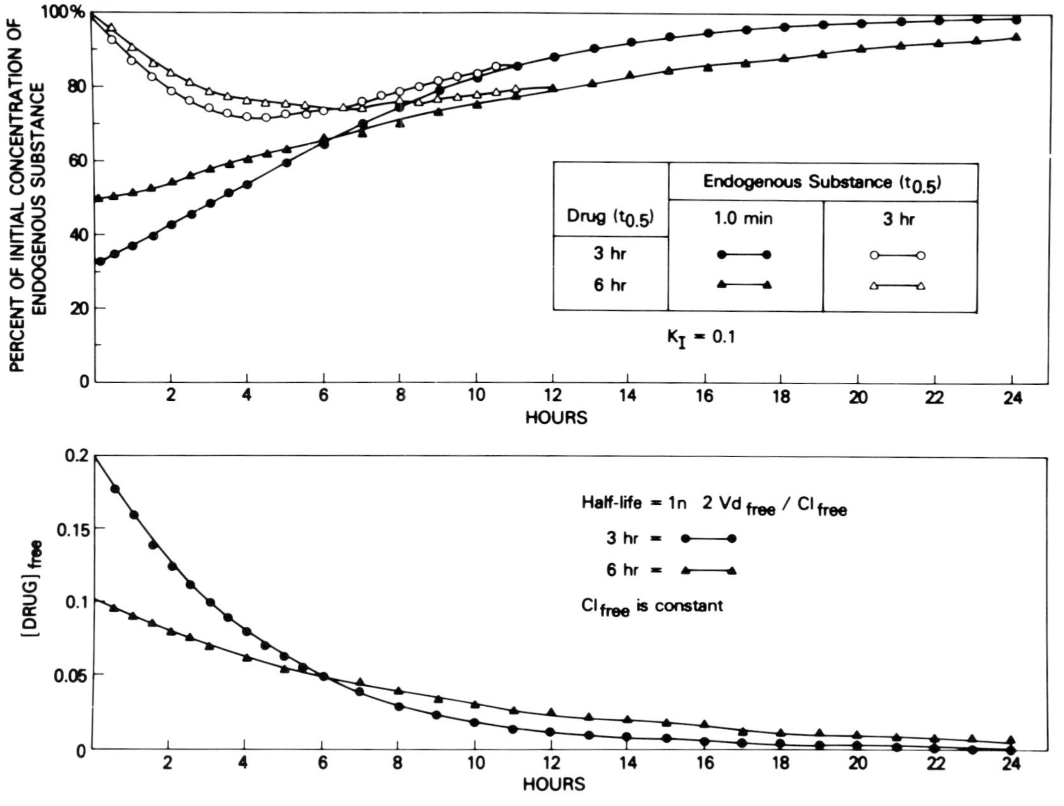

FIG. 8. Noncompetitive inhibition of the synthesis of an endogenous substance: the importance of the turnover rate of the endogenous substance and the volume of distribution of the inhibitor. In these simulations, the clearances of elimination of unbound drug were identical.

in the amount of the endogenous substance will be greater, but the rate of return to the control amount will be faster. In this situation, therefore, the intensity of the effect will appear to be closely related to the concentration of the inhibitor in the compartment in which the endogenous substance is synthesized.

By contrast, when the turnover rate of the endogenous substance is slow, its nadir concentration will be delayed. Moreover, the decrease in the amount of the endogenous substance may be sustained long after most of the inhibitor has left the body, but eventually the amount of the substance will return to the initial values. If the volume of distribution of the inhibitor were decreased, the maximum decrease would appear sooner, but the return to the initial values of the endogenous substance would be faster. Thus, the effects of altering the volume of distribution on the intensity and duration of action would be similar regardless of the turnover rate of the endogenous substance, even though the relationship between the concentration of the inhibitor and the intensity of the effect at any given time might not seem obvious.

If the inhibitor were administered repeatedly until a steady state occurred, however, seemingly paradoxical effects would occur. With this dosage schedule, the decrease in the amount of the endogenous substance would become greater as the number of doses of the inhibitor increased, until a steady state is reached (Fig. 9). However, a decrease in

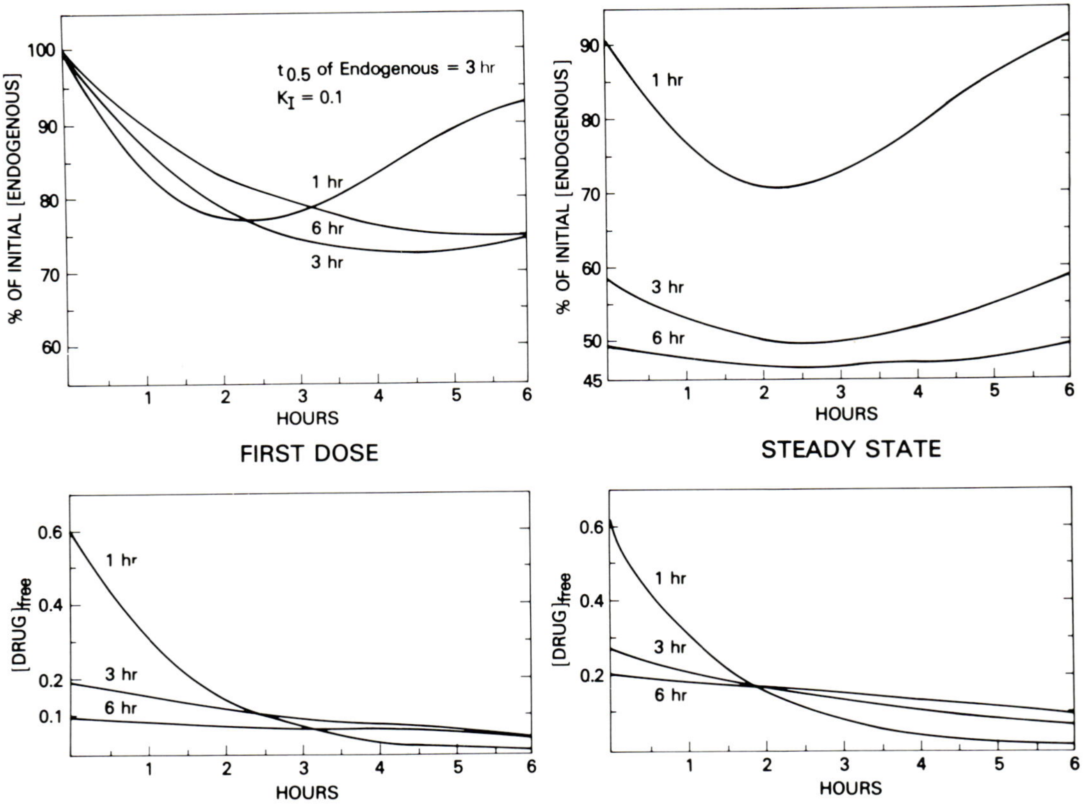

FIG. 9. Differences in effects of a single dose and multiple doses of a noncompetitive inhibitor of the synthesis of an endogenous substance: the effects of differences in the half-life (1 hr, 3 hr, and 6 hr) of the distribution. In these simulations, the clearances of elimination of unbound drug were identical.

the volume of distribution of the inhibitor would diminish the effect on the endogenous substance even though the decrease in the volume of distribution would have increased the initial concentration of the inhibitor. The difference in effects caused by alterations in the volume of distribution cannot be caused by a change in the average concentration of the inhibitor in the body because changes in volume of distribution do not change the area under the curve of the inhibitor when the inhibitor is eliminated by first-order processes. Instead, the intensity of the effect would appear to be superficially related to the minimum rather than the maximum concentration of the inhibitor during multidose therapy. Moreover, the effects of such drugs would be greater when they are given in small divided doses than when they are given as a single large dose.

In deriving equation 48, we have assumed that the formation of the endogenous substance represents only a minor pathway of elimination of the precursor (S). If the formation of the endogenous substance had been a major pathway, the maximum effect would appear rather early and then would have diminished with time even during multidose therapy. The reason for this becomes clear when it is realized that the concentration of the precursor will increase until the rate of formation of the precursor equals its rate of elimination from the body. If the formation of the endogenous substance were the sole pathway of elimination of the precursor, the concentration of the precursor would increase until the rate of synthesis of the endogenous substance was the same as it was in the absence of the inhibitor, and the effect would disappear. In other words, the animal would become tolerant to the inhibitor. However, if the inhibitor were suddenly withdrawn, a superabundance of the endogenous substance would be synthesized, and the animal might exhibit toxicities caused by high concentrations of the endogenous substance.

Drugs that Act Irreversibly

Several drugs evoke their action by combining irreversibly with enzymes that catalyze the synthesis or catabolism of endogenous substances in organs of the body. In this mechanism, the intensity and duration of the effect would depend not only on the initial concentration and kinetics of elimination of the inhibitor but also on the rate constant of reaction of the inhibitor with the enzyme and the rate of synthesis and catabolism (and repair) of the enzyme and the endogenous substance. In addition, irreversible inhibitors that act competitively will depend on the concentration of the precursor of the endogenous substance and on the relative affinities of the enzyme for the precursor and the inhibitor.

If the catabolism of the enzyme were first order, and the reaction of the inhibitor with the enzyme were second order and independent of the concentration of the precursor, the rate of change in the amount of the enzyme might be expressed as follows:

$$\frac{\mathrm{d}E}{\mathrm{d}t} = \mathrm{Rate}_{\mathrm{syn(E)}} - E(k_{\mathrm{E}} + k[\mathrm{I}]) \qquad (49)$$

where $\mathrm{Rate}_{\mathrm{syn(E)}}$ is the rate of synthesis of the enzyme, E is the amount of enzyme at any given time, Ek_{E} is the rate of catabolism of the enzyme, and $Ek[\mathrm{I}]$ is the rate of inactivation of the enzyme by the inhibitor I. Under the initial steady-state conditions, however, the rate of synthesis will equal the initial rate of catabolism. Thus,

$$\frac{\mathrm{d}E}{\mathrm{d}t} = E_0 k_{\mathrm{E}} - E(k_{\mathrm{E}} + k[\mathrm{I}]) \qquad (50)$$

If the inhibitor were mainly eliminated from the body by first-order processes,

$$[\mathrm{I}] = [\mathrm{I}_0]\mathrm{e}^{-k_{\mathrm{e}}t} \qquad (51)$$

where k_{e} is the rate constant of elimination of the inhibitor from the body. Substitution of equation 51 into equation 50 gives

$$\frac{\mathrm{d}E}{\mathrm{d}t} = E_0 k_{\mathrm{E}} - E(k_{\mathrm{E}} + kI_0\mathrm{e}^{-k_{\mathrm{e}}t}) \qquad (52)$$

Meanwhile, the rate of change in the amount of the endogenous component (P) formed from precursor (S) may be expressed as

$$\frac{\mathrm{d}P}{\mathrm{d}t} = \frac{Ek_{\mathrm{P}}[\mathrm{S}]}{[\mathrm{S}] + K_m} - k_{\mathrm{d}}P \qquad (53)$$

where Ek_{P} is the rate of synthesis of P at infinite concentrations of [S].

From these equations, we may develop simulations of the time course of the effects of changes in the volume of distribution of the inhibitor on the concentration of the endogenous substance. Such simulations with single doses of the inhibitor would reveal that the nadir amount of endogenous substance would occur at some time after the maximum concentration of the inhibitor. The amount of endogenous substance would then return to normal values as the inhibitor is eliminated from the body. However, the effect may persist long after virtually all of the inhibitor has been eliminated, depending on the value of k_{d}. A decrease in the volume of distribution of the inhibitor would accelerate both the decrease in the endogenous substance and the initial rate of the return to normal values and thereby shorten the time required to achieve the nadir amount of endogenous substance. Thus, the effect of a single dose of the inhibitor will superficially resemble that of the reversible noncompetitive inhibitor. With multiple doses of the inhibitor under steady-state conditions, however, the average amount of the endogenous substance will be related to the area under the curve of the inhibitor. Thus, the average magnitude of the effect will be independent of changes in the volume of distribution of the inhibitor.

OTHER MECHANISMS OF DRUG ACTION

Drugs may, of course, evoke their effects by even more complex mechanisms. Some of the metabolites of drugs may also evoke pharmacologic actions by combining reversibly with the receptor sites that also combine with the drug and thus either potentiate or antagonize the action of the drug. During the time course of the metabolism of the drug, the relative amounts of the complexes formed between the receptor sites and the drug and between the receptor sites and the metabolite may change in ways that are virtually impossible to predict from *in vivo* data alone. Studies *in vitro,* however, frequently provide estimates of the affinity constants and the intrinsic activities of the drugs and metabolites, which would be required in simulations of these combinations *in vivo.*

Some of the metabolites of drugs evoke effects by reacting irreversibly with cellular components. The magnitude of the effect of such drugs will depend in part on the fraction of the dose of the compound that is converted to the metabolite and the fraction of the amount of metabolite that combines with the endogenous components.

Many of the mechanisms of action of drugs and their metabolites depend on the properties and the kinetics of metabolism of endogenous substances. If these properties and kinetics of the relevant endogenous substances as well as the pharmacokinetics of the drug and its metabolite were known, however, it might be possible to predict the relative effects of various doses of drugs in different animal species and strains. Clearly, however, much needs to be accomplished before we reach this panacea. To find a needle in a haystack, one first must be able to identify a needle. To understand the relationships between drug concentrations in blood and drug responses in organs, we must first understand the mechanism and kinetics of the responses.

REFERENCES

1. Beeken, W. L., Volwiler, W., Goldsworthy, P. D., Garby, L. E., Reynolds, W. E., Stogsdill, R., and Stemler, R. S. (1962): Studies on I-131 albumin catabolism and distribution in normal young male adults. *J. Clin. Invest.,* 41:1312–1333.
2. Brodie, B. B., and Reid, W. D. (1972): The value of determining the plasma concentration of drugs in animals and man. In: *Fundamentals of Drug Metabolism and Drug Disposition,* edited by B. N. La Du, H. G. Mandel, and E. L. Way, pp. 328–339. Williams & Wilkins, Baltimore.
3. Conney, A. H. (1972): Environmental factors influencing drug metabolism. In: *Fundamentals of Drug Metabolism and Drug Disposition,* edited by B. N. La Du, H. G. Mandel, and E. L. Way, pp. 253–278. Williams & Wilkins, Baltimore.
4. Gibaldi, M., and Perrier, D. (1975): *Pharmacokinetics,* pp. 208–211. Marcel Dekker, New York.
5. Kalow, W. (1962): *Pharmacogenetics, Heredity and Response to Drugs.* W. B. Saunders, Philadelphia.
6. Levy, G., and Nelson, E. (1965): Theoretical relationships between dose, elimination rate and duration of pharmacologic effects of drugs. *J. Pharm. Sci.,* 54:812.
7. Mantel, N., and Bryan, W. R. (1961): "Safety" testing of carcinogenic agents. *J. Natl. Cancer Inst.,* 27:455–470.
8. Waddell, W. J., and Butler, T. C. (1959): Calculation of intracellular pH from the distribution of 5,5-dimethyl-2,4-oxazolidimedione (DMO). Application to skeletal muscle of the dog. *J. Clin. Invest.,* 38:720–729.
9. Whittemore, A. S. (1978): Quantitative theories of oncogenesis. *Adv. Cancer Res.,* 27:55–88.
10. Williams, R. T. (1972): Species variations in drug biotransformation. In: *Fundamentals of Drug Metabolism and Drug Disposition,* edited by B. N. La Du, H. G. Mandel, and E. L. Way, pp. 187–205. Williams & Wilkins, Baltimore.

Drug Metabolism and Drug Toxicity,
edited by J. R. Mitchell and M. G. Horning.
Raven Press, New York © 1984.

Role of Sodium and Calcium Regulation in Toxic Cell Injury

Benjamin F. Trump and Irene K. Berezesky

Department of Pathology, University of Maryland School of Medicine, Baltimore, Maryland 21201

The initiating events and the putative final common pathway in toxic cell injury and cell death have long eluded description by both experimental pathologists and toxicologists. During the last several years, the introduction of a variety of new morphological and functional techniques to the study of toxicologic cell injury has yielded considerable new information of a descriptive nature, the synthetic analysis of which has evolved less rapidly. During this period of time, our laboratory has been engaged in characterizing the effects of a variety of injuries on several cell types with the ultimate goal of attempting to reduce the information to one, or at least a few, final common pathways (91,94–96,98,99,101,105–107,110–112). The situation has always appeared complex because of the diversity of toxic and injurious agents and the apparent diversity of cellular and subcellular effects and initial interactions as seen either chemically or morphologically. Morphologic changes range from those involving the ribosomes and the endoplasmic reticulum (ER) to changes in the cell membrane, changes in nuclei, changes in lysosomes, and changes in the mitochondria. An equal complex series of biochemical and functional events results, including modified cellular ion shifts, modification of respiration and oxidative phosphorylation, alterations in protein and DNA synthesis, and changes in secretion, phagocytosis, autophagocytosis, and motility (10).

Can these seemingly diverse effects be synthesized into a coherent view of the events that occur following cell injury? Clearly, such a synthesis could be important not only for a basic understanding of the pathobiology involved but also to facilitate the design of preventive and/or therapeutic interventions that could ameliorate or eliminate the effects of lethal injury with wide consequences to disease in humans, other animals, and plants.

It is the purpose of this chapter to review these events as they are presently understood and to present our current hypothesis regarding the role of ion shifts as a final common pathway in cell injury.

STAGES OF CELL INJURY

It has long been evident that following an injury that will ultimately lead to the death of a cell (lethal injury), there is a series of reasonably reproducible ultrastructural changes that occur prior to the point of cell death ("point of no return") (reversible phase) and a series of events that occur after that event, termed the phase of necrosis (irreversible phase). Although the rate of progression varies in many different cell types and many different types of injury, the endpoint remains the same.

What has not been as frequently recognized is that the events during the reversible phase following cell injury are very similar to the events that occur in a variety of physiologic and pathologic processes ranging from fertilization of an ovum to the events that occur following binding of a bacterium to a ligand on the surface of a polymorphonuclear cell (PMN), which initiates the process of phagocytosis. These include a depolymerization of the cell membrane followed by influx of sodium, sometimes accompanied by an ejection of protons; further, the events characteristic of the point of cell death in the irreversible phase are commonly characterized by failure to control intracellular calcium.

We have observed in animal cells of several phyla and in many organs, as well as in plant cells, that these events appear to be remarkably similar. We have, therefore, designated these morphological changes as "stages" of cell injury, both reversible and irreversible. For the purpose of convenience of notation, these stages have been documented in several previous publications (91,106,109,111). However, additional data have necessitated some modifications, and although these have been recently described in detail elsewhere (96), we again review them briefly below in order to provide the reader with sufficient detail to facilitate easy comprehension of our concepts concerning cell injury.

Stage I is a normal cell with normal appearance and relationships of organelles (Fig. 1). Following lethal injury, progression through stages II to VII occurs. In the first stage, an injury such as ischemia results in a sudden decrease in the oxygen tension within the extracellular fluid and the cell. Because of the rapid fall in oxygen tension, the cell seems to "attempt" to maintain its homeostasis by using very rapid feedback control mechanisms.

Such control mechanisms involve changes in ion concentrations as well as in various coenzymes and regulating enzyme activities. As the oxygen concentration falls, mitochondrial phosphorylation decreases rapidly, and contraction of the inner mitochondrial compartment begins. The drop in cellular ATP is believed to stimulate the activity of phosphofructokinase (PFK) in many cells, and this results in an increased rate of anaerobic glycolysis, assuming an ample supply of glycogen is present. This accelerated glycolysis leads to the accumulation of lactate which, together with the increased inorganic phosphate from ATP hydrolysis, soon reduces the intracellular pH. Since the circulation has ceased, metabolites such as lactate and hydrogen ions also tend to accumulate as well in the extracellular microenvironment, depressing the extra- as well as the intracellular pH. This decreased pH appears to be protective in that it has a "stabilizing" effect on the cell membrane (67–71). The change in

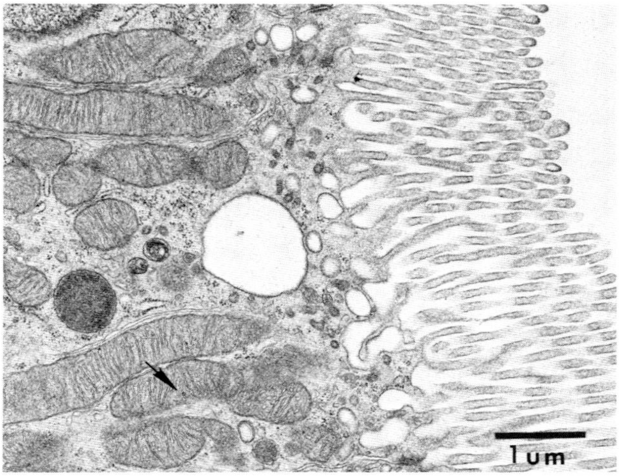

FIG. 1. Portion of a control proximal convoluted tubule cell (PCT) from rat kidney exhibiting elongated mitochondria in orthodox conformation. Note the presence of normal mitochondrial granules (*arrow*) in some profiles. Stage I. (From Trump et al., ref. 96, with permission.)

intracellular pH is probably reflected by the rapid clumping of nuclear chromatin (stage IA), which occurs very rapidly, but which is clearly reversible. This could also result from loss of bound potassium, which also occurs very quickly. Clumping of nuclear chromatin is known to be associated with decreased nuclear RNA synthesis. However, this is of no immediate consequence to the cell since if circulation is not restored, the cell will die and undergo necrosis long before the decreased RNA synthesis has any significant effect.

In addition to nuclear chromatin clumping and the reduction in glycogen, cells in stage IA also show the disappearance of mitochondrial matrix granules, as seen after glutaraldehyde/osmium fixation and Epon® embedment. Meanwhile, the cell also begins to show the effects of the reduced ATP concentration. Among the consequences of the fall in ATP concentration is a decrease in the activity of the ion pumps at the cell membrane, which leads to movements of Na^+, K^+, Ca^{2+}, and Mg^{2+} down their concentration gradients. With X-ray microanalysis, such ion shifts are seen as early as 10 min following ischemia (62) and probably occur even prior to that.

One of the earliest ultrastructural changes that can be seen in cells after a variety of acute lethal injuries is enlargement in the volume of the endoplasmic reticulum, which is reflected in electron micrographs as dilatation of the cisternae (stage II) (Fig. 2). This initial change can be correlated with increased sodium and decreased potassium content of the cell and often with increased water content, although studies by Laiho and Trump (42,43) indicate that significant dilatation of the ER can sometimes occur even with decreased total cell volume. The implied mechanism is intracellular redistribution of ions and water. This stage is clearly reversible and occurs before the "point of no return."

Also in stage II, cell surface changes in the form of protrusions or "blebs" commonly begin to appear. These alterations in cell shape appear to reflect acute changes in the microtubules and microfilaments whose normal function is to maintain cell shape. Recent data have implied that lack of control of cell calcium levels during this phase, probably through effects on the cytoskeleton, may result in these changes (97,101,102). In addition, alterations in the inner membrane-associated Mg^{2+}-dependent ATPase can be seen (55). As the pH continues to drop in the cytosol, it is probable that inhibition of PFK occurs, with a gradual decrease in the rate of glycolysis, tending to stabilize the glycogen levels at low but significantly greater than zero values. The fall in cellular ATP concentration continues, and ADP rises. This de-

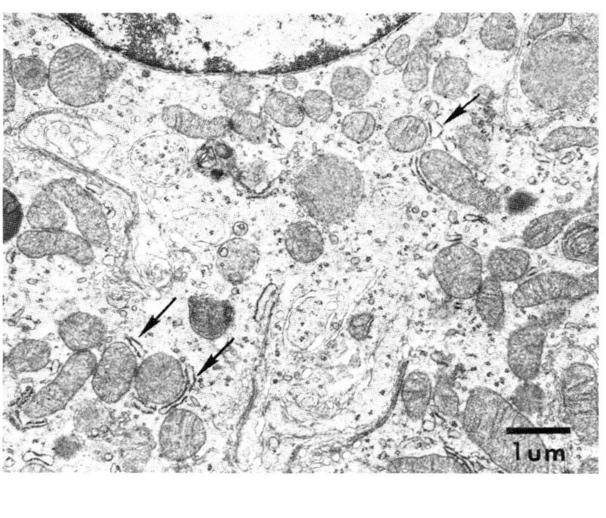

FIG. 2. Portion of a proximal pars recta tubule cell from rat kidney following 15 min of ischemia. Note slight enlargement in the volume of the rough ER (*arrows*). Stage II. (From Glaumann and Trump, ref. 26, with permission.)

creased ATP concentration begins to be reflected by decreased functions of the various energy-requiring systems such as protein synthesis, ion pumps at the cell surface, and most probably ion accumulation by mitochondria, which begin to undergo shrinkage of the inner compartment.

In stage III, which can occur rapidly, the mitochondria appear dense, showing marked condensation of the inner compartment and enlargement of the space between the inner and outer membranes of the envelope and the intracristal space (Fig. 3). This is associated with dilatation of the ER and the cell sap, both of which correlate with the gradual increases in sodium and water content as well as with decreases in potassium and magnesium. Loss of potassium and calcium from mitochondrial inner compartments could result in shrinkage of that structure, and movements into the ER could explain the dilatation of those cisternae. Decreased potassium content is also a factor that can be associated with inhibited protein synthesis, although at this stage the membrane-bound polysomes usually appear unaltered and maintain both their ordered arrangements and their membrane attachments. The increased water content at this stage is often reflected by the presence of blebs at the cell surface, although the latter may also involve modulations of the cytoskeleton. Mitochondrial function is inhibited because of the continued lack of oxygen, and, as a consequence, ATP and now ADP levels are low (36).

If cells in this stage are restored to normal conditions, the mitochondrial inner compartments reexpand, the ER cisternae contract, and the cells extrude sodium and calcium along with water and chloride. Therefore, although the mitochondria are temporarily albeit dramatically changed in form, they retain their ability to respire and phosphorylate as well as the ability to regain their normal internal compartment volume following restitution of a normal microenvironment both *in vivo* and in *in vitro.* At this stage, protein synthesis remains severely inhibited, and both free and bound polysomes are present as monosomes, some of which maintain their membrane attachments. The cell sap is swollen because of the increased water content. The lysosomes have a clear matrix and are often swollen, although significant macromolecular-sized leaks in the lysosomal membranes apparently do not occur. At present, it is not clear whether the release of lysosomal hydrolases to the cytosol plays a significant role in this or later stages.

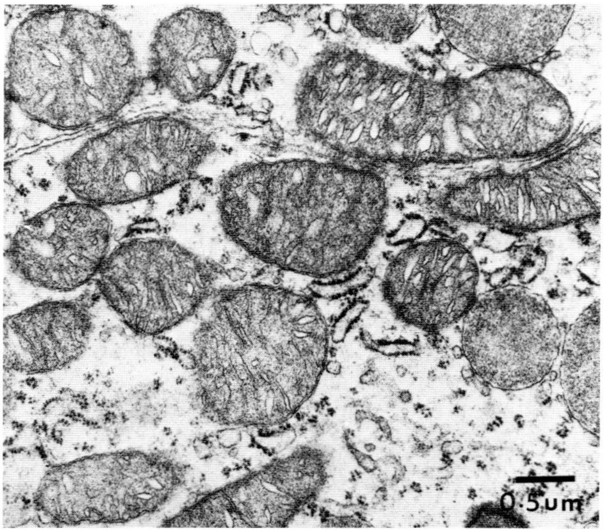

FIG. 3. Portion of a PCT cell from rat kidney following 15 min of ischemia. Mitochondria show condensation of inner compartments with increased matrix density and expansion of intracristal spaces. The rough ER is slightly dilated. Stage III.

In stage IV, the transition across the "point of no return" appears to begin. Here, some mitochondria begin to show high-amplitude swelling, which seems to indicate initially reversible and later irreversible loss of the inner membrane function. As a result, some mitochondrial profiles show high-amplitude inner compartment swelling, although others remain condensed (Fig. 4). In some cells, such as renal tubular epithelium, where two or more inner compartments are present in a given mitochondrion, one compartment may be condensed while others are swollen (23,26,36,116). The remaining organelles resemble those seen in stage III. This series of membrane permeability changes involving both the mitochondria and the cell membrane probably reflects basic chemical as well as structural modifications in the molecular architecture. The mitochondrial swelling is probably associated with the increased content of sodium and calcium in the inner compartments, although the precise ionic composition of the mitochondria probably depends on that of the cytoplasm. Among the factors that may result in this structural damage to the mitochondrial inner membrane is the continued magnesium deficiency and the destruction of phospholipids with release of fatty acids. The role of changes in membrane fluidity is not known but may be important. Mitochondrial membranes possess endogenous phospholipases that can be activated by factors such as the increased levels of calcium known to be present at this time (27).

In stage IVA, in addition to the alterations mentioned above, all mitochondria are swollen, with inner compartments expanded (Fig. 5). In stage IVB, not only are all mitochondria swollen, but also some contain tiny dense aggregates (Fig. 6). These may represent early, reversible protein denaturation (47). This stage was recently described by Glaumann et al. (24,25) in proximal tubules from the pars convoluta of rat kidney following 30 and 60 min of ischemia. Both of these stages, however, are still capable of being resuscitated. Also, some membrane intracristal densities may be seen (see below). We still do not know whether all mitochondria are reversible or whether only the ones that do not have the tiny dense aggregates are. In any case, the cells do survive.

In stage V, all mitochondria exhibit massive swelling and show marked increases in inner membrane permeability associated with loss of proteins, including matrix enzymes and cofactors, to the cell sap and ultimately through the cell membrane to the extracel-

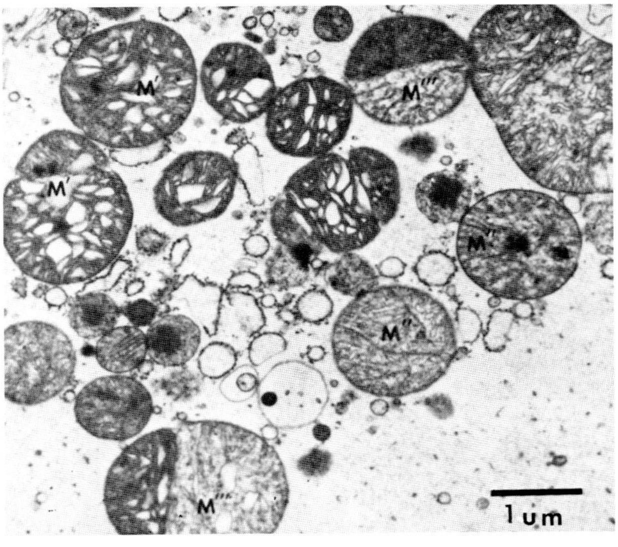

FIG. 4. Portion of a rat PCT cell from a kidney slice incubated in Robinson's buffer at 4°C for 48 hr, illustrating three types of mitochondria. In the first type (M′), the matrix is markedly condensed with expansion of intracristal spaces and flocculent densities. In the second type (M″), the inner compartments are expanded and contain flocculent densities. In the third type (M‴), both types of changes are present in the same mitochondrion, indicative of stage IV, although those with flocculent densities probably are not reversible. (From Trump et al., ref. 116, with permission.)

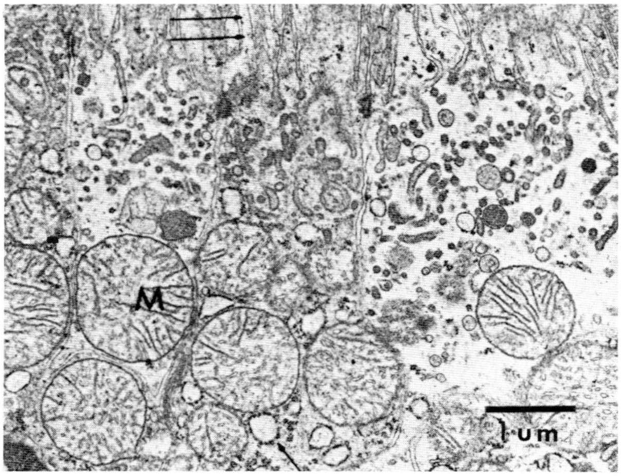

FIG. 5. Rat PCT cell following 30 min of ischemia. Mitochondria (M) are rounded and show swelling of inner compartments. The rough ER is dilated (*arrow*), the microvilli swollen (*double arrow*), and the cytosol is less electron dense. Stage IVa. (From Glaumann et al., ref. 23, with permission.)

lular space. Cell sap enzymes are probably lost before mitochondrial or other organelle enzymes, and the sum of adenosine nucleotides is only a small fraction of normal (36). Also at this stage, prominent, large flocculent densities appear in the inner compartment, presumably the result of denaturation of matrix proteins (Fig. 7). Cells are swollen, and the membranes of the cytocavitary network are fragmented. Distortion of intracellular membrane systems with whorl-like configurations often can be seen at the cell surfaces. Chromatin begins to undergo enzymatic attack and in later stages is completely dissolved (karyolysis), presumably by the combined action of proteolytic enzymes and DNase. Lysosomes continue to swell as evidenced by increased size, clarification of the matrix, and condensation of the contents. The lysosomal swelling may result in leak of acid hydrolases. In some cells, calcification of the inner mitochondrial compartments can be seen, consisting of amorphous calcium phosphate or crystalline deposits of hydroxyapatite along the inner membrane.

In stage VI, the changes are mainly characterized by a rapid acceleration in the rate of digestion of intracellular constituents, as

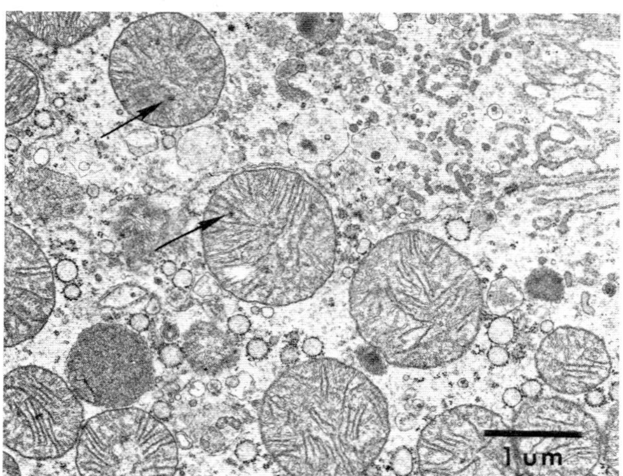

FIG. 6. Rat PCT cell following 60 min of ischemia. Mitochondria are swollen, and some contain tiny dense aggregates (*arrows*). Stage IVb.

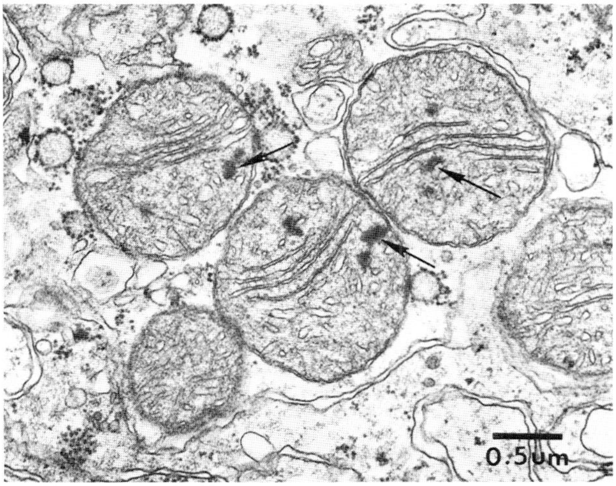

FIG. 7. Rat PCT cell following 120 min of ischemia. All mitochondria exhibit marked swelling, and most contain large flocculent densities (*arrows*), the hallmark of irreversibility. Stage V. (From Trump et al., ref. 96, with permission.)

measured by marked increases in free fatty acids, free amino acids, and inorganic phosphorous and decreases in phospholipids, triglycerides, protein, DNA, and RNA. This is reflected morphologically by continuing karyolysis and changes in the staining pattern of the cytoplasm. There is evidence that, at this stage, the lysosomal contents can escape into the cytosol, and, indeed, the disappearance of the macromolecular components of the cell as well as the persistence of lysosomal hydrolases as compared with the many other enzymes strongly indicates that lysosomal leakage is followed by digestion. Other membrane systems show dramatic rearrangements, including vesiculation, wrappings, formation of tubular forms in the inner compartment of the mitochondria, disappearance of ribosomes from the ER membrane surface, alterations in the nucleolus, disappearance of microbody matrices, and frequent visible breaks in plasma membrane contours (Fig. 8).

In stage VII, in spite of the fact that the cell is virtually completely degraded, new structures in the cytoplasm occur as large dense inclusions composed of dense, homogeneous, osmiophilic material with la-

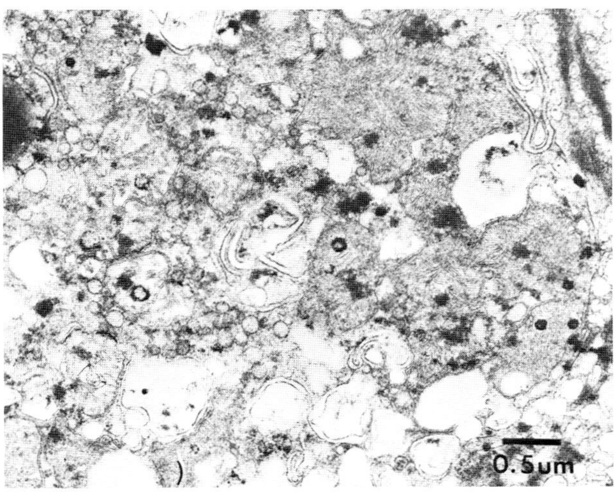

FIG. 8. Rat PCT cell after 60 min ischemia followed by 24 hr reflow. Disrupted organelles are seen with swollen mitochondria containing flocculent densities. Stage VI. (From Glaumann and Trump, ref. 26, with permission.)

mellar regions in lacunae within bodies or at the margins of the bodies. These periodic regions resemble stacks of membranes, although the fine structure within the bodies has not been discerned. However, they probably correspond to the myelin of Virchow, so-named because of the resemblance to the bodies that Virchow described following autolysis in various cell types, especially the CNS. In general, at this stage, most enzymatic activity has approached zero. Unless other sources of enzymes such as those produced by microorganisms are present, the cells are stabilized for long periods of time in this state. However, equilibration once again occurs during this phase when the extracellular fluid pH approaches physiological levels. Greater and greater calcium binding by these cells is observed, possibly related to the change in pH as well as to changes in reactive protein sites. How much of the calcium binding is mitochondrial is not known. At this stage, this type of calcification is often, however, extensive (dystrophic calcification), and it is almost certainly not energy dependent (Fig. 9).

Comments on the Stages

As mentioned above, the rate of progression through these stages varies dramatically in different cell types and with different types of injury. We do not yet know all of the reasons for this variation. For example, stage III is extremely variable. In hypoxic Ehrlich ascites tumor cells (EATC) (108) or renal cortical slices at 0 to 4°C (36,116), stage III is prominent, as it also is with acute cell membrane damage by organic mercurials (69,71) or complement (30). On the other hand, this stage is absent or very transient in acute total ischemia of rat kidney (23,26), dog (94,112) or rat myocardium (60), human or rat pancreas (34), and human or hamster bronchus (1).

Also, different cell types do not reach the irreversible stage V at the same time interval. For example, totally ischemic rat renal proximal tubule cells require approximately 1 to 2 hr (23,26), whereas hamster and human bronchial epithelia require over 3 hr (1). The ambient temperature of the cells during the injurious process also has obvious relevance to the rate of change through these stages. Kidney cells at 37°C progress to stage V in 1 to 1.5 hr, whereas at 4°C, this same progression requires over 48 hr (36). Similarly, at 0 to 4°C, human bronchus and mammary epithelia survive for over 1 week (1).

Both smooth and skeletal muscle also represent special cases, possibly based on their

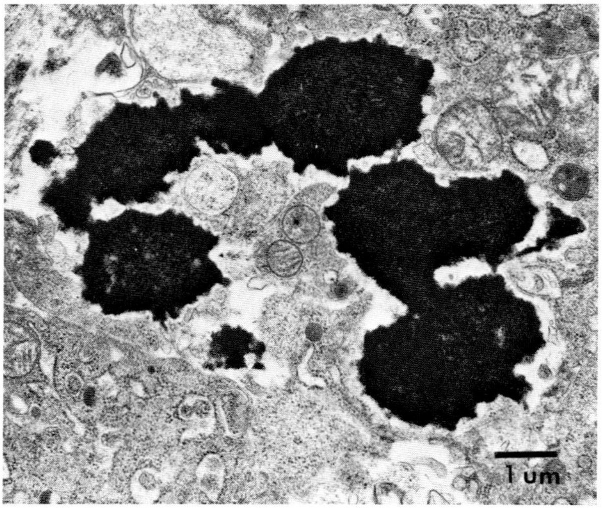

FIG. 9. An area from a 7-day rat myocardial infarct illustrating extensive areas of dense deposits surrounded by cellular debris and fibroblasts. X-ray microanalysis over this area reveals significant peaks for Ca and P. Stage VII. (From Trump et al., ref. 96, with permission.)

remarkable capacity for anaerobic glycolysis (66). We are currently investigating the latter for its possible relationship to hypertension and atherosclerosis. Hochachka (32) has recently reexamined some remarkable adaptations to anoxia in lower forms. In some situations, flocculent densities and, presumably, irreversibility can occur in this stage.

In addition, recent studies in our laboratories have necessitated modifications of stages IV and V. In proximal tubules from the pars convoluta of rat kidney following 30 and 60 min of ischemia, all mitochondria appeared swollen (indicative of stage IVA), and some contained tiny dense aggregates (24). These alterations were classified into stage IVB. Since these changes were compatible with the apparently complete recovery seen in the cortex, it was inferred that this stage was also a reversible one. The tiny dense aggregates are believed to represent reversible denaturation of matrix proteins in the mitochondria; it is well known that protein denaturation is initially reversible (47). Moreover, Majno et al. (51) reported reversibility of protein denaturation prior to the "point of no return" in light-scattering studies of tissue slices following ischemic injury.

In stages III, IV, and V, under certain conditions, altered cells do occur in which there is calcification of mitochondria in addition to the other changes mentioned. This modification does not occur with total ischemia or with chemicals that inhibit respiration or oxidative phosphorylation but does appear after ischemia followed by reflow (24,25) (Figs. 10 and 11) or after lethal injury with membrane-damaging agents such as complement and antibody (30), amphotericin B (78), penetrating or nonpenetrating mecurials (28,76), inhibition of the Na^+–K^+ ATPase with ouabain (21) (Fig. 12), and direct mechanical damage (116).

Another stage modification is that of mitochondrial intracristal densities (ICDs). In acute myocardial infarction in the rat, and to some extent also in acute ischemia of the rat kidney, the mitochondrial inner membranes exhibit such densities, resulting in the formation of intracristal or intramembrane helical arrays with a periodicity of 15 nM (60,63,64,98). These ICDs typically appear in large numbers during early time intervals following occlusion and tend to decline and disappear in the later intervals (Fig. 13). Although the nature of these ICDs is not presently known, we speculate that they represent partial or beginning membrane fusion, possibly the effect of a calcium-induced phospholipase action with the release of fusogenic agents such as fatty acids or lysophosphatides or some direct action of calcium itself. In

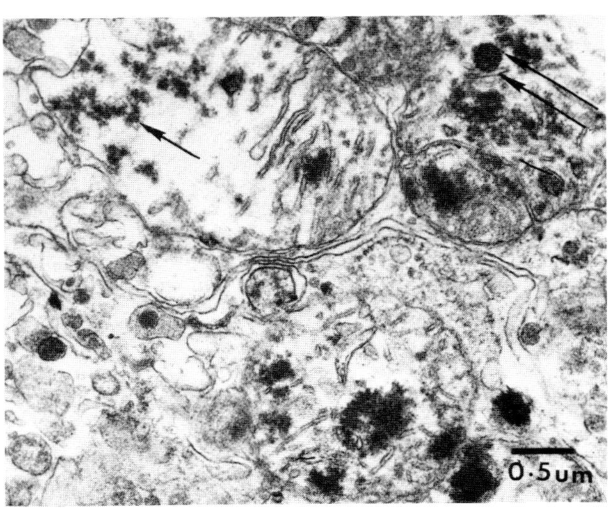

FIG. 10. Rat PCT cell after 120 min of ischemia followed by 24 hr of reflow. Mitochondria are swollen and contain large flocculent densities (*arrow*) and calcifications (*double arrow*). Stage IVc. (From Glaumann et al., ref. 23, with permission.)

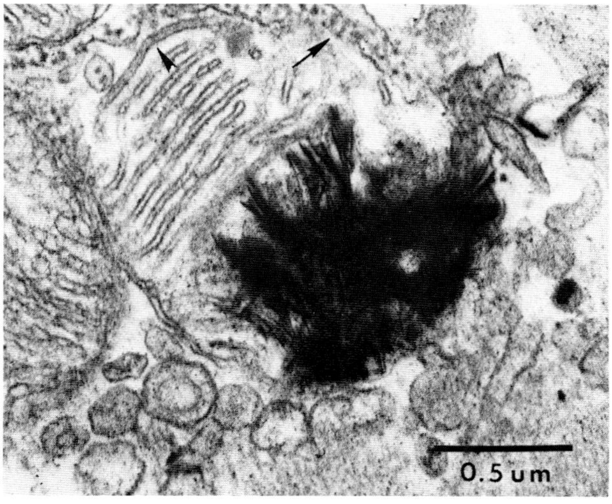

FIG. 11. A mitochondrion in a rat myocardial cell following a 60-min infarction. Needle-shaped inclusions are seen, which reveal significant Ca and P peaks when analyzed with the electron probe. Note also the mitochondrial outer membrane disruption (*arrow*) and the inner membrane fusion (*arrowhead*). (From Trump et al., ref. 96, with permission.)

muscle, inner membrane mitochondrial inclusions have been observed in several diverse conditions such as ischemia (29,37), postmortem aging (13,77), and anoxia (83). However, the exact nature of these inclusions and the factors responsible for their formation remain to be determined. Recently, Hanzlikova and Schiaffino (29) reported that they were protein in nature as shown by enzyme digestion experiments and suggested that they may result from the polymerization of enzymes such as creatine kinase present in the mitochondrial intermembrane space. A diagrammatic representation of mitochondrial profiles following each of the various stages of cell injury is shown in Fig. 14.

Stage V, which can only be recognized by electron microscopy, seems to be a hallmark of irreversible injury. Its definition has meant the difference between recognizing significant lesions in patients and animals using modern methods and failure to recognize such irreversible injury using the methods of the past. This, therefore, represents a mile-

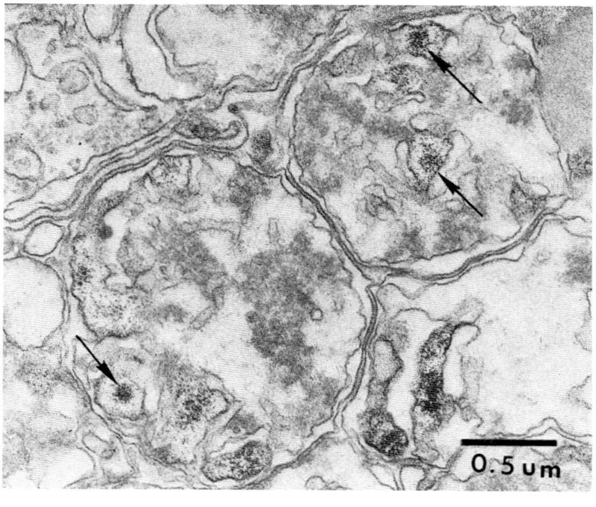

FIG. 12. PCT cell from an isolated flounder nephron treated with 10^{-5} M ouabain for 4 hr. Mitochondria are swollen and contain calcifications (*arrows*).

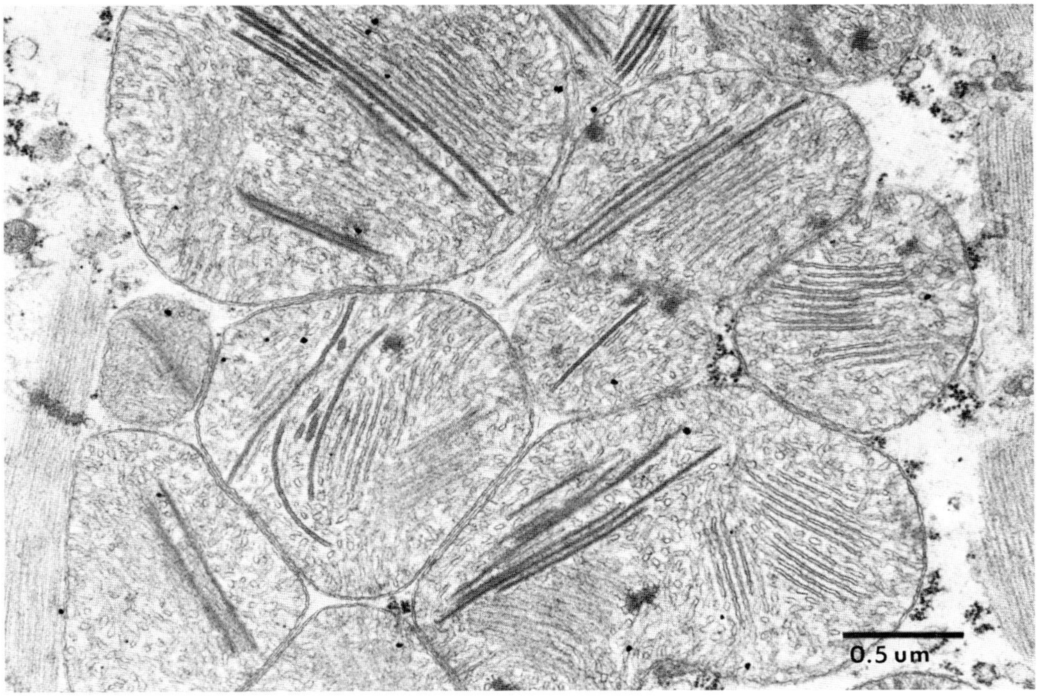

FIG. 13. Mitochondria from a rat myocardial cell following a 60-min infarct illustrating abundant intracristal densities (ICDs).

stone in the progression of knowledge concerning the nature of cell injury. The problem is especially acute in humans because following somatic death all organs become acutely ischemic and progress over a period of minutes and hours to stage V. Therefore, unless an autopsy is performed virtually immediately following death (117), recognition of the reversible or irreversible nature of cell injury becomes impossible. The same obviously applies to experimental animals; however, in these cases, it is ordinarily possible to control the initiation of studies.

GENERAL EFFECTS OF ION AND MEMBRANE REGULATION

The above formulation of these events implies that the principal cell modulations following lethal cell injury involve membrane effects, including the cell membrane, the mitochondrial inner membrane, and the membranes of the endoplasmic reticulum. This is to be contrasted with effects on other macromolecules including those of protein, RNA, and DNA, which, although known to have important side effects and primary effects in some cases, e.g., neoplasia, do not ordinarily participate directly in acute cell death. At the same time, it must be kept in mind that membrane effects such as those seen in fertilization, regeneration, or neoplasia can modulate macromolecular syntheses if the effects are sublethal. Thus, lesser degrees of such injury may result in phenomena ranging from tumor promotion to initiation of neoplasia (80).

These events involving the cell membrane also have close and important relationships with another very important subcellular system, namely, the cytoskeleton. Therefore, the following formulation involves both of these

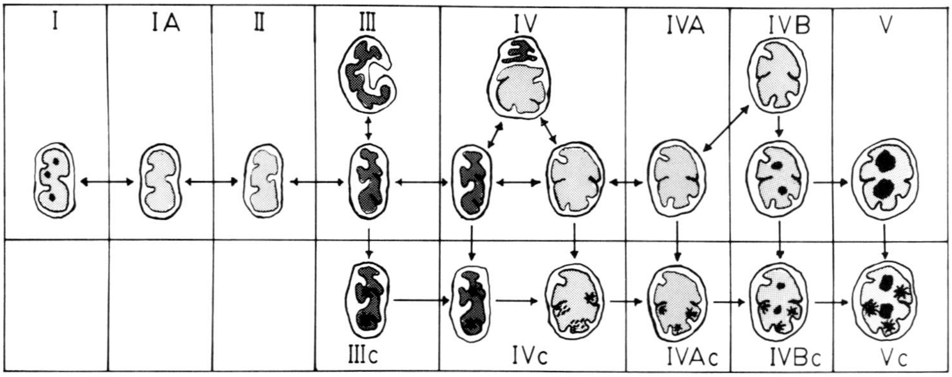

FIG. 14. A diagrammatic representation of mitochondrial profiles following cell injury. This figure shows the configuration of mitochondria in each of the various stages of cell injury. The numbering on the stages is as defined in the text. In stage I, the mitochondria are in orthodox conformation with normal, electron-dense matrix granules. In stage IA, the mitochondria are unaltered except for the disappearance of the normal matrix granules; the same occurs in stage II. In stage III, the mitochondria assume a condensed configuration with increased density of the matrix and the beginning of fusions and adhesions of the inner membrane. When this is severe, the mitochondria can assume curved donut configurations, and when the matrix condensations are extremely severe, adhesion of cristae on the matrix side develops. Calcifications can also occur in this phase under some conditions (IIIc); also, in some conditions, flocculent densities may develop. In stage IV, some mitochondria remain in the condensed configuration while others show inner compartment swelling. Still other mitochondria, in some cells in which there are several inner compartments, may show one compartment condensed and the other swollen. This stage may also have each of the conformations also showing calcifications (IVc). In the next stage, IVA, all of the mitochondria have swollen inner compartments. The matrix space is pale, presumably because of increased water content. In IVAc, calcific deposits occur, especially in proximity to cristae. In IVB, some mitochondria retain the appearance of IVA, whereas others show the appearance of tiny dense aggregates. In IVBc, in addition to the tiny dense aggregates, small calcific deposits occur. In stage V, large flocculent densities appear within the matrix compartment, whereas in Vc, they occur together with large calcific deposits. It is to be emphasized that the progression of stages I through V is characteristic of certain types of injury, specifically anoxia and ischemia. With reflow into ischemic areas, stages IIIc, IVc, IVAc, IVBc, and Vc may also occur. The c series can also occur with direct membrane injury. Flocculent densities can occur not only in stage V but in stages III and IV as well. This is a rare occurrence and may indicate irreversibility, although we do not presently know the factors responsible for it. (From Trump et al., ref. 95, with permission.)

systems, which appear to mutually interact, resulting in a series of changes following both lethal and sublethal injury.

ION REGULATION IN NORMAL AND INJURED CELLS

It is not the purpose of this chapter to exhaustively review current knowledge concerning ion regulation in normal cells; however, a few basic phenomena in this area need review to establish the premise of the investigation. It should also be borne in mind by the reader that these phenomena are undergoing constant investigation and that in the immediate future new facts concerning their normal regulation will be forthcoming.

Figure 15 shows a schematic diagram of a normal cell limited by the plasma membrane. Intra- and extracellular ions are in constant exchange through transplasmalemma diffusion. This diffusion is complex, involves several mechanisms, and, in many cases, may involve specific ionophorous channels including specific proteins; in excitable cells, it often involves voltage-acti-

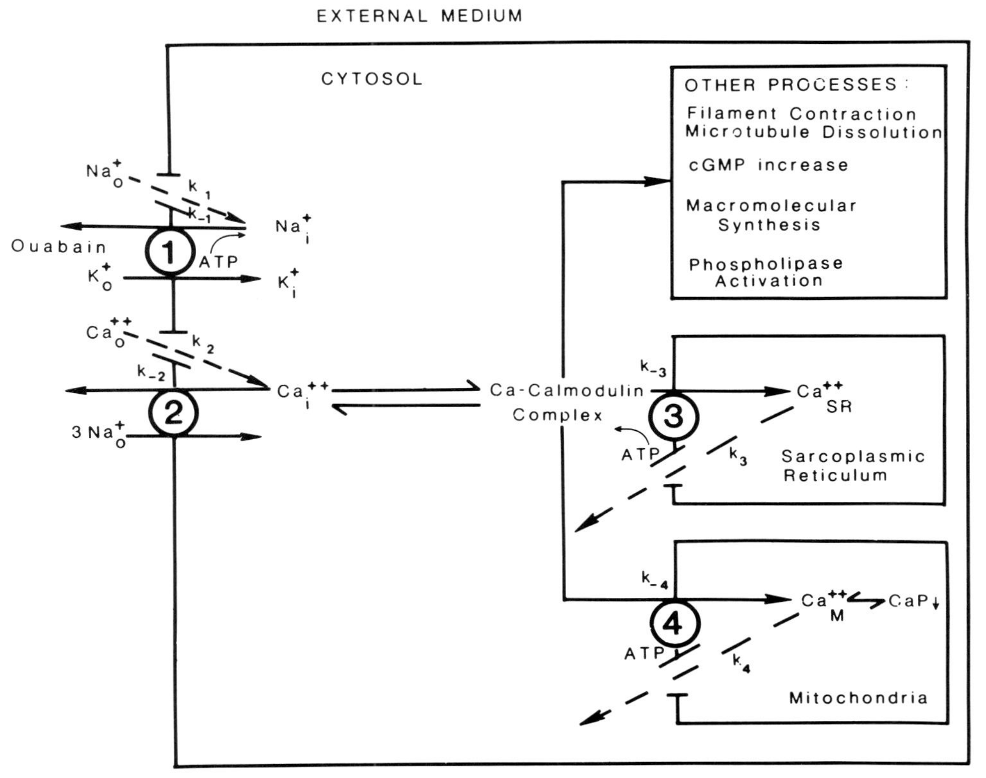

FIG. 15. Diagram illustrating the predominant pathways for sodium and calcium movements (see text for discussion). (From Trump et al., ref. 101, with permission.)

vated gated channels. The ions passively "leak" down their concentration gradient through channels, some but not all of which are electrically gated. Thus, sodium tends to leak into the cell along with calcium, whereas potassium and magnesium tend to leak out.

To maintain homeostasis within the cell, mechanisms must exist that control ionized calcium and sodium at low levels while maintaining high levels of potassium and magnesium, all of which are important in many cell processes. Sodium and potassium appear to be regulated at the plasmalemma in animal cells through the action of a specific protein, the sodium–potassium, ouabain-sensitive ATPase, which extrudes sodium and accumulates potassium. The significance of this vectorial transport system undoubtedly transcends its effect on sodium and potassium in that it also indirectly regulates calcium and, in some transporting epithelium, chloride secretion. Thus, through sodium–calcium exchange (3,4), if the sodium–potassium ATPase fails to operate, sodium and calcium both accumulate within the cell. Any condition that lowers extra- or raises intracellular sodium will favor the accumulation of calcium.

It has also been suggested that changes in cytosolic calcium regulate epithelial sodium transport (90). Any injury that results in increased leak or decreased extrusion of sodium will, at the same time, also favor the accumulation of calcium. Calcium and possibly sodium are also regulated by membranes of intracellular organelles. Thus, mitochondria in organs such as liver and kidney and ER (especially in muscle) can accumulate calcium and buffer the cytosol ion concentrations in the presence of energy, even under conditions that alter the activity of the sodium–potassium ATPase, or increase sodium permeability at the cell membrane. Modification of the buffering function of mitochondria and/or ER will quickly result in failure to control calcium.

The hypothesis developed in this chapter can be summarized by stating that, during the reversible phase after a lethal injury, a common characteristic is failure to regulate sodium. In the irreversible phase, the failure additionally involves calcium. Although calcium precipitates in cells have long been recognized by pathologists as a secondary accompaniment of cell death (dystrophic calcification), it is only recently that the role of calcium in initiating cell death has been suspected (95,96,98,99,101,102). We, for example, noted some years ago that there was a moderate correlation between cell calcium and cell death (43) and that the irreversible stages of cell injury could be correlated with total levels of cell calcium. Other investigators (12,82) have confirmed these results, and experiments in our laboratory (39,40) and those of Casini and Farber (12) tend to support the concept that modification of extracellular calcium can ameliorate or delay toxic injury. Eventually, however, cell death occurs with or without added extracellular calcium. This could imply that calcium immobilized from intracellular stores could also play an important role. For example, Ehrlich ascites tumor cells can tolerate marked increases in cell calcium if they are aerated and have a substrate source. Anoxic cells, however, die very rapidly when exposed to A23187 in media containing 1 mM calcium.

The effects of modifying extracellular calcium on acute cell injury are, however, complex. Experiments *in vitro* indicate that reduction of extracellular calcium prolongs the survival time of CCl_4-treated hepatocytes if cultured in monolayer (12) but not if cultured in suspension (33,85). Schanne et al. (82), using primary cultures of adult rat hepatocytes, showed that killing of rat liver cells by various toxins involved two clearly definable steps. The first step involved disruption of plasma membrane integrity and was independent of extracellular calcium, whereas the second step represented an influx of calcium across the damaged plasma membrane and was dependent on extracellular calcium. They concluded that toxic cell death is a specific consequence of a disturbance in intracellular calcium homeostasis.

Smith et al. (85), using isolated hepatocytes, showed that three differently acting liver cell toxins (CCl_4, bromobenzene, ethylmethanesulfonate) were more toxic to the cells in the absence of extracellular calcium than in its presence. They suggested that a change in intracellular calcium, not an influx of extracellular calcium, was responsible for the surface alterations (blebbing) noted after exposure to the toxic substrates. This was recently confirmed by the same group (33) from studies in which they concluded that interference with intracellular calcium homeostasis was more important for toxicity and, furthermore, that the concentration of extracellular calcium appeared to be controlled by the thiol status of the cells and possibly also by the mitochondria.

In direct contradiction to the above studies (85), Casini and Farber (12), using primary cultures of adult rat hepatocytes exposed to CCl_4, found that in the presence of extracellular calcium, initially nonlethal cell injury became irreversible; i.e., killing of cultured hepatocytes by CCl_4 was dependent on extracellular calcium.

To determine whether the cytotoxicity of copper and cadmium was related to the presence of calcium, Stacey and Klaassen (89) studied cell viability and lipid peroxidation of isolated hepatocytes exposed to these metal ions in the absence of extracellular calcium. Their studies did not support the hypothesis that calcium plays a ubiquitous role in the death of liver cells. Also of interest is the fact that their data contradicted those of Schanne et al. (82) in that neither copper nor cadmium showed any signs of reduced toxicity in the absence of extracellular calcium. However, they did find agreement in that calcium-free medium did ameliorate the toxic effects of the calcium ionophore A23187.

Although the reason for the discrepancy between the above results is unclear, a major difference between the studies is the use of primary adult hepatocyte cultures (12,82) versus isolated hepatocytes (33,85,89). The results using suspensions are compatible with our results using EATC, as mentioned above. Hepatocytes in suspension may well be damaged and already have increased calcium, so that the level of cytosolic calcium is not limiting. Edmondson and Bang (19) showed that freshly isolated hepatocytes exhibit rapid cell death if suspended in calcium-deficient media; this is apparently not true of hepatocytes in monolayer culture. Thus, such experiments may not be possible to interpret; however, it should be noted that hepatocytes are not adapted to living in suspension, which is in marked contrast to EATC. At the same time, it also should be pointed out that in our experiments with calcium-free media, injured EATC show only partial protection from cell death (39,40). Death is really delayed if one observes the cells for 6 hr, at which time the results are similar. In the experiments of Smith et al. (85), however, this is only relevant to extracellular calcium.

If a toxin or injury blocks calcium uptake but not release by mitochondria, rapid increases of calcium occur in the cytosol (e.g., ruthenium red). Although this may not be important in cells such as squid axons (7) where mitochondria are few, it is clearly very important in many important target organs including liver and kidney. In liver cells, for example, mitochondria contain 60 to 70% of the calcium (59). Recent results in our laboratory (81,115a) using anoxic rat proximal tubule cells in suspension showed that calcium-deficient medium resulted in some prolongation of viability; however, it was observed that the amount of washing of the cells also had an effect. In the absence of calcium, both viability and NAD reduction were higher in the cells washed three times than in cells washed three times and incubated in the presence of calcium. In cells washed six times, viability and NAD reduction were approximately of the same low levels both in the absence and presence of extracellular calcium. These data suggest that increased washing may possibly have the effect of removing membrane-bound calcium and thus destabilizing cell membranes. Also, the results point out that in *in vitro* studies the methods of cell isolation need to be standardized before any final conclusions on the role of extracellular calcium in cell injury can be reached.

In summary, many types of cell injury result in modification of intracellular sodium followed by diminished sodium–calcium exchange, increased intracellular calcium, and, probably through calcium–calmodulin, a variety of effects occurs (92,93,100). The major categories of lethal cell injury can be generally categorized as follows, although in some cases overlap occurs and, in the late stages, the situation becomes more complex as secondary effects develop.

1. Conditions that primarily affect ATP synthesis. These include anoxia and ischemia, inhibitors of respiration, e.g., CN^-, CO, and antimycin, and uncouplers of oxidative phosphorylation, e.g., halogenated phenols (2,4-DNP) and substituted hydrazines (FCCP).
2. Inhibitors of the Na–K ATPase. This includes specific inhibitors, e.g., the cardiac glycosides, as well as nonspecific inhibitors, e.g., heavy metals including Hg.
3. Conditions that modify cell membrane permeability. (a) Modification of lipids, proteins, or lipid–protein interactions. This is a large category, which includes agents associated with lipid and peroxidation formation including free-radical-generating compounds such as CCl_4, $CHCl_3$, PAH; toxicity from ozone, O_2,

superoxide; phosphorlipases and lipid solvents; physical agents including UV light; and mechanical trauma to the membrane. (b) Conditions associated with channel formation.[1] These include chemical toxins, e.g., amphotericin B, and also apparently include membrane damage by complement activation. (c) Ionophores. Although these hydrophobic compounds do not directly modify membrane permeability, they do result in rapid equalization of ionic gradients across membrane barriers.

It appears that most conditions resulting in acute lethal injury do so by modulating one or more of the above mechanisms. As we discuss later in this chapter, they appear to do so primarily by modulating cell ion regulation.

CONSIDERATIONS OF THE CYTOSKELETON

Very important to the arguments to be developed is the interaction of elements of the cytoskeleton with the cell membrane (Fig. 16). At the present time, the cytoskeleton includes the following major elements (6): thin filaments of actin, which interact with myosin and other proteins in a variety of cell types; microtubules consisting of the polymer tubulin; intermediate filaments termed keratin in epithelial cells; and an incompletely characterized three-dimensional system recently described by Porter (73) and known as the "microtrabecular network" (Fig. 17), which gives structure to the cytosol and may provide orientation and functional alignment of several so-called cytosol proteins ranging from free polysomes to glycolytic enzymes. These polymers interact with membranes of the cell surface and organelles and modulate many important cell phenomena including cell shape, cell movement, phagocytosis, secretion, autophagocytosis, cell division, movement of receptors in the cell membrane, and organization and movement of intracellular cytoplasmic and nuclear structures.

The relationship of the cytoskeleton components with each other and with the cell membrane can be rapidly and dramatically altered by modulation of cell ion regulation. For example, the intermediate filament, keratin, present in virtually all epithelial cells, often varies in concentration depending on cell injury and bears a particular relationship to calcium (31). In cultured epithelial cells from both the bronchus and the epidermis, additional keratin is vividly expressed in the presence of high extracellular calcium and suppressed with low or absent extracellular calcium. In hamster tracheal rings studied *in vitro,* addition of the calcium ionophore A23187 also results in squamous metaplasia and is accompanied by keratin accumulation (79). Altered expression of keratin is also related to concentration of vitamin A and related retinoids (88). In the absence or deficiency of vitamin A, keratin expression is intensified; this is part of the squamous or epidermoid metaplasia that occurs in a variety of end organs in such deficient states. Expression of keratin may be a preneoplastic change in the bronchus, cervix, and other organs and may also represent a typical response to tumor promotors. Keratin filaments also interact with desmosomes at lateral cell membranes and with hemidesmosomes along basilar membranes (Fig. 18). In the absence of extracellular calcium, many epithelial cells detach from each other and from the basal lamina.

Tubulin also bears a definite relationship to a variety of cell functions including shape, movement of secretory and phagocytic vacuoles, and autophagy. Interference with the integrity of tubulin results in marked cell shape changes at the surface and along the elements of the ER and other cytoplasmic organelles. These involve the formation of protrusions that extend either to the extracellular space in the case of the cell surface or into internalized potential extracellular

[1] It is recognized that the distinction between categories b and c is somewhat arbitrary and possibly nonsubstantive.

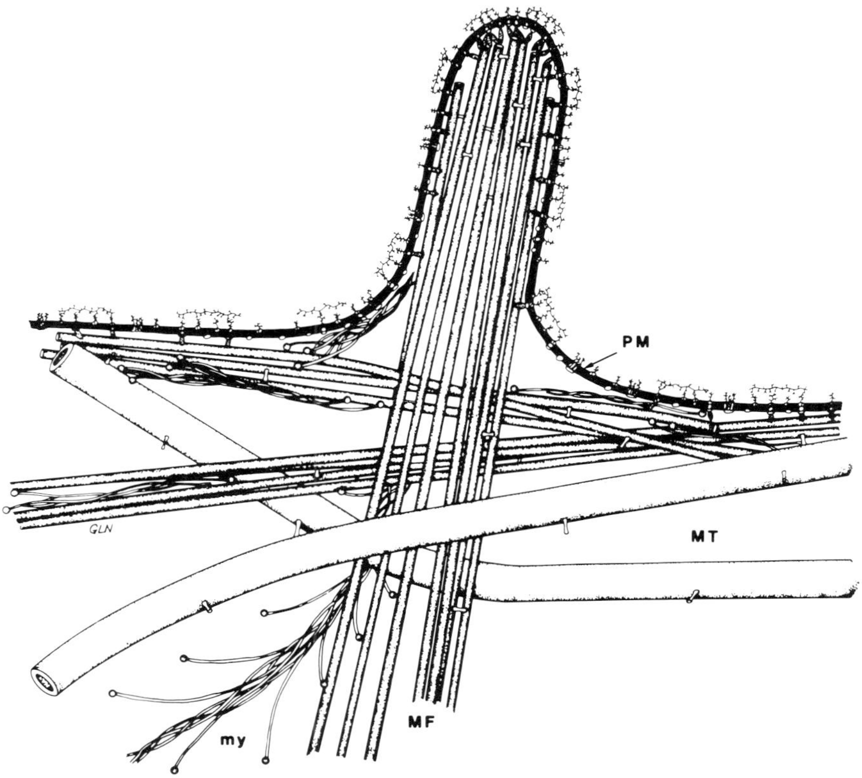

FIG. 16. Model illustrating the relationship of cytoskeletal components and the cell membrane. The model demonstrates hypothetical interactions between membrane-associated microtubule (MT) and microfilament (MF) systems involved in transmembrane control over cell surface receptor mobility and distribution. This model envisages opposite but coordinated roles for microfilaments (contractile) and microtubules (skeletal) and suggests that that they are linked to one another or to the same plasma membrane (PM) inner surface components. This linkage may occur through myosin molecules either in small bundles or the larger filaments (my), or through cross-bridging molecules such as α-actin. In addition, peripheral membrane components linked at the inner or outer plasma membrane surface may extend this control over specific membrane domains. (From Nicolson et al., ref. 59a, with permission.)

space in the case of ER or phagosomes (autophagy). Modification and depolymerization of microtubules may also represent a stimulus for cell division. Many agents are known to modify the structure of microtubules; among these is an elevation of intracellular calcium, which causes depolymerization.

The thin actin filaments bear obvious relationships to cell movement, including tumor invasion. Changes in the distribution of these filaments characterize both preneoplastic and neoplastic lesions and have been invoked to explain or characterize invasive versus noninvasive cancers of the skin. Differences in actin patterns have been noted in transformed cells and are being investigated in cells with sublethal and lethal injuries.

The high-affinity calcium-binding protein calmodulin, although not part of the defined cytoskeleton, plays an important role in the modulation of those structures as well as in the execution of many other calcium-mediated events. This protein has been partially characterized by immunocytochemistry (54) and well characterized biochemically (14,15).

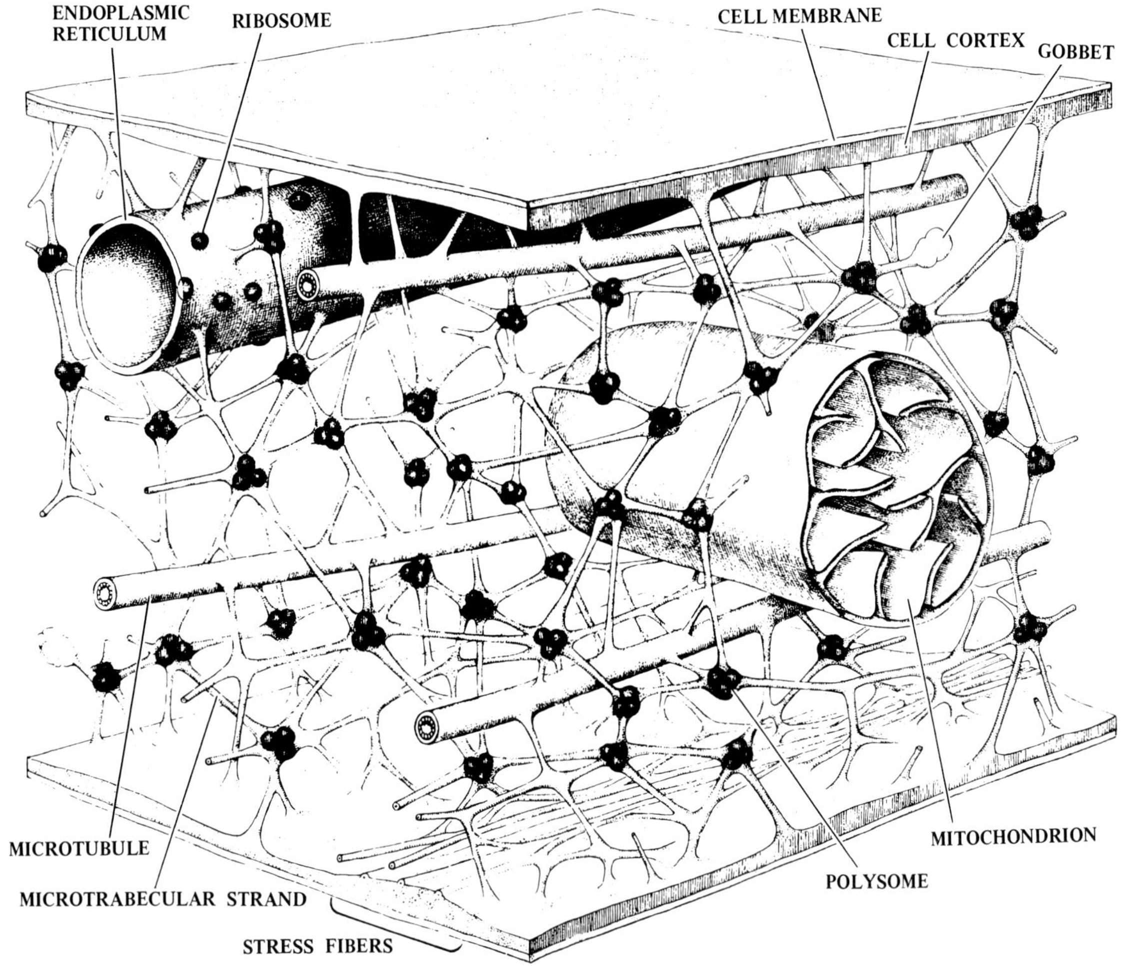

FIG. 17. Model of the microtrabecular lattice, magnified over 300,000 times its actual size, was derived from hundreds of images of cultured cells viewed in the high-voltage electron microscope. The model illustrates how the microtrabecular filaments are related to the other components of the cytosol. The microtrabeculae suspend the elongated structures of the endoplasmic reticulum, the mitochondria, the microtubules, and the microfilaments. At junctions of the lattice are polysomes. (From Porter, ref. 73, with permission.)

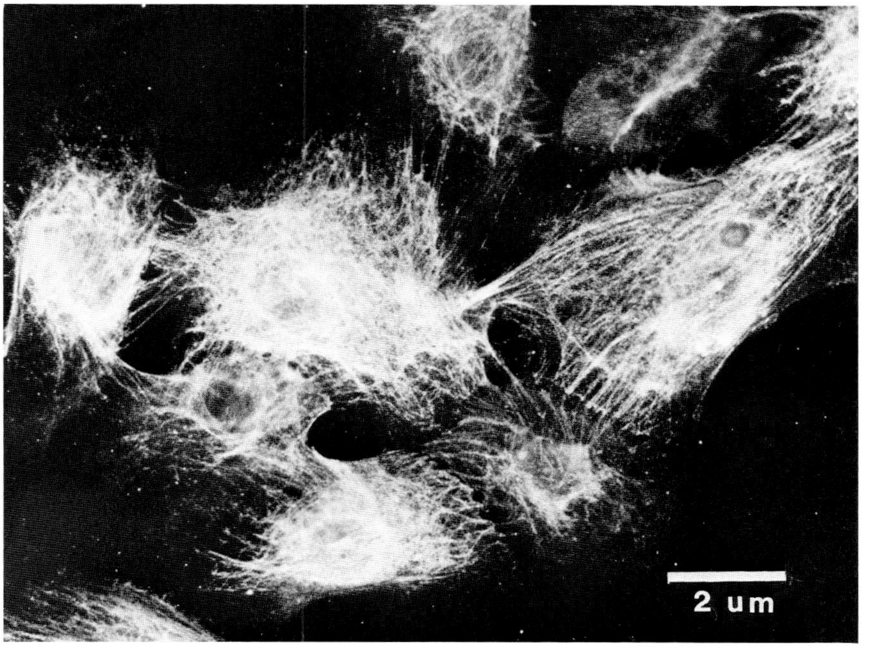

FIG. 18. Indirect immunofluorescent staining of keratin filaments in normal human bronchus outgrowth cells (keratin antibody courtesy of T.-T. Sun, Johns Hopkins University, Baltimore, MD). Abundant filaments are seen in individual cells and also at intercellular attachment areas. Cells were grown in standard media with calcium. (Courtesy of P. C. Phelps).

Localization varies with cell type, but in some interphase cells, mitochondrial localization has been reported, and in mitotic cells, calmodulin alignment along the spindles has been frequently assessed. Marcum et al. (52) postulated a role for calcium–calmodulin complexes in the microtubule depolymerization that occurs during anaphase. Localizations and/or redistributions of this protein in cell injury have not been well studied. Welsh et al. (119) observed calmodulin binding to gap junctions in lens epithelium and suggested a regulatory role for calcium in gap junction function.

EXAMPLES OF THE PRINCIPAL CATEGORIES OF ACUTE LETHAL INJURY

It is not our intention to cover in detail the total literature on acute lethal injury. Instead, we consider only the several principally known mechanisms mentioned above, focusing on the roles of the plasma membrane and the cytoskeleton.

Inhibition of ATP Synthesis

Acutely injurious agents that, like anoxia or ischemia, act initially through reduction or cessation of oxidative phosphorylation include a variety of metabolic inhibitors including cyanide (103,104), carbon monoxide, halogenated phenols, and antibiotics such as antimycin. Such models have been extensively studied in a variety of organ systems including heart, kidney, brain, pancreas, and bronchus as well as in single cell models. Moreover, studies have been carried out in a variety of vertebrate and invertebrate species as well as in explants. Two examples are discussed here: myocardial infarction and anoxia of Ehrlich ascites tumor cells *in vitro*.

Myocardial Infarction

Both human and animal models of myocardial infarction ordinarily result from occlusion of a major branch of the coronary artery. Although many studies have been carried out in man, the most detailed studies from the mechanistic point of view have been performed in rats, dogs, and rabbits. Allowing for differences in the details of the blood supply, the results appear to be similar in all of these species at the cellular level. In most of the models, the "point of no return" is somewhere between 30 min and 1 hr.

During the first 30 min, changes in myocardial cells can be characterized as passing through stages II, III, and IV. Stage V is ordinarily reached between 30 min and 1 hr. During the early stages of mitochondrial swelling, peculiar adhesions or putative fusions of mitochondrial inner membranes are commonly seen in human, rat (60,63,64,98), and dog models (112). These fusions are presently being characterized in our laboratory and appear to contain both lipid and protein (63,64). Mitochondrial calcification in the form of hydroxyapatite crystals can be seen in stage V of myocytes beginning between 30 min and 1 hr and increasing later. These are not uniform throughout the infarct but appear mainly at the periphery and in scattered regions throughout, possibly at the edges of areas supplied by collateral circulation. As mentioned elsewhere, it appears that totally ischemic cells do not exhibit mitochondrial calcification. On the other hand, if reflow is started into a previously ischemic necrotic area in the myocardium or kidney, rapid calcification occurs, predominantly in the mitochondria, often very rapidly.

We have previously shown that mitochondria, even in necrotic cells, are able to actively accumulate calcium phosphate (56). All of these early events are difficult or impossible to define by light microscopy. In addition to the above, there is depletion of glycogen and relaxation of monofilaments. Between 12 and 24 hr, inflammatory cells begin to appear at the periphery, and typical coagulation necrosis can be seen at this time even by light microscopy. Measurements of ATP and energy charge show rapid decrements during the first few minutes with acceleration of anaerobic glycolysis (55,57,58). It has been postulated that the consequent reduction in pH ultimately limits the action of phosphofructokinase and that anaerobic glycolysis cannot maintain function after that time.

Studies of cellular ion content by analytical microscopy following experimental myocardial infarction show early increases in sodium and chlorine beginning by 5 min and progressively increasing thereafter (62) (Fig. 19). Significant increases are seen prior to the "point of no return." Calcium levels, however, are within normal limits prior to 30 min in the rat model; at 30 min and thereafter, marked increases in calcium content occur. Thus, in this model, increases in sodium and chlorine precede increases in total cell calcium. Total calcium increases proceed with and parallel the onset of irreversible injury. It should not be construed from such measurements, however, that cytosolic calcium is not modified prior to cell death. In the absence of mitochondrial function, cytosolic calcium cannot be regulated and is presumably increased very early.

Reimer and Jennings (74) have also studied the ability of myocardial slices to regulate volume during the early stages of cell injury. Their data are consistent with the above analytical data, as the ischemic slices exhibit decreased ability to extrude sodium and accumulate potassium.

Studies are currently under way in this laboratory to investigate this more thoroughly. We hypothesize that the early ICDs or fusions of mitochondrial membranes seen following myocardial occlusion may be, in fact, the result of fusegenic agents resulting from calcium activation of phospholipase (63,64). Modification of mitochondrial phospholipids, e.g., cardiolipin, prior to the "point of no return" has been noted in ischemic kidney

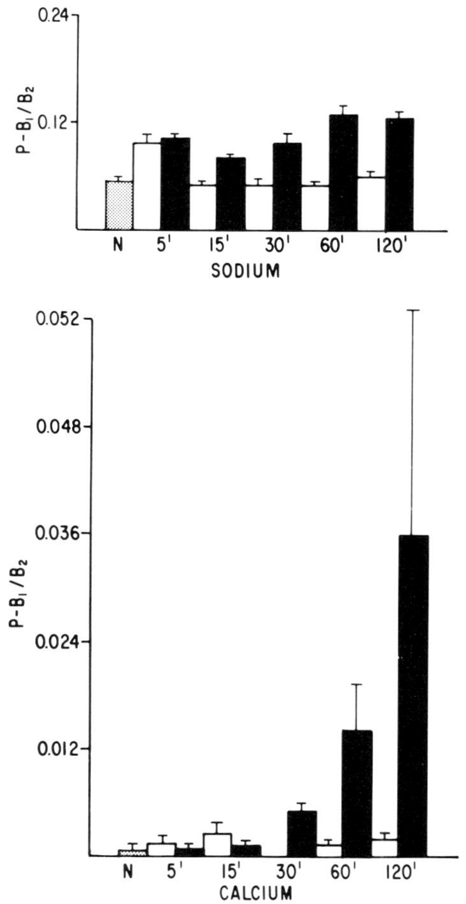

FIG. 19. *Bar graphs* illustrating peak-to-background ratios ($P - B_1/B_2$) for sodium and calcium from X-ray microanalysis measurements obtained over 4-μm freeze-dried cryosections of rat myocardium following 5, 15, 30, 60, and 120 min occlusion of the coronary artery. N, normal, unoperated animals; *white bars,* control; *black bars,* ischemic regions. (From Osornio-Vargas et al., ref. 62, with permission.)

(86). A number of intracellular phospholipases, in particular phospholipase A_2, release both fatty acids and lysophosphatides that are capable of modifying cell membranes. Sobel et al. (87) and Corr et al. (17) both reported lysophosphatide accumulation in ischemic myocardium. These two types of products or enzymatic hydrolase itself could render the membrane nonfunctional. During stage II, normal mitochondrial matrix granules disappear. As these granules are believed to represent phospholipid cardiolipin, this may also be a reflection of calcium-activated phospholipase(s).

Modification of myocardial ischemia.

Numerous attempts are under way in various laboratories to modify the consequences of myocardial ischemia. Several such attempts have involved the use of calcium entry blockers such as verapamil and nifedipine. The positive results obtained in several such studies are compatible with a role of calcium in mediating the necrosis, although it is difficult presently to determine whether such effects are exerted on the vasculature, including the microvasculature, or the myocytes themselves. Recent studies in our laboratory (61,65) as well as from others (18,35,46,50) indicate that administration of the nonsteroidal antiinflammatory agent ibuprofen also reduces the size of myocardial infarctions. The explanation for this is presently not clear, although data have recently been forthcoming that some of the products of the cyclooxygenase pathway may, in fact, act as calcium ionophores. Similar studies have been performed on the brain following anoxia or ischemia. Agents used as calcium entry blockers and associated with improved cerebral function following reperfusion include flunarizine, $MgSO_4$, verapamil, and lidoflazine (120).

Comments on other organs.

The effects of ischemia have been studied on many other organs including kidney, brain, liver, pancreatic duct and acinar cells, and bronchus. Although the time to the "point of no return" varies markedly in these different organs, for example 30 min to 1 hr in the case of the liver and 3 hr in the case of pancreas and bronchus (1,34), the progression of change is similar in principle through the several stages mentioned in the heart; other details vary, depending on the specializations in a particular cell. The mitochondrial membrane ICDs, so prominent in ischemic myocardium, are present but much less numerous in other organs. In cells with free luminal surfaces, such as kidney tubules, bile canaliculi, and pancreatic duct, the early reversible changes typically include the formation of large bleb-like protrusions that extend into the lumen and sometimes detach (24). These are discussed in more detail below. Another variant is the extent of mitochondrial condensation in stage III. Ordinarily, with total ischemia, this is relatively slight and transient. We infer that this condition, which may involve ion loss, probably potassium from the inner compartment, is dependent on maintenance of the integrity of the inner membrane and is totally reversible. If permeability changes occur in the inner membrane very rapidly, then, according to this concept, the formation of condensed mitochondria would be retarded or very transient. It is much more prominent in cells made anoxic or treated with mitochondrial inhibitors in the presence of excess extracellular fluid, e.g., perfused anoxic preparations or cells suspended in media and then treated. This is probably because exchange of ions, e.g., potassium, is much more extensive.

Ehrlich Ascites Tumor Cells

This well-characterized model from the biochemical and metabolic points of view has been used extensively in our laboratories to investigate the mechanism of acute cell injury (38–45,108). The cell model has importance not only in the study of general cell injury but also in carbohydrate metabolism and in the actions of cancer chemotherapeutic agents.

If EATC are made anoxic by gassing with purified nitrogen in the absence of glucose, they very rapidly lose potassium, and their ATP levels decrease very rapidly (43,45). The "point of no return" at 37°C is estimated to be approximately 2 to 3 hr for the population. That is, if the cells are reoxygenated, and glucose is added prior to these times, the morphologic changes reverse, the ion changes reverse, and the ATP levels return. In this anoxic system, if glucose is present at all times during anoxia, the cells are partially protected and survive for a much longer period of time, presumably because of anaerobic glycolysis. It must be remembered that anoxia differs from ischemia in that in anoxia, in addition to having the cells bathed with extracellular medium, they can also receive substrates, exchange products of catabolism, etc.

Ultrastructural changes in anoxic EATC include the very rapid formation of blebs or protrusions at the surface replacing the normal microvilli (114) (Figs. 20 and 21). This is associated with modification of the feltwork of microfilaments, which normally occurs at the cell periphery and within the microvilli. It also involves modification of the microtubules. Also, during the reversible phase, the cells rapidly pass through stages II, III, and IV, although stage III is much more prolonged, with marked condensation of mitochondria; this can even become sufficiently severe so that ring-like configurations exist. Between 2 and 3 hr, the cells pass through stage IV and then into stage V, the "point of no return." Calcifications in mitochondria are never noted, although cytosolic calcium levels do increase. Potassium loss is very rapid in the system, accompanied by gradual increase of sodium during the reversible phase. Measurements of cell calcium show a good correlation with cell death, and plots of viability and calcium content show a reciprocal relationship (43) (Fig. 22).

Modification of Ehrlich ascites tumor cells. In this system, partial protection with prolongation of viability can be obtained in calcium-free Krebs–Ringer phosphate solution. Similar results can be obtained by adding a calcium-chelating agent, such as EDTA, to the medium (40). On the other hand, addition of the calcium ionophore A23187 in the presence of normal extracellular calcium concentrations in the presence of anoxia synergistically causes explosive cell death (39) (Fig. 23). It is probably quite significant that

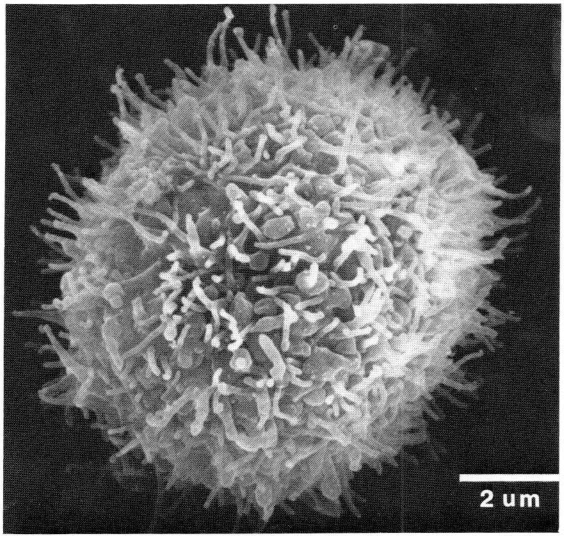

FIG. 20. Scanning electron micrograph (SEM) of a control Ehrlich ascites tumor cell (EATC) illustrating the many delicate, closely packed microvilli. (From Trump et al., ref. 114, with permission.)

addition of the calcium ionophore to oxygenated cells can be associated with marked increases in cell calcium content without significant cell death, presumably because intracellular systems, including the mitochondria, are able to buffer the increased cytosolic concentration. This result differs from that of Segal and Inbar (84) who noted that physiological concentrations of the calcium ionophore A23187 did result in cell death, whereas 10^{-6} M did not, therefore suggesting a nonspecific effect. Thus, in this system, it appears that extracellular calcium influx from the extracellular space contributes to but does not totally explain the cell death following anoxia. Failure of mitochondrial regulation does, however, appear to be very significant, as the cells can tolerate much

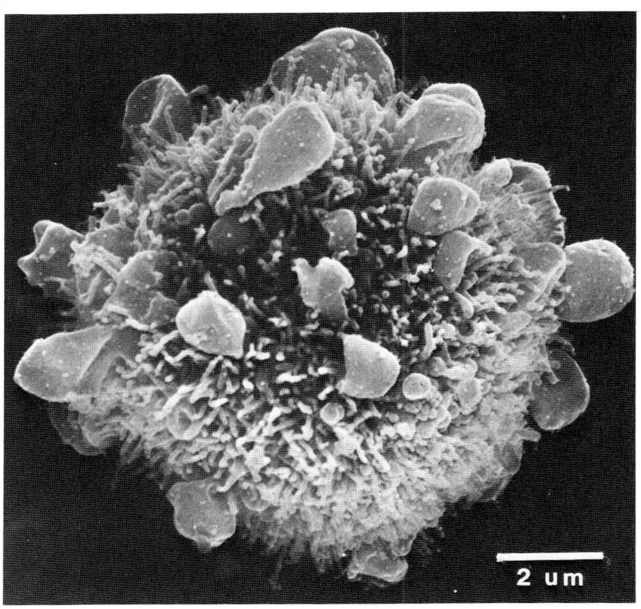

FIG. 21. Scanning EM of an EATC following 1 hr of anoxia. Although numerous microvilli are still present, some areas of the cell surface contain large blebs. (From Trump et al., ref. 102a, with permission.)

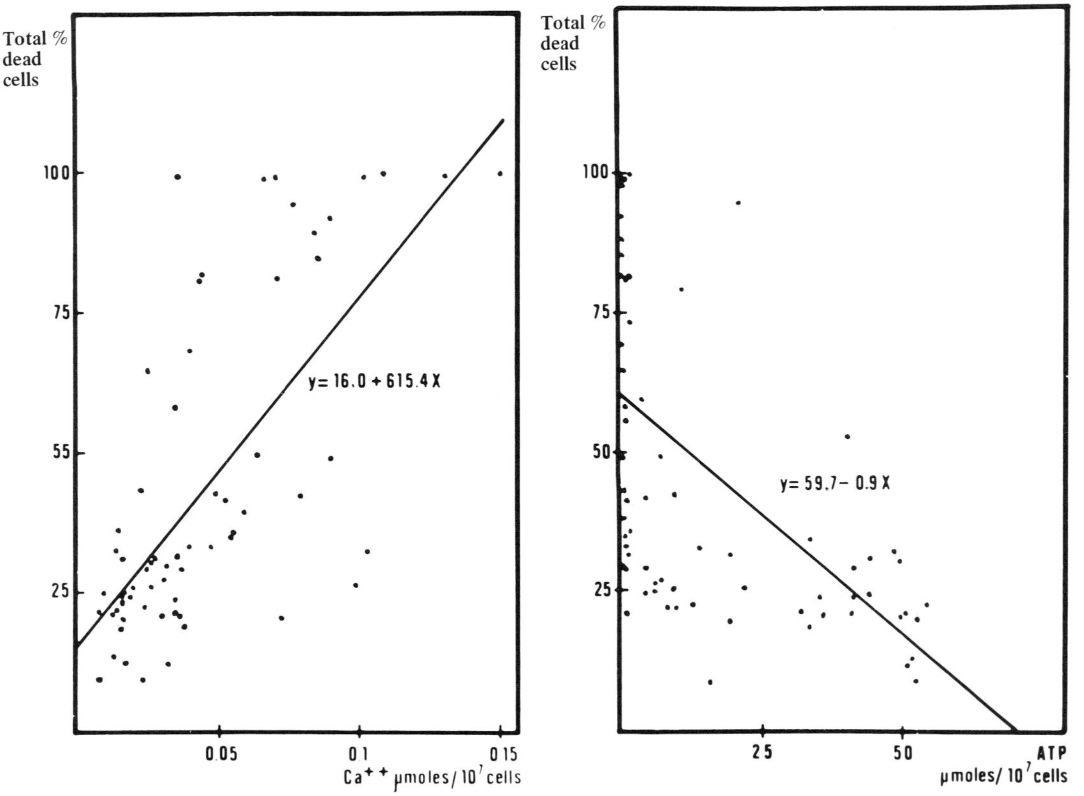

FIG. 22. Left: Scatter plot with *regression line* showing a good positive correlation between Ca^{2+} content of cells and the total percentage of dead cells. Cellular injury was produced by an inhibitor of function of the plasma membrane (*p*-chloromercuribenzene sulfonic acid) or by inhibitors of respiration (antimycin A), glycolysis (iodoacetic acid), or oxidative phosphorylation (2,4-dinitrophenol), or by combinations of the latter (r = 0.68, $p < 0.001$, N = 62). (From Laiho and Trump, ref. 43, with permission.) **Right:** Scatter plot with *regression line* showing a moderate correlation between ATP content of the cells and the total percentage of dead cells. Cellular injury was produced as in Fig. 23A (r = 0.58, $p < 0.001$, N = 72). (From Laiho and Trump, ref. 43, with permission.)

more total calcium in the presence of intact mitochondrial function. We infer that in this system, failure of oxidative phosphorylation is associated with calcium influx from the extracellular space and that failure of mitochondria and other systems to control such influx results in events leading to cell death.

Compatible with this conclusion is a series of experiments conducted in our laboratory on the modifying effects of reduced extracellular pH (67–71). Reductions of pH from 7.4 to 6.4 or lower are associated with doubling of the survival time after acute total anoxia (Fig. 24). On the other hand, slight increases in pH from 7.4 to 7.5 or 7.6 are associated with marked acceleration of cell death. We interpret this as proton protection from calcium-mediated effects, possibly through antagonism with calcium–calmodulin binding.

In many other cellular systems, H^+ has been reported to antagonize calcium-mediated effects, whereas OH^- ions tend to augment the effects (75). Additionally, Philipson et al. (72) recently showed that reduction of pH inhibits sodium–calcium exchange in canine cardiac sarcolemmal vesicles. Clarkson and Amole (16) have recently reported that calcium ions are synergistic with salicylhydroxamic (SHAM) in killing trypanosomes;

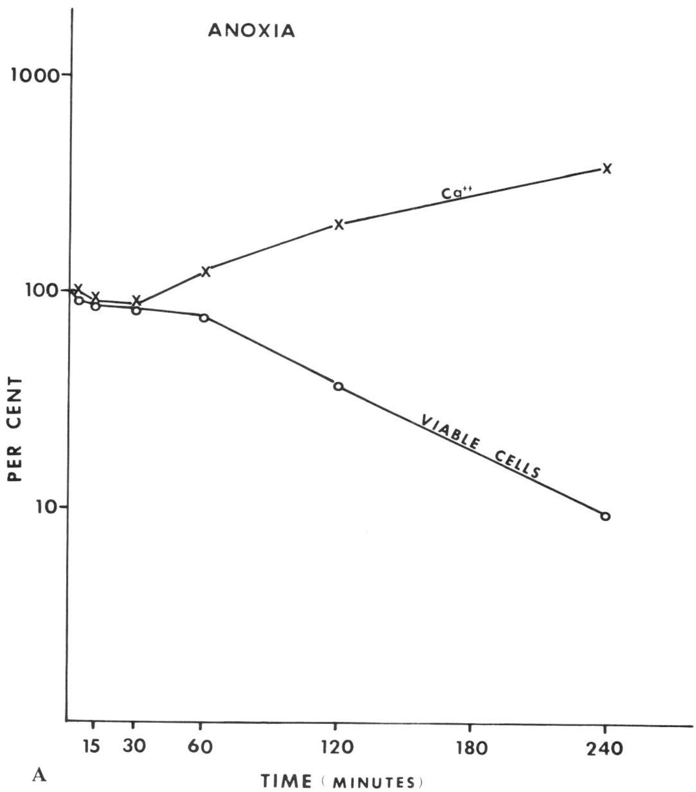

A

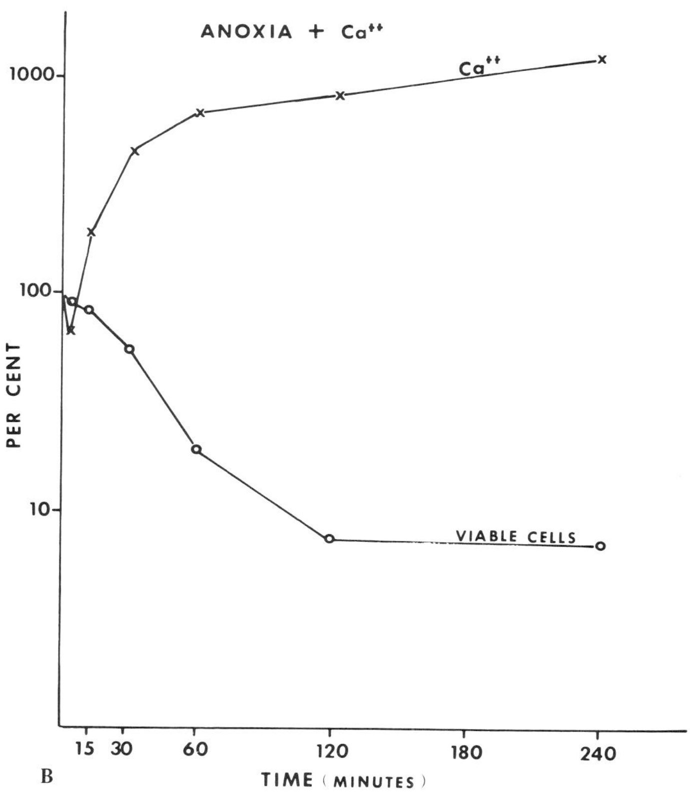

B

FIG. 23. A: Graph illustrating percent of viable cells and Ca^{2+} uptake in EATC following 0 to 240 min of anoxia. Cells were preincubated in Krebs–Ringer phosphate buffer (pH 7.4) for 10 min prior to the experiments, and at 0 time, the gasing phase was changed to purified nitrogen. Cell viability was determined by nigrosin staining. **B:** Graph illustrating percent of viable cells and Ca^{2+} uptake in anoxic EATC following 0 to 240 min treatment with 10 μM ionophore A23187. Experimentation was performed as in Fig. **A.** Cell Ca^{2+} levels were determined by atomic absorption spectrophotometry using ^{14}C-inulin to estimate extracellular space. (From Trump et al., ref. 96, with permission.)

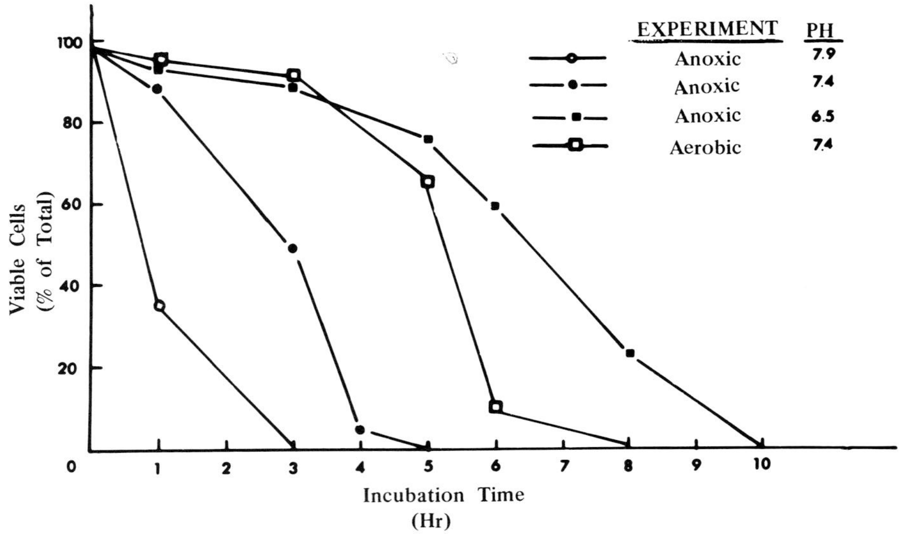

FIG. 24. Viability of EATC incubated aerobically and anaerobically at various pH values. (From Penttila and Trump, ref. 70, with permission.)

SHAM is known to block glucose metabolism (8). In this system, calcium hydroxide was much more active than calcium lactate, indicating the importance of ionized calcium. Calcium is also synergistic with other trypanocidal agents including melarsoprol and iodoacetamide (16). Calcium is even more critical for melarsoprol. In this regard, it was also suggested that calcium influx provides the trigger for release of surface coat glycoprotein, a process enhanced by modifying glycolysis with 2-deoxyglucose (118).

Many other experiments have been performed with inhibitors of respiration or uncouplers of oxidative phosphorylation with or without inhibitors of glycolysis (42,43). Antimycin with or without glucose in the medium yields results similar to anoxia with or without glucose. If iodoacetic acid is added, however, the addition of glucose gives little or no protection.

Inhibition of ATPase

Specific inhibition of the plasma membrane sodium–potassium ATPase with ouabain has been carried out in a series of experiments using isolated flounder kidney tubules (21). Addition of ouabain to such tubules leads to progression of the cells through the stages mentioned above. Again, stage III is very prominent, with marked condensation of mitochondria. Ouabain, however, has little initial effect on mitochondrial function, and as sodium accumulates in the cells, calcification, in the form of calcium phosphate precipitates, is prominent in the mitochondria (see Fig. 12). This, we infer, results from greatly diminished sodium–calcium exchange at the plasmalemma. Similar effects of ouabain have been noted in isolated cultured cardiac myocytes (48). These experiments again emphasize the fact that mitochondrial calcification is noted only under conditions in which cytosolic calcium increases in the presence of relatively intact mitochondrial function.

Alterations in Membrane Permeability

A variety of agents specifically or nonspecifically modify plasma membrane permeability. At sufficient doses, such modifications are ordinarily lethal. Possible mechanisms include formation of ion channels, membrane lipid peroxidation, mechanical damage, and modification of membrane proteins. Only a few examples are discussed.

Membrane Lipid Peroxidation

A variety of physical and chemical agents result in peroxidation of membrane lipids. These include a variety of organic and inorganic compounds whose metabolites are associated with formation of free radicals or superoxide ions and physical agents such as ultraviolet or ionizing irradiation (22).

One of the best studied models is carbon tetrachloride (CCl_4) toxicity, which is extremely hepatotoxic both *in vivo* and *in vitro.* Carbon tetrachloride is known to be metabolized in the hepatic microsomal oxygenase system to form highly reactive free radicals which result in membrane peroxidation. This is associated with cell swelling, increased cell sodium, and decreased cell potassium. Morphologically, there is dilatation of ER, dissociation of polysomes, and mitochondrial swelling. Again, as mentioned above, the initial effects do not appear to involve the mitochondria, and mitochondrial calcification is a very prominent feature. The effects of extracellular calcium in CCl_4-treated hepatocytes was discussed above.

Modification of Membrane Protein Sulfhydryl Groups

Many experiments, both *in vivo* and *in vitro,* have been carried out with both organic and inorganic mercurials, which are classic modifiers of protein sulfhydryl groups. *In vivo,* mercuric chloride has been extensively studied as a model of acute renal failure and produces acute cell death and necrosis predominantly within the pars recta of the proximal tubule both in the medullar rays of the cortex and in the outer stripe of the outer medulla (28). These changes progress rapidly over a period of 6 to 12 hr, beginning with alterations in membrane marker enzymes such as 5′-nucleotidase and involving dilatation of the ER with detachment of polysomes, mitochondrial condensation, aggregation of ER, mitochondrial swelling, and mitochondrial calcification. In addition to the effects on protein sulfhydryl groups, recent evidence indicates that mercury may also facilitate membrane peroxidation through inactivation of detoxification pathways, e.g., glutathione peroxidase. Again, the primary effect is not on the mitochondria, and, therefore, the marked calcium phosphate accumulation in mitochondria would be predicted.

Studies with mercury have also been carried out in EATC in which both penetrating and nonpenetrating mercurials have been used. Mitochondria have a relatively low affinity (10 μM) but a large capacity for calcium uptake (11,90), which implies, in these experiments, that cytosolic calcium reached or exceeded this concentration. Nonpenetrating mercurials such as *p*-chloromercuribenzene sulfonic acid (PCMBS) are perhaps better for such studies because they do not readily penetrate the cell membrane and, therefore, seem to initially interact only with surface ligands. In contrast to conditions that inhibit ATP synthesis, compounds that modify cell membrane permeability are associated with extremely rapid cell swelling and membrane blebs (Fig. 25), marked increases in sodium, chloride, and total cations, and marked decreases in potassium. Calcium levels increase in parallel with cell death, and, unless extremely high doses are utilized, mitochondrial calcification can readily be demonstrated. These effects of PCMBS can be greatly diminished by addition of mannitol to the medium (38) or by reduction of medium pH (69,71). Although the mechanism of mannitol is not totally understood, at least two effects seem possible: one is the obvious effect of balancing intracellular colloid osmotic pressure, the other, perhaps more interesting, is the fact that mannitol is a free radical scavenger.

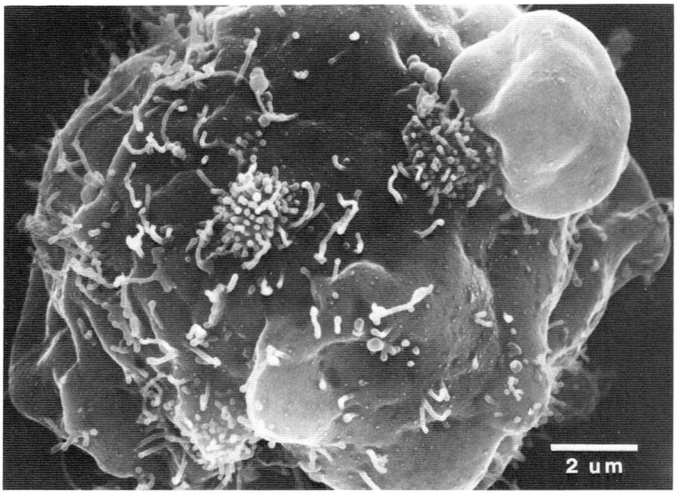

FIG. 25. Scanning EM of EATC following 20 min incubation with 1 mM PCMBS. Note large protruding bleb, smooth-surfaced areas, and small areas of closely packed microvilli. (From Trump et al., ref. 113, with permission.)

Membrane Channel Formers

A few studies have been carried out with membrane channel formers that have effects essentially similar to those of PCMBS. The antibiotic amphotericin B, which forms channels in high-cholesterol membranes, has been studied in hamster tracheal epithelium (115) and in the isolated toad bladder (78).

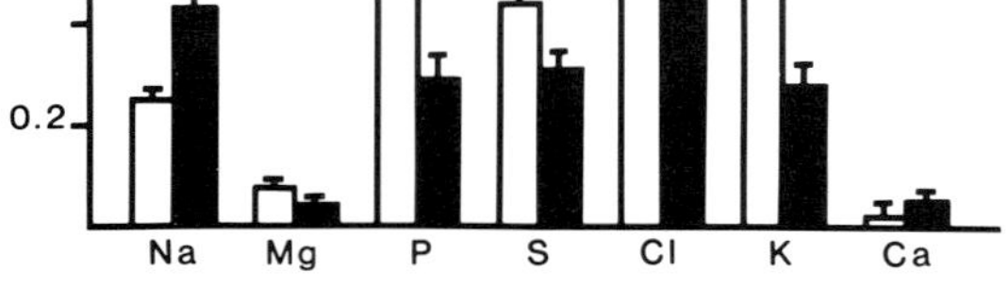

FIG. 26. *Bar graph* illustrating peak-to-background ratios ($P - B_1/B_2$) for Na, Mg, P, S, Cl, K, and Ca from X-ray microanalysis measurements obtained over 4-μm freeze-dried cryosections of hamster tracheobronchial epithelium following 3 days in culture. *White bars,* control; *black bars,* 2 hr treatment with amphotericin B.

In both cases, it results in marked increases in cellular sodium and water and decreases in potassium; calcium increases in parallel with sodium (Fig. 26). Some selectivity is typically seen in the tracheal epithelium, where the ciliated cells are most susceptible, whereas in the toad bladder, mitochondria-rich cells are most susceptible. During the early phase of cell swelling in both systems, the cells enter a pronounced stage III with dilated cytosol, swollen ER, and markedly condensed mitochondria (Figs. 27 and 28). If amphotericin B is utilized in the toad bladder in low-sodium media, calcification is greatly intensified, and numerous mitochondrial calcifications are noted. The interpretation, again, is one of diminished sodium–calcium exchange.

Complement

Activation of complement is known to produce acute cytolysis in a variety of cell types. It is known from the work of Mayer (53) and others to form ionophorous channels in the plasma membrane (Fig. 29). The results, then, are similar to those with PCMBS in that rapid cell swelling, initial mitochondrial condensation followed by swelling, and

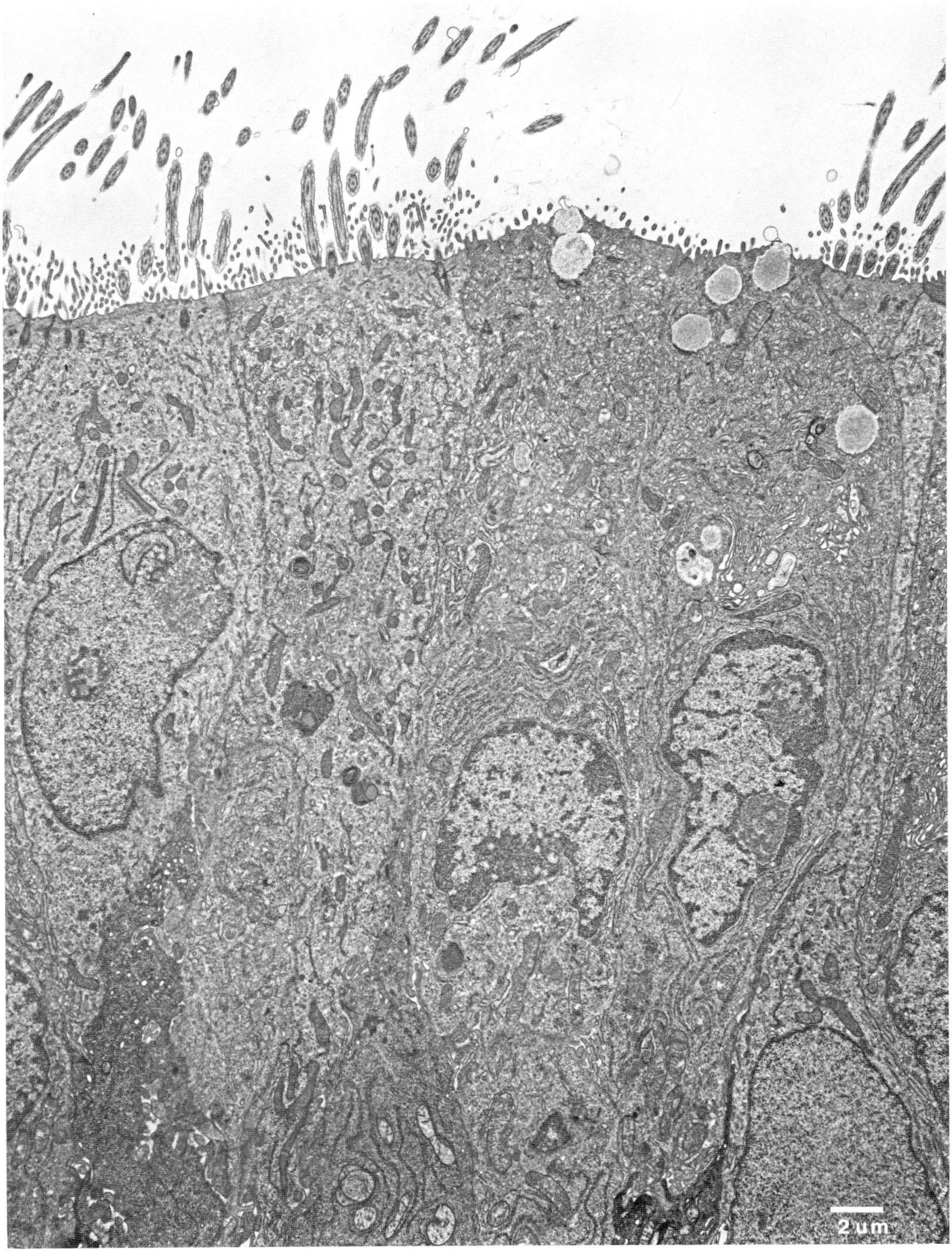

FIG. 27. Normal hamster tracheal epithelium after 3 days in culture showing ciliated, mucous, intermediate, and basal cells.

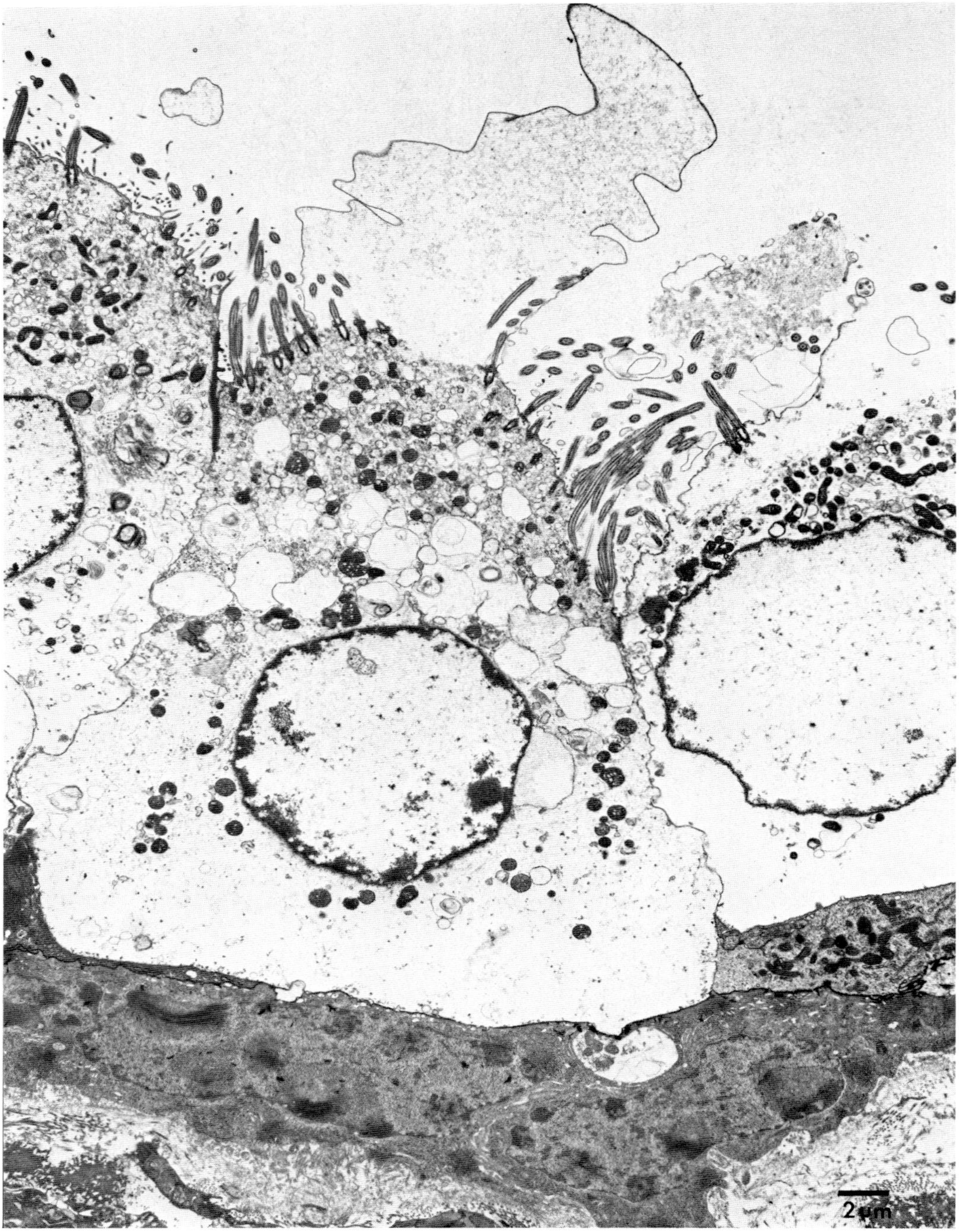

FIG. 28. Hamster tracheal epithelium in culture following 2-hr exposure to amphotericin B. Note the marked swelling of the cytosol and ER. Mitochondria are condensed, the nuclei show chromatin margination, and large blebs occur at the apical surfaces. Note that the basal and mucous cells are not swollen.

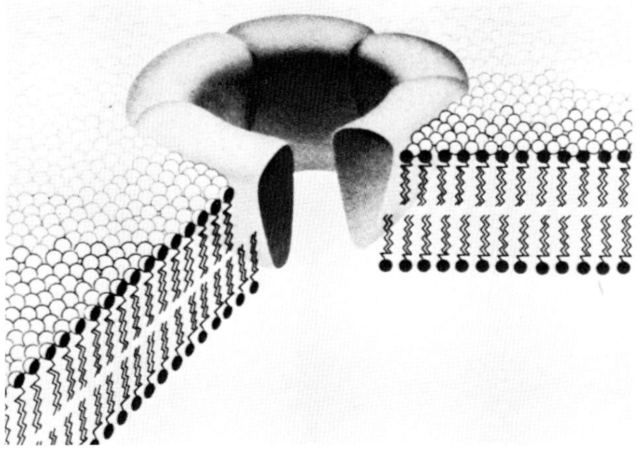

FIG. 29. Model of the structure of complement lesion. The structure is believed to consist of the five late-acting complement components C5b, C6, C7, C8, and C9, which are thought to attach themselves to the lipid bilayer of the cell membrane. The bilayer consists of lipid molecues stacked side by side with their polar heads pointing outward and their nonpolar fatty acid tails pointing inward. The complement components, which are proteins, are believed to assemble themselves into a doughnut or funnel shape that penetrates the bilayer. The hollow core of the structure could form the lesion through which water and ions flow into the cell until it bursts. (From Mayer, ref. 53, with permission.)

mitochondrial calcification occur (30). A similar conclusion was reached by Campbell and Luzio (9), who, using the protein oblein trapped in erythrocyte ghosts as a model system, proposed that the earliest intracellular event induced by the action of complement is an increase in cytosolic calcium. Of even greater interest is their observation that a rise in free calcium within the range of 0.1 to 1.0 μM leads to changes without lysis whereas rises to 10 μM lead to membrane damage. As mentioned above, 10 μM approximates the K_m for mitochondrial calcium uptake, and, therefore, precipitates of calcium in mitochondria would imply such a concentration. This may explain why calcium precipitates in mitochondria are seen virtually only in dead cells.

Ionophores

A number of studies have been performed using the calcium ionophore A23187; some of these were mentioned above. Depending on the dose, addition of the calcium ionophore has a wide range of effects from acute cell death at high concentrations to stimulation of cell division at lower concentrations (5). In the hamster tracheal epithelium (Fig. 30), addition of high doses (10^{-4} M) results in rapid cell swelling and massive dilatation of the ER (79). The ions responsible for the dilatation are not known but could include calcium as well as sodium. The cells rapidly detach from each other, which is consistent with the studies of Loewenstein and Rose (49) and others who observed that increased intracellular calcium is associated with cell–cell detachment. Eventually, mitochondrial swelling and cell death occur. In EATC, similar changes occur (Fig. 31). However, in these cells, little cell killing occurs in the presence of oxygen; rather, marked shape changes occur at the periphery as well as formation of autophagocytic vacuoles.

HYPOTHESIS AND SUMMARY

Figure 32 illustrates our current working hypothesis of the sequence of events following acute toxic lethal cell injury. The events above the broken line are considered to be reversible; the events accompanying cell death are shown below the broken line. The diagram summarizes several important events involving primary interactions with ATP

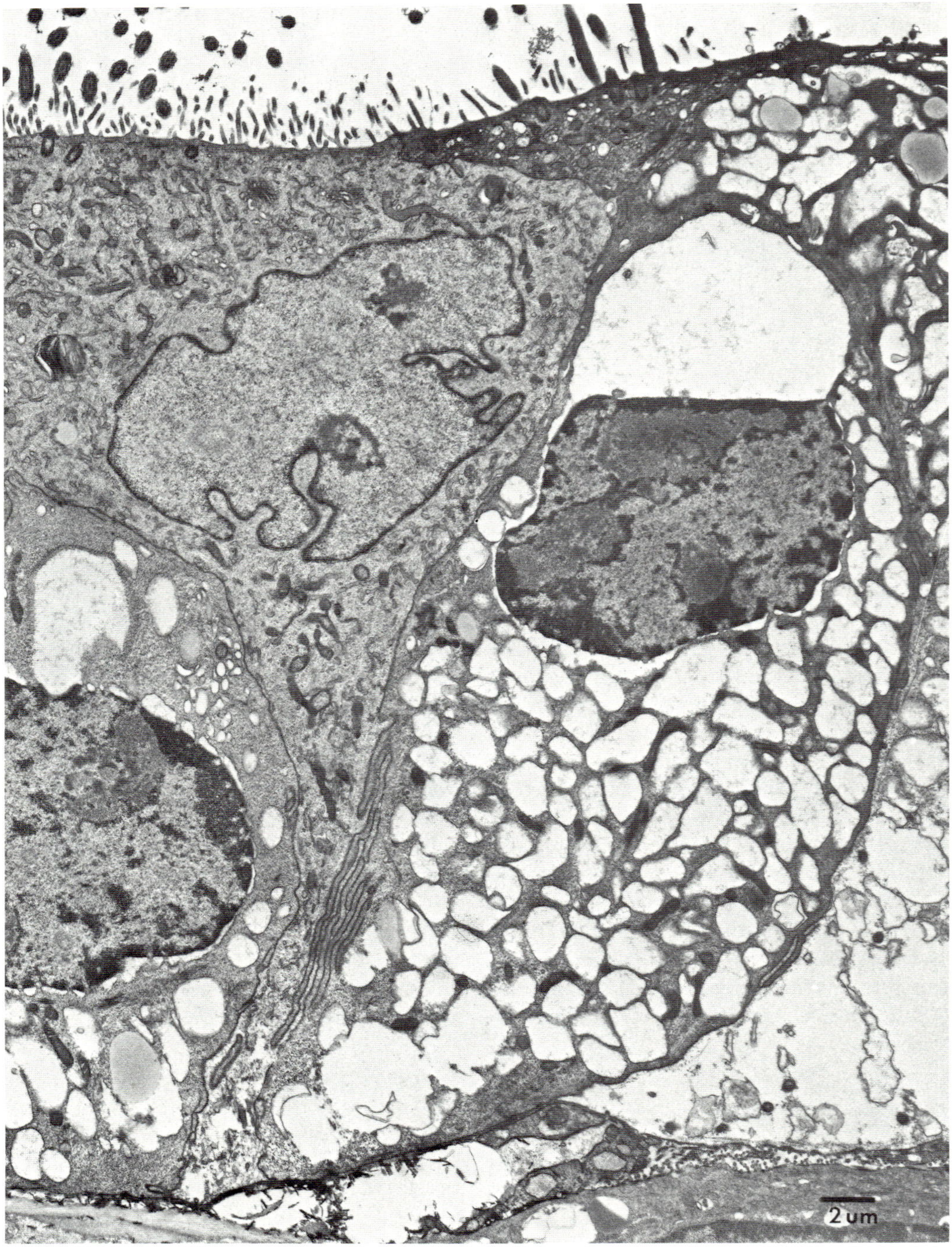

FIG. 30. Hamster tracheal epithelium in culture following 48-hr continuous exposure to 10^{-5} M A23187. Note marked vacuolization and distension of smooth endoplasmic reticulum, possibly suggesting calcium sequestration.

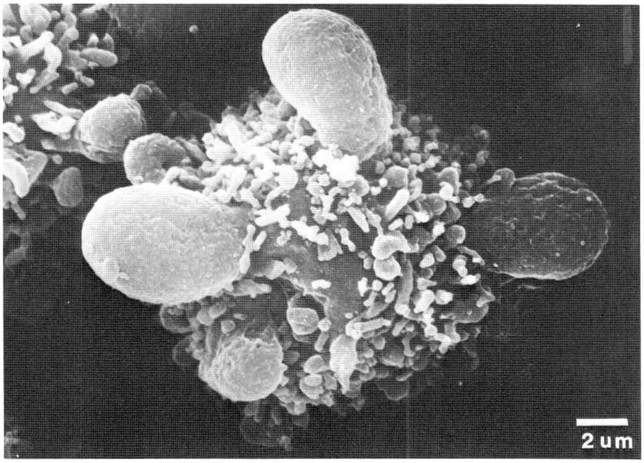

FIG. 31. Scanning EM of EATC following 60-min incubation with 10^{-3} M ionophore A23187 illustrating large surface blebs. (From Trump et al., ref. 102a, with permission.)

synthesis or cell membrane structure and function. The initial events focus on the control of sodium, calcium, and calcium–calmodulin complexes. The next series of events during the irreversible phase includes the early effects of calcium–calmodulin complexes, and the final events include irreversible steps accompanying cell death.

Inhibition of ATP Synthesis

Inhibition of ATP synthesis by various combinations of inhibition or uncoupling of mitochondrial oxidative phosphorylation and/or inhibition of glycolysis, depending on the cell type, results in rapid ATP deficiency. This has a number of immediate effects relevant to the hypothesis. The activity of the Na^+–K^+ ATPase in the cell membrane quickly diminishes through limitation of ATP synthesis. This results in increased concentrations of sodium in the cytosol as a function of time, decreased sodium–calcium exchange, increased cytosolic calcium, and activation of calcium–calmodulin complexes. The cytosolic calcium cannot be effectively buffered since both mitochondrial sequestration and ER uptake require substrate energy and/or oxygen. The effects of the calcium–calmodulin complex, as shown below, are, therefore, activated. ATP deficiency may also result in efflux of calcium from mitochondria and possibly other intracellular stores in the cytosol, thereby augmenting the effect. It should be reemphasized that calcium phosphate precipitates within the mitochondria cannot occur with total ischemia or total inhibition of mitochondrial function and, thus, are not features of totally ischemic areas of efflux. Note also that ATP deficiency in some cells may deactivate plasmalemmal calcium ATPases; these may be important in some cells, and this would also directly result in increased cytosolic calcium.

Plasma Membrane Integrity

Three types of primary injury to the plasma membrane structure and function are indicated: (a) direct inhibition of ATPase; (b) general increase in permeability; and (c) modification of channels, permitting entry of sodium. Also shown are calcium ionophores as compounds that facilitate entry of calcium from the extracellular fluid.

Rather general increases in membrane permeability can result from a variety of agents or conditions that modify cell membrane lipid and/or protein. These include membrane lipid peroxidation, common to many xenobiotic compounds and physical agents; modification of membrane protein sulfhydryl groups, e.g., with mercurials; activation of complement; and possibly direct

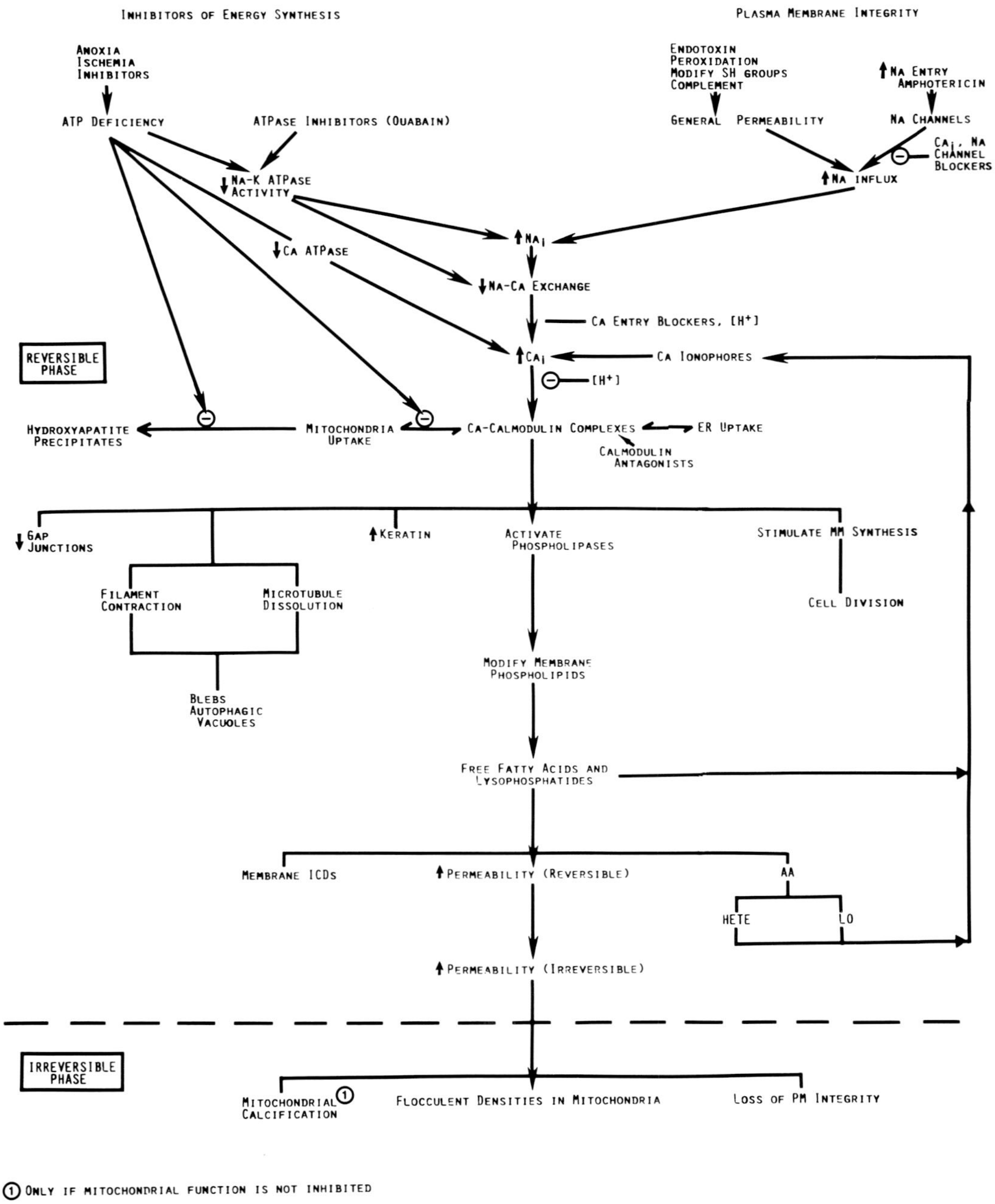

FIG. 32. Diagram illustrating our conceptualization of the relationships among sodium and calcium regulation, the cytoskeleton, and a number of pathological processes (see text for discussion).

effects of endotoxin. Again, this results in increased sodium influx and potassium efflux, from which point the stages proceed as indicated above. It should be noted, however, that with these modifications of permeability at the cell surface, cell death often proceeds much more rapidly and is accompanied by more dramatic volume changes. Another difference from energy deficiency is the fact that, in this case, as with treatment with ouabain or other cardiac glycosides, mitochondrial function is at least initially preserved, so the increased cytosolic calcium is quickly reflected by calcium phosphate precipitates in mitochondria.

The third case includes agents or conditions that more or less specifically increase sodium entry through channels, e.g., the antibiotic amphotericin. Again, the changes proceed rapidly and may be accompanied by mitochondrial calcification. In several of these cases, sodium entry may be modified by compounds such as amiloride, which retard sodium entry and thus may alleviate the rate of exchange (2).

With a calcium ionophore such as A23187, it is possible to bypass several of these steps and increase cell calcium directly. Calcium ionophores in oxygenated cells may not result in acute cell death because of mitochondrial or other buffering within the cytosol; at the same time, calcium ionophores in the presence of energy deficiency greatly accelerate the process. Other modifiers include calcium entry blockers, which may be able to modify calcium entry from the extracellular space and thus prevent or delay cell injury. One native calcium entry blocker may be metabolic acidosis, which is shown to be protective in several toxic types of cell injury. It has been rather well demonstrated in several cell types that protons are capable of blocking sodium–calcium exchange.

Consequences of Calcium–Calmodulin Activation

Many consequences obviously result in the cell following increased cytosolic calcium. We have selected several that seem to be of relevance in reversible and irreversible cell injury.

Reversible Phase

One of the early consequences of increased cytosolic calcium is decreased cell–cell communication through effects on gap junctions. This has been interpreted as a possible protective effect, especially in epithelia, since changes in one cell are not transmitted to the community. These changes in gap junctions may also be related to changes in membrane fluidity and redistribution of intramembranous particles, as has been described in some toxic injuries.

Another very early consequence is the formation of protrusions or blebs at the membrane surface, which may pinch off (113,114). Since agents capable of modifying microfilaments and/or microtubules are sufficient to produce this, it is our hypothesis that cytoskeletal modifications, including thin filaments and microtubules, result in these blebs. A similar phenomenon occurs within the cell, where blebs containing organelles and/or cytosol protrude into parts of the cytocavitary network, including the ER. These are termed autophagic vacuoles; they ultimately fuse with lysosomes, resulting in increased proteolysis and other types of organelle catabolism in the turnover period. These also represent irreversible changes occurring prior to cell death. If sublethal injury is prolonged, other cytoskeletal changes occur, including increased keratin synthesis in the presence of higher calcium levels, especially in epithelia.

Another sublethal effect that is rapidly stopped if the cell dies but which continues in marginally sublethal injured cells at the edge of the lesion includes stimulation of macromolecular synthesis and cell division. There are many studies implicating increased sodium and/or calcium as a possible trigger in such cell division.

The most significant change leading to cell death in our hypothesis is calcium activation of phospholipases such as phospholipase A_1 and phospholipase C. This results in modification of membrane phospholipid, resulting in modification and release of free fatty acids and lysophosphatides among other events, and has a number of important consequences through the cell. Some of these products may themselves act as ionophores, further perpetuating the change. In addition, some of the products may also result in the characteristic intracristal densities (ICDs) within mitochondria, which may represent inner membrane adhesions and/or fusions. Products such as arachidonic acid are metabolized through the HETE pathway or cyclooxygenase pathway to form a variety of mediators. Some of these may be protective, and others injurious, in addition to having ionophorous activity. Finally, modification of phospholids leads to total breakdown of permeability barriers, resulting in irreversible damage. The characteristics of the irreversible phase include mitochondrial calcium phosphate precipitates (in systems in which mitochondrial function is not totally inhibited) and mitochondrial flocculent densities. These seem to represent the denatured matrix and/or membrane proteins and typify irreversible change in a variety of cell types, including loss of cell membrane integrity characterized by vital dye uptake and loss of macromolecules from the cytosol, e.g., lactic dehydrogenase.

Although many more studies are needed on these phenomena in order to completely understand all of the processes involved, we feel that our model, as presented here, could eventually establish the fact that a wide variety of pathological processes are actually all a common series of reactions linked with volume regulation and sodium modification through mechanisms such as sodium–calcium exchange and, furthermore, that these processes are coupled with interactions of the cytoskeleton and the cell membrane. In addition, it is evident that therapeutic interventions designed to manipulate these processes could potentially result in the control and possible prevention of many human diseases.

ACKNOWLEDGMENT

B. F. Trump is an American Cancer Society Professor of Oncology. Research supported in part by NIH Grants AM 15540 and NOICP15738.

REFERENCES

1. Barrett, L. A., McDowell, E. M., Harris, C. C., and Trump, B. F. (1977): Studies on the pathogenesis of ischemic cell injury. XV. Reversal of ischemic cell injury in hamster trachea and human bronchus by explant culture. *Beitr. Pathol.*, 161:109–121.
2. Benos, D. J. (1982): Amiloride: A molecular probe of sodium transport in tissues and cells. *Am. J. Physiol.*, 242:C131–C145.
3. Blaustein, M. P. (1974): The interrelationship between Na and Ca fluxes across cell membranes. *Rev. Physiol. Biochem. Pharmacol.*, 70:33–82.
4. Blaustein, M. P. (1977): Sodium ions, blood pressure regulation and hypertension: A reassessment and a hypothesis. *Am. J. Physiol.*, 232:C165–C173.
5. Borle, A. B., and Studer, R. (1978): Effects of calcium ionophores on the transport and distribution of calcium in isolated cells and in liver and kidney slices. *J. Membr. Biol.*, 38:51–72.
6. Brinkley, B. R. (1982): The cytoskeleton: A perspective. In: *Methods in Cell Biology, Vol. 24, The Cytoskeleton. Part A: Cytoskeletal Proteins, Isolation and Characterization,* edited by L. Wilson, pp. 1–8. Academic Press, New York.
7. Brinley, F. J., Jr. (1978): Calcium-buffering in squid axons. *Annu. Rev. Biophys. Bioeng.*, 7:363–392.
8. Brohn, F. H., and Clarkson, A. B. (1978): Quantitative effects of salycylhydroxamic acid and glycerol on *Trypanosoma brucci* glycolysis *in vitro* and *in vivo. Acta Trop.*, 35:23–33.
9. Campbell, A. K., and Luzio, J. P. (1981): Intracellular free calcium as a pathogen in cell damage initiated by the immune system. *Experientia,* 37:1110–1112.
10. Carafoli, E. (1982): Membrane transport and the regulation of cell calcium levels. In: *Pathophysiology of Shock, Anoxia and Ischemia,* edited by R. A. Cowley and B. F. Trump, pp. 95–111. Williams & Wilkins, Baltimore.
11. Carafoli, E., and Crompton, M. (1976): Calcium ions and mitochondria. *Soc. Exp. Biol. Symp.*, 30:89–115.
12. Casini, A. F., and Farber, J. L. (1981): Dependence of the carbon tetrachloride-induced death of cultured hepatocytes on the extracellular calcium concentration. *Am. J. Pathol.*, 105:138–148.
13. Cheah, K. S., and Cheah, A. M. (1977): Inclusions in aged mitochondria. *J. Bioenerg. Biomembr.*, 9:105–115.
14. Cheung, Y. W. (1980): Calmodulin plays a pivotal role in cellular regulation. *Science,* 207:19–27.
15. Cheung, W. Y. (1982): Calmodulin: An overview. *Fed. Proc.*, 41:2253–2256.
16. Clarkson, A. B., Jr., and Amole, B. O. (1982): Role of calcium in trypanocidal drug action. *Science,* 216:1321–1323.
17. Corr, P. B., Cain, M. E., Witkowski, F. X., Price, D. A., and Sobel, B. E. (1979): Potential arrhythmogenic electrophysiological derangements in canine Purkinje fibers induced by lysophosphoglycerides. *Circ. Res.*, 44:822–832.
18. Darsee, J. R., and Kloner, R. A. (1981): Depen-

dency of location of salvageable myocardium on type of intervention. *Am. J. Cardiol.*, 48:702–710.
19. Edmonson, J. W., and Bang, N. U. (1981): Deleterious effects of calcium deprivation on freshly isolated hepatocytes. *Am. J. Physiol.*, 241:C3–C8.
20. Gerson, D. F., Kiefer, H., and Eufe, W. (1982): Intracellular pH of mitogen-stimulated lymphocytes. *Science*, 216:1009–1010.
21. Ginn, F. L., Shelburne, J. D., and Trump, B. F. (1968): Disorders of cell volume regulation. I. Effects of inhibition of plasma membrane adenosine triphosphatase with ouabain. *Am. J. Pathol.*, 53:1041–1071.
22. Ginn, F. L., and Trump, B. F. (1970): Ultrastructural changes after ultraviolet irradiation of isolated flounder kidney tubules. *Lab. Invest.*, 22:496.
23. Glaumann, B., Glaumann, H., Berezesky, I. K., and Trump, B. F. (1975): Studies on the pathogenesis of ischemic cell injury. II. Morphological changes of the pars convoluta (P_1 and P_2) of the proximal tubule of the rat kidney made ischemic *in vivo*. *Virchows Arch.* [*Cell Pathol.*], 19:281–302.
24. Glaumann, B., Glaumann, H., Berezesky, I. K., and Trump, B. F. (1977): Studies on cellular recovery from injury. II. Ultrastructural studies on the recovery of the pars convoluta of the proximal tubule of the rat kidney from temporary ischemia. *Virchows Arch.* [*Cell Pathol.*], 24:1–18.
25. Glaumann, B., Glaumann, H., and Trump, B. F. (1977): Studies of cellular recovery from injury. III. Ultrastructural studies of the recovery of the pars recta of the proximal tubule (P_3 segment) of the rat kidney from temporary ischemia. *Virchows Arch.* [*Cell Pathol.*], 25:281–308.
26. Glaumann, B., and Trump, B. F. (1975): Studies on the pathogenesis of ischemic cell injury. III. Morphological changes of the proximal pars recta tubules (P_3) of the rat kidney made ischemic *in vivo*. *Virchows Arch.* [*Cell Pathol.*], 19:303–323.
27. Goracci, G., Porcellati, G., and Woelk, H. (1979): Subcellular localization and distribution of phospholipases A in liver and brain tissue. *Adv. Prostaglandin Thromboxane Res.*, 3:55–67.
28. Gritzka, T. L., and Trump, B. F. (1968): Renal tubular lesions caused by mercuric chloride. Electron microscopic observations: Degeneration of the pars recta. *Am. J. Pathol.*, 52:1225–1277.
29. Hanzlikova, V., and Schiaffino, S. (1977): Mitochondrial changes in ischemic skeletal muscle. *J. Ultrastruct. Res.*, 60:121–133.
30. Hawkins, H. K., Ericsson, J. L. E., Biberfeld, P., and Trump, B. F. (1972): Lysosome and phagosome stability in lethal cell injury. *Am. J. Pathol.*, 68:255–287.
31. Hennings, H., Michael, D., Cheng, C., Steinert, P., Holbrook, K., and Yuspa, S. H. (1980): Calcium regulation of growth and differentiation of mouse epidermal cells in culture. *Cell*, 19:245–254.
32. Hochachka, P. W. (1980): *Closed and Open Systems in Hypoxia Tolerance.* Harvard University Press, Cambridge.
33. Jewell, S. A., Bellomo, G., Thor, H., Orrenius, S., and Smith, M. (1982): Bleb formation in hepatocytes during drug metabolism is caused by disturbances in thiol and calcium ion homeostasis. *Science*, 217:1257–1259.
34. Jones, R. T., Garcia, J. H., Mergner, W. J., Pendergrass, R. E., Valigorsky, J. M., and Trump, B. F. (1975): Effects of shock on the pancreatic acinar cell. Cellular and subcellular effects in humans. *Arch. Pathol.*, 99:634–644.
35. Jugdutt, B. I., Hutchins, G. M., Bulkley, B. H., and Becker, L. C. (1980): Salvage of ischemic myocardium by ibuprofen during infarction in the conscious dog. *Am. J. Cardiol.*, 46:74–82.
36. Kahng, M. W., Berezesky, I. K., and Trump, B. F. (1978): Metabolic and ultrastructural response of rat kidney cortex to *in vitro* ischemia. *Exp. Mol. Pathol.*, 29:183–198.
37. Karpati, G., Carpenter, S., Melmed, C., and Eisen, A. A. (1974): Experimental ischemic myopathy. *J. Neurol. Sci.*, 23:129–161.
38. Laiho, K. U., Berezesky, I. K., and Trump, B. F. (1983): Studies on the modification of the cellular response to injury. Effect of mannitol on Ehrlich ascites tumor cells following injury by anoxia or *p*-chloromercuribenzene sulfonic acid (PCMBS). *Exp. Mol. Pathol.*, 13.
39. Laiho, K. U., Berezesky, I. K., and Trump, B. F. (1982): Studies on the modification of the cellular response to injury. Effect of the ionophore A23187 on Ehrlich ascites tumor cells following injury by anoxia or *p*-chloromercuribenzene sulfonic acid (*in press*).
40. Laiho, K. U., Berezesky, I. K., and Trump, B. F. (1983): The role of calcium in cell injury. Studies in Ehlich ascites tumor cells following anoxia and organic mercurials. *Surv. Synth. Pathol. Res.* (*in press*).
41. Laiho, K. U., Shelburne, J. D., and Trump, B. F. (1971): Observations on cell volume, ultrastructure, mitochondrial conformation and vital-dye uptake in Ehrlich ascites tumor cells: Effects of inhibiting energy production and function of the plasma membrane. *Am. J. Pathol.*, 65:203–230.
42. Laiho, K. U., and Trump, B. F. (1974): Relationship of ionic, water, and cell volume changes in cellular injury of Ehrlich ascites tumor cells. *Lab. Invest.*, 31:207–215.
43. Laiho, K. U., and Trump, B. F. (1974): The relationship between cell viability and changes in mitochondrial ultrastructure, cellular ATP, ion and water content following injury of Ehrlich ascites tumor cells. *Virchows Arch.* [*Cell Pathol.*], 15:267–277.
44. Laiho, K. U., and Trump, B. F. (1975): Studies on the pathogenesis of cell injury. Effects of inhibitors of metabolism and membrane function on the mitochondria of Ehrlich ascites tumor cells. *Lab. Invest.*, 32:163–182.
45. Laiho, K. U., and Trump, B. F. (1975): Mitochondrial changes, ion and water shifts in the cellular injury of Ehrlich ascites tumor cells. *Beitr. Pathol.*, 155:237–247.
46. Lefer, A. M., and Crossley, K. (1980): Mechanisms of the optimal protective effects of ibuprofen in acute myocardial ischemia. *Adv. Shock Res.*, 3:133–141.

47. Lehninger, A. (1970): *Biochemistry,* p. 59. Worth, New York.
48. Lieberman, M., Adam, W. J., and Bullock, P. N. (1980): The cultured heart cell: Problems and prospects. In: *Methods in Cell Biology, Vol. 21,* edited by C. C. Harris, B. F. Trump, and G. D. Stoner, pp. 187–204. Academic Press, New York, London.
49. Loewenstein, W. R., and Rose, B. (1978): Calcium in (junctional) intercellular communication and a thought on its behavior in intracellular communication. *Ann. N.Y. Acad. Sci.,* 307:285–307.
50. Maclean, D., Fishbein, M. C., Blum, R. I., Braunwald, E., and Maroko, P. R. (1978): Long-term preservation of ischemic myocardium by ibuprofen after experimental coronary artery occlusion. *Am. J. Cardiol.,* 41:394.
51. Majno, G., Lagattuta, M., and Thompson, T. (1960): Cellular death and necrosis; chemical, physical and morphological changes in rat liver. *Virchow Arch.* [*Pathol. Anat.*], 333:421–465.
52. Marcum, J. M., Dedman, J. R., Brinkley, B. F., and Means, A. R. (1978): *Proc. Natl. Acad. Sci. U.S.A.,* 75:3771–3775.
53. Mayer, M. M. (1973): The complement system. *Sci. Am.,* 229:54–66.
54. Means, A. R., and Dedman, J. R. (1980): Calmodulin—An intracellular calcium receptor. *Nature,* 285:73–77.
55. Mergner, W. J., Chang, S. H., Marzella, L., Kahng, M. W., and Trump, B. F. (1979): Studies on the pathogenesis of ischemic cell injury. VIII. ATPase of rat kidney mitochondria. *Lab. Invest.,* 40:686–694.
56. Mergner, W. J., Smith, M. W., Sahaphong, S., and Trump, B. F. (1977): Studies on the pathogenesis of ischemic cell injury. VI. Accumulation of calcium by isolated mitochondria of ischemic rat kidney cortex. *Virchows Arch.* [*Cell Pathol.*], 26:1–16.
57. Mergner, W. J., Smith, M. W., and Trump, B. F. (1977): Studies on the pathogenesis of ischemic cell injury. XI. P/O ratio and acceptor control. *Virchows Arch.* [*Cell Pathol.*], 26:17–26.
58. Mergner, W. J., Smith, M. W., and Trump, B. F. (1977): Studies on the pathogenesis of ischemic cell injury. IV. Alteration of ionic permeability of mitochondria from ischemic rat kidney. *Exp. Mol. Pathol.,* 26:1–12.
59. Murphy, E., Coll, K., Rich, T. L., and Williamson, J. R. (1980): Hormonal effects on calcium homeostasis in isolated hepatocytes. *J. Biol. Chem.,* 255:6600–6608.
59a. Nicholson, G. L., Giotta, G., Lotan, R., Neri, A., and Poste, G. (1977): Modifications in transformed and malignant cells. In: *International Cell Biology,* edited by B. R. Brinkley, and K. R. Porter, pp. 138–148. Rockefeller University Press, New York.
60. Osornio, A. R., Berezesky, I. K., Mergner, W. M., and Trump, B. F. (1980): Mitochondrial membrane fusions in experimental myocardial infarction. *Fed. Proc.,* 39:634.
61. Osornio-Vargas, A. R., Berezesky, I. K., and Trump, B. F. (1981): Effects of the nonsteroidal anti-inflammatory drug ibuprofen on the pathogenesis of acute myocardial infarction in the rat. *Fed. Proc.,* 40:751.
62. Osornio-Vargas, A. R., Berezesky, I. K., and Trump, B. F. (1981): Progression of ion movements during acute myocardial infarction in the rat. An X-ray microanalysis study. *Scan. Electron Microsc.,* 2:463–472.
63. Osornio-Vargas, A. R., Berezesky, I. K., and Trump, B. F. (1983): Mitochondrial intracristal densities. An early ultrastructural change in the evolution of myocardial infarction in the rat (*in press*).
64. Osornio-Vargas, A. R., Berezesky, I. K., and Trump, B. F. (1983): Mitochondrial intracristal densities. Their nature and possible significance in myocardial ischemia (*in press*).
65. Osornio-Vargas, A. R., Berezesky, I. K., and Trump, B. F. (1983): Modification of myocardial infarction. Ameliorating effects of ibuprofen in the rat (*in press*).
66. Paul, R. J., Bauer, M., and Prease, W. (1979): Vascular smooth muscle: Aerobic glycolysis linked to sodium and potassium transport processes. *Science,* 206:1414–1416.
67. Penttila, A., Glaumann, H., and Trump, B. F. (1976): Studies on the modification of the cellular response to injury. IV. Protective effect of extracellular acidosis against anoxia, thermal, and *p*-chloromercuribenzene sulfonic acid treatment of isolated rat liver cells. *Life Sci.,* 18:1419–1430.
68. Penttila, A., and Trump, B. F. (1974): Extracellular acidosis protects Ehrlich ascites tumor cells and rat renal cortex against anoxic injury. *Science,* 185:277–278.
69. Penttila, A., and Trump, B. F. (1975): Studies on modification of the cellular response to injury. I. Protective effect of acidosis on *p*-chloromercuribenzene sulfonic acid-induced injury of Ehrlich ascites tumor cells. *Lab. Invest.,* 32:690–695.
70. Penttila, A., and Trump, B. F. (1975): Studies on modification of the cellular response to injury. II. Electron microscopic studies on the protective effect of acidosis on anoxic injury of Ehrlich ascites tumor cells. *Virchows Arch.* [*Cell Pathol.*], 18:1–16.
71. Penttila, A., and Trump, B. F. (1975): Studies on the modification of the cellular response to injury. III. Electron microscopic studies on the protective effect of acidosis on *p*-chloromercuribenzene sulfonic acid-(PCMBS) induced injury of Ehrlich ascites tumor cells. *Virchows Arch.* [*Cell Pathol.*], 18:17–34.
72. Philipson, K. D., Bersohn, M. M., and Nishimoto, A. Y. (1982): Effects of pH on Na^+–Ca^{2+} exchange in canine cardiac sarcolemmal vesicles. *Circ. Res.,* 50:287–293.
73. Porter, K. R. (1981): The ground substance of the living cell. *Sci. Am.,* 244:56–67.
74. Reimer, K. A., and Jennings, R. B. (1982): Ion and water shifts, cellular. In: *Pathophysiology of Shock, Anoxia, and Ischemia,* edited by R. A. Cowley and B. F. Trump, pp. 132–146. Williams & Wilkins, Baltimore.
75. Roos, A., and Boron, W. F. (1981): Intracellular pH. *Physiol. Rev.,* 61:296–434.
76. Sahaphong, S., and Trump, B. F. (1971): Studies of cellular injury in isolated kidney tubules of the

flounder. V. Effects of inhibiting sulfhydryl groups of plasma membrane with the organic mercurials PCMB (parachloromercuribenzoate) and PCMBS (parachloromercuribenzenesulfonate). *Am. J. Pathol.*, 63:277–298.

77. Saito, A., Smigel, M., and Fleisher, S. (1974): Membrane junctions in the intermembrane space of mitochondria from mammalian tissues. *J. Cell Biol.*, 60:653–663.
78. Saladino, A. J., Bentley, P. J., and Trump, B. F. (1969): Ion movements in cell injury. Effect of amphotericin B on the ultrastructure and function of the epithelial cells of the toad bladder. *Am. J. Pathol.*, 54:421–466.
79. Saladino, A. J., Berezesky, I. K., Resau, J. H., and Trump, B. F. (1982): Ionophore A23187 causes hyperplasia in hamster tracheal epithelium. *Fed. Proc.*, 41:740.
80. Sasaki, Y., and Hidaka, H. (1982): Calmodulin and cell proliferation. *Biochem. Biophys. Res. Commun.*, 104:451–456.
81. Sato, T., Berezesky, I. K., Nakatani, T., and Trump, B. F. (1982): The role of extracellular (EC) calcium on isolated rat proximal tubule cells. *J. Cell Biol.*, 95:466a.
82. Schanne, F. A. X., Kane, A. B., Young, E. E., and Farber, J. L. (1979): Calcium dependence of toxic cell death: A final common pathway. *Science*, 206:700–702.
83. Schiaffino, S., Severin, E., and Hanzlikova, V. (1979): Intermembrane inclusions induced by anoxia in heart and skeletal muscle mitochondrial. *Virchows Arch.* [*Cell Pathol.*], 31:169–179.
84. Segal, J., and Ingbar, S. H. (1982): A postulated mechanism for the coordinate effects of ionophore A23187 on calcium uptake and cell viability in rat thymocytes. *Biochim. Biophys. Acta*, 684:7–11.
85. Smith, M. T., Thor, H., and Orrenius, S. (1981): Toxic injury to isolated hepatocytes is not dependent on extracellular calcium. *Science*, 213:1257–1259.
86. Smith, M. W., Collan, Y., Kahng, M. W., and Trump, B. F. (1980): Changes of fatty acids and phospholipids in ischemic rat kidney. *Biochim. Biophys. Acta*, 168:192–201.
87. Sobel, B. E., Corr, P. B., Robison, A. K., Goldstein, R. A., Witkowski, F. X., and Klein, M. S. (1978): Accumulation of lysophosphoglycerides with arrhythmogenic properties in ischemic myocardium. *J. Clin. Invest.*, 62:546–553.
88. Sporn, M. B., and Newton, D. L. (1979): Chemoprevention of cancer with retinoids. *Fed. Proc.*, 38:2528–2534.
89. Stacey, N. H., and Klaassen, C. D. (1982): Lack of protection against chemically induced injury to isolated hepatocytes by omission of calcium from the incubation medium. *J. Toxicol. Environ. Health*, 9:267–276.
90. Taylor, A., and Windhager, E. E. (1979): Possible role of cytosolic calcium and Na–Ca exchange in regulation of transepithelial sodium transport. *Am. J. Physiol.*, 236:F505–F512.
91. Trump, B. F., and Arstila, A. U. (1975): Cellular reaction to injury. In: *Principles of Pathobiology*, second edition, edited by M. F. LaVia, and R. B. Hill, Jr., pp. 9–96. Oxford University Press, New York.
92. Trump, B. F., Berezesky, I. K., Chang, S. H., and Bulger, R. E. (1976): Detection of ion shifts in proximal tubule cells of the rat kidney using X-ray microanalysis. *Virchows Arch.* [*Cell Pathol.*], 22:111–120.
93. Trump, B. F., Berezesky, I. K., Chang, S. H., Pendergrass, R. E., and Mergner, W. J. (1979): The role of ion shifts in cell injury. *Scan. Electron. Microsc.*, 3:1–14.
94. Trump, B. F., Berezesky, I. K., Collan, Y., Kahng, M. W., and Mergner, W. J. (1976): Recent studies on the pathophysiology of ischemic cell injury. *Beitr. Pathol.*, 158:363–388.
95. Trump, B. F., Berezesky, I. K., and Cowley, R. A. (1982): The cellular and subcellular characteristics of acute and chronic injury with emphasis on the role of calcium. In: *Pathophysiology of Shock, Anoxia and Ischemia*, edited by R. A. Cowley and B. F. Trump, pp. 6–46. Williams & Wilkins, Baltimore.
96. Trump, B. F., Berezesky, I. K., Laiho, K. U., Osornio, A. R., Mergner, W. J., and Smith, M. W. (1980): The role of calcium in cell injury. A review. *Scan. Electron Microsc.*, 2:437–462.
97. Trump, B. F., Berezesky, I. K., Mergner, W. J., and Phelps, P. C. (1978): The role of calcium in cell injury. *Micron*, 9:5–6.
98. Trump, B. F., Berezesky, I. K., and Osornio-Vargas, A. R. (1981): Role of Na^+ and Ca^{2+} regulation in the initiation of membrane changes in myocardial cell injury. *J. Cell Biol.*, 91:282a.
99. Trump, B. F., Berezesky, I. K., and Osornio-Vargas, A. R. (1981): Cell death and the disease process. The role of calcium. In: *Cell Death*, edited by I. D. Bowen and R. A. Lockshin, pp. 209–242. Chapman and Hall, London.
100. Trump, B. F., Berezesky, I. K., Pendergrass, R. E., Chang, S. H., Bulger, R. E., and Mergner, W. J. (1978): X-ray microanalysis of diffusible elements of scanning electron microscopy of biological thin sections. Studies of pathologically altered cells. *Scan Electron Microsc.*, 2:1027–1039.
101. Trump, B. F., Berezesky, I. K., and Phelps, P. C. (1981): Sodium and calcium regulation and the role of the cytoskeleton in the pathogenesis of disease. A review and hypothesis. *Scan Electron Microsc.*, 2:435–545.
102. Trump, B. F., Berezesky, I. K., and Phelps, P. C. (1981): The role of altered sodium and calcium regulation and the cytoskeleton in the pathogenesis of human disease. *J. Clin. Electron Microsc.*, 14:366–369.

102a. Trump, B. F., Berezesky, I. K., Phelps, P. C., and Jones, R. T. (1983): An overview of the role of membranes in human disease. In: *Cellular Pathology of Human Disease*, edited by B. F. Trump, R. J. Jones, and A. Laufer, pp. 3–48. Gustav Fischer, New York.

103. Trump, B. F., and Bulger, R. E. (1968): Studies of cellular injury in isolated flounder tubules. III. Light microscopic and functional changes due to cyanide. *Lab. Invest.*, 18:721–730.
104. Trump, B. F., and Bulger, R. E. (1968): Studies of

cellular injury in isolated flounder tubules. IV. Electron microscopic observations of changes during the phase of altered homeostasis in tubules treated with cyanide. *Lab. Invest.*, 18:731–739.

105. Trump, B. F., Croker, B. P., and Mergner, W. J. (1971): The role of energy metabolism, ion, and water shifts in the pathogenesis of cell injury. In: *Cell Membranes: Biological and Pathological Aspects*, edited by G. W. Richter and D. G. Scarpelli, pp. 84–128. Williams & Wilkins, Baltimore.
106. Trump, B. F., and Ginn, F. L. (1969): The pathogenesis of subcellular reaction to lethal injury. In: *Methods and Achievements in Experimental Pathology, Vol. IV*, edited by E. Bajusz, and G. Jasmin, pp. 1–29. S. Karger, Basel.
107. Trump, B. F., Jesudason, M. L., and Jones, R. T. (1978): Ultrastructural features of diseased cells. In: *Diagnostic Electron Microscopy, Vol. I*, edited by B. F. Trump and R. T. Jones, pp. 1–88. John Wiley & Sons, New York.
108. Trump, B. F., and Laiho, K. U. (1975): Studies of cellular recovery from injury. I. Recovery from anoxia in Ehrlich ascites tumor cells. *Lab. Invest.*, 33:706–711.
109. Trump, B. F., Laiho, K. U., Mergner, W. J., and Arstila, A. U. (1974): Studies on the subcellular pathophysiology of acute lethal cell injury. *Beitr. Pathol.*, 152:243–271.
110. Trump, B. F., McDowell, E. M., and Arstila, A. U. (1980): Cellular reaction to injury. In: *Principles of Pathobiology*, Third Edition, edited by R. B. Hill, Jr. and M. F. LaVia, pp. 20–111. Oxford University Press, New York.
111. Trump, B. F., and Mergner, W. J. (1974): Cell injury. In: *The Inflammatory Process, Vol. I*, Second Edition, edited by B. W. Zweifach, L. Grant, and R. T. McClusky, pp. 115–257. Academic Press, New York.
112. Trump, B. F., Mergner, W. M., Kahng, M. W., and Saladino, A. J. (1976): Studies on the subcellular pathophysiology of ischemia. *Circulation*, 53(Suppl. I):17–26.
113. Trump, B. F., Pentilla, A., and Berezesky, I. K. (1979): Studies on cell surface conformation following injury. I. Scanning and transmission electron microscopy of cell surface changes following p-chloromercuribenzene sulfonic acid (PCMBS)-induced injury of Ehrlich ascites tumor cells. *Virchows Arch.* [*Cell Pathol.*], 29:281–296.
114. Trump, B. F., Pentilla, A., and Berezesky, I. K. (1979): Studies on cell surface conformation following injury. II. Scanning and transmission electron microscopy of cell surface changes following anoxic injury in Ehrlich ascites tumor cells. *Virchows Arch.* [*Cell Pathol.*], 29:297–307.
115. Trump, B. F., Saladino, A. J., Berezesky, I. K., and Resau, J. H. (1982): A Na ionophore results in metaplasia and hyperplasia in the hamster tracheobronchial epithelium (HTBE). *Fed. Proc.*, 41:491.

115a. Trump, B. F., Sato, T., Berezesky, I. K., and Laiho, K. U. (1983): Cell calcium (Ca_i) and anoxic cell death. *Fed. Proc.*, 42:661.

116. Trump, B. F., Strum, J. M., and Bulger, R. E. (1974): Studies on the pathogenesis of ischemic cell injury. I. Relation between ion and water shifts and cell ultrastructure in rat kidney slices during swelling at 0–4°C. *Virchows Arch.* [*Cell Pathol.*], 16:1–34.
117. Trump, B. F., Valigorsky, J. M., Jones, R. T., Mergner, W. J., Garcia, J. H., and Cowley, R. A. (1975): The application of electron microscopy and cellular biochemistry to the autopsy. Observations on cellular changes in human shock. *Hum. Pathol.*, 6:499–516.
118. Voorheis, H. P., Bowles, D. J., and Smith, G. A. (1982): Characteristics of the release of the surface coat protein from bloodstream forms of *Trypanosoma brucei*. *J. Biol. Chem.*, 257:2300–2304.
119. Welsh, M. J., Aster, J. C., Ireland, M., Alcala, J., and Maisel, H. (1982): Calmodulin binds to chick lens gap junction protein in a calcium-independent manner. *Science*, 216:642–643.
120. White, B. C., Gadzinski, D. S., Hoehner, P. J., Krome, C., Hoehner, T., White, J. D., and Trombley, J. H., Jr. (1982): Effect of flunarizine on canine cerebral cortical blood flow and vascular resistance post cardiac arrest. *Ann. Emerg. Med.*, 11:119–126.

Drug Metabolism and Drug Toxicity,
edited by J. R. Mitchell and M. G. Horning.
Raven Press, New York © 1984.

Reactive Metabolites and the Pathophysiology of Acute Lethal Cell Injury

J. R. Mitchell, C. V. Smith, B. H. Lauterburg, H. Hughes, G. B. Corcoran, and E. C. Horning

Department of Medicine and Institute for Lipid Research, Baylor College of Medicine, Houston, Texas 77030

Drug-induced tissue lesions are nearly always of grave concern to the physician and often lead to organ failure or even death of the patient. These toxic drug reactions are also the major impediment to the rapid development of new chemical entities into useful therapeutic agents. Elucidation of their underlying pathogenetic mechanisms has not been possible in the past and attempts to explain them on the basis of the chemical structure of the parent drug have failed, as is readily apparent from a quick comparison of such strikingly different compounds as paraquat and nitrofurantoin which nevertheless appear to share similar pulmonary toxicities. The discovery that many drug-induced tissue lesions are initiated by the formation of chemically reactive metabolites from the drugs has made it possible to begin to classify and arrange the reactions into general groups. Thus, many of the drug-induced tissue lesions might best be understood, categorized, and ultimately predicted on the basis of the nature of the chemically reactive intermediate that is initiating the drug injuries. However, an interdisciplinary, highly integrated approach is necessary in order to correlate the formation of chemically reactive metabolites with the incidence, types, and severities of toxicities caused by drugs and other foreign compounds. One needs to correlate the findings of several different kinds of studies, including the measurement of the biological half-life of the drug, the quantitative isolation of urinary drug metabolites, the determination of the amount of covalent binding of reactive metabolites both *in vivo* and *in vitro*, and the measurement of tissue peroxidative reactions. Determination of the effects of various pretreatments concomitantly on these parameters is essential. Careful consideration of the types of electrophilic and radical metabolites of drugs that might be formed, and their likely chemical reaction mechanisms with tissue molecules, should provide an understanding of the molecular basis for many drug-induced tissue injuries. An understanding of the biochemical mechanisms of human drug toxicity is requisite for rational risk-benefit decision-making and for any approaches to prevention of toxicity or the development of new nontoxic analogs to replace currently toxic agents.

PEROXIDATION MECHANISMS AND LETHAL CELL INJURY

Some chemicals show no discernible change in their tissue damage on manipulation of target tissue glutathione (GSH) *in vivo*. For other substances, manipulation of GSH or GSH-dependent enzyme systems will remarkably alter the toxicity, thereby providing strong biological evidence that GSH is responsible for protection against the toxicity of that substance.

Conclusions concerning mechanism of toxicity, however, cannot confidently be drawn without additional investigations correlating biological data with chemical studies in a highly integrated research effort. Such studies of the biological nature (Table 1) and chemical nature (Table 2) of reactive metabolites have led to the current view (44,45) that several categories of reactive species causing tissue lesions can be postulated: (a) electrophilic species not showing significant GSH conjugation *in vivo* and minimal, if any, potentiation of toxicity by prior GSH depletion (e.g., furosemide, dimethylnitrosamine); (b) electrophilic intermediates showing significant GSH conjugation *in vivo* and potentiation of toxicity by prior depletion of GSH (e.g., 2-furamide, acetaminophen, bromobenzene); (c) alkylating radicals not showing GSH depletion *in vivo* and minimal potentiation of toxicity by GSH depletion or by vitamin E deficient diets (e.g., carbon tetrachloride, halothane, hydrazine drugs); and (d) nonalkylating reactive metabolites that generate reactive oxygen species and show marked potentiation of toxicity by either GSH deficiency or by vitamin E deficient diets (e.g., paraquat, diquat, nitrofurantoin).

The experimental data supporting the proposed assignments in Table 1 and for the first 3 parameters in Table 2 have evolved from multiple laboratories over the last several years and have been reviewed elsewhere (7,15,23,24,32,42,44,45,54, and Smith and Orrenius, *this volume*). This discussion will be restricted to recent toxicologic studies concerning GSH, lipid peroxidation and the chemical nature of reactive metabolites obtained under the last 3 parameters of Table 2, i.e., alkane expiration, lipid hydroperoxides and hydroxy acids (LOOH and LOH), and oxidized glutathione (GSSG) excretion.

Alkane Expiration

Hepatocytes and most other cells show a somewhat stereotyped pattern of cellular and organelle response when dying from acute lethal injury regardless of the inciting agent or event, e.g., chemical injury or acute anoxia. Thus, it has been attractive to toxicologists and pathologists over the last two decades to look for a single, common mechanism initiating the stereotypical events of cell death (32,44). In earlier periods, the "model hepatotoxin" available for studies of acute chemical injury was carbon tetrachloride, a compound that clearly is converted to a radical metabolite which peroxidizes (and alkylates) tissue macromolecules. The dominant hypothesis that arose from such studies was that peroxidation is the common mechanism initiating the stereotypical events of acute lethal cell injury.

However, the measurement of peroxidation

TABLE 1. *Biological nature of reactive metabolites*

Parameter	Class A Strong electrophile or nonsubstrate for GSH–*S*-transferase	Class B Weak electrophile or substrate for GSH-*S*-transferase	Class C Organic free radical	Class D[a] Generator of oxygen intermediates
Necrosis increased by prior GSH depletion	0	++++	0	++
Necrosis decreased by prior treatment with GSH precursors	0	++++	0	++
Necrosis increased by selenium deficiency	0 or −	0 or −	+(?)	++++
Necrosis increased by vitamin E deficiency	−	−	+(?)	++++

[a] Data obtained mainly from studies with lung toxins.

TABLE 2. *Chemical nature of reactive metabolites*

Parameter	Class A Strong electrophile or nonsubstrate for GSH-*S*-transferase	Class B Weak electrophile or substrate for GSH-*S*-transferase	Class C Organic free radical	Class D Generator of oxygen intermediates
Protein alkylation	++++	++++	++++	0
Lipid alkylation	0	0	++++	0
Preferential GSH depletion	0	++++	0	++
Alkane expiration	0	+++	++++	+++[a]
LOOH and LOH[c]	0	0	++++	(?)[b]
Stimulation of GSSG excretion	0	−	0	++++

[a] Selenium and vitamin E deficient animals.
[b] Availability of hepatic glutathione never exceeded in normal animals; selenium or vitamin E deficient animals have not yet been examined.
[c] Lipids that have been oxidized to hydroperoxy or hydroxy derivatives, respectively; particularly the alkyl portions of polyunsaturated fatty acid groups.

reactions *in vivo* was, and is, a tedious and difficult proposition. For this reason, experiments were often carried out with microsomal *in vitro* systems so that it would be possible to obtain indirect measurements of peroxidation by methodology, such as the thiobarbituric acid technique. No recognition was taken of the aberrantly large (22) endogenous microsomal formation of superoxide and hydrogen peroxide during the normal metabolism of many xenobiotics by monooxygenases or of the ultimate, innocuous conversion of these oxidants released in intact cell systems to water by glutathione peroxidase. Recent studies of the oxidation of GSH to GSSG in complete systems, such as the isolated perfused liver (23), isolated hepatocyte preparation (51,68, and Smith and Orrenius, *this volume*), and biliary fistula rat model (29), have documented this process.

Fortunately, advances in methodology in recent years have led to the use of new and sensitive, although still indirect, assays of lipid peroxidation suitable for studies *in vivo*. The measurement of expired hydrocarbons (ethane, pentane, etc.) from beta-scission of lipid hydroperoxides is becoming widely and occasionally indiscriminantly employed as an index of lipid peroxidation *in vivo*. [For more details, the reader is referred to thoughtful analyses of carbon tetrachloride by Recknagel et al. (54) and of halothane by Sipes and Gandolfi (61).] However, a brief perusal of the conditions determining the expiration of ethane and pentane (Fig. 1) makes it apparent that several factors must be carefully considered in studies of chemical-induced lipid peroxidation by this technique: (a) the availability of GSH and glutathione peroxidase for prevention of peroxidation through detoxification of cellular oxygen species (major effect) and

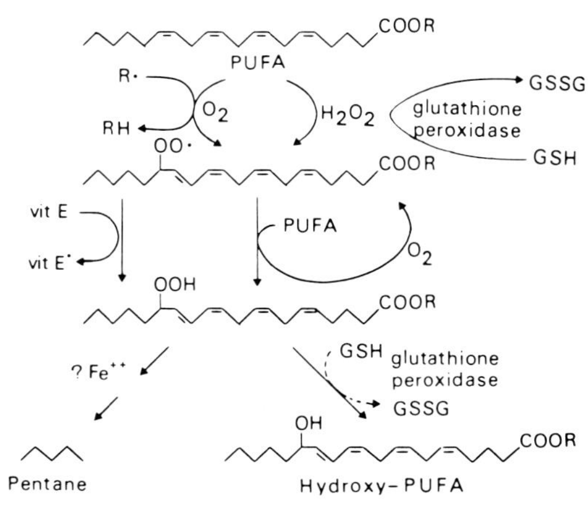

FIG. 1. Schematic outline of reactions involved in peroxidation of polyunsaturated fatty acids (PUFA) by organic radicals ($R^{\cdot}$) or H_2O_2.

possibly through reduction of membrane lipid hydroperoxides (minor effect); (b) the availability of vitamin E to stop the propagation of peroxidation; and possibly (c) the availability of trace metal ions to accelerate decomposition of membrane lipid hydroperoxides via the beta-scission rather than the reductive pathway in Fig. 1, thereby propagating lipid peroxidation when R$^{\bullet}$ (pentyl radical, which is not shown in the simplified scheme in Fig. 1) reacts with another polyunsaturated fatty acid (PUFA) to propagate the peroxidation cycle. The importance of these factors in interpreting the results of studies of chemical-induced pentane and ethane expiration are illustrated in investigations (Table 3) with acetaminophen, 2-furamide, bromobenzene, and thiophene (class B in Table 2—electrophilic metabolites with GSH toxic dose threshold); with furosemide (class A in Table 2); with carbon tetrachloride (class C in Table 2); and with diquat (class D in Table 2).

For acetaminophen a large body of data exists that supports the hypothesis that acetaminophen initiates hepatocellular necrosis in laboratory animals and in man by its conversion into a highly electrophilic metabolite, *N*-acetyl-*p*-benzoquinoneimine, which arylates liver macromolecules. GSH is thought to protect susceptible cytochrome P-450-containing target cells by preferentially adding to or reducing the quinoneimine metabolite to prevent initiation of arylation damage (11). The generation of *N*-acetyl-*p*-benzoquinoneimine from synthetic *N*-hydroxyacetaminophen (11), or by electrochemical (36) or silver oxide (4) oxidation of acetaminophen, has shown that the chemical and toxicologic characteristics are consistent with its originally

TABLE 3. *Drug-induced expiration of ethane and pentane*

				Ethane		Pentane	
Compound	Dose	Class	Pretreatment	Time (hr)[a]	pmole[b]/kg·min	Time (hr)[a]	pmole/kg·min
Furosemide	400 mg/kg	A	—	No increase[c]		No increase[c]	
Furosemide	400 mg/kg	A	400 DEM[d]	3	2,113 ± 684	3	1,369 ± 391
2-Furamide	275 mg/kg	B	—	2	1,146 ± 370	2	575 ± 156
Thiophene	250 mg/kg	B	—	3	1,035 ± 395	4	453 ± 223
Acetaminophen	400 mg/kg	B	—	3	1,539 ± 259	2	922 ± 260
Acetaminophen	400 mg/kg	B	fat diet 3 days[e]	3	2,045 ± 693	3.5	2,237 ± 994
Bromobenzene	314 mg/kg	B	phenobarbital[f]	2	182 ± 42	2	2,057 ± 854
CCl_4	2 ml/kg	C	—	0.5	764 ± 145	0.5	479 ± 77
CCl_4	2 ml/kg	C	400 DEM[d]	0.5	770 ± 121	0.5	671 ± 126
CCl_4	0.6 ml/kg[g]	C	—	0–6 hr[h]	103[i]	n.d.[j]	n.d.
CCl_4	0.6 ml/kg[g]	C	Vit E deficient	0–6 hr[h]	128[i]	n.d.	n.d.
CCl_4	0.6 ml/kg[g]	C	Se deficient	0–6 hr[h]	139[i]	n.d.	n.d.
Diquat	230 μmole/kg[g]	D	—	0–6 hr[h]	9[i]	n.d.	n.d.
Diquat	19.5 μmole/kg[g]	D	Se deficient	0–6 hr[h]	323[i]	n.d.	n.d.

[a] Time in hours post i.p. dose to animal when maximal expiration observed.
[b] Peak rate of expiration; mean ± SE of 3 to 10 experiments.
[c] No elevation above basal rates of ~50 pmole/kg·min.
[d] Mice given 400 mg/kg diethyl maleate, i.p., in corn oil 1 hr prior to drug.
[e] Mice fed a 10% corn oil supplemented diet for 3 days prior to experiment.
[f] Male Sprague-Dawley rats were induced with 80 mg/kg sodium phenobarbital for 3 days and fasted 18 hr prior to i.p. administration of bromobenzene in corn oil.
[g] Data from rats Burk et al. (6a,7).
[h] Measurements of total ethane accumulated over 6 hr post dose.
[i] Data recalculated as average rates of expiration in pmole/kg·min.
[j] n.d., Not determined.

postulated role as the toxic metabolite formed by P-450 monooxygeneses from acetaminophen *in vivo.*

Nevertheless, recent studies have provided support for the hypothesis that acetaminophen could be initiating necrosis by peroxidative reactions rather than by arylation. The peroxidative hypothesis was originally considered and rejected (69) because the chemical and toxicologic characteristics of the acetaminophen metabolite could not be distinguished from other hepatotoxins thought to produce electrophilic metabolites that undergo two-electron addition reactions with tissue macromolecules, such as furosemide, dimethylnitrosamine, bromobenzene, thiophene, and 2-furamide (44,45). The electrophilic characteristics of the acetaminophen metabolite were markedly different from the reaction properties with sulfhydryl nucleophiles and tissue macromolecules of hepatotoxic metabolites thought to produce one-electron radical attack on tissue macromolecules, such as those from carbon tetrachloride or isopropyl hydrazine. Moreover, we found no evidence of tissue peroxidation such as an increase in diene conjugation in membrane phospholipids after hepatotoxic doses of acetaminophen or furosemide (69), in contrast to carbon tetrachloride (54,69).

Thus, the surprising finding by Wendel et al. (76,77) that acetaminophen-intoxicated mice exhale large amounts of ethane, which presumably arise from beta-scission of lipid hydroperoxides, led to our reexamination of the peroxidation hypothesis. In preliminary experiments, we found that hydrocarbon expiration occurred after administration of a variety of hepatotoxins whenever hepatic GSH is coincidentally depleted either by the compound itself or by prior treatment with another compound, such as diethyl maleate (Table 3) (44,63). We concluded that the lipid peroxidation was produced by the release of reactive oxygen species in the glutathione-deficient cell (44); most importantly, however, the peroxidation reactions could clearly be dissociated from the hepatic necrosis produced by hepatotoxins, such as furosemide, since pretreatment with diethyl maleate (Table 3) or phenobarbital (77) markedly stimulates the expiration of ethane and pentane but does not increase either the incidence or severity of furosemide-induced hepatic necrosis (41).

In addition, an examination of the time courses showed that the expiration of ethane and pentane (Table 3) produced by electrophilic metabolites in classes A and B of Table 2 occurred rather late when cells were dying (2–4 hr after poisoning), in contrast to the early onset (0.5 hr) for organic radical metabolites in class C, such as carbon tetrachloride. Similar observations were recently reported with studies of chemical-induced ethane and pentane formation in isolated hepatocytes (66).

In a further set of experiments, the influence of a high-fat diet on alkane expiration and acetaminophen hepatotoxicity was examined (Table 3). Similar to the dissociation of peroxidation reactions and necrosis seen in the experiments with furosemide with and without diethyl maleate (Table 3), a 3-day feeding of a corn oil supplemented diet enriched with linoleic acid (a potential precursor of pentane during peroxidation reactions) strikingly increased the relative amount of pentane expired after administration of acetaminophen without changing the incidence or severity of necrosis. Analysis of the changes in the composition of fatty acids in hepatic triacylglycerols versus membrane phospholipids following the 3-day feeding of the corn oil diet showed large increases in pentane precursors (mainly linoleic and arachidonic acids) in the triacylglycerol fraction but no change in the phospholipid fraction; as expected, the membrane phospholipids were unlikely to be the site of the peroxidation reactions.

It is well known that GSH performs many functions within the hepatocyte. In addition to its protective role in detoxifying electrophilic substances via glutathione transferase-catalyzed conjugation reactions, the participation of GSH as a cofactor for the glutathione peroxidase enzyme system is also a primary cellular protection function. In the latter system GSH provides reducing equivalents, enabling the enzyme to metabolize hydrogen peroxide (major effect) and possibly to convert radical-producing lipid hydroperoxides to nontoxic lipid alcohols (minor effect) (Fig. 1).

This role of glutathione peroxidase raises the possibility that the increased ethane and pentane evolution after administration of hepatotoxins that coincidentally deplete GSH might arise from the formation of rancid fats (lipid hydroperoxides) within dying cells by the release of oxygen species from mono-reduced oxycytochrome P-450, oxygenated hemoglobin, xanthine oxidase, eicosanoid metabolites, and so on. When GSH has been removed from the cell by an alkylating metabolite, such as the one formed from acetaminophen or similar agents, hydrogen peroxide and possibly lipid peroxides formed by the release of oxygen within dying cells can no longer be metabolized by glutathione peroxidase. Nonselective chemical peroxidation of tissue lipids then occurs with subsequent one-electron, homolytic cleavage reactions of the lipid hydroperoxides, thus giving rise to enhanced ethane and pentane expiration. Obviously, an alternative explanation of these results would be an inhibition of either glutathione peroxidase or reductase by the alkylating metabolites from these hepatotoxins. Indeed, Babson et al. (1) have shown that peroxidation after adriamycin can be demonstrated when one adds an alkylating agent (BCNU) that inhibits glutathione reductase. Moreover, Thor et al. (68) and Orrenius et al. (51) have shown that bromobenzene metabolites inhibit reductase activity presumably as a result of effects on free thiol groups required for enzyme activity. Nevertheless, this mechanism would not appear to be quantitatively significant *in vivo* because acetaminophen does not result in an increased efflux of GSSG in the rat (29) and bromobenzene minimally increases efflux of GSSG from isolated hepatocytes (68).

Lipid Hydroperoxy and Hydroxy Acids

It was apparent that direct chemical measurements of membrane lipid hydroperoxides and hydroxy acids formed *in vivo* were needed to document our suspicions that the apparent peroxidation occurring late after acetaminophen and other compounds was taking place in nonmembrane sites. For the direct assay of lipid hydroperoxy and hydroxy acids *in vivo* (19), lipids were extracted (Folch procedure) from liver homogenates prepared from animals treated with vehicle control or with hepatotoxic doses of acetaminophen or carbon tetrachloride. The phosphatidylcholine fractions were separated by thin layer chromatography and hydrolyzed with phospholipase A2. The resulting fatty acids were methylated with diazomethane, reduced with triphenylphosphine and separated by high pressure liquid chromatography (HPLC). The fractions collected on HPLC were derivatized to *O*-trimethylsilyl ethers and subjected to analysis by gas chromatography–mass spectrometry (GC-MS) (Table 4). After administration of carbon tetrachloride, large amounts of lipid hydroxy acids were formed. The major products were hydroxysubstituted isomers of linoleic, arachidonic, docosahexaenoic acids. In stark contrast, the administration of hepatotoxic doses of acetaminophen failed to increase membrane hydroperoxy or hydroxy fatty acids at any of the time points examined from 0.25 to 4 hr. These data support the hypothesis that the expired ethane and pentane observed after administration of a hepatotoxic dose of acetaminophen are not coming from membrane phospholipids.

The ability to measure both expired hydrocarbons and hydroxy fatty acids also has enabled us to study the role of glutathione peroxidase in lipid peroxidation *in vivo* by examining the effects of diethyl maleate pretreatment on the biological and chemical consequences of carbon tetrachloride administration. No significant differences were found in mice receiving diethyl maleate and carbon tetrachloride when compared with mice re-

TABLE 4. *GC–MS Data for trimethylsilyl derivatives of hydroxy fatty acid methyl esters isolated by HPLC*

Retention time (min)	Position of OH group	Methyl ester	MU[a]	m/z[b] (relative intensities) of characteristic ions: Molecular ion	Fragment ions
19.5	14	22:6	26.2		321(83), 283(17), 181(34), 129(100), 119(83), 105(66)
20.3	12	20:4	24.4		375(2), 316(2), 295(100), 229(14), 131(78)
21.5	15	20:4	24.4	406(2),	311(1), 335(14), 316(7), 295(7), 225(100), 129(75), 117(76)
23.4	13	18:2	22.9	382(10),	367(1), 311(48), 259(12), 225(45), 143(48), 130(100)
	13	22:6	26.2		223(100), 157(21), 129(17), 105(24)
26.5	11	20:4	24.4		391(0.3), 316(0.3), 257(1), 225(100), 155(7)
	11	22:6	26.2		281(100), 249(6), 159(13), 131(51), 117(69), 105(27)
28.3	10	22:6	26.2	430(2)	263(52), 243(11), 155(45), 129(100), 117(69), 105(64)
33.5	9	18:2	22.9	382(5)	367(1), 311(7), 225(100), 155(16), 143(27), 130(39)
	8 + 9	20:4	24.4		391(1), 265(11, 8-OH), 255(74, 9-OH), 181(13), 133(36), 105(100)
36.8	9	18:2	22.9	382(5)	311(7), 225(100), 155(16), 143(27), 130(39)
	7	22:6	26.2		303(6), 155(25), 129(100), 117(32), 105(34)
43.3	8	22:6	26.2	430(1)	415(7), 241(32), 143(54), 129(81), 117(82), 105(100)
56.5	5	20:4	24.4	406(2)	305(11), 255(26), 203(31), 155(47), 129(85), 117(70), 105(100)

[a] Methylene units ± 0.1 on 3% S.E. 30.
[b] Mass/charge ratio.
HPLC analysis of the hydroxy fatty acid methyl esters was carried out on μ-Porasil columns with mobile phase: hexane/isopropanol/acetic acid (995:4:1) and a flow rate of 2.4 ml/min. Fractions eluting between 19 and 60 min were derivatized with BSTFA prior to GC–MS analysis. The position of hydroxylation was confirmed by further GC–MS analysis of the corresponding hydrogenated samples.
Data from Hughes et al. (19), with permission.

ceiving vehicle control and carbon tetrachloride by employing the criteria of ethane and pentane expiration, hydroxy fatty acids in hepatic phosphatidylcholines, plasma transaminases, or histologically evaluated necrosis in the liver (62). If the major role of glutathione peroxidase were the reduction of lipid hydroperoxides to the chemically more stable hydroxy acids, an increase in hydrocarbon production would have been expected, possibly at the expense of a decrease in lipid hydroxy acids. The results, however, support our belief that the major effect of glutathione peroxidase is the prevention of peroxidation reactions by potentially toxic oxygen species rather than the detoxification of lipid hydroperoxides (Fig. 1). They also document the strikingly different interaction between GSH and glutathione peroxidase in peroxidation reactions initiated by oxygen species for the chemical metabolites in classes A, B, and D of Table 3 versus those in class C (organic radicals) when the protective GSH detoxification systems are compromised.

Glutathione Disulfide Excretion: Index of Intracellular Oxidant Stress

As another approach to the determination of peroxidative events *in vivo,* any significant oxidative stress intracellularly should be accompanied by an increased oxidation of GSH to its disulfide. The interaction of glutathione peroxidase with an oxidant substrate generates GSSG, most of which will be reduced back to GSH by glutathione reductase. However, a fraction of the excess GSSG generated within hepatocytes is excreted into the bile and can be measured as an index of intracellular oxidant stress (23,29,51,68). Since this method, in principle, provides a measure of the amount of potential toxicant detoxified, an increased biliary excretion of GSSG could reflect either a greater production or a more efficient detoxification of a constant amount of that toxicant. Nevertheless, the method does provide information on the general cellular exposure to oxidative stress, which should be a more suitable index than alkane expiration of the exposure to oxidative damage of nonlipid cellular components, such as proteins and nucleic acids.

The biliary excretion of GSSG increases severalfold and does so in a dose-response manner following administration of increasing doses of *t*-butylhydroperoxide to rats with a biliary fistula. Similarly, the administration of aminopyrine, and particularly of nitrofurantoin and diquat, markedly increase the biliary excretion of GSSG. The former is metabolized rapidly by the hepatic mixed-function monooxygenases, a process generating hydrogen peroxide, whereas the last two compounds appear to undergo NADPH-dependent, redox-cycling generation of superoxide anions (Table 5). In contrast, carbon tetrachloride does not increase biliary excretion of GSSG (Table 5) and does not stimulate the fractional turnover of hepatic GSH (29), even though it certainly produces hydroperoxy and hydroxy fatty acids *in vivo.* The most likely reason for this difference is that CCl_4 produces lipid peroxidation by trichloromethyl radical abstraction of bisallylic hydrogen atoms in fatty acids rather than by generation of reactive oxygen intermediates, as previously discussed. Apparently very little GSH is oxidized *in vivo* by reduction of membrane lipid peroxides relative to the large amount consumed by reduction of intracellular reactive oxygen intermediates. Moreover, these data would appear to explain why organic radicals from such compounds as carbon tetrachloride can produce lipid peroxidation in the presence of normal intracellular concentrations of glutathione and glutathione peroxidase: They bypass the major protective site of action of glutathione peroxidase (Fig. 1). Finally, as was expected, administration of acetaminophen not only failed to increase biliary excretion of both glutathione and glutathione disulfide, it actually decreased their biliary excretion as well (29).

We have recently developed reliable assays for the measurement of GSH and GSSG excretion into plasma after administration of the above hepatotoxins (30). The results have been similar and are reviewed by Lauterburg et al. (*this volume*).

ALKYLATION MECHANISMS AND ACUTE LETHAL INJURY

In many studies of chemical-induced toxicity, emphasis has been placed on the use of the toxins as metabolic probes of cellular function. When the critical target macromolecules responsible for chemical-induced injury are known, such studies have proved to be

TABLE 5. *Increment in biliary excretion of GSSG following various compounds*[a]

Diquat (0.09 mmole/kg)	1.420 ± 0.058
Nitrofurantoin (0.2 mmole/kg)	0.036 ± 0.007
Paraquat (0.3 mmole/kg)	0.012 ± 0.001
t-Butyl hydroperoxide (1.4 mmole/kg)	0.004 ± 0.0004
Aminopyrine (0.8 mmole/kg)	0.004 ± 0.001
Ethylmorphine (0.08 mmole/kg)	No increment in GSSG
Iproniazid (0.4 mmole/kg)	No increment in GSSG
Carbon tetrachloride (10 mmole/kg)	No increment in GSSG
Dimethylnitrosamine (0.4 mmole/kg)	No increment in GSSG
Furosemide (1.2 mmole/kg)	No increment in GSSG
Chloroform (12 mmole/kg)	Decrement in GSSG
Acetaminophen (6.6 mmole/kg)	Decrement in GSSG

[a] Micromoles of GSSG, expressed as GSH equivalents, per micromole of the administered compound excreted during each experiment.

Data from Lauterburg et al. (29), with permission.

useful approaches to an understanding of how the biological system responds to such derangement. Elegant examples of this successful approach include the pioneering work of the Millers demonstrating that alkylation of DNA was responsible for the initiation of the carcinogenicity of many chemical compounds (35) and the studies by Farber (12) elucidating the relationship between metabolism of *S*-adenosylmethionine and *S*-adenosylethionine in ethionine-induced hepatic injury.

But when the critical target molecules responsible for chemical injury are unknown, which is the unfortunate situation for chemical-induced acute lethal injury, it is difficult to determine whether the myriad changes in cell function result from a single initial biochemical lesion (e.g., plasma membrane damage) or from the concerted action of a number of different initial biochemical lesions. Thus, if one's choice of a putative target macromolecule is inappropriate or incorrect, then a great investment of research time and effort can be channeled into the pursuit of fallacious leads, which may be occurring presently in studies of exaggerated oxidative stress in isolated hepatocyte systems (*vide infra*).

This viewpoint led to the development of an alternative research approach to the broad problem of chemical-induced acute lethal injury, the purpose of which has been misunderstood by many investigators. The realization that the enzyme pathways responsible for the metabolic activation of many carcinogens are the same microsomal monooxygenases that metabolize most drugs led to the hypothesis that most drug-induced tissue lesions might also be initiated by a common underlying mechanism, i.e., the metabolic activation of drugs to chemically reactive metabolites (6,15,37). It was recognized that rapid evaluation of this hypothesis with a large number of drugs and chemicals would be impossible if the conventional search for the critical "target" macromolecule was the research approach that was pursued. Alternatively, it seemed equally slow and unlikely to be successful to pursue the classical pharmacological approach of examining the relationship between the plasma (or urine) concentration of a putative toxic metabolite and the severity of the tissue lesion. The toxic metabolite might be formed only in minor quantities relative to nontoxic metabolites, and for highly reactive metabolites little or none would even reach the plasma or urine.

On the other hand, it was reasoned that the severity of the tissue lesion and the amount of reactive metabolite that became covalently bound would be roughly proportional to the number of critical target macromolecules attacked. Moreover, kinetic changes in the amount of reactive metabolite within the tissue should be reflected by changes in the rate of covalent binding not only to the target macromolecules but also to the other nontarget macromolecules. Thus the covalent binding of the reactive metabolite to nonspecific macromolecules could be used as an index of the formation of the metabolite. Furthermore, this parameter could well be the most reliable kinetic estimate of the overall availability of the metabolite *in situ* for initiating tissue damage, since the metabolite often decomposes or is further metabolized before it can be isolated in body fluids or urine. According to this view, therefore, it would not be necessary to identify either the reactive metabolite or the target macromolecule to determine whether the tissue injury was initiated by a chemically reactive alkylating metabolite or by the inert parent compound or inert metabolites. In addition, in many cases the target substance would not have to be present in the sample being assayed for covalent binding.

The theoretical, kinetic, and practical considerations of this approach for the study of liver injury were extensively discussed in several reviews by Gillette (13,14, and *this volume*), Mitchell (40), and Gillette and Mitchell (16). These considerations subsequently were extended to include the kidney and lung as target organs in reviews by Mitchell et al. (43) and Boyd (5). The success of this approach is evident both from the large number of chemicals now known to initiate tissue injury via chemically reactive metabolites (81) and from the development of specific antidotes for human poisoning by toxic drugs, such as acetaminophen (39). As summarized recently by others (9), the results have been quite consistent and have produced two major conclusions. First, most toxic drugs are not biologically active but must be metabolically activated by the target cell itself. Target cell specificity and the actual extent of cell injury are, in turn, dependent on this metabolism. Second, the critical metabolites apparently initiate their biological action by covalently binding to cellular macromolecules since a persistent correlation occurs between the extent of binding and the severity of the accompanying cell necrosis.

Nevertheless, despite the obvious usefulness of this approach for demonstrating the involvement of reactive metabolites in chemical-induced acute lethal injury, such studies are not designed to test the hypothesis per se that covalent binding to macromolecules produces cell injury that results in necrosis. First, measurable covalent binding of reactive metabolites to tissue protein is not always accompanied by tissue necrosis (21,33,52). Second, the molecular targets that interact with reactive metabolites and lead to cell death have not been identified. Third, the functional consequences of such interactions between the chemical toxin and key cellular targets *in vivo* have rarely been considered, as noted in our 1976 review (42). These and other considerations have led some investigators, particularly advocates of the oxidant stress hypothesis of lethal cell injury, to question the role of alkylation in the generation of membrane or of any other form of cell injury. Thus, the peroxidation camp points to the preferential depletion of "protective antioxidant" glutathione by electrophilic metabolites of some toxins (e.g., bromobenzene, acetaminophen) and to the valid assumption that the alkylated protein measured in covalent binding studies may be mostly nontarget macromolecules and therefore not critical to the mechanism of cell death. Ignored is the *singular fact* that many alkylating toxins, such as furosemide, 2-furoic acid, and dimethylnitrosamine, form electrophilic metabolites indistinguishable in studies *in vitro* from the metabolites of bromobenzene or acetaminophen except that they neither preferentially deplete cellular glutathione *in vivo* nor increase diene conjugation (peroxidation) in cells (44,69). At the present time no viable alternative hypothesis to an alkylation mechanism as the initiator of acute lethal injury is available for these compounds.

We have attempted to reconcile these facts regarding peroxidation and alkylation concepts (44,45,63) because we do not view them as mutually exclusive or competing hypotheses and for chemicals converted to radical metabolites, they might even be additive. Therefore, fundamental to further progress, the chemical nature (organic radical, generator of oxygen species, type of electrophile) of each reactive metabolite must be recognized as the key determinant of its toxicological interactions and these reaction mechanisms must be defined on an individual drug basis. Our scientific data base now is at a point where an examination of the cellular products of these alkylating reactions is technically feasible, particularly with the advent of effective methods for mass spectral examination of highly polar substances, such as amino acid and peptide adducts.

The association between covalent binding and acute lethal injury produced by administration of acetaminophen and bromobenzene has been known for over a decade (21,38,57); changes in experimental procedures that produce increased levels of covalent binding are accompanied by increases in toxicity. The observations that analogs of these substances, namely *m*-hydroxyacetanilide (58) and *p*-bromophenol (46,56), produce measurable amounts of covalent binding to hepatic proteins yet fail to produce hepatic necrosis presently represent possible contradictions to hypotheses invoking binding to tissue protein in a causal role for necrosis. However, since the covalent binding reported for the nontoxic compounds was less than that produced by its toxic analog, and since treatments that produced comparable levels of binding were not compared, these possible contradictions remain untested. Important studies carried out on ortho-substituted bromobenzenes by Hanzlik and Wiley and co-workers (17,18,71,78) confirm a lack of correspondence between relative hepatotoxicity and covalent binding to protein in microsomal or postmitochondrial preparations (cf. 41,52). Similar studies that compare *in vivo* covalent binding with hepatotoxicity are required to clarify the anomaly.

Nevertheless, the very clear demonstrations of substantial covalent binding in the absence of tissue necrosis exist (Fig. 2) (18,21,33,46,52,57,58), and any hypothesis that invokes covalent binding as a cause of acute lethal injury must explain these observations. Since it is not expected that all alkylation events are equally damaging to the cell (13,14,16,18), determination of the differences between the binding produced by toxic and nontoxic treatments is needed.

If equivalent levels of binding of the analogs discussed above were found to produce dissimilar degrees of necrosis, then the binding would need to be evaluated on a more precise basis, chemically and/or biologically. If, however, such studies do not show differential tissue toxicity at equivalent binding, then the distinction between critical and noncritical targets may be approached by a study of the targets alkylated by toxic versus nontoxic doses of acetaminophen and bromobenzene. Both acetaminophen (see Fig. 2) and bromobenzene (57) have been studied in models where substantial covalent binding to hepatic protein (in the range of 0.6 nmole/kg protein) is produced at a given time post dose in an animal that will not subsequently develop extensive necrosis. However, increases in peak covalent binding to 1 nmole/mg protein or higher are normally accompanied by substantial necrosis.

Thus, for the nontoxic analog and/or for the subtoxic dose of the hepatotoxin, a set of macromolecular targets exists whose alkylation by these substances is noncritical. Whether their repair (see Fig. 2 and Table VI of ref. 57) is true repair or degradation or a mixture of both is not known. What is known is that their chemical modification for the period of time required for this repair does not measurably compromise the viability of the cell.

The binding patterns produced by the toxic and nontoxic treatments can be examined to determine whether the progression is accompanied by a change in chemical or biological target or is simply an extrapolation of the nontoxic patterns. This requires the identification and quantitation of the major products of binding, although it is recognized that minor products may be of great importance. Namely,

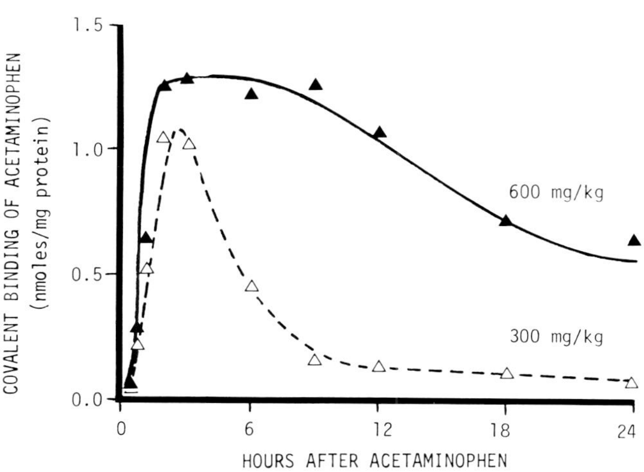

FIG. 2. Time course of covalent binding to hepatic protein of toxic and nontoxic doses of acetaminophen. Adult male ICR mice (TIMCO, Houston, Texas) were given 300 (*open triangle*) or 600 (*solid triangle*) mg/kg [^{3}H]-acetaminophen, i.p. in saline, and covalent binding to hepatic protein measured at indicated time points as described in text. Mean ± S.E. of 6 animals per point.

is the crossover to toxic binding a result of saturation of noncritical sites with resultant reaction of the electrophilic metabolite at kinetically less favorable yet more critical sites? Or is the toxicity simply a function of total alkylation?

In this regard Lau and Zannoni (28) have reported interesting studies suggesting the specificity of binding may be part of the explanation for the difference in toxicity of bromobenzene in the 3-methylcholanthrene versus the phenobarbital-induced rat. Microsomes from the 3-methylcholanthrene-pretreated rat produced relatively more 2,3-epoxide from bromobenzene than the 3,4-epoxide characteristic of the microsomes from the phenobarbital-induced animal, a relationship which applies *in vivo* as well (27,56,80). Similarly, these same authors found that BALB/cJ mice were much more susceptible to bromobenzene hepatotoxicity than were C57BL/J mice; this relationship correlated with the markedly greater activity of microsomes from the former strain to produce products of the 3,4-epoxide pathway (27). In studies of the fate of these 2 reactive intermediates in microsomal incubations of bromobenzene with added hemoglobin beta-protein, they showed that binding in the phenobarbital-pretreated animals was confined primarily to the microsomal protein. And by preferential alkylation of cysteine or histidine nucleophilic sites, they showed that the electrophilic metabolites that did bind to hemoglobin revealed a modest preference for histidine as a site of binding. Conversely, much of the 2,3-epoxide seemed to escape from the microsomes and bind to the hemoglobin, with a marked preference for cysteine residues.

Similar studies for the chemical specificity of acetaminophen binding to polymeric nucleophiles have not been reported; the subcellular binding has been examined, although not in great detail (21). However, in some recent studies we measured the covalent binding to hepatic protein and lipid of hepatotoxic doses of carbon tetrachloride, dimethylnitrosamine, acetaminophen, bromobenzene, 2-furamide, and furosemide (64). In these studies we observed an apparent covalent binding to lipid by a metabolite of dimethylnitrosamine; since these adducts were not produced via carbon–carbon bond formation with aliphatic or alicyclic residues (therefore radical addition or combination products), this suggested that the radioactivity did not remain with the lipid fraction upon transesterification. Formation of lipid phosphotriesters and/or alkylation of phosphatidylethanolamines are possible explanations of this observation (34). Carbon tetrachloride did bind covalently to alkyl portions of the lipid fraction (4.34 nmole/mg), further supporting the well-documented role of the trichloromethyl radical in the interaction of this hepatotoxin with tissue molecules. Significantly, none of the other toxins showed measurable binding to transesterified lipid. Once again, we feel that there is much to be learned about the relationship of covalent binding to initiation of cell injury by a careful study of the extent and persistence of covalent binding that accompanies toxic versus nontoxic treatments with acetaminophen and bromobenzene, just as the studies of chemical carcinogenesis were greatly facilitated by a recognition of the importance of site specificity and repair of the molecular lesions produced by binding to DNA (31,60).

The need for identification of the specific adducts formed *in vitro* was recognized early in the studies of covalent binding and toxicity, but attempts to identify these products in 1970 and 1971 came to a halt because of an inability to apply the analytical methodologies available at that time to successful structural elucidation (25). Subsequent advances in chromatography, coupled with recent advances in mass spectrometry, however, combine to make these vitally important investigations now possible.

CALCIUM HOMEOSTASIS AND ACUTE LETHAL INJURY

Current concepts about the pathogenesis of lethal cell injury have come mainly from cell culture studies of toxic conditions *other than* the lethal injury caused by chemically reactive drug metabolites. Thus, direct extrapolation of the concepts to drug-induced lethal injury is uncertain.

The major conditions resulting in lethal cell injury have been categorized recently by Trump and colleagues (72–74, and Trump et al., *this volume*) who have carried out important studies on ischemic lethal injury and on direct plasma membrane damage by complement or heavy metals. These investigations include conditions that (a) primarily inhibit ATP synthesis (e.g., anoxia, ischemia, mitochondrial uncouplers) or oxidize mitochondrial NADPH, (b) inhibit Na^+-K^+-ATPase (e.g., mercury, ouabain), or (c) modify cell membrane permeability (e.g., complement activation, ionophores). They propose that acute lethal injury is modulated primarily through cell ion regulation involving membrane and ion pump effects, including plasma membranes, mitochondrial membranes, and the membranes of the endoplasmic reticulum (microsomes). This is in contrast to effects on other cell macromolecules, such as DNA and RNA, which do not ordinarily participate directly in acute cell death despite their important role in other toxicities, such as mutagenicity and neoplasia. Their hypothesis then is that a common characteristic during the *reversible* phase following the initiation of lethal injury is a failure of the plasma membrane to regulate sodium ion accumulation. In the *irreversible* phase, the failure additionally involves calcium ions, as these investigators showed several years ago in studies with Ehrlich tumor cells (26). Farber and colleagues (8,59) also have provided evidence that modulating the concentration of extracellular calcium ions in primary hepatocyte cultures can ameliorate or delay toxic injury and hence also have provided support for the view that an increased influx of calcium, or a decreased efflux, through a damaged plasma membrane is indeed a pivotal event in lethal injury. Eventually, however, cell death occurs with or without added extracellular calcium in the incubation medium, and several investigators therefore have speculated that calcium mobilized from intracellular stores might also play an important role in lethal injury (20,65).

The original discovery in 1975 by Moore et al. (47) of a calcium sequestration system in microsomal membranes greatly extended interest in the concept of intracellular calcium ion regulation and lethal injury. Moore subsequently has shown that the liver necrosis produced by carbon tetrachloride (48), carbon disulfide (49), and 1,1-dichloroethylene (50) is associated with a marked inhibition of this microsomal calcium pump activity. Thus, the concepts originally derived from cell culture studies of ischemia and other toxic conditions have now been shown to be compatible with *in vivo* studies of lethal injury caused by chemically reactive metabolites, with the additional caveat that intracellular regulation of calcium by hepatic microsomes (containing 40% of intracellular calcium ions) and mitochondria (containing 60% of calcium ions) might be as important as plasma membrane calcium regulation for lethal injury.

In this regard, Orrenius and his colleagues (20,65) have shown in isolated hepatocytes that three differently acting liver cell toxins (CCl_4, bromobenzene, ethylmethanesulfonate) are more toxic to isolated hepatocytes in the absence of extracellular calcium than in its presence. They suggest that an efflux of intracellular calcium from subcellular organelles, not an influx of extracellular calcium, is responsible for the toxicity. Stacey and Klaassen (67) also failed to find a role for extracellular calcium in the cytotoxicity produced by copper and cadmium in isolated hepatocytes. Additionally, Bellomo et al. (3) have shown intracellular release of mitochondrial calcium caused by NADPH oxidation during reduction of peroxides by the mitochondrial glutathione peroxidase system or by reduction of menadione by mitochondrial oxidoreductases. When mitochondrial release exceeds the buffering capacity of the microsomal calcium uptake system, they speculate that cytotoxicity then occurs (3).

Obviously, resolution of these differences will require a careful comparison not only of the effects of selected hepatotoxins on subcellular calcium stores and on membrane calcium "transport" function in isolated hepatocytes but especially of their effects on free cytosolic calcium levels, which have not been determined by any of the investigators. In addition, studies of the effects of the same hepatotoxins on membrane calcium transport function in plasma and in mitochondrial and microsomal membranes after toxin administration *in vivo* are requisite for an evaluation of the significance of the data obtained with isolated hepatocytes. Preliminary investigations *in vivo* already have provided results different from those obtained with isolated cells and indicate that inhibition of the plasma membrane calcium pump *in vivo* could be of particular importance in reactive metabolite-induced acute lethal injury (75).

COMMENTARY

Chemicobiological Interactions Between Toxin and Tissue

The processes by which covalent binding or peroxidation by reactive drug metabolites leads to cell death remain unknown. It seems almost axiomatic that the initial interactions between a toxin and tissue should be described in physiochemical terms. Examples of such interactions are rare, however, and have been defined for only a few toxins, e.g., fluoroacetate poisoning of the citric acid cycle via incorporation into fluorocitrate (32).

In the 1960s, studies demonstrating alterations in the composition and function of the endoplasmic reticulum after various model hepatotoxins (e.g., carbon tetrachloride) led to the view that these changes result from the destruction of this organelle by reactive metabolites and that this injury plays a causal role in the subsequent development of hepatic necrosis (10,32,54). By this concept all hepatotoxins would produce a similar biochemical derangement that proceeds to hepatocellular death, independent of the damaging agent. As we have discussed elsewhere (40), the difficulty here is that the significance of many of the cellular changes is unknown. Cell necrosis is primarily a histologist's definition of cellular changes recognized to be irreversible and is influenced by dynamic processes *in vivo,* such as intraorgan blood flow and cellular repair (53,81). At present it is not possible to recognize the irreversible biochemical and ultrastructural changes of cell necrosis with equal certainty. Moreover, many of the biochemical alterations induced in the endoplasmic reticulum by hepatotoxins are reproduced by partial hepatectomy in animals, even though the residual liver is not injured at all (Fig. 3). In fact, the liver itself need not be manipulated. Sham hepatectomy alone decreases cytochrome P-450 by 35% within 6 hr and decreases dimethylaniline *N*-demethylation by 50% after 24 hr (2).

Similarly, it is easy to visualize how a chemically reactive metabolite of acetaminophen, furosemide, carbon tetrachloride, or dimethylnitrosamine formed *de novo* by cytochrome P-450 enzymes in the endoplasmic reticulum might severely damage the organelle by electrophilic or free radical attack, thereby leading to the observed biochemical changes and possibly to cell death. This would explain the centrilobular localization of necrosis, since histochemical evidence has shown that the endoplasmic reticulum of central hepatocytes is especially active in metabolizing drugs and other foreign compounds. Yet the same pattern of biochemical change is seen after furosemide (69) (Fig. 3), which produces a midzonal necrosis; more importantly, the pattern is seen after *N*-hydroxy-2-acetylaminofluorene (70) and allyl alcohol (70) (Fig. 3), both of which cause periportal lesions. If the target organelle is the endoplasmic reticulum containing cytochrome P-450 monooxygenases located primarily in the centrilobular hepatocytes, why should toxic damage by electrophilic or radical metabolites formed in periportal hepatocytes produce the same biochemical changes as metabolites formed in centrilobular hepatocytes? Furthermore, why

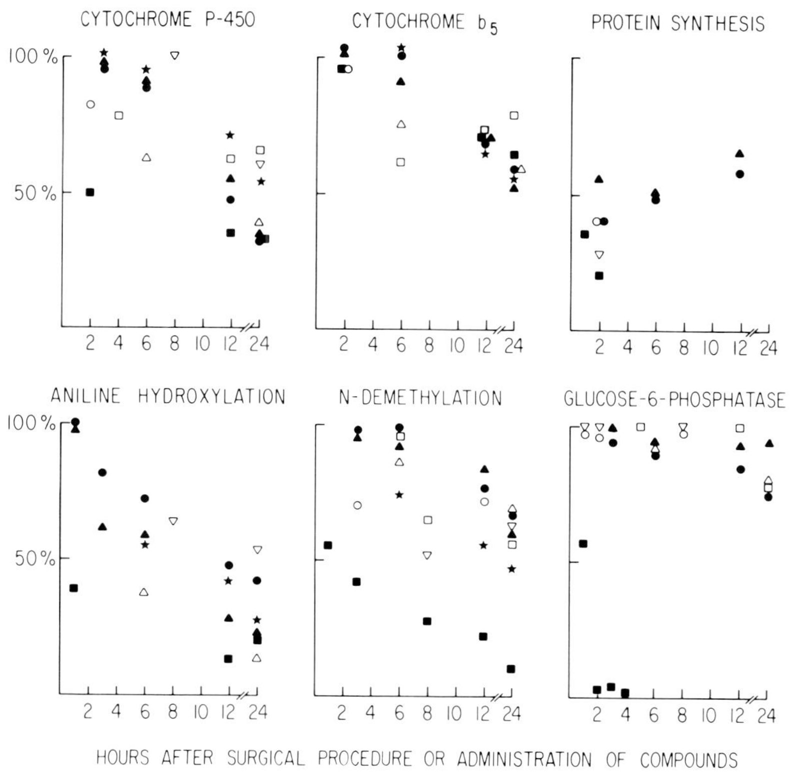

FIG. 3. Effects of several hepatotoxins and of surgical partial hepatectomy on microsomal composition and function from rat liver. *Solid circle,* acetaminophen; *solid square,* CCl_4; *solid triangle,* furosemide; *open circle,* dimethylnitrosamine; *star,* allyl alcohol; *open triangle,* N-OH-AAF; *open square,* partial hepatectomy. (From Thorgeirsson et al., ref. 70, with permission.)

should allyl alcohol and *N*-hydroxy-2-acetylaminofluorene severely alter the endoplasmic reticulum? Allyl alcohol is converted to its presumed reactive metabolite acrolein by an alcohol dehydrogenase localized in the soluble fraction of periportal hepatocytes. *N*-Hydroxy-2-acetylaminofluorene is thought to react after sulfation in the soluble fraction of periportal hepatocytes. Thus these hepatotoxins would not have been expected to damage the endoplasmic reticulum to a similar degree as would reactive metabolites formed *in situ* in this organelle.

In summary, several patterns of biochemical and structural alterations in the endoplasmic reticulum are apparent from the effects of several hepatotoxins: (a) haloalkane radicals from compounds such as CCl_4 produce direct structural changes (lipid diene conjugation, lipid hydroxy acid formation, and microsomal protein loss) as well as functional changes both *in vivo* and *in vitro* shortly after administration, (b) alkylating electrophilic metabolites from such compounds as acetaminophen cause loss of microsomal protein but no lipid hydroxy acid formation, or lipid diene conjugation *in vivo;* (c) most other hepatotoxins that have been studied produce functional alterations in the endoplasmic reticulum similar to acetaminophen. These functional changes appear later than the above structural changes (Fig. 3) and result in a similar pattern of biochemical derangements irrespective of the mechanism of action or the intraorgan target for each hepatotoxin. It is apparent that the initiation of liver injury physically may affect targets other than the endoplasmic reticulum even though the end results, such as fatty liver and necrosis, may be quite similar. It is imperative that changes directly attributable to the chemical lesion be distinguished from those resulting from efforts of the liver to repair and regenerate itself because many of the late changes (>12 hr) seen after administration of hepatotoxins also occur in the normal noninjured liver during periods of growth, after treatment of animals with growth hormone (79), and during liver regeneration after surgical partial hepatectomy (2) (Fig. 3).

Recently, interest in the concept of the endoplasmic reticulum being the physiochemical target for hepatotoxins has been regenerated because of evidence that organic radical metabolites impair calcium sequestration by the endoplasmic reticulum (47–50,54,55). However, the latter is not inhibited by electrophilic metabolites from acetaminophen and bromobenzene or by oxidizing metabolites from diquat, whereas acetaminophen, bromobenzene, and CCl_4 all inhibit plasma membrane calcium transport (75). For these reasons it seems appropriate to question whether or not toxicant-induced alterations in the endoplasmic reticulum necessarily have any causal relationship to the subsequent development of hepatocellular necrosis. Perhaps more attention needs to be paid to the effects of covalently bound metabolites or to radical metabolite-initiated oxidative changes on the function of plasma membranes, mitochondria, and other cell structures, including Mg-Ca-ATPase and calmodulin. Recent developments in bioanalytical methodology and techniques may make it possible to answer these vital questions in the near future (see chapters by Trump et al., Smith and Orrenius, and Horning et al., *this volume*).

Extrapolation of *In Vitro* Observations to *In Vivo* Significance

It is apparent that many drugs and foreign substances are converted to chemically reactive metabolites since they either are covalently bound to enzyme protein when incubated *in vitro* with cytochrome P-450 monooxygenases or generate superoxide and hydrogen peroxide. However, such studies should be interpreted carefully. Although they can be very useful in biochemical studies of the enzyme pathway leading to a chemically reactive metabolite, they do not necessarily predict the occurrence of necrosis *in vivo* (13–16,40,42). The manifestation of toxicity caused by reactive metabolites depends on several critical kinetic factors—namely, the rate of formation, the inherent reactivity, the rate of detoxification (e.g., by glutathione), the availability of cosubstrates, the maintenance of intraorgan blood flow, and the rate of tissue repair—which are not reflected in studies with isolated cells. Because of better control of experimental variables, the use of *in vitro* model systems will always play a vital role in research on mechanisms. However, the dominant influence that studies *in vitro* are beginning to have on the type of research approaches undertaken to elucidate mechanisms of acute lethal injury may be cause for future concern. Significant differences in the mechanisms by which isolated cells die versus mechanisms of cell necrosis *in vivo* are apparent. Studies elucidating these differences are necessary, particularly investigations of the excessive oxidative reactions occurring in many *in vitro* systems (22).

REFERENCES

1. Babson, J. R., Abell, N. S., and Reed, D. J. (1981): Protective role of glutathione redox cycle against adriamycin mediated toxicity in isolated hepatocytes. *Biochem. Pharmacol.,* 30:2299–2304.
2. Barker, E. A., Arcasory, M., and Smuckler, E. A. (1969): A comparison of the effect of partial surgical and partial chemical (CCl_4) hepatectomy on microsomal cytochrome b_5 and cytochrome P-450 and oxidative N-demethylation. *Agents Actions,* 1:27–35.
3. Bellomo, G., Jewell, S. A., and Orrenius, S. (1982): The metabolism of menadione impairs the ability of rat liver mitochondria to take up and retain calcium. *J. Biol. Chem.,* 274:11558–11562.
4. Blair, I. A., Boobis, A. R., and Davies, D. S. (1980): Paracetamol oxidation: synthesis and reactivity of N-acetyl-*p*-benzoquinoneimine. *Tetrahedron Lett.,* 21:4947–4950.

5. Boyd, M. R. (1980): Biochemical mechanisms in chemical-induced lung injury: Role of metabolic activation. *CRC Crit. Rev. Toxicol.*, 7:103–176.
6. Brodie, B. B., Reid, W. D., Cho, A. K., Sipes, G., Krishna, G., and Gillette, J. R. (1971): Possible mechanisms of liver necrosis caused by aromatic organic compounds. *Proc. Natl. Acad. Sci. USA*, 68:160–164.
6a. Burk, R. F., and Lane, J. M. (1979): Ethane production and liver necrosis in rats after administration of drugs and other chemicals. *Tox. Appl. Pharmacol.*, 50:467–478.
7. Burk, R. F., Lawrence, R. A., and Lane, J. M. (1980): Liver necrosis and lipid peroxidation in the rat as the result of paraquat and diquat administration. *J. Clin. Invest.*, 65:1024–1031.
8. Casini, A. F., and Farber, J. L. (1981): Dependence of the carbon tetrachloride-induced death of cultured hepatocytes on the extracellular calcium concentration. *Am. J. Pathol.*, 105:138–148.
9. Casini, A., Giorli, M., Hyland, R. J., Serroni, A., Gilfor, D., and Farber, J. L. (1982): Mechanisms of cell injury in the killing of cultured hepatocytes by bromobenzene. *J. Biol. Chem.*, 257:6721–6728.
10. Clifford, J., and Rees, K. R. (1966): Biochemical changes in the endoplasmic reticulum in liver injury. *J. Pathol. Bacteriol.*, 91:215–222.
11. Corcoran, G. B., Mitchell, J. R., Vaishnav, Y. N., and Horning, E. C. (1980): Evidence that acetaminophen and N-hydroxy-acetaminophen form a common arylating intermediate, N-acetyl-*p*-benzoquinoneimine. *Mol. Pharmacol.*, 28:3285–3290.
12. Farber, E. (1971): Biochemical pathology. *Ann. Rev. Pharmacol.*, 11:71–96.
13. Gillette, J. R. (1974): A perspective on the role of chemically reactive metabolites of foreign compounds in toxicity—I. Correlation of changes in covalent binding of reactive metabolites with changes in the incidence and severity of toxicity. *Biochem. Pharmacol.*, 23:2785–2794.
14. Gillette, J. R. (1974): A perspective on the role of chemically reactive metabolites of foreign compounds in toxicity—II. Alterations in the kinetics of covalent binding. *Biochem. Pharmacol.*, 23:2927–2938.
15. Gillette, J. R., Mitchell, J. R., and Brodie, B. B. (1974): Biochemical basis for drug toxicity. *Ann. Rev. Pharmacol.*, 14:271–288.
16. Gillette, J. R., and Mitchell, J. R. (1975): Drug actions and interactions: Theoretical considerations. In: *Handbook of Experimental Pharmacology*, Vol. 38, Part 3, edited by J. R. Gilette and J. R. Mitchell, pp. 359–382. Springer-Verlag, New York.
17. Gotschall, D. W., Wiley, R. A., and Hanzlik, R. P. (1983): Toxicity of *o*-substituted bromobenzenes in isolated rat hepatocytes: Comparison to *in vivo* results. *Toxicol. Appl. Pharmacol.*, 69:55–65.
18. Hanzlik, R. P. (1982): Effects of substituents on reactivity and toxicity of chemically reactive intermediates. *Drug. Metab. Rev.*, 13:207–234.
19. Hughes, H., Smith, C. V., Horning, E. C., and Mitchell, J. R. (1982): HPLC and GC-MS determination of specific lipid peroxidation products *in vivo*. *Anal. Biochem.*, 130:431–436.
20. Jewell, S. A., Bellomo, G., Thor, H., Orrenius, S., and Smith, M. T. (1982): Bleb formation in hepatocytes during drug metabolism is caused by disturbances in thiol and calcium ion homeostasis. *Science*, 217:1257–1259.
21. Jollow, D. J., Mitchell, J. R., Potter, W. Z., Davis, D. C., Gillette, J. R., and Brodie, B. B. (1973): Acetaminophen-induced hepatic necrosis. II. Role of covalent binding *in vivo*. *J. Pharmacol. Exp. Ther.*, 187:195–202.
22. Jones, D. P., Thor, H., Andersson, B., and Orrenius, S. (1978): Detoxification reactions in isolated hepatocytes. *J. Biol. Chem.*, 253:6031–6037.
23. Kappus, H., and Sies, H. (1981): Toxic drug effects associated with oxygen metabolism: redox cycling and lipid peroxidation. *Experientia*, 37:1233–1358.
24. Ketterer, B. (1982): The role of nonenzymatic reactions of glutathione in xenobiotic metabolism. *Drug Metab. Rev.*, 13:161–187.
25. Krishna, G., Eichelbaum, M., and Reid, W. D. (1971): Isolation and characterization of liver proteins containing covalently bound ^{14}C-bromobenzene. *Pharmacologist*, 13:196.
26. Laiho, K. U., and Trump, B. F. (1974): Relationship of ionic, water and cell volume changes in cellular injury of Ehrlich ascites tumor cells. *Lab. Invest.*, 31:207–215.
27. Lau, S. S., Abrams, G. D., and Zannoni, V. G. (1980): Metabolic activation and detoxification of bromobenzene leading to cytotoxicity. *J. Pharmacol. Exp. Ther.*, 214:703–708.
28. Lau, S. S., and Zannoni, V. G. (1982): Bromobenzene epoxidation leading to binding on macromolecular sites. *J. Pharmacol. Exp. Ther.*, 219:563–572.
29. Lauterburg, B. H., Smith, C. V., Hughes, H., and Mitchell, J. R. (1983): Biliary excretion of glutathione and glutathione disulfide in the rat: regulation and response to oxidative stress. *J. Clin. Invest.*, (*in press*).
30. Lauterburg, B. H., Adams, J. D., and Mitchell, J. R. (1983): Plasma glutathione and glutathione disulfide in the rat: regulation and response to oxidative stress. *J. Pharmacol. Exp. Ther.* (*in press*).
31. Lutz, W. K. (1979): *In vivo* covalent binding of organic chemicals to DNA as a quantitative indicator in the process of chemical carcinogenesis. *Mut. Res.*, 65:289–356.
32. McLean, A. E. M., McLean, E., and Judah, J. D. (1965): Cellular necrosis in the liver induced and modified by drugs. *Int. Rev. Exp. Pathol.*, 4:126–157.
33. McMurtry, R. J., Mitchell, J. R. (1977): Renal and hepatic necrosis after metabolic activation of γ-substituted furans and thiophenes, including furosemide and cephalondine. *Toxicol. Appl. Pharmacol.*, 42:285–300.
34. Margison, G. P., and O'Connor, P. G. (1979): Nucleic acid modification by N-nitroso compounds. In: *Chemical Carcinogens and DNA*, Vol. 1, edited by P. L. Grover, pp. 111–159. CRC Press, Boca Raton, Florida.
35. Miller, E. C., and Miller, J. A. (1966): Mechanisms of chemical carcinogenesis: Nature of proximate carcinogens and interactions with macromolecules. *Pharmacol. Rev.*, 18:805–838.
36. Miner, D. J., and Kissinger, P. T. (1979): Evidence for the involvement of N-acetyl-*p*-quinoneimine in acetaminophen metabolism. *Biochem. Pharmacol.*, 28:3285–3290.

37. Mitchell, J. R., Jollow, D. J., Gillette, J. R., and Brodie, B. B. (1973): Drug metabolism as a cause of drug toxicity. *Drug Metab. Dispos.,* 1:418–423.
38. Mitchell, J. R., Jollow, D. J., Potter, W. Z., Davis, D. C., Gillette, J. R., and Brodie, B. B. (1973): Acetaminophen-induced hepatic necrosis. I. Role of drug metabolism. *J. Pharmacol. Exp. Ther.,* 187:185–194.
39. Mitchell, J. R., Thorgeirsson, S. S., Potter, W. Z., Jollow, D. J., and Keiser, H. (1974): Acetaminophen-induced hepatic injury: Protective role of glutathione in humans and rationale for possible therapy. *Clin. Pharmacol. Therap.,* 16:676–684.
40. Mitchell, J. R. (1974): Covalent binding: Useful index of the formation of chemically reactive metabolites. *Biochem. Soc. Trans.,* 3:622–626.
41. Mitchell, J. R., Nelson, W. L., Potter, W. Z., Sasame, H. A., and Jollow, D. J. (1976): Metabolic activation of furosemide to a chemically reactive, hepatotoxic metabolite. *J. Pharmacol. Exp. Ther.,* 199:41–52.
42. Mitchell, J. R., Nelson, S. D., Thorgeirsson, S. S., McMurtry, R. J., and Dybing, E. (1976): Metabolic activation: biochemical basis for many drug-induced liver injuries. In: *Progress in Liver Disease, Vol. 5,* edited by H. Popper, and F. Schaffner, pp. 259–276. Grune & Stratton, New York.
43. Mitchell, J. R., McMurtry, R. J., Statham, C. N., and Nelson, S. D. (1977): Molecular basis for several drug-induced nephropathies. *Am. J. Med.,* 62:518–526.
44. Mitchell, J. R., Corcoran, G. B., Smith, C. V., Hughes, H., and Lauterburg, B. H. (1981): Alkylation and peroxidation injury from chemically reactive metabolites. In: *Biological Reactive Intermediates II,* edited by R. Snyder et al., pp. 199–224. Plenum Press, New York.
45. Mitchell, J. R., Hughes, H., Lauterburg, B. H., and Smith, C. V. (1982): Chemical nature of reactive intermediates as determinant of toxicologic responses. *Drug. Metab. Rev.,* 13:527–541.
46. Monks, T. J., Lau, S. S., and Gillette, J. R. (1982): Further evidence against the role of *p*-bromophenol in bromobenzene toxicity. *Pharmacologist,* 24:144.
47. Moore, L., Chen, T., Knapp, H. R., and Landon, E. J. (1975): Energy dependent calcium sequestering activity in rat liver microsomes. *J. Biol. Chem.,* 250:4562–4568.
48. Moore, L., Davenport, G. R., and Landon, E. J. (1976): Calcium uptake of a rat liver microsomal subcellular fraction in response to *in vivo* administration of carbon tetrachloride. *J. Biol. Chem.,* 251:1197–1201.
49. Moore, L. (1982): Carbon disulfide hepatotoxicity and inhibition of liver microsome calcium pump. *Biochem. Pharmacol.,* 31:1465–1467.
50. Moore, L. (1982): 1,1-Dichloroethylene inhibition of liver endoplasmic reticulum calcium pump. *Biochem. Pharmacol.,* 31:1465–1467.
51. Orrenius, S., Thor, H., Eklow, L., Moldeus, P., and Jones, D. P. (1982): Drug-stimulated H_2O_2 formation in hepatocytes. Possible toxicological implications. In: *Biological Reactive Intermediates II,* edited by R. Snyder et al., pp. 395–405. Plenum Press, New York.
52. Potter, W. Z., Thorgeirsson, S. S., Jollow, D. J., and Mitchell, J. R. (1974): Acetaminophen-induced hepatic necrosis V. Correlation of hepatic necrosis, covalent binding and glutathione depletion in hamsters. *Pharmacology,* 12:129–143.
53. Rappaport, A. M. (1979): Physioanatomical basis of toxic liver injury. In: *Toxic Injury of the Liver,* Part A, edited by E. Farber and M. M. Fisher, pp. 1–57. Marcel Dekker, New York.
54. Recknagel, R. O., Glende, A. A., Jr., Waller, R. L., and Lowrey, K. (1982): Lipid peroxidation: Biochemistry, measurement, and significance in liver cell injury. In: *Toxicology of the Liver,* edited by G. L. Plaa and W. R. Hewitt, pp. 213–241. Raven Press, New York.
55. Recknagel, R. O. (1983): A new direction in the study of carbon tetrachloride hepatotoxicity. *Life Sci.,* 33:401–408.
56. Reid, W. D., Christie, B., Eichelbaum, M., and Krishna, G. (1971): 3-Methylcholanthrene blocks hepatic necrosis induced by administration of bromobenzene or carbon tetrachloride. *Exp. Mol. Pathol.,* 15:363–372.
57. Reid, W. D., Krishna, G., Gillette, J. R., and Brodie, B. B. (1973): Biochemical mechanisms of hepatic necrosis induced by aromatic hydrocarbons. *Pharmacology,* 10:193–214.
58. Roberts, S. A., and Jollow, D. J. (1979): Acetaminophen structure-toxicity studies: *in vivo* covalent binding of a nonhepatotoxic analog, 3-hydroxyacetanilide. *Fed. Proc.,* 38:426.
59. Schanne, F. A. X., Kane, A. B., Young, E. E., and Farber, J. L. (1979): Calcium dependence of toxic cell death: a final common pathway. *Science,* 206:700–703.
60. Singer, B. (1979): N-Nitroso alkylating agents: formation and persistence of alkyl derivatives in mammalian nucleic acids as contributing factors in carcinogenesis. *J.N.C.I.,* 62:1329–1339.
61. Sipes, I. G., and Gandolfi, A. J. (1982): Role of reactive intermediates in halothane associated liver injury. In: *Biological Reactive Intermediates II,* edited by R. Snyder et al., pp. 603–618. Plenum Press, New York.
62. Smith, C. V., Hughes, H., Lauterburg, B. H., Corcoran, G. B., and Mitchell, J. R. (1982): Function of GSH in CCl_4-induced peroxidation and necrosis *in vivo. Pharmacologist,* 24:147.
63. Smith, C. V., Hughes, H., Lauterburg, B. H., and Mitchell, J. R. (1983): Chemical nature of reactive metabolites determines their biological interactions with glutathione. In: *Functions of Glutathione: Biochemical, Physiological and Toxicological Aspects,* edited by A. Larsson, S. Orrenius, A. Holmgrën, and B. Mannervik, pp. 125–138. Raven Press, New York.
64. Smith, C. V., Hughes, H., and Mitchell, J. R. (1983): Measurement of covalent binding to lipids as index of free radical metabolites: studies with hepatotoxic doses of carbon tetrachloride, dimethylnitrosamine, furosemide, 2-furamide, and acetaminophen. *Fed. Proc.,* 42:890.
65. Smith, M. T., Thor, H., and Orrenius, S. (1981): Toxic injury to isolated hepatocytes is not dependent on extracellular calcium. *Science,* 213:1257–1259.
66. Smith, M. T., Thor, H., Hartzell, P., and Orrenius, S. (1982): The measurement of lipid peroxidation in isolated hepatocytes. *Biochem. Pharmacol.,* 31:19–26.

67. Stacey, N. H., and Klaassen, C. D. (1982): Lack of protection against chemically-induced injury to isolated hepatocytes by omission of calcium from the incubation medium. *J. Toxicol. Environ. Health,* 9:267–276.
68. Thor, H., Svensson, S.-Å., Hartzell, P., and Orrenius, S. (1982): Biotransformates of bromobenzene to reactive metabolites by isolated hepatocytes. In: *Biological Reactive Intermediates II,* edited by R. Snyder et al., pp. 287–299. Plenum Press, New York.
69. Thorgeirsson, S. S., Sasame, H. A., Mitchell, J. R., Jollow, D. J., and Potter, W. Z. (1976): Biochemical changes after hepatic injury from toxic doses of acetaminophen or furosemide. *Pharmacology,* 14:205–217.
70. Thorgeirsson, S. S., Mitchell, J. R., Sasame, H. A., and Potter, W. Z. (1976): Biochemical changes after hepatic injury by allyl alcohol and N-hydroxy-2-acetylaminofluorene. *Chem. Biol. Interact.,* 15:139–147.
71. Toranzo, E. G., Gillesse, T., Mendehall, M., Traiger, G. J., Riley, P. G., Hanzlik, R. P., and Wiley, R. A. (1977): Effect of substituents on arene oxide-mediated liver toxicity amount substituted bromobenzenes. *Toxicol. Appl. Pharmacol.,* 40:415–425.
72. Trump, B. F., Berezesky, I. K., Laiho, K. U., Osornio, A. R., Mergner, W. J., and Smith, M. W. (1980): The role of calcium in cell injury. A Review. *Scan. Electron Microsc.,* 2:437–462.
73. Trump, B. F., McDowell, E. M., and Arstila, A. U. (1980): Cellular reaction to injury. In: *Principles of Pathobiology,* 3rd Ed., edited by R. B. Hill, Jr. and M. F. LaVia, pp. 20–111. Oxford University Press, New York.
74. Trump, B. F., Berezesky, I. K., and Phelps, P. C. (1981): Sodium and calcium regulation and the role of the cytoskeleton in the pathogenesis of disease. A review and hypothesis. *Scan. Electron Microsc.,* 2:435–545.
75. Tsokos-Kuhn, J. O., Todd, E. L., McMillin-Wood, J. and Mitchell, J. R. (1983): Plasma membrane Ca^{++} pump inhibition: final common pathway for tosic cell death? *Clin. Res.* (*in press*).
76. Wendel, A., Feuerstein, S., and Konz, K.-H. (1979): Acute paracetamol intoxication of starved mice leads to lipid peroxidation *in vivo. Biochem. Pharmacol.,* 28:2051–2055.
77. Wendel, A., and Feuerstein, S. (1981): Drug-induced lipid peroxidation in mice I. Modulation by monooxygenase activity, glutathione and selenium status. *Biochem. Pharmacol.,* 30:2513–2520.
78. Wiley, R. A., Hanzlik, R. P., and Gillesse, T. (1979): Effects of substituents on *in vitro* metabolism and covalent binding of substituted bromobenzenes. *Toxicol. Appl. Pharmacol.,* 49:249–255.
79. Wilson, J. J., and Frohman, L. A. (1974): Concomitant association between high plasma levels of growth hormone and low hepatic mixed-function oxidase activity in the young rat. *J. Pharmacol. Exp. Ther.,* 189:255–263.
80. Zampaglione, N., Jollow, D. J., Mitchell, J. R., Stripp, B., Hamrick, M., and Gillette, J. R. (1973): Role of detoxifying enzymes in bromobenzene-induced liver necrosis. *J. Pharmacol. Exp. Ther.,* 187:218–227.
81. Zimmerman, H. J. (1978): *Hepatotoxicity: The Adverse Effects of Drugs and Other Chemicals on the Liver.* Appleton-Century-Crofts, New York.

Drug Metabolism and Drug Toxicity,
edited by J. R. Mitchell and M. G. Horning.
Raven Press, New York © 1984.

Regulation of Hepatic Glutathione Homeostasis

Bernhard H. Lauterburg, Charles V. Smith, and Jerry R. Mitchell

Department of Internal Medicine, Baylor College of Medicine, Houston, Texas 77030

Glutathione plays a critical role in the detoxification of electrophilic metabolites and reactive oxygen intermediates generated during the metabolism of xenobiotics (10,40,44). The redox couple glutathione:glutathione disulfide, moreover, is a major determinant of the intracellular sulfhydryl:disulfide ratio, which may regulate the activity of many vitally important cellular processes (15,26). Because of its importance, cells can maintain adequate intracellular concentrations of glutathione by rapidly increasing the rate of synthesis in order to compensate for losses of glutathione from the cell via efflux, catabolism, or conjugate formation.

Since the liver is both the major site of detoxification reactions and also the major source of extracellular glutathione, the regulation of hepatic glutathione homeostasis is of particular importance. The main focus of this chapter is therefore on the dynamics of hepatic glutathione homeostasis. The complex interplay of intra- and extrahepatic factors regulating hepatic turnover of glutathione and its precursors is considered. An understanding of these interactions is essential for a critical analysis of biochemical events involving glutathione. Misinterpretations of the complex kinetics of hepatic glutathione have led to erroneous models of glutathione compartmentalization. In addition, the loss of regulatory mechanisms in *in vitro* systems may result in *in vitro* artifacts, requiring cautious interpretation of the biological relevance of many *in vitro* studies.

DYNAMICS OF HEPATIC GLUTATHIONE TURNOVER

Determination of Hepatic Glutathione Turnover

The determination of glutathione turnover *in vivo* is complex but must be the standard of reference in order to evaluate the biological significance of *in vitro* data. The administration of an inhibitor of glutathione synthesis will result in a progressive decrease in hepatic glutathione (17). Provided that the inhibition of synthesis is complete and that the inhibitor does not have any effect on glutathione metabolism other than inhibition of synthesis, the rate of consumption of hepatic glutathione can be calculated from the rate at which the concentration of glutathione declines. The validity of these assumptions is difficult to prove, however, and this approach is not optimal for studying the regulation of glutathione synthesis *in vivo* since it provides an estimate only of the rate of consumption of glutathione.

Because it interferes least with glutathione homeostasis, the use of tracer methodology is probably best suited to study glutathione turnover *in vivo*. Early estimates of glutathione synthesis were based on the incorporation of labeled precursor amino acids into glutathione (21,61). However, because of methodologic limitations at that time, these investigators could not appropriately deal with the complex kinetics of the precursor–

product relationship involved with the tracer approach.

Intact glutathione does not enter the cell (20), and the hepatic glutathione pool therefore has to be labeled via one of its precursor amino acids. Besides being used for glutathione synthesis, the precursor amino acids also will be incorporated into other peptides and proteins. On catabolism of a labeled protein or peptide, including glutathione itself, the labeled amino acids will reenter the precursor pool for glutathione synthesis. It has been estimated that in the isolated rat hepatocyte, approximately 50% of the cysteine used for glutathione synthesis originates from the catabolism of intracellular proteins (47).

The above tracer methods for measurement of hepatic glutathione turnover *in vivo* rely on the isolation of glutathione from liver homogenates. Glutathione turnover thus cannot be determined in individual animals, because each animal provides only one time point. Moreover, such an approach is obviously not feasible in man. Our laboratory has therefore developed and validated another approach, which is based on the formation of an adduct between glutathione and the reactive metabolite of acetaminophen, a technique that we call acetaminophen probe analysis (35). Following the administration of a labeled precursor amino acid and a small dose of acetaminophen, labeled acetaminophen–glutathione will appear in bile, and, provided that labeled cysteine was used to pulse-label the glutathione pool, labeled acetaminophen–mercapturic acid will appear in urine. The specific activity of the acetaminophen adducts reflects the specific activity of the intrahepatic glutathione (35), and the fractional rate of glutathione turnover can be calculated for individual animals or for man from the specific activity–time curves of the adducts in bile or urine, respectively. In order to estimate the rate of glutathione synthesis, the hepatic concentration of glutathione still has to be determined. An analysis of the specific activity–time curve of free plasma glutathione should provide similar information. Because the plasma concentration of glutathione is rather low (15–20 μM in the rat), however, it is difficult to achieve sufficient incorporation of label for accurate measurements of the specific activity.

As estimated by acetaminophen probe analysis, the fractional rate of turnover in male Sprague–Dawley rats weighing an average of 200 g is 0.186 ± 0.042 hr^{-1}. Other laboratories have reported values between 0.17 and 0.41 hr^{-1} (21,22,61). Assuming that there is just one hepatic glutathione pool, the rate of synthesis can be estimated from the intrahepatic concentration of glutathione of 4.7 ± 0.9 μmole/g and this rate constant. This calculation yields a value of 0.86 ± 0.17 μmole glutathione synthesized/g liver per hour.

Using a similar tracer method, the fractional rate of glutathione turnover in the liver of the mouse has been estimated at 0.29 hr^{-1}, and hepatic glutathione synthesis at 1.8 μmole/hr per g liver (50). In these studies, the rate constant for renal turnover of glutathione was estimated at 1.44 hr^{-1}, and the renal synthesis of glutathione at 3.9 μmole/hr per g.

In man, the half-life of glutathione in the liver is much longer, averaging 23 hr compared to 145 min in the mouse and 3.7 hr in the rat (33). In addition, the hepatic concentration of glutathione appears to be lower in man. Average values between 1.1 and 3.5 μmole glutathione/g liver have been reported in apparently normal human liver biopsy specimens (46,51,52). One laboratory, however, has reported an average of 7.4 mM in three brain-dead subjects (49). Based on these values, hepatic glutathione synthesis in normal man can be estimated at approximately 0.1 μmole/g liver per hour.

Efflux of Glutathione from the Liver

Even in the absence of any stress on the glutathione pool by detoxification reactions that consume glutathione via either the formation and excretion of glutathione adducts or of glutathione disulfide, hepatic glutathione synthesis is very active. Most of this basal turnover is accounted for by efflux of glutathione into blood and bile.

In the perfused rat liver, approximately 0.9 μmole glutathione/g liver per hr and 60 nmole glutathione disulfide/g liver per hr (8,54) are released into the perfusate. *In vivo,* the concentration of glutathione in hepatic vein plasma of rats is about 12 nmole/ml higher than the concentration in arterial plasma (5,27). From the hepatic plasma flow and this concentration difference, the sinusoidal efflux can be estimated at 0.8 μmole/hr per g liver *in vivo* (27). Together with the biliary excretion, which amounts to 0.1 to 0.2 μmole/hr per g liver, efflux thus accounts for virtually all hepatic turnover under physiologic conditions.

The efflux from the liver into blood, moreover, accounts for over 90% of total glutathione inflow into the circulation. Thus, the liver is the major source of plasma glutathione (27). Consequently, the plasma concentration of glutathione, which is 15 to 20 μM in normal rats, reflects the intrahepatic concentration of glutathione if renal function is normal. Depletion of intracellular glutathione by fasting or the administration of diethylmaleate or acetaminophen is associated with proportional decreases in the plasma concentration of glutathione (2). In the absence of an oxidant stress, virtually all glutathione released into the circulation is in the reduced form (8). In contrast to earlier reports (19), most of the circulating glutathione is also in the reduced form (18 μM) and not as the disulfide (0.3 μM). Plasma glutathione undergoes rapid autooxidations to the disulfide and mixed disulfides *in vitro* (6), and spuriously high values for plasma glutathione disulfide are obtained unless careful attention is paid to sample preparation.

Although the percentage of glutathione disulfide is higher in bile, biliary glutathione is also mostly in the reduced form. The biliary excretion measured *in vivo* (13,31) or in the perfused rat liver (3) is approximately 2.5 nmole glutathione/min per g liver and 0.5 nmole glutathione disulfide/min per g liver. The fraction of the originally secreted glutathione that is metabolized by γ-glutamyltransferase during its passage through the biliary tree may be as high as 50% (1).

The biliary excretion of reduced glutathione and glutathione disulfide both depend on the hepatic concentration of the two compounds. For glutathione, the concentration in bile averages 30% of the intrahepatic concentration (6 mM). In contrast, a steep concentration gradient exists for glutathione disulfide, where the biliary concentration is about 20-fold higher than the intrahepatic concentration of 18 μM (3). This concentration gradient persists during oxidative stress, when significant extrahepatic oxidation of glutathione can be excluded as a significant contributor to biliary glutathione disulfide, suggesting the presence of an active transport system for glutathione disulfide. Further evidence for a carrier-mediated transport of glutathione disulfide is provided by experiments demonstrating competition between the biliary excretion of glutathione disulfide and the glutathione adducts of chloro-2,4-dinitrobenzene (4) and sulfobromophthalein (28). Although most of the glutathione disulfide generated in the liver will be reduced by glutathione reductase, and only about 3% of the flux of glutathione disulfide through the glutathione reductase system will appear in bile (55), intracellular increases in glutathione disulfide will be amplified in bile as a result of the concentrating transport mechanism such that the biliary excretion of glutathione disulfide is a sensitive index of oxidant stress.

Thus, the analysis of biliary glutathione may provide important information regarding the mechanism of toxic reactions produced by reactive metabolites of chemicals. Diquat, nitrofurantoin, and paraquat markedly stimulate the biliary excretion of glutathione disulfide, presumably through their generation of active oxygen intermediates. On a molar basis, these compounds generate much more glutathione disulfide than a direct substrate for glutathione peroxidase such as *t*-butylhydroperoxide, indicating that the compounds undergo redox cycling with concomitant production of hydrogen peroxide. In hepatic microsomal preparations, other compounds such as aminopyrine and ethylmorphine generate hydrogen peroxide, apparently by the release of superoxide anion from monoreduced oxycytochrome P-450 (for review, see R. W. Estabrook, *this volume*). Although the administration of aminopyrine increases the biliary excretion of glutathione disulfide *in vivo,* this increase is associated with a proportional increase in biliary glutathione such that the glutathione disulfide:glutathione ratio in bile does not change. This small increase in biliary glutathione disulfide therefore appears to arise from a constant rate of extrahepatic oxidation of glutathione, which in turn is excreted in greater amounts because of the choleresis produced by aminopyrine administration. Aminopyrine thus produces no biologically significant oxidative stress intrahepatically *in vivo* in noninduced, normal rats. This view is supported by data obtained in the perfused rat liver (45,53).

In contrast to chemicals that may produce hydrogen peroxide intracellularly, compounds generating electrophilic metabolites that deplete intrahepatic glutathione, such as acetaminophen and chloroform, lead to a progressive decrease in the biliary excretion of glutathione and glutathione disulfide. These data indicate that oxygen radical-induced lipid peroxidation probably does not contribute significantly to the toxicity of acetaminophen, as has been postulated (63; see also J. R. Mitchell, C. V. Smith, B. H. Lauterburg, H. Hughes, G. B. Corcoran, and E. C. Horning, *this volume*). Other chemicals such as furosemide and dimethylnitrosamine, the electrophilic metabolites of which do not deplete hepatic glutathione, minimally alter biliary glutathione and glutathione disulfide. Similarly, carbon tetrachloride and iproniazid, which yield organic radical metabolites that can peroxidize membrane lipids, do not increase the biliary excretion of glutathione disulfide, indicating that membrane-bound lipid hydroperoxides may not be good substrates for glutathione peroxidases (37). The measurement of the biliary excretion of glutathione disulfide and of the glutathione disulfide:glutathione ratio in bile therefore is a sensitive index of oxidative stress *in vivo* and thus complements other *in vivo* parameters for the study of reactive intermediates of xenobiotics such as the determination of covalent binding, the formation of lipid hydroxy acids, and the depletion of intracellular glutathione (39).

Plasma glutathione disulfide is likewise a highly sensitive index of oxidant stress. Compounds such as paraquat, diquat, and *t*-butyl hydroperoxide lead to 20-fold increases in plasma glutathione disulfide, although the intracellular concentration of the disulfide rises by less than threefold. Even such massive oxidant stresses, however, do not significantly decrease the intracellular concentration of glutathione because of the compensatory mechanisms stimulating glutathione synthesis that are operative *in vivo* (2).

REGULATION OF HEPATIC GLUTATHIONE SYNTHESIS *IN VIVO*

Glutathione regulates its own synthesis by feedback inhibition of the rate-limiting step, the formation of γ-glutamylcysteine by γ-glutamylcysteine synthetase (12,48). Not surprisingly, therefore, a decrease in the hepatic glutathione concentration *in vivo* is associated with a prompt increase in the fractional rate of glutathione turnover, indicating that a similar feedback regulation is operative *in vivo* (30,35,60). In addition to activation of the rate-limiting enzymatic step, the availability of precursor amino acids is obviously a key determinant of the ability to increase glutathione synthesis. The one amino acid most likely to play a rate-limiting role is cysteine because its intrahepatic concentration is just about equal to the K_m of cysteine for γ-glutamylcysteine synthetase (11,48,60). Thus, the amount of free cysteine within the liver can sustain glutathione synthesis for only a brief period of time, and glutathione synthesis therefore depends heavily on the mobilization of cysteine from other pools. The dependence of a normal glutathione synthesis on extrahepatic sources of cysteine is clearly demonstrated in isolated hepatocytes, the glutathione concentration of which gradually decreases unless the incubation medium contains precursor amino acids (9).

Both *in vivo* and *in vitro,* methionine can be utilized for glutathione synthesis via its conversion to cysteine through the cystathionine pathway (47). Cystathionase is absent in human fetal liver (57), but glutathione concentrations are not decreased in human fetal liver (49). Moreover, patients with cystathionine synthetase deficiency do not have symptoms readily attributable to glutathione deficiency such as hemolytic anemia (43). Under basal conditions, generation of cysteine via the cystathionine pathway thus does not appear to be crucial to maintenance of normal glutathione concentrations. However, the contribution of this pathway to glutathione synthesis may be more important when the cysteine pool is stressed. A further source of cysteine is the catabolism of proteins. Protein catabolism can probably not satisfy an acutely increased demand for cysteine such as occurs following a large dose of acetaminophen. In contrast, under basal physiologic conditions, protein turnover provides as much as 50% of the cysteine used for glutathione synthesis (47). Tracer studies *in vivo* also suggest that proteins are an important source of cysteine for glutathione synthesis. When the hepatic glutathione pool is pulse-labeled with radioactive cysteine, the specific activity–time curve of glutathione is biphasic (22,38), and the late phase of the curve is best explained by recirculation of labeled cysteine originating from protein catabolism, as discussed in a later section.

In order to maintain even basal glutathione concentrations intracellularly, it is essential to recover the cysteine originating from the catabolism of glutathione itself (18,38). Most of the glutathione turnover in liver *in vivo* under basal conditions is accounted for by efflux on the sinusoidal side of the hepatocyte into plasma and to a lesser extent by biliary excretion (27). Glutathione in plasma is rapidly catabolized, mainly in the kidneys (20), and in view of the high activity of γ-glutamyltransferase in the brush border membrane of small bowel mucosa and in pancreatic secretions, it is likely that biliary glutathione is also rapidly metabolized to its constituent amino acids by the intestinal transferase and peptidases (16). The cysteine originating from glutathione catabolism is effectively recovered by the kidneys and probably also by intestinal absorption and reenters the precursor pool for glutathione synthesis.

Inhibition of γ-glutamyltransferase results in glutathionuria and thus a loss of cysteine. This loss of cysteine is associated with a progressive decrease in the hepatic glutathione concentration, suggesting that recovery of the cysteine moiety of glutathione is essential to maintain hepatic glutathione levels (18,38). The cysteine moiety of glutathione is also lost when glutathione is utilized for detoxification of electrophiles such as the reactive metabolite of acetaminophen or when cysteine is consumed to support sulfation reactions with drugs such as acetaminophen. The decreased availability of cysteine resulting from the formation of glutathionyl-*S*-acetaminophen and sulfoacetaminophen may be responsible for the decreased synthesis of glutathione in rats following a large dose of acetaminophen (34). In support of this interpretation, supplementation of cysteine by the administration of *N*-acetylcysteine promptly increases glutathione synthesis after a large dose of acetaminophen (29). Furthermore, the administration of diethylmaleate, which also forms a glutathione adduct, is followed by a prompt increase in glutathione synthesis (32). In contrast to acetaminophen, however, diethylmaleate does not undergo sulfation and therefore does not doubly drain the cysteine pool for generation of sulfate in addition to glutathione.

Dietary factors also play an important role in glutathione homeostasis, as first recognized by Leaf and Neuberger (36). Short-term fasting is associated with a decrease in free hepatic glutathione, which in part is accounted for by an increase in glutathione–protein mixed disulfides (23). The decreased concentrations of glutathione have generally been attributed to a lack of cysteine resulting in a decreased synthesis of glutathione. However, the hepatic concentrations of cysteine do not fall during a fast of 48 hr duration (11), and the fractional rate of glutathione turnover actually increases (30,60), resulting in an increase in hepatic glutathione synthesis from 0.86 to 1.5 μmole/g per hour. Since the liver weight decreases by approximately 35% during a fast of 48 hr duration, total hepatic production of glutathione remains essentially unchanged.

As in the basal state, the hepatic turnover during fasting is also accounted for by efflux. In spite of an unchanged rate of efflux, the plasma concentration of glutathione decreases markedly during fasting, indicating an increased extrahepatic catabolism of glutathione. This may reflect the increased activity of γ-glutamyltransferase, which is essential to recover the constituent amino acids of glutathione since the intact tripeptide is not taken up. By utilizing methionine for glutathione synthesis and exporting glutathione, the liver can thus make more cysteine available to other organs when the dietary supply of cysteine decreases. Hepatic glutathione thereby in a sense functions as a reservoir for cysteine (59). If the diet lacks cysteine, there is indeed an increased incorporation of methionine into hepatic glutathione (58). In addition, cysteine catabolism decreases, thus making more cysteine available for glutathione and protein synthesis.

It is obvious that the maintenance of adequate glutathione concentrations is a highly dynamic process regulated by a complex interplay of intra- and extrahepatic factors. The high capacity to stimulate glutathione turnover provides abundant glutathione in most situations in which the glutathione pools are stressed. Consequently, the availability of glutathione will rarely become rate limiting *in vivo*. With the exception of electrophilic compounds that form adducts with glutathione and therefore result not only in the consumption of glutathione but also the loss of precursor cysteine for resynthesis, biologically important depletion of glutathione (i.e., a 60–70% decrease in the intracellular concentration) does not occur. This degree of depletion appears to be the critical threshold at which toxic events against which glutathione protects become manifest (42).

COMPARTMENTALIZATION OF GLUTATHIONE

Of course, it can be argued that minor decreases in total organ glutathione reflect critical localized depletion within an organ or depletion at crucial subcellular target sites and therefore may still be toxicologically relevant. This argument would imply intraorgan or subcellular compartmentalization of glutathione.

Kinetic Homogeneity of the Hepatic Glutathione Pool

Based on nutritional studies, the presence of a labile and a stable pool of glutathione in the liver was first proposed 30 years ago (14). Fasting decreases the hepatic concentration of glutathione by approximately 30%, the size of the proposed labile or metabolizable pool of glutathione. However, these early studies failed to take into account the dynamics of hepatic glutathione turnover. Every change in either the rate of synthesis or the rate of consumption of glutathione will lead to a new steady-state concentration. This new plateau concentration reflects a new balance between production and consumption and does not necessarily imply that a compartment has been drained of its glutathione. During fasting, for example, the hepatic synthesis of glutathione increases, and the decrease in the hepatic concentration reflects increased efflux rather than depletion of a labile pool.

However, preliminary kinetic analyses of later tracer studies were construed as further evidence for the presence of two kinetically distinct pools of glutathione (22). After pulse-labeling of hepatic glutathione with radioactive cysteine, the specific activity of glutathione shows a biphasic time course. During the first phase, the specific activity declines with an apparent half-life of approximately 2 hr, reflecting the fractional rate of turnover of the proposed "labile" pool. During the second phase, the specific activity declines with an apparent half-life of approximately 30 hr, which was interpreted as evidence for an additional glutathione pool with slow turnover (22,38). However, simulations of the flux of tracer through the proposed two intrahepatic glutathione compartments by integrating the corresponding differential equations demonstrate that the proposed intrahepatic pool with slow turnover would have to be substantially larger than the pool with rapid turnover if it were to explain the specific activity–time curve of glutathione in the whole liver (B. H. Lauterburg and J. R. Mitchell, *unpublished data*).

Several experiments speak strongly against the presence of such a large pool of glutathione with slow turnover that could explain the specific activity–time curve found by Higashi et al. (22) and confirmed by Meredith and Reed (38). As mentioned earlier, our laboratory has measured hepatic glutathione turnover by acetaminophen probe analysis. Because this analysis yields a glutathione half-life corresponding to the proposed glutathione pool with rapid turnover, the specific activity of free intrahepatic glutathione should be lower than the specific activity of glutathione in the acetaminophen adduct excreted in bile if a sizable pool with slow turnover and thus a lower specific activity were present. However, the specific activity of free glutathione in liver homogenates and of the acetaminophen–glutathione adduct in bile were the same (30). In addition, inhibition of glutathione synthesis by buthionine sulfoximine results in a monophasic, and not biphasic, decline of the intrahepatic glutathione concentration to 20% of control values (17).

Based on these experimental data, and taking into account the complex precursor–product relationship between the labeled precursor amino acid and the specific activity of intrahepatic glutathione, it is much more likely that the apparent glutathione pool with slow turnover is an artifact resulting from recirculation of tracer, as previously discussed. Indeed, in the studies of Higashi et al. (22), the specific activity of plasma proteins declined at a rate similar to the late phase of their glutathione specific activity–time curve. The apparent fractional rate of turnover of all pools containing labeled cysteine will eventually approach the fractional rate of turnover of the pool with the slowest turnover. If the recirculation of cysteine originating from the catabolism of glutathione is prevented by the administration of an inhibitor of γ-glutamyltransferase, the protein pool will attain a lower specific activity, and the late phase of the specific activity–time curve of glutathione will be shifted downward with a more or less identical slope (38).

It cannot be overemphasized that hepatic glutathione kinetics are not an isolated phenomenon but must be analyzed in the context of intra- and extrahepatic factors determining the kinetics of the precursor amino acids. These experiments, however, do not rule out the presence of a lobular gradient or a small, kinetically distinct pool of glutathione as might exist in mitochondria.

Lobular Gradient of Hepatocellular Glutathione Concentration

The hepatic necrosis produced by compounds that are metabolically activated to reactive electrophilic intermediates and that deplete hepatic glutathione tends to be located in the central part of the hepatic lobule, sparing the periportal areas (41). This may be because of increased activation in the perivenous zone, where the NADPH-dependent hydroxylases are more abundant than in the periphery of the lobule (for review, see 25). A reciprocal gradient of glutathione and cytochrome P-450 resulting in increased activation and decreased detoxification in the perivenous zone might contribute to the increased susceptibility of the central part of the hepatic lobule to the toxic effects of compounds such as bromobenzene and acetaminophen. Recent data have indeed suggested that the centrilobular concentration of glutathione is lower than the periportal concentration (56). Earlier studies using a different histochemical approach have failed to demonstrate a similar concentration gradient (7).

All the histochemical methods reported so far are based on the reactivity of the sulfhydryl group of glutathione and therefore are not specific. Consequently, the interpretation of the data depends on a number of assumptions, the validity of which are difficult to prove. So far, localized depletion of glutathione by the toxins within the hepatic lobule has not been documented. Better techniques for separating isolated hepatocytes in periportal and perivenous cell fractions or more specific histochemical methods should confirm the presence of a lobular concentration gradient for glutathione.

Subcellular Localization of Glutathione

Ten to 15% of rat hepatic glutathione is within mitochondria, where the concentration of glutathione is 8 to 11 mM (24,62). Because this is a calculated value based on reported water content of mitochondria, the difference from the simultaneously determined cytoplasmic concentration of 5 to 8 mM may be more apparent than real. The glutathione disulfide:glutathione ratio is similar in cytoplasm and mitochondria.

Isolated rat liver mitochondria do not appear to take up glutathione from the incubation medium, suggesting that they might synthesize their own glutathione. In isolated hepatocytes, the turnover of mitochondrial glutathione is indeed much slower than the turnover of cytoplasmic glutathione, and diethylmaleate depletes cytoplasmic but not mitochondrial glutathione (38). *In vivo,* however, decreases in cytosolic glutathione produced by fasting or the administration of acetaminophen or diethylmaleate are associated with proportional decreases in mitochondrial glutathione. Moreover, the specific activities of mitochondrial and cytosolic glutathione are identical between 1 and 5 hr after pulse-labeling glutathione with ^{35}S-cysteine, indicating that the two pools turn over at a similar rate (B. H. Lauterburg and J. R. Mitchell, *unpublished data*). If the rate of turnover of mitochondrial glutathione *in vivo* were as slow as the rate found in isolated hepatocytes, the specific activity of glutathione within mitochondria should be at least one order of magnitude lower than that in cytosol. These *in vivo* data indicate that a segregated mitochondrial glutathione pool with slow rate of turnover may be an *in vitro* artifact. More definitive studies are needed to define the significance of mitochondrial glutathione.

CONCLUSIONS

The maintenance of hepatic glutathione homeostasis is a highly dynamic process regulated by an interplay of many intrahepatic and extrahepatic factors. These dynamics must be considered before conclusions regarding the mechanism of toxicity of a xenobiotic can be drawn from a static assessment of the intracellular glutathione status. Methods are now available to estimate the rate of synthesis, the rate of consumption, and the pathways by which glutathione is utilized by and lost from the cell. These approaches should not only provide critical mechanistic information about toxic compounds but also help to elucidate many of the still poorly understood functions of glutathione and of glutathione regulation.

REFERENCES

1. Abbott, W. A., and Meister, A. (1982): Biliary glutathione; hepatic and pancreatic contributions. *Fed. Proc.,* 41:1430.
2. Adams, J. D., Lauterburg, B. H., and Mitchell, J. R.: Plasma glutathione and glutathione disulfide in the rat: Regulation and response to oxidative stress. *J. Pharmacol. Exp. Ther. (in press).*
3. Akerboom, T. P. M., Bilzer, M., and Sies, H. (1982): The relationship of biliary glutathione disulfide efflux and intracellular glutathione disulfide content in perfused rat liver. *J. Biol. Chem.,* 257:4248–4252.
4. Akerboom, T. P. M., Bilzer, M., and Sies, H. (1982): Competition between transport of glutathione disulfide (GSSG) and glutathione *S*-conjugates from perfused rat liver into bile. *FEBS Lett.,* 140:73–76.
5. Anderson, M. E., Bridges, R. J., and Meister, A. (1980): Direct evidence for inter-organ transport of glutathione and that the non-filtration renal mechanism for glutathione utilization involves γ-glutamyl transpeptidase. *Biochem. Biophys. Res. Commun.,* 96:848–853.
6. Anderson, M. E., and Meister, A. (1980): Dynamic state of glutathione in blood plasma. *J. Biol. Chem.,* 255:9530–9533.
7. Ashgar, K., Reddy, B. G., and Krishna, G. (1975): Histochemical localization of glutathione in tissues. *J. Histochem. Cytochem.,* 23:774–779.
8. Bartoli, G. M., and Sies, H. (1978): Reduced and oxidized glutathione efflux from liver. *FEBS Lett.,* 86:89–91.
9. Beatty, P., and Reed, D. J. (1981): Influence of cysteine upon the glutathione status of isolated rat hepatocytes. *Biochem. Pharmacol.,* 30:1227–1230.
10. Chance, B., Sies, H., and Boveris, A. (1979): Hydroperoxide metabolism in mammalian organs. *Physiol. Rev.,* 59:527–605.
11. Cho, E. S., Sahyoun, N., and Stegink, L. D. (1981): Tissue glutathione as a cyst(e)ine reservoir during fasting and refeeding of rats. *J. Nutr.,* 111:914–922.
12. Davis, J. S., Balinksy, J. B., Harington, J. S., and Shepherd, J. B. (1973): Purification, properties and mechanism of action of γ-glutamylcysteine synthetase from the liver of the rat and *Xenopus laevis. Biochem. J.,* 133:667–678.
13. Eberle, D., Clarke, R., and Kaplowitz, N. (1981): Rapid oxidation *in vitro* of endogenous and exogenous glutathione in bile of rats. *J. Biol. Chem.,* 256:2115–2117.
14. Edwards, S., and Westerfield, W. W. (1952): Blood and liver glutathione during protein deprivation. *Proc. Soc. Exp. Biol. Med.,* 79:57–59.
15. Fahey, R. C. (1977): Biologically important thiol–disulfide reactions and the role of cyst(e)ine in proteins: An evolutionary perspective. *Adv. Exp. Med. Biol.,* 86A:1–20.
16. Grafström, R., Stead, A.-H., and Orrenius, S. (1980): Metabolism of extracellular glutathione in rat small intestinal mucosa. *Eur. J. Biochem.,* 106:571–577.
17. Griffith, O. W., and Meister, A. (1979): Glutathione: Inter-organ translocation, turnover and metabolism. *Proc. Natl. Acad. Sci. U.S.A.,* 76:5606–5610.
18. Griffith, O. W., and Meister, A. (1979): Translocation of intracellular glutathione to membrane-bound γ-glutamyl transpeptidase as a discrete step in the γ-glutamyl cycle: Glutathionuria after inhibition of transpeptidase. *Proc. Natl. Acad. Sci. U.S.A.,* 76:268–272.
19. Haeberle, D., Wahllaender, A., and Sies, H. (1979): Assessment of the kidney function in maintenance of plasma glutathione concentration and redox state in anesthetized rats. *FEBS Lett.,* 108:335–340.
20. Hahn, R., Wendel, A., and Flohé, L. (1978): The fate of extracellular glutathione in the rat. *Biochim. Biophys. Acta,* 359:324–337.
21. Henriques, S. B., Henriques, O. R., and Mandelbaum, F. R. (1957): Incorporation of glycine into glutathione and fibrinogen of rats under adrenaline treatment. *Biochem. J.,* 66:222–227.
22. Higashi, T., Tateishi, N., Naruse, A., and Sakamoto, Y. (1977): A novel physiologic role of liver glutathione as a reservoir of L-cysteine. *J. Biochem. (Tokyo),* 82:117–124.
23. Isaacs, J. T., and Binkley, F. (1977): Glutathione dependent control of protein disulfide–sulfhydryl content by subcellular fractions of hepatic tissue. *Biochim. Biophys. Acta,* 497:192–204.
24. Jocelyn, P. C., and Kamminga, A. (1974): The nonprotein thiol of rat liver mitochondria. *Biochim. Biophys. Acta,* 343:356–362.
25. Jungermann, K., and Katz, N. (1982): Functional hepatocellular heterogeneity. *Hepatology,* 2:385–395.
26. Kosower, N. S., and Kosower, E. M. (1978): The glutathione status of cells. *Int. Rev. Cytol.,* 54:109–160.
27. Lauterburg, B. H., Adams, J. D., and Mitchell, J. R. (1983): Efflux of glutathione from the liver accounts for total hepatic production *in vivo. Fed. Proc.,* 42:890.
28. Lauterburg, B. H., Smith, C. V., Hughes, H., and Mitchell, J. R.: Biliary excretion of glutathione and glutathione disulfide in the rat: Regulation and response to oxidative stress. *J. Clin. Invest. (in press).*
29. Lauterburg, B. H., Corcoran, G. B., and Mitchell, J. R. (1983): Mechanism of action of *N*-acetylcysteine in the protection against the hepatotoxicity of acetaminophen in rats *in vivo. J. Clin. Invest.,* 71:980–991.
30. Lauterburg, B. H., and Mitchell, J. R. (1981): Regulation of hepatic glutathione turnover in rats *in vivo* and evidence for kinetic homogeneity of the hepatic glutathione pool. *J. Clin. Invest.,* 67:1415–1424.
31. Lauterburg, B. H., and Mitchell, J. R. (1981): Biliary excretion of oxidized glutathione: An index of the *in vivo* generation of reactive oxygen intermediates by xenobiotics. *Hepatology,* 1:525.
32. Lauterburg, B. H., and Mitchell, J. R. (1981): *In vivo* regulation of hepatic glutathione synthesis: Effects of food deprivation or glutathione depletion by electrophilic compounds. In: *Second International Symposium on Biological Reactive Intermediates,* edited by R. Snyder, G. Gibson, and D. Parke, pp. 453–461. Plenum Press, New York.
33. Lauterburg, B. H., and Mitchell, J. R. (1981): Therapeutic doses of acetaminophen stimulate hepatic glutathione turnover in man. *Clin. Res.,* 29:273.
34. Lauterburg, B. H., and Mitchell, J. R. (1982): Toxic

doses of acetaminophen suppress hepatic glutathione synthesis in rats. *Hepatology,* 2:8–12.

35. Lauterburg, B. H., Vaishnav, Y., Stillwell, W. G., and Mitchell, J. R. (1980): The effect of age and glutathione depletion on hepatic glutathione turnover *in vivo* determined by acetaminophen probe analysis. *J. Pharmacol. Exp. Ther.,* 213:54–58.
36. Leaf, G., and Neuberger, A. (1947): The effect of diet on the glutathione content of the liver. *Biochem. J.,* 41:280–287.
37. McCay, P. B., Gibson, D. D., Fong, K. L., and Hornbrook, K. R. (1976): Effect of glutathione peroxidase activity on lipid peroxidation in biological membranes. *Biochim. Biophys. Acta,* 431:459–468.
38. Meredith, M. J., and Reed, D. J. (1982): Status of the mitochondrial pool of glutathione in the isolated hepatocyte. *J. Biol. Chem.,* 257:3747–3753.
39. Mitchell, J. R., Hughes, H., Lauterburg, B. H., and Smith, C. V. (1982): Chemical nature of reactive intermediates as determinant of toxicologic responses. *Drug Metab. Rev.,* 13:539–553.
40. Mitchell, J. R., and Jollow, D. J. (1975): Metabolic activation of drugs to toxic substances. *Gastroenterology,* 68:392–410.
41. Mitchell, J. R., Jollow, D. J., Potter, W. Z., David, D. C., Gillette, J. R., and Brodie, B. B. (1973): Acetaminophen-induced hepatic necrosis. I. Role of drug metabolism. *J. Pharmacol. Exp. Ther.,* 187:185–194.
42. Mitchell, J. R., Jollow, D. J., Potter, W. Z., Gillette, J. R., and Brodie, B. B. (1973): Acetaminophen-induced hepatic necrosis. IV. Protective role of glutathione. *J. Pharmacol. Exp. Ther.,* 187:211–217.
43. Mudd, S. H., and Levy, H. L. (1978): Disorders of transsulfuration. In: *The Metabolic Basis of Inherited Disease,* fourth edition, edited by J. B. Stanbury, J. B. Wyngaarden, and D. S. Fredrickson, pp. 458–503. McGraw-Hill, New York.
44. Orrenius, S., and Jones, D. P. (1978): Functions of glutathione in drug metabolism. In: *Functions of Glutathione in Liver and Kidneys,* edited by H. Sies and A. Wendel, pp. 164–175. Springer, New York.
45. Oshino, N., and Chance, B. (1977): Properties of glutathione release observed during reduction of organic hydroperoxide, demethylation of aminopyrine and oxidation of some substances in perfused rat liver and their implication for the physiological function of calase. *Biochem. J.,* 162:509–525.
46. Poulsen, H. E., Ranek, L., and Andreasen, P. B. (1981): The hepatic glutathione content in liver disease. *Scand. J. Clin. Lab. Invest.,* 41:573–576.
47. Reed, D. J., and Orrenius, S. (1977): The role of methionine in glutathione biosynthesis by isolated hepatocytes. *Biochem. Biophys. Res. Commun.,* 77:1258–1264.
48. Richman, P. G., and Meister, A. (1975): Regulation of γ-glutamylcysteine synthetase by nonallosteric feedback inhibition by glutathione. *J. Biol. Chem.,* 250:1422–1426.
49. Rollins, D., Larsson, A., Steen, B., Krishnaswamy, K., Hagenfeldt, L., Moldeus, P., and Rane, A. (1981): Glutathione and γ-glutamyl cycle enzymes in human fetal liver. *J. Pharmacol. Exp. Ther.,* 217:697–700.
50. Sekura, R., and Meister, A. (1974): Glutathione turnover in the kidney: Considerations relating to the glutamyl cycle and the transport of amino acids. *Proc. Natl. Acad. Sci. U.S.A.,* 71:2969–2972.
51. Shi, E. C. P., Fisher, R., McEvoy, M., Vantol, R., Rose, M., and Ham, J. M. (1982): Factors influencing hepatic glutathione concentrations: A study in surgical patients. *Clin. Sci.,* 62:279–283.
52. Siegers, C. P., Bossen, K. H., Younes, M., Mahlke, R., and Oltmanns, D. (1982): Glutathione and glutathione-*S*-transferases in the normal and diseased human liver. *Pharmacol. Res. Commun.,* 14:61–71.
53. Sies, H., Bartoli, G. M., Burk, R. F., and Waydhas, C. (1978): Glutathione efflux from perfused rat liver after phenobarbitol treatment, during drug oxidations, and in selenium deficiency. *Eur. J. Biochem.,* 89:113–118.
54. Sies, H., Gerstenecker, C., Menzel, H., and Flohe, L. (1972): Oxidation in the NADPH system and release of GSSG from hemoglobin-free perfused rat liver during peroxidatic oxidation of glutathione by hydroperoxides. *FEBS Lett.,* 27:171–175.
55. Sies, H., and Summer, K. H. (1975): Hydroperoxide metabolizing systems in rat liver. *Eur. J. Biochem.,* 57:503–512.
56. Smith, M. T., Loveridge, N., Wills, E. D., and Chayen, J. (1979): The distribution of glutathione in the rat liver lobule. *Biochem. J.,* 182:103–108.
57. Sturman, J. A., Gaull, G., and Räihä, N. C. R. (1970): Absence of cystathionase in human fetal liver: Is cysteine essential? *Science,* 169:74–76.
58. Tateishi, N., Higashi, T., Naruse, A., Hikita, K., and Sakamoto, Y. (1981): Relative contributions of sulfur atoms of dietary cysteine and methionine to rat liver glutathione and proteins. *J. Biochem. (Tokyo),* 90:1603–1610.
59. Tateishi, N., Higashi, T., Naruse, A., Nakashima, K., Shiozaki, H., and Sakamoto, Y. (1977): Rat liver glutathione: Possible role as a reservoir of cysteine. *J. Nutr.,* 107:51–60.
60. Tateishi, N., Higashi, T., Shinya, S., Naruse, A., and Sakamoto, Y. (1974): Studies on the regulation of glutathione level in rat liver. *J. Biochem. (Tokyo),* 75:93–103.
61. Waelsch, H., and Rittenberg, D. (1942): Glutathione. II. The metabolism of glutathione studied with isotopic ammonia and glutamic acid. *J. Biol. Chem.,* 144:53–58.
62. Wahlländer, A., Soboll, S., and Sies, H. (1979): Hepatic mitochondrial and cytosolic glutathione content and the subcellular distribution of GSH-*S*-transferases. *FEBS Lett.,* 97:138–140.
63. Wendel, A., and Feuerstein, S. (1981): Drug-induced lipid peroxidation in mice. I. Modulation by monooxygenase activity, glutathione and selenium status. *Biochem. Pharmacol.,* 30:2513–2520.

Drug Metabolism and Drug Toxicity,
edited by J. R. Mitchell and M. G. Horning.

Liver Perfusion Studies in Drug Metabolism and Drug Toxicity

K. Sandy Pang

Faculty of Pharmacy, University of Toronto, Toronto, Ontario M5S 1A1, Canada

The liver has long been recognized as the major organ for all phases of intermediary metabolism (24,25). Moreover, its metabolizing ability extends not only to endogenous compounds but also to exogenously administered xenobiotics. Because of the diverse nature of these hepatic drug-metabolizing enzymes, which act rather nonspecifically on a great variety of compounds (166), the liver is the largest drug-metabolizing organ in the body.

The biotransformation of an exogenous compound to its metabolites is usually accompanied by a modification of the inherent pharmacological and toxicological properties of the xenobiotic. The liver is involved in detoxication/deactivation mechanisms in which metabolic reactions transform xenobiotics to nontoxic or nonpharmacologic entities. Alternatively, hepatic biotransformation may generate toxic metabolites that usually attack macromolecules such as proteins or DNA in liver and, if they are sufficiently stable, escape to the systemic circulation to reach other organs to exert their toxic effects. Also, through bioactivation, the liver transforms "inert" xenobiotics to more potent pharmacologic molecules, a principle used in prodrug therapy.

The liver is also unique in its anatomical placement. It receives a *dual* supply of blood via the hepatic artery, arising from the aorta (25%), and via the portal vein (75%), which is a conglomerate of venous returns from the intestines, spleen, and mesenteries. By lying between the portal and systemic circulation, the liver will receive drugs entering via the portal system during oral absorption and may dispose of a major portion of the dose, a phenomenon known as the "first-pass" effect of drugs (51).

Because of the importance of the liver in bioactivation or termination of pharmacological activity of xenobiotics, and because the liver is also the major organ responsible for drug-mediated toxicity through activation, much attention is paid to various aspects of drug metabolism and drug toxicity. For this reason, *in vivo* and *in vitro* techniques, the latter including perfusion systems, liver homogenates, liver slices, isolated hepatocytes, and membrane fractions as well as purified enzyme preparations, are widely used. Needless to say, each *in vitro* approach has its distinctive design and pertains to specific questions on metabolic processes or mechanisms that cannot be answered by *in vivo* experimentation. Occasionally, however, the contribution of one metabolic pathway is exploited over others, especially when an *in vitro* system is compromised by the exclusion of competing pathways, and the metabolism is shunted towards a manipulated and planned pathway.

The perfused liver preparation, however, allows only for xenobiotic removal by the liver, be it metabolic or excretory, and is a preparation that incorporates flow dynamics similar to those in the *in vivo* situation, be it metabolic or excretory. In contrast to homogenates, hepatocytes, and membrane fractions or purified enzymes preparations, organ structure, spatial heterogeneity, and architecture are preserved in this technique. The portal tracts, sinusoids, and space of Disse, which are channels that facilitate material exchange, remain unperturbed. Moreover, as discussed later in the text, the technique has widespread applications in all facets of drug metabolism and drug toxicity studies.

Although liver perfusion techniques have been applied to many animal species such as the cow (37), pig (1), guinea pig (78), dog (58), frog (39), mouse (74), rabbit (7), and rat (88), the most prevalent animal species used is the rat. The rat offers advantages over other animal species in that the gall bladder is absent (140), and hence bile flow is continuous. Moreover, its small size, low cost, and the ease of handling allow for preservation of perfusate because flow rate need not be high. Because of its extensive use, the ensuing discussion pertains largely to rat liver perfusion. The technique described, however, also applies to most animal species and to the perfusion of other organs.

METHODS

Liver perfusion techniques have been extensively reviewed (6,82,84,122,124). The initial usage in the characterization of biochemical mechanisms is now expanded to include drug metabolism and drug toxicity studies.

Liver Perfusion Apparatus

The essentials of a liver perfusion apparatus provide the necessary components that support viability and stability of the liver preparation (Fig. 1). The original home-built apparatus by Miller (87,88) and Brauer (29) and modifications thereof (5) include a reservoir unit, which stores the perfusion medium, an artificial "heart and lung" in the form of an oxygenator and pump or a hydrostatic overflow reservoir above the liver, a heating unit, usually in the form of a heating bath, and a chamber to maintain temperature (37°C). Usually a bubble trap and filter device are placed between the reservoir and liver to remove undesired debris or emboli from the perfusate. The oxygenators range from expensive units such as the multifilament gas exchangers used for dialysis or organ preservation to inexpensive "lungs" comprised of coils of silastic tubing that channel blood intraradially in a perspex cylinder and allow for permeability of oxygen (usually flowing at 1 liter/min; O_2:CO_2, 95:5, vol/vol) from the enriched and enclosed atmosphere of oxygen (9,36).

Artificial "hearts" for delivery of the perfusate in home-built apparati usually operate via a roller or peristaltic pump that brings

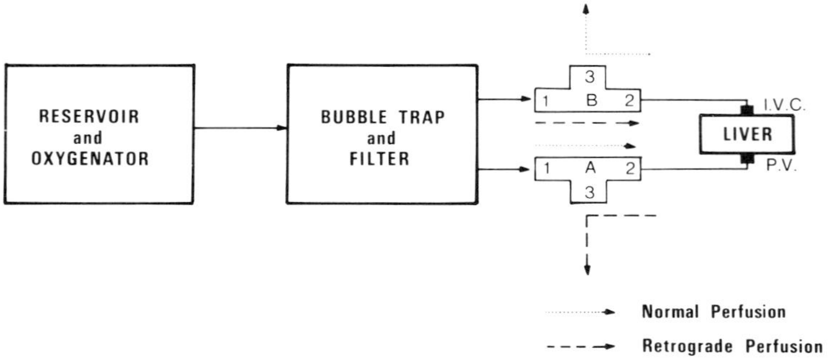

FIG. 1. Schematic representation of the liver perfusion apparatus. A and B denote three-way stopcocks that facilitate the change from anterograde to retrograde perfusion. Symbols pv and ivc denote the portal vein and inferior vena cava (hepatic vein), respectively.

perfusate to a hydrostatic reservoir placed above the plane of the liver preparation. The height of the hydrostatic overflow reservoir (usually 10–20 cm above liver) determines the perfusion pressure and, therefore, flow. This constant-pressure device for flow delivery allows for fluctuations in flow to be induced either by intrahepatic pressure changes or by the vasodilatory or vasoconstrictive actions of the administered xenobiotics. Flow changes in the perfusion systems were observed for chloroform (27), which increases perfusate flow, and vanadate, ouabain (149), and chlorpromazine (146), which decrease perfusate flow in the constant-pressure delivery system. Direct pumping of perfusate to liver, however, has been found to provide constant flow rates because changes in intrahepatic pressure induced by drugs during perfusion are overcome by the direct pumping action. Other added features include pressure, pH, and Po_2 monitoring devices and elaborations such as dialyzing units for removal of metabolic products from venous blood (5). These devices are interconnected by tubing (tygon or silastic) that serves as the circulation. The home-built perfusion setups are usually very cumbersome. Commercially available units (TWO/TEN Perfuser, MX International, Aurora, CO), which are both compact and functional, are now used more extensively than home-built perfusion apparati (43,99).

Perfusion Medium

Perfusion medium usually varies from laboratory to laboratory, but the common features entail an oxygen carrier such as red cells and an oncotic agent in the form of protein or a plasma expander such as dextran. The medium is fortified with nutrients such as glucose, essential amino acids, and vitamins in a buffer solution that provides the necessary elements to support cosubstrate syntheses (93,117); the solution is buffered to pH 7.4.

The addition of an oxygen carrier in perfusate is desirable because of the high oxygen capacity at the reduced flow rates (0.8–2.0 ml/min per g liver) required of liver perfusion. Studies on oxygen requirements indicate that a minimum of 45 mm Hg is required for rat liver perfusion (40), and the usual consumption of oxygen is around 0.62 ml/min per g liver or 2.3 μmole/min per g liver (9,44,60). To this end, pooled, heparinized, and defibrinated blood from donors of the same species diluted with Krebs Ringer bicarbonate solution (hematocrit of 20–30%) (5,88) or semisynthetic media of washed outdated human red blood cells (1,60,105), sheep erythrocytes (102), pig (169), or ox erythrocytes (127) are often employed. Comparative morphology studies on hemoglobin and hemoglobin-free perfusate have shown that although a reduced flow rate (15 ml/min per liver) maintained cellular integrity for perfusion systems that entailed red cells, the same flow rate did not provide adequate oxygenation for hemoglobin-free systems. The latter condition led to anoxia with endothelial cell injury, the absence of hepatic microvilli, and intensive vacuolization (129). The extent of injury was partially reduced with higher flow rates (45, 60, 72 ml/min per liver) in the hemoglobin-free system, but the sensitivity of centrilobular cells to injury still persisted (129).

Flow rates of 0.6 ml/min per g liver with hemoglobin, however, were found to be anoxic to the liver (128). Similar findings were obtained in our laboratory for reduced flow rates (0.4 ml/min per g liver) (105). Reduced metabolic activities of the liver under these instances are attributed not only to inadequate oxygenation but to a reduction in pressure because of the reduced flow rate, because a critical pressure flow is required to support and sustain the opening of the vascular channels according to Brauer (28).

Fluorocarbons substituted for red cells in perfusion medium have met with varying success. Equivalence between the red cell and fluorocarbon media was found in some instances (33,54), and a longer duration of viability (10 hr) was provided with fluorocarbon perfusion (73). Fluorocarbons, however, may act as uncouplers of monooxygenation

(154) and as dead-end inhibitors because of high lipid solubility; fluorocarbons were also found to interact with amino acids and proteins and, unless the perfusate is filtered, may cause ballooning of sinusoids near the portal areas (158).

The addition of an oncotic agent such as protein or dextran aids in exerting a hydrostatic pressure to prevent perfusate water from entering cells. The fortification with glucose and nutrients aids in functional intermediary metabolism, and liver stores in the liver are not depleted. These nutrients, together with metal ions and cationic groups present in buffer, support most enzymatic reactions whose actions require bivalent ions for activation and precursors in the synthesis of cosubstrates. Examples of the latter are glucose for UDPGA (117) and inorganic sulfate for PAPS syntheses (93). Occasionally, bile salts such as taurocholate are added to support bile flow. Vitamins are included to aid in metabolic reactions, and antibiotics to prevent bacterial growth during long-term perfusions.

A hemoglobin- and protein-free perfusate, when utilized at high flow rates (3–4 ml/min per g liver), often presents a desirable alternative in perfusion systems because the system allows for a direct monitoring of biochemical events. For example, spectrophotometry of light transmitted through a lobe of the perfused liver permits a direct measurement of absorbances for enzymes (136); surface fluorimetry monitors redox changes of flavin and pyridine nucleotides (130,131). Microlight guides, when placed on the periportal or pericentral regions of the liver surface, will detect fluorescence changes of pyridine nucleotides (67) and substrate disappearance coincidental to metabolite production (38). Effluent perfusate may be assayed directly for oxygen content or for substrate and metabolic concentrations so that kinetic and continuous monitoring are provided (150). In these systems, the course of a metabolic reaction can be followed, and often the rate-limiting step can be identified. The disadvantages of this type of perfusate are the high flow rates required to sustain adequate oxygenation such that the test compounds are utilized at higher amounts (for single-pass experiments) and the relatively shorter duration of the experiment because of the rapid onset of deleterious effects with perfusion of buffer solutions (129).

The composition of the perfusion medium strongly influences organ functionality: the absence or presence of red cells (and perfusate flow), the absence or presence of proteins, the presence or absence of nutrients and of precursors. For this reason, data obtained from different laboratories may not be strictly comparable because of differences in the composition of the medium.

The semisynthetic perfusate employed in our laboratory for the past 10 years is similar to that proposed by Schimassek (127) and Hems et al. (60). Human outdated red cells (obtained from local blood banks or the Red Cross) are repetitively washed (two or three times) with equal volumes of physiological saline and lactated Ringers solution and centrifuged. The supernatant after each washing is suctioned off by vacuum, together with deposits of proteins and ghost cells at the interphase. The prepared cells are filtered through a thin mesh prior to their addition to "plasma" perfusate. "Plasma" perfusate is prepared as follows: Krebs–Henseleit bicarbonate (see Table 1) is used to dissolve dextran (3%), and

TABLE 1. *Perfusate for isolated liver*

Krebs–Henseleit bicarbonate	
NaCl 0.9% (0.154 M)	100 parts
KCl 1.15% (0.154 M)	4
$CaCl_2$ 1.22% (0.11 M)	3
KH_2PO_4 2.11% (0.154 M)	1
$MgSO_4 \cdot 7H_2O$ 3.82% (0.154 M)	1
$NaHCO_3$ 1.3% (0.154 M)	21
To prepare	
Gas $NaHCO_3$ 1 hr with CO_2 prior to use	
Perfusate composition	
Bovine serum albumin (Tyrode solution, Sigma Chemical Co.)	1%
Dextran T-40 (Pharmacia Fine Chemicals)	3%
Glucose (Travenol Labs) 50% solution	300 mg%
Krebs–Henseleit carbonate	75.6%
Washed human red cells	20%

the resulting solution is filtered through Whatman No. 1 filter paper. After the addition of glucose and the test substrate, the entire solution is thoroughly mixed. Bovine serum albumin (1%) is added to the dextran–glucose–buffer and is buffered to a pH of 7.4. At this stage, washed red cells (20%) are added to the "plasma" solution (formula of semisynthetic medium is seen in Table 1). A perfusate flow of 10 ml/min per liver is customarily used in rat liver perfusion studies in the commercial TWO/TEN Perfuser.

Surgical Procedure

Although there are minor differences in the operative procedure, the basic steps are essentially the same. After treatment of the animal with an anesthetic (pentobarbital, 50 mg/kg i.p.), the following steps are performed:

1. An incision is made at the midpoint of the lower abdomen, and a V section is made from the point of entry to the two sides of the rat just below the diaphragm. Caution is exercised not to puncture the diaphragm.
2. The V section of the abdomen is flipped back to the thorax of the animal and secured into place with a hemostat.
3. With the use of a wetted cotton gauze, the intestines of the animal are displaced to the right (of the operator) to expose portal areas.
4. The bile duct is identified by following the juncture of the stomach to the duodenum. The intestines are held loosely between the fingers with gentle tension, and a small duct that contains a straw-colored fluid is displayed. This is the bile duct. A loose ligature (surgical silk, size 0-0) is placed around a cleared upper portion of the bile duct proximal to the liver, and an incision is made at a distal position. A wedged cannula (PE 20) is inserted through the cut and the tip advanced to the bifurcations of the bile duct. After the first ligature is tied off, another tie is made to secure the bile duct in place.
5. The pyloric vein, a small venous branch that enters the upper portal vein from the left of the animal, is also tied (surgical silk, 0-0).
6. The lower right liver lobe, which lies on top of the vena cava, is freed of connecting ligatures to the vena cava, and a loose ligature (silk, size 1) is placed around the vena cava above the entry of the right renal vein.
7. The celiac artery, identified as a thick-walled pulsating artery which branches to the hepatic artery, is tied.
8. Loose ligatures (three) are placed around the portal vein. A catheter placement unit (16G, $2\frac{1}{4}''$, Jelco Labs, Raritan, NJ), which comprises an inner needle and an outer Teflon® sheath, is used to puncture the portal vein. After insertion, the inner needle is withdrawn, leaving the Teflon® catheter in place for advancement to the tip of the liver. The backflow of rat blood fills the catheter, and the middle ligature is tied. The outflow from the perfusion apparatus is immediately connected to the portal catheter to initiate perfusion. The remaining ligatures are then tied.
9. The ligature around the vena cava is tied, and the abdominal inferior vena cava and aorta are severed to allow animal blood and perfusate to exit.
10. The diaphragm is cut, exposing the thorax. By means of a pair of curved scissors, the rib cage is completely removed, and the right atrium cut. Another Teflon® catheter (14G; $2\frac{1}{4}''$) is placed through the right atrium into the inferior vena cava, with the tip of the catheter advanced to the entry of the hepatic vein. Ties (two or three) are made around the catheter to secure its placement.

During the surgical procedure, there is no prolonged period of anoxia (<5 sec) because perfusion is started immediately after cannulation of the portal vein. The entire surgical procedure should take about 10 to 15 min to insure the success of the preparation.

Cannulation of both the hepatic artery and the portal vein is sometimes carried out in larger animal species such as pig liver perfusion (169) or bovine liver perfusion (37). No differences in intermediary metabolism between the perfusion of the portal versus portal and arterial perfusion are found (156). The perfusion of the hepatic artery is not essential for normal function of the liver.

Methods of Perfusion

There are two commonly used methods of liver perfusion: the isolated perfused liver (88) and the perfused liver *in situ* (92). In the latter, the organ remains *in situ* in the body, and the surgical procedure is completed as described in the above procedure. For the isolated perfused liver technique, the lobes of the liver are freed from the loose ligaments that attach it to structures such as the stomach, intestines, and abdominal wall. Care is exercised in removal of the organ, particularly for the small lobe that lies beneath the stomach. From right to left (of the operator), and with the fingers encasing and protecting the liver, liver lobes are freed from the esophagus, stomach, aorta, intestines, and vena cava (cut made below the ligature on the vena cava). The isolated organ is (a) placed into a bath of perfusate, (b) suspended in air with catheters supported by prongs such that the surface of the liver is not in contact with any surface, or (c) placed onto a dish that supports the liver. A comparison of both isolated organ and *in situ* techniques showed equivalence in intermediary metabolism (124).

A third, yet underutilized technique is the method of retrograde perfusion. As implied by the nomenclature, retrograde perfusion (155) entails the entry of perfusate via the hepatic vein and exit by the portal vein and/or hepatic artery. The surgical procedure for this method is similar to that for anterograde perfusion as described above. A recently published procedure for retrograde perfusion (107) employs the use of two three-way stopcocks to facilitate the change from anterograde perfusion to retrograde perfusion (Fig. 1). Despite the fact that long-term (3 hr) retrograde perfusion is deemed detrimental to liver function (121), short-term (50 min) perfusion with this technique is without deleterious effects as confirmed by the monitoring of K^+, SGOT, SGPT, and LDH and by examination of ultrastructure by light and electron microscopy in our laboratory (101).

Recirculating and Nonrecirculating Designs

Two modes of perfusion experiments, (a) the recirculation of perfusate with venous blood leaving the liver returned to the reservoir or (b) the once-through design, synonomous with single-pass or nonrecirculating, provide a choice for different experimental conditions.

Advantages for the once-through design as outlined by Lindros (77) include the provision of sampling of large volumes of perfusate (inflow and outflow), a direct assessment of material balance for substrate loss across the liver, and the accrual of metabolic events at steady-state conditions. Other advantages include the ease of varying experimental conditions such as input concentrations, cosubstrates and their precursors, and, most importantly, return to control conditions with the same liver preparation. These advantages appear to justify the large volume of perfusate required in single-pass perfusions. A drawback in the design, however, lies in the possible depletion of cosubstrates or endogenous compounds that are repetitively "washed out" of the liver.

Recirculating designs mimic more closely the circulation *in vivo,* and only small volumes of perfusate are required. But recirculating experiments accumulate endogenous metabolites, which sometimes inhibit or influence organ function. The repetitive circulation of perfusate via pumping brings increased hemolysis to red cells in the medium. Moreover, an added inconvenience lies in the limited volume that can be removed from the system (reservoir or hepatic venous perfusate) without affecting material balance and volume changes. In recirculating experiments, reservoir perfusate should be of sufficiently large volume such that the "dead volume" occupied by the tubing, bubble trap, and other devices do not present a major percentage of the total volume of the reservoir. Or else, high perfusate flow should circumvent inadequate mixing with the reservoir.

Liver Viability and Stability

Assessment of liver function should be performed to establish good viability and functionality of the liver prior to utilization of the technique in drug metabolism and drug toxicity studies. These include physical tests such as pressure (5,28,33), pH (31), Po_2 (54,127,156), and Pco_2 monitoring, biochemical tests for K^+ and enzymes (SGOT, SGPT, LDH) in hepatic venous blood (1,5,74,127,156), and histological examination of ultrastructure by light and electron microscopy (73,96). Endogenous indices such as lactate/pyruvate ratio (54,128,156), ATP/ADP ratio (41,60), glucose (5,36, 60,73), and urea production (5,36,60,74), and exogenous markers such as hepatic extraction of bromosulfophthalein (1,74) and galactose (73,156) have also been used.

The rate of bile production is no longer an acceptable criterion to assess metabolic function of the liver. Reasons are that bile flow (usually at 1 ml/hr) fluctuates with perfusion flow rate (29), temperature (26), and the presence of bile acids that promote bile flow (20). Moreover, bile flow tends to decrease with perfusion time and is subjected to the choleretic (123) and cholestatic (32,71,146,164) actions of administered xenobiotics. Gross deterioration of the liver often precedes cessation of bile flow.

For the experienced experimenter, however, the gross appearance of the liver, the constancy of observations in the identical first and last perfusion periods during the experiment, the degree of oxygenation of arterial and venous blood (visual detection of color difference in red cell perfusate), and the smoothness of the operative procedure are the more routine and preferred markers for liver viability. Moreover, liver weight should remain at 3 to 4% of total body weight at the end of the perfusion experiment.

CHARACTERISTIC FEATURES OF LIVER PERFUSIONS

Suitability of Liver Perfusion

Because the liver is enriched with enzymes capable of carrying out most phases of metabolic reactions, the literature is replete with applications of the technique in studies of drug metabolism and drug toxicity. The suitability of the technique depends greatly on (a) a lack of binding or loss of substrate to the perfusion apparatus, e.g., tubings and catheters, and (b) the duration of experimental conditions. In drug metabolism studies, the method can be used as a "metabolite factory" for the examination of patterns of metabolism and excretion when test substrates are inert to the perfusion apparatus. The technique, however, is not suitable for toxicity studies that require chronic procedures and long incubation periods for the manifestations of toxicity.

Experimental Conditions

It is noteworthy that the conditions of liver perfusion drastically influence the type and quantity of metabolites formed. The composition of perfusate (absence or presence of cells and proteins) determines not only flow rates but also the degree of reversible binding to perfusate components (unbound substrate is considered as the species that traverses membranes into hepatocytes for elimination).

Other controlling factors include concentration of cofactors to support metabolic reactions, the degree and adequacy of oxygenation (40,94,164), temperature (26,138), perfusate flow rate, which influences hepatic extraction efficiency (28,105,106,134), and the dose or concentration of the substrate in perfusate entering the liver, which influences the degree of saturability of metabolic pathways. Pretreatment with inducers such as phenobarbital (66,113), 3-methylcholanthrene (59,66), with inhibitors such as diethylstilbesterol (91), SKF-525A (43), or with depleting agents such as diethylmaleate (115), and predisposing factors of liver donors such as age (142), sex (18,79), diet (34,137), and nutritional status (fasted versus fed) (117) are additional considerations.

The choice of experimental design, whether recirculating or single pass, is also of key importance. The recirculation of medium allows for the reentry of substrates and metabolites into the liver for further metabolism, and because of the absence of the kidneys for excretion of polar metabolites, glucuronides and sulfates will be excreted to a greater extent into bile than *in vivo*. First-, second-, or multistage metabolites emerge as a result of repetitive biotransformation processes by the liver. For this reason, the recirculating design is often employed to generate metabolites in perfusate and bile for isolation and identification purposes. This design is also more appropriate for drug toxicity studies, which depend on bioactivation and the accumulation of toxic entities. Moreover, the design is favored for substrates whose extractability (hepatic extraction ratio) by the liver is low; that is, only a small fraction of the substrate is removed during a single delivery through the liver. Examples of these compounds include antipyrine (105) and carbamazepine (113). But in studies in which only a limited amount of precursor of cosubstrate synthesis is present in the finite volume in recirculating studies, depletion of cosubstrate easily arises because of an insufficiency of precursor, and a concentration dependence as well as a time dependence develops. Additionally, end products accumulate and occasionally cause unwanted interactions (inhibition of metabolism of parent compound).

In contrast, the single-pass design permits flow of perfusate through the liver only once, thereby eliminating subsequent metabolism and the accumulation of metabolites. Steady-state conditions are attained readily, however, at which time the binding processes that influence loss of substrate in addition to eliminatory processes are essentially completed; rate of loss at steady state is attributed to rates of metabolism and excretion. Precursors for cosubstrate synthesis are replenished easily and constantly in single-pass designs, and the concentration and time dependence in recirculating experiments are circumvented. More importantly, the metabolic reaction is identified by the loss of substrate, which reflects enzymatic activity and not synthesis of cosubstrate as the limiting condition. For this reason, the design is most suitable for kinetic considerations of enzymatic reactions. Input conditions are interchanged to accommodate other substrates or precursors. Kinetic constants such as K_m and V_{max} (Michaelis–Menten constant and maximum velocity) are readily assessed within the system (45,69,70,102,168). Also, because of the ease of maneuverability of input conditions, controls are easily set within the same liver.

Sampling and Quantitation

After the choice of the experimental design (composition of perfusate and recirculating or single pass), judicious planning of sampling sites and sampling times facilitates the maximization of information that can be gained from liver perfusion studies. Besides the extensive information that is obtained on substrate and metabolites, the liver may be removed for the examination of reversible binding (43,132) to subcellular fractions or irreversible binding such as covalent binding to tissue macromolecules (18,79). The liver, removed after perfusion studies, may be tested for metabolic activity after homogenization, and metabolism may be examined from a different aspect and under varying conditions (an abundance of cosubstrate). The effects of substrate and its metabolites on intermediary metabolism, oxygen consumption, leakage of hepatic enzymes, and K^+, which are indicative of liver damage, and histology of organ after treatment will furnish additional information on the biochemical mechanism in drug metabolism, drug toxicity, and drug–drug interactions.

APPLICATIONS OF LIVER PERFUSION TECHNIQUE

Drug Metabolism and Drug Toxicity

Because the liver is replete with enzyme systems capable of supporting both phase I and phase II reactions (Table 2), the liver perfusion techniques are often used for the synthesis of metabolites. Phase I products usually undergo sequential metabolism (100) prior to their emergence into hepatic venous circulation. Phase II products, usually glucuronides that have "favorable" molecular weights (62), are excreted predominantly into bile rather than into the perfusate and are accompanied by sulfate and glutathione conjugates. Liver perfusion has been utilized to demonstrate differences in metabolic disposition of enantiomers. Examples are ±hexobarbital (30) and *d*- and *l*-methadone (48,80). On the other hand, toxicity studies with liver perfusion have demonstrated the covalent binding of ^{3}H-benzo(a)pyrene (66), ^{3}H-benzo(a)pyrene-4,5-oxide (139), ^{14}C-styrene oxide (159), and 2,6-dinitro-[^{14}C]toluene (79) to proteins, DNA, and RNA.

The perfused liver preparation is a useful tool in the examination of drug–drug interactions (Table 3). Because drug-induced and secondary physiological changes that occur *in vivo* may be circumvented, this technique frequently provides insight into the mode of interaction. An example of such a study is the interaction between *dl*-propranolol and lidocaine. Although hepatic flow to the perfused liver preparation was maintained constant by pump action, lidocaine clearance was decreased by pretreatment with *dl*-propranolol (165), suggesting that the mechanism of interaction between lidocaine and propranolol as reported in the *in vivo* dog (23) was not a simple interaction via induced changes in hepatic blood flow with propranolol.

Another application of this technique lies in the use of retrograde perfusion of the liver. There has been renewed interest in this technique for the examination of problems related to the heterogeneous distribution of drug-metabolizing enzymes. Retrograde perfusion, as originally proposed by Trowell (155), presented merely an alternative to liver perfusion. The flow of substrate during retrograde flow, however, allows the substrate to be exposed to enzyme systems in an opposite direction with respect to their delivery via anterograde flow. The first application was in a study of the distribution of enzyme activities for *O*-deethylation and sulfation of phenacetin to acetaminophen and acetaminophen sulfate (99). The comparative metabolism of ^{14}C-phenacetin and ^{3}H-acetaminophen delivered simultaneously to the liver preparation revealed that the distribution of sulfation activity was periportal, whereas the distribution of *O*-deethylation activity was centrilobular. Confirming evidence on the distribution of *O*-deethylase activity was provided by a fluorimetric technique for measuring 7-hydroxycoumarin production from 7-ethoxycoumarin with microlight guides placed in the periportal and pericentral regions of the rat liver surface (65).

The probe into the distribution of sulfation and glucuronidation activities of the rat liver preparation with anterograde and retrograde perfusion was carried out with phenolic substrates such as 7-hydroxycoumarin (38) and harmol (103). Despite the different approaches employed, microlight guides in the former and metabolic data and computer

TABLE 2. *Widespread use of liver perfusion techniques in all phases of drug metabolism*

Examples	Comments on metabolite formed	References
Hydroxylation		
Acetanilide	Acetaminophen	110
Allopurinol	Oxipurinol	98
Cyclazocine	Hydroxylated metabolite	81
Diphenylhydantoin	4-Hydroxydiphenylhydantoin	49,64
Hexobarbital	Hydroxylated metabolite	148
Imipramine	2-Hydroxyimipramine	10,42
Lidocaine	3-Hydroxylidocaine	147
(+)Lysergic acid diethylamide	13-Hydroxy, 14-hydroxy metabolite	135
Metacyclazone	Hydroxylated metabolite	81
MEGX	3-Hydroxy MEGX	147
Pentazocine	Hydroxylated metabolite	81
Phenobarbital	Hydroxylated metabolite	148
Procainamide	3-Hydroxy-*N*-acetylprocainamide	157
Quinidine	3-Hydroxyquinidine	172
Volazocine	Hydroxylated metabolite	81
N-dealkylation		
Imipramine	Desmethylimipramine	10
MEGX	GX	101
Lidocaine	MEGX	105
Procainamide	Desethylprocainamide	157
Naltrexone	*N*-Dealkylated metabolite	123
O-Dealkylation		
7-Ethoxycoumarin	7-Hydroxycoumarin	65
p-Nitroanisole	*p*-Nitrophenol	89,150
Phenacetin	Acetaminophen	99,107,110
Quinidine	*O*-Desmethylquinidine	172
Epoxidation		
Acrolein	Glycialdehyde	111
Carbamazepine	10,11-Epoxide	113
Oxidation		
Ethanol	Acetaldehyde	77
Reduction		
7-Nitrazepam	7-Aminonitrazepam	5,7
N-Oxidation		
Imipramine	Imipramine *N*-oxide	90
Hydrolysis		
Mestranol	Ethynylestradiol	17
MK-421	MK-422	109
Hydration by epoxide hydratase		
Styrene oxide	Styrene glycol	159
Benzo(a)pyrene-4,5-oxide	Benzo(a)pyrene-4,5-dihydrodiol	139
Sulfation and glucuronidation		
Acetaminophen	Sulfate conjugation	99,107,110
Acetaminophen	Sulfate and glucuronide conjugation	57
4-Dimethylaminophenol	Sulfate and glucuronide conjugation	45
Harmol	Sulfate and glucuronide conjugation	93
N-Hydroxy-2-acetylaminofluorene	*N*-Sulfation	83
7-Hydroxycoumarin	Sulfate and glucuronide conjugation	38
Naltrexone	Naltrexone-3-glucuronide	123
N-Acetylation		
7-Aminonitrazepam	7-Acetylamino derivative	7
Procainamide	*N*-Acetylprocainamide	151
Styrene oxide cysteine conjugate	Styrene oxide mercapturic acid	143
Glutathione conjugation		
Acetaminophen	Acetaminophen glutathione conjugate	57
Beonzo(a)pyrene-4,5-oxide	Glutathione adduct	139
Styrene oxide	Styrene oxide glutathione conjugate	159

TABLE 3. *Interactions between substrates as studied in perfused liver preparations*

Interactants	Comments	References
Acetanilide with phenacetin	Inhibition of metabolism mutually	110
Acetaldehyde with *p*-nitroanisole	Inhibition of *O*-demethylation	116
t-Butylhydroperoxide with hexobarbital	Inhibition of hexobarbital metabolism	50
Desmethylimipramine with imipramine	DMI inhibits hydroxylation and *N*-oxidation of imipramine	90
2,6-Dichloro-4-nitrophenol with harmol	Inhibition of harmol sulfation	71,72
Ethanol with *p*-nitroanisole	Stimulation of O-demethylation of *p*-NA at ethanol (0.2 mM) in fasted rats; inhibition at high ethanol (20 mM) concentrations	118,119
Galactosamine with 1-naphthol and bilirubin	Decreased glucuronidation of 1-naphthol with UDPGA, but failed to decrease glucuronidation of bilirubin	97
MEGX with lidocaine	MEGX inhibited *N*-deethylation of lidocaine	106
SKF-525A, ethylmorphine, chlorpromazine, codeine, levomethorphan, morphine with hexobarbital	Inhibited metabolism of hexobarbital	144
Xylitol and sorbital with *p*-nitroanisole	NADH produced from metabolism of xylitol and sorbital stimulated *O*-demethylation in fasted rats	116,120

modeling in the latter, both studies assigned an anterior distribution for sulfation activity (periportal) and a more posterior distribution for glucuronidation activity. It should be noted, however, that anterograde and retrograde delivery of substrate reveals only the distributions of metabolic activity of enzyme systems and does not identify the rate-limiting step of the metabolic reaction. In contrast, immunohistochemical and staining techniques for enzyme localization point to the presence of enzymes that partake in the coupling reaction with designed antibodies and do not reveal metabolic activity. These two methods, however, complement each other in the understanding of the complex architecture of the liver, especially in the uneven distribution of enzymes.

The anterograde and retrograde perfusion technique is also used in the examination of ethanol metabolism in the rat liver preparation. The coupled measurements of fluorescence of NADH in the periportal and pericentral areas and ethanol uptake in the presence and absence of 4-methylpyrazole, an inhibitor of alcohol dehydrogenase, led to the conclusion that NADH concentrations in the liver correlated closely with ethanol uptake and the distribution of NAD^+ rather than with the distribution of alcohol dehydrogenase (67).

Intermediary Metabolism and Interactions

The application of liver perfusion in studies of intermediary metabolism and chemical toxicity has recently been reviewed by Thurman and Reinke (151). With an understanding of the factors governing drug metabolism and intermediary metabolism and the effects of xenobiotic administration on perturbations of intermediary metabolism, the underlying mechanisms of induced toxicity and the basis of drug–drug interactions become more apparent. Changes in intermediary metabolism were observed during the following treatments in liver perfusion studies: a reduction in the utilization of oxygen as a result of alterations of mitochondrial respiratory chain and uncoupling of oxidative phosphorylation is observed with cyanide (153), halothane (13), and *p*-nitrophenol (68); gluconeogenesis, which depends on such key intermediates as pyruvate, triose phosphate, NADPH, and cellular energetics, is inhibited by aminopyrine (130), salicylate (171), phenformin (78), and ethanol (151), whereas stimulation of gluconeogenesis is seen with glucagon (163); glycolysis is inhibited by ethanol when NAD^+ needed by the glycolytic enzyme 3-glyceraldehyde phosphate dehydrogenase is used during ethanol oxidation (151); lipogenesis, which requires NADPH, is inhibited by aminopyrine (153), whose oxidation interfered with NADPH; ethanol is found to inhibit β-oxidation of acetyl-CoA compounds and lipid metabolism; carbon tetrachloride reduced urea production from ammonium chloride (112). Glucagon effects are inhibited by (+)decanoyl-carnitine (167).

Regulation of mixed-function oxidation in the perfused liver has been studied extensively. In contrast to the *in vitro* homogenate system, in which the NADPH-generating system is in abundance, NADPH is found to be the regulating factor in the metabolism of aminopyrine (152) and *p*-nitroanisole in liver perfusion studies with rats that were fasted, fed, or induced with phenobarbital. Fasted and phenobarbital-treated rats lacked NADPH to support the metabolism of these compounds, but on addition of ethanol (0.2 mM), which produced NADH and xylitol or sorbitol, which produced NADPH, improved *O*-demethylation of *p*-nitroanisole was observed (119,120). High concentrations of ethanol (20 mM) in fasted livers, however, inhibited *p*-nitroanisole *O*-demethylation because NADH produced during ethanol metabolism inhibited the citric acid cycle and led to decreased cytosolic NADPH (116,118).

Other studies of conjugation reactions carried out in the perfused liver showed that fasted, fed, and fasted–refed states influenced glucuronidation of the phenolic substrate *p*-nitrophenol (117); a correlation was found between the glycogen content, UDP-glucose, and UDP-glucuronic acid induced by these states and glucuronidation. Compounds that increased $NADH/NAD^+$ ratio, such as ethanol, or decreased ATP/ADP ratio (potassium cyanide and dinitrophenol) also decreased glucuronidation. This finding indicated that the supply of UDP-glucuronic acid is rate limiting in glucuronidation.

Liver perfusion has also been employed in the study of enzymes regulating hepatic glutathione levels. Phenobarbital pretreatment increased glutathione (mostly reduced) in the perfusate. However, during drug oxidation (aminopyrine, ethylmorphine, and hexobarbital) or paraquat infusion (31), oxidized glutathione (GSSG) was released, possibly because of the oxidation of NADPH (137). When phenobarbital pretreatment was combined with dietary measures (selenium-supplemented or selenium-deficient diets), subsequent liver perfusion with *t*-butyl hydroperoxide or hydrogen peroxide produced different patterns in GSSG efflux; *t*-butyl hydroperoxide stimulated the release of GSSG into perfusate for both diets, whereas hydrogen peroxide was unable to cause a release of GSSG in the selenium-deficient diet, suggesting that a selenium-independent glutathione peroxidase was present (34).

Kinetic Studies

Liver perfusion techniques have been used to illustrate some of the principles underlying substrate disappearance as initially characterized by Brauer (28). Shand et al. (134) and Pang and Rowland (105,106) extended these studies to elucidate the effect of hepatic flow on hepatic clearance: when hepatic extraction is high, hepatic clearance changes are directly proportional to flow, and flow is devoid of effects on the hepatic extraction ratio; when the hepatic extraction is low, hepatic clearance is unperturbed by changes in flow, but hepatic extraction ratio changes inversely with hepatic flow (104,134). The highly cleared compounds propranolol and lidocaine (105,134) and the poorly cleared compounds diphenylhydantoin and antipyrine (105,134) were used to demonstrate these principles.

The effects of binding on clearance and extraction ratio of highly and poorly cleared compounds in liver perfusion studies indicated that the clearance of highly cleared compounds is independent of changes in binding, whereas the clearance for poorly cleared compounds will change in direct proportion to the unbound fraction in perfusate. Examples of the former and latter are propranolol and diphenylhydantoin (133).

Additionally, the saturability of enzyme systems with respect to dose (recirculating) and input concentration (single pass) are amply demonstrated in liver perfusion studies. Examples for the recirculating design are procainamide (157), propranolol (22,132), acetaminophen (35,57), diphenylhydantoin (49,164), ethanol (55), *p*-nitroanisole (89); examples for the single pass are ethanol (67,77,141), *p*-nitroanisole (150), lidocaine and its metabolite MEGX (105,106), acetaminophen (108), quinidine (172), galactose (69,70), 7-ethoxycoumarin and its metabolite 7-hydroxycoumarin (65), harmol (102), and 4-dimethylaminophenol (45).

Important information is obtained from these kinetic experiments. In recirculating studies and under first-order conditions, deviations from monoexponential characteristics indicate extensive binding to liver components (126). The plot of concentration of parent drug or area under the curve, when divided into the dose, provides the clearance of the compound. Subsequent division of clearance by hepatic flow furnishes the hepatic extraction ratio. Regarding metabolite data, a longer apparent half-life ($t_{1/2}$) for a metabolite in perfusate when compared to that for parent compound is indicative of elimination of metabolite as the rate-limiting step.

Biliary excretion data can also be utilized for confirmation and substantiation of perfusate data. The rate plot, or semilogarithmic plot of the biliary excretion rate of metabolite versus the midpoint time of the collecting interval, provides similar information on the rate-limiting step. Moreover, the plot of excretion rate versus perfusate concentration at the midpoint of the interval provides the biliary clearance.

When the cumulative amount excreted into bile is summed, the extent of excretion (% dose) can be calculated. The total amount of metabolite in the reservoir (volume of reservoir × metabolite concentration at end of perfusion) plus the total amount of metabolite excreted in bile represents the total sum of metabolite at the end of perfusion, and when this amount is normalized to dose, it provides an estimate of the fraction of dose that is converted into the metabolite. This calculation, however, will underestimate the fraction because the metabolite may undergo sequential metabolism during its time of formation or may be metabolized on subsequent recirculation through the liver. Similarly, the total amount of metabolite in bile divided by the total amount in perfusate and bile will furnish an estimate of the fraction of metabolite formed that is excreted in bile. Again, this estimate is an underestimation of the true value when further metabolism of metabolite occurs.

Of little value is the plot of concentration in bile versus time. The concentration of parent compound and metabolite in bile is strongly influenced by bile volume or bile flow, which in turn is influenced by factors outlined previously such as temperature, perfusate flow, and the choleretic or cholestatic actions of the test compounds and its metabolites. Of more value is the ratio of the concentration in bile and plasma (11,164);

this ratio may provide some insight into the "concentrating" ability of bile and the mechanism of transport.

The absolute meanings of clearance and $t_{1/2}$ in the liver perfusion system should be treated carefully. Clearance is not only influenced by the metabolizing capabilities of the liver but is also dependent on perfusate composition, hepatic flow, and binding. It should also be noted that the $t_{1/2}$ in the perfusate is strongly dependent on the initial volume used in the reservoir in recirculating experiments.

Data from single-pass studies, however, are easier to interpret. With steady-state conditions, the loss of a compound is accounted for by the rates of metabolism and excretion. The sum of the rate of efflux in bile and perfusate provides the total efflux rate. Under prevailing first-order conditions, hepatic extraction ratio is calculated by the drop in concentration across the liver divided by the input concentration and is a constant. Multiplication of hepatic flow by hepatic extraction ratio provides hepatic clearance. With increasing input concentrations of substrate, the Michaelis–Menten parameters V_{max} and K_m can be assessed (126,170).

Metabolic patterns are drastically simplified during single-pass perfusions. Phase I products are usually conjugated to glucuronide and sulfate prior to their entry into bile and perfusate. Enzymatic hydrolysis usually provides a complete recovery for the amount of phase I product formed. The summation of rate of efflux in perfusate and bile after enzymatic hydrolysis will provide an estimate of the rate of formation. When the rate of formation of a metabolite is expressed in terms of the rate of loss of parent compound, the fractional clearance conducive to metabolite formation (99) may be calculated. Biliary excretion data may be described by a "rate plot," and the cumulative amount in bile can be expressed as a function of dose (flow rate × infusion time × input concentration) during steady-state conditions.

Nonlinear conditions of metabolite formation are easily apparent when the disappearance rate of a substrate or the appearance rate of a metabolite (summed perfusate and bile) changes out of proportion to the input concentration or input rate. Saturability of enzymatic reaction can be inferred only if binding of the substrate of metabolite is independent of changes in substrate concentration (172). Estimates of K_m and V_{max} are provided in this system. Care should be exercised, however, to account for sequential metabolite metabolism. If a phase I product is conjugated, hydrolysis of the samples usually furnishes the total amount of metabolite formed (64). Moreover, estimates of K_m and V_{max} are highly dependent on the concentration chosen as the concentration in liver (102,170) because it is virtually impossible to assess the substrate concentration around the locale of the enzyme. The transport maximum for biliary excretion is readily apparent in the "rate plots" (172).

A better understanding of metabolite kinetics is provided by data obtained from perfusion studies. As a result of observations made during the single pass of ^{14}C-phenacetin and ^{3}H-acetaminophen in perfused rat liver, sequential first-pass metabolism of a primary metabolite was observed (100); that is, ^{14}C-acetaminophen formed in liver during the single pass of ^{14}C-phenacetin was further metabolized to ^{14}C-acetaminophen sulfate conjugate before the primary metabolite left the liver.

This finding led to the kinetic treatment of the phenomenon in *in vivo* systems (106). The extent of sequential metabolism during the genesis of the nascently formed primary metabolite, however, was different from that of the preformed metabolite, ^{14}C-acetaminophen and ^{3}H-acetaminophen (99). The discrepancy between the extents of sequential metabolism was initially attributed to the uneven distribution of drug-metabolizing activities in the liver for *O*-deethylation and sulfation (107). Determinants of metabolite kinetics were further elucidated by the combined use of acetaminophen precursors as ^{14}C-acetanilide and ^{3}H-phenacetin. The fast acetaminophen precursor, phenacetin, provided acetaminophen that was sulfated to a greater extent than that generated from the slow acetaminophen precursor acetanilide (110). Interpretation of these data was based on the concept of "transit time" of the metabolite in liver: the faster metabolite-forming precursor will furnish the metabolite rapidly after the parent drug enters the liver and allows more time for the metabolite to be further metabolized, whereas the opposite will hold for the slower metabolite-forming precursor.

Another aspect that will influence metabolite kinetics is the presence of diffusional barriers that retard the entry of a substrate or its metabolites. ^{3}H-MK-422 (*N*-[1-(*S*)-carboxy-3-phenylpropyl]-L-alanyl-L-proline), a new angiotensin-converting enzyme inhibitor, and its precursor, ^{14}C-MK-421, a maleate salt of the monoethyl ester of MK-422, were perfused simultaneously into the rat liver preparation. Because of the marked polarity of the dicarboxylic acid, ^{3}H-MK-422 does not enter hepatocytes readily, and only 5% was excreted into bile. The more lipophilic precursor ^{14}C-MK-421, however, entered in hepatocytes, and the generated ^{14}C-MK-422 was excreted to a greater extent (18%) in bile (109).

Biliary Excretion and Transport

Biliary excretion represents another component in the elimination of endogenous and exogenous substrates and may contribute significantly in some instances to the removal of these compounds by the liver. The processes involved in biliary excretion are hepatic uptake, intracellular transport, biotransformation, and excretion into the biliary tree. These processes have been studied with liver perfusion techniques for endogenous substrates such as bile acids/salts and bilirubin and for xenobiotics. The entire complement of bile salts *in vivo* are found in liver perfusion studies (145).

The formation of bile and the mechanisms of its secretion have been reviewed in detail (20,46), and bile is considered to originate from bile ductules or canaliculi. A bile-salt-independent fraction, in contrast to a bile-salt-dependent fraction, was initially identified by Boyer et al. (21) who found, in perfusion studies, that a large fraction of bile flow and bile secretory pressure was independent of the amount of bile salt secreted into bile.

Bile acids are formed in liver from cholesterol by at least two pathways involving enzymes in the mitochondria and microsomal fraction. Specific receptors for cholic acid and taurocholate uptake have been identified in isolated liver surface membranes. These receptors demonstrate saturability and are competed for by the organic cation bromosulfophthalein (2) Gonzalez et al. (53) also identified a carrier-mediated membrane complex that initiates translocation of bile salts. This carrier-mediated process is between the sinusoidal and canalicular membrane and is inhibited by cycloheximide, which decreases cholic acid binding sites concomitantly. Reichens and Paumgartner (114) demonstrated in liver perfusion studies that taurocholate exhibited a similar distribution space as albumin in liver and that cholate and taurocholate mutually inhibited the uptake of each other into liver via a mechanism dependent on Na^{+} ions. Blitzer and Boyer (14) confirmed the presence of a Na^{+}–K^{+} ATPase system in the sinusoidal and lateral membranes with the classical dependence on K^{+} and Mg^{2+} as well as inhibition by ouabain.

Another endogenous substrate, bilirubin, was studied in perfused liver preparations. Proportional increases in biliary excretion rate, liver concentrations, and bile flow were observed for increases in infusion rates of bilirubin (3). Hepatic uptake of bilirubin, however, was found to be dependent on unbound bilirubin concentrations (16). A detailed description of bilirubin uptake kinetics was recently provided by Gollan et al. (52) who incorporated the effects of uptake, biotransformation, and reversible conjugation of bilirubin in the liver perfusion model.

The technique of segmented retrograde intrabiliary injection was recently introduced by Olson and Fujimoto (95) to examine the modes of transfer of solutes across the biliary tree epithelium in the reabsorption direction so as to elucidate the pattern of transit of compounds through the liver into venous perfusate (63). The technique is similar in principle to that described by Goresky et al. (56) for tissue distribution spaces of marker compounds in the liver. The segmented retrograde intrabiliary injection entails the injection of a marker compound or substrate solution through retrograde biliary injection, followed by saline-wash injection. Efflux of the marker in bile and venous perfusate demonstrates the extent of transfer as well as the transfer mechanisms in liver.

Biliary excretion of xenobiotics has been extensively reviewed in perfusion systems. Most compounds are readily excreted into bile, including quaternary ammonium compounds (75). The ratio of the concentration in bile to that in plasma, if greater than unity, denotes the concentrating ability of cholephiles in bile, possibly through micelle formation (11,12).

The excretion of the organic anion bromosulfophthalein (BSP) and its transport maximum were found to be similar in animals *in vivo* and in the perfused liver preparations (61). The clearance for uptake of dibromosulfophthalein (DBSP), another organic anion, was found to be virtually identical *in vivo* and in perfused livers (15). Similar findings were obtained for the nonionic compound ouabain and for the quaternary organic cation *d*-tubocurarine in perfused liver preparations and *in vivo* (15). Uptake of quaternary compounds, however, was found to be highly dependent on lipophilicity, as shown by the comparison between *d*-tubocurarine and its more polar counterpart, trimethyltubocurarine (85). The hepatic uptake of the organic anions DBSP (86) and rose bengal (47) was found to be influenced by plasma albumin concentration. Dissociation of the anion with albumin at the liver cell surface may occur prior to uptake. The dissociation mechanism, however, displayed saturation kinetics as albumin concentration increased (47). The transport of DBSP was found to be associated with both Y and Z proteins in liver cytosol; induction with phenobarbital, which increased the Y protein, decreased the efflux of DBSP in liver (86).

The influence of bile salts on hepatic transport mechanisms was investigated for various compounds in liver perfusion systems and at different doses of bile salts. A stimulation of DBSP excretion into bile was seen at low taurocholate and dehydrocholate infusion rates, whereas inhibition was observed for high bile salt infusion rates (161). High bile salt infusion also decreased the hepatic uptake of the organic cations *d*-tubocurarine and N^4-acetyl procainamide ethobromide (162), but taurocholate failed to alter the hepatic transport of ouabain and strophanthoside, two uncharged compounds (163). Free fatty acid uptake by perfused liver, however, was inhibited by cholephilic anions (121).

CONCLUSIONS

The applications of liver perfusion techniques have been reviewed. The widespread utility and versatility of liver perfusion techniques have extended to the lung (125), kidney (19), and intestines (4). Besides the use of liver perfusion for metabolic data, the preparation can also be used to model disease states, for example, jaundice through bile duct ligation (76) or decreased flow as in diseased states of the liver. Correlations between this *in vitro* approach and *in vivo* are often attempted (160) because of the closeness of this approach to the *in vivo* situation. But care must be exercised in corroborating data because limitations still exist in the *in vitro* preparation that differ from those of the organ *in situ*.

ACKNOWLEDGMENTS

This work was supported by the Faculty Development Award from the Medical Research Council of Canada (#DG-262, 263, and 264).

REFERENCES

1. Abouna, G. M. (1968): Pig liver perfusion with human blood. The effect of preparing and flushing the liver with various balanced solutions on its subsequent viability and function. *Br. J. Surg.*, 55:761–768.
2. Accatino, L., and Simon, F. R. (1976): Identification and characterization of a bile acid receptor in isolated liver surface membranes. *J. Clin. Invest.*, 57:496–508.
3. Barnhart, J. L., and Clarenburg, R. (1973): Factors determining clearance of bilirubin in perfused rat liver. *Am. J. Physiol.*, 225:497–508.
4. Barr, W., and Riegelman, S. (1970): Intestinal drug absorption and metabolism I: Comparison of methods and models to study physiological factors of *in vitro* intestinal absorption. *J. Pharm. Sci.*, 59:154–163.
5. Bartosěk, I., Guaitani, A., and Garattini, S. (1972): Long-term perfusion of isolated rat liver. *Pharmacology,* 8:244–258.
6. Bartosěk, I., Guaitani, A., and Miller, L. L. (1973): In: *Isolated Liver and Its Applications.* Raven Press, New York.
7. Bartosěk, I., Kvetina, J., Guaitani, A., and Garattini, S. (1970): Comparative study of nitrazepam metabolism in perfused isolated liver of laboratory animals. *Eur. J. Pharmacol.*, 11:378–382.
8. Bartosěk, I., Mussini, E., and Garattini, S. (1969): Reduction of nitrazepam by rat liver. *Biochem. Pharmacol.*, 18:2263–2264.
9. Berry, M. N., Hamilton, R. L., Severinghams, E. M., and Williams, M. C. (1974): A simple and inexpensive membrane "lung" for rat liver perfusion. In: *Alfred Benzoin Symposium VI. Regulation of Hepatic Metabolism,* edited by F. Lundqvist and N. Tygstrup, pp. 790–795. Munksgaard, Copenhagen.
10. Bickel, M. H., and Börner, H. (1974): Uptake, subcellular distribution and transfer processes of imipramine and its metabolites formed in rat liver perfusion systems. *Naunyn Schmiedebergs Arch. Pharmacol.*, 284:339–352.
11. Bickel, M. H., and Minder, R. (1970): Metabolism and biliary excretion of the lipophilic drug molecules, imipramine and desmethylimipramine in the rat-I. *Biochem. Pharmacol.*, 19:2425–2435.
12. Bickel, M. H., and Minder, R. (1970): Metabolism and biliary excretion of the lipophilic drug molecules, imipramine and desmethylimpramine in the rat-II uptake into bile micelles. *Biochem. Pharmacol.*, 19:2437–2443.
13. Biebuyck, J. F., Lund, P., and Krebs, H. A. (1972): The effects of halothane (2-bromo-2-chloro-1,1,1-trifluoroethane) on glycolysis and biosynthetic processes of the isolated perfused rat liver. *Biochem. J.*, 128:711–720.
14. Blitzer, B. L., and Boyer, J. L. (1978): Cytochemical localization of Na^+,K^+-ATPase in the rat hepatocyte. *J. Clin. Invest.*, 62:1104–1108.
15. Blom, A., Scaf, S. H. J., and Meijer, D. K. F. (1982): Hepatic drug transport in the rat. A comparison between isolated hepatocytes, the isolated liver and the liver in vivo. *Biochem. Pharmacol.*, 31:1553–1565.
16. Bloomer, J. R., Berk, P. D., Vergalla, J., and Berlin, N. I. (1973): Influence of albumin on the hepatic uptake of unconjugated bilirubin. *Clin. Sci. Molec. Med.*, 45:505–516.
17. Bolt, H. M., and Remmer, H. (1973): The fate of mestranol (17α-ethynylestradiol-3-methyl ether) in the isolated perfused rat liver. *Horm. Metab. Res.*, 5:101–105.
18. Bond, J. A., Medinsky, M. A., Dent, J. G., and Rickert, D. E. (1981): Sex-dependent metabolism and biliary excretion of [2,4-^{14}C] dinitrotoluene in isolated perfused rat livers. *J. Pharmacol. Exp. Ther.*, 219:598–603.
19. Bowman, R. H., and Maack, T. (1972): Glucose transport by isolated perfused rat kidney. *Am. J. Physiol.*, 222:1499–1504.
20. Boyer, J. L. (1980): New concepts of mechanisms of hepatocyte bile formation. *Physiol. Rev.*, 60:303–326.
21. Boyer, J. L., and Klatskin, G. (1970): The paracellular pathway and bile formation. *Gastroenterology,* 59:853–859.
22. Branch, R. A., Nies, A. S., and Shand, D. G. (1973): The disposition of propranolol VII. General implications of the effects of liver blood flown elimination from the perfused rat liver. *Drug Metab. Dispos.*, 1:677–690.
23. Branch, R. A., Shand, D. G., Wilkinson, G. R., and Nies, A. S. (1973): The production of lidocaine clearance by *dl*-propranolol: An example of hemodynamic drug interaction. *J. Pharmacol. Exp. Ther.*, 184:515–519.
24. Brauer, R. W. (1956): Liver. *Annu. Rev. Physiol.*, 18:253–278.
25. Brauer, R. W. (1963): Liver Circulation and Function. *Physiol. Rev.*, 43:115–213.
26. Brauer, R. W., Holloway, R. J., and Leong, G. F. (1957): Temperature effects on radiocolloid uptake by the isolated rat liver. *Am. J. Physiol.*, 189:24–30.
27. Brauer, R. W., Leong, G. F., and Holloway, R. J. (1960): Liver injury in isolated perfused rat liver preparation exposed to chloroform. *Am. J. Physiol.*, 200:548–550.
28. Brauer, R. W., Leong, G. F., McElroy, R. F., Jr., and Holloway, R. J. (1956): Hemodynamics of the

vascular tree of the isolated rat liver preparation. *Am. J. Physiol.,* 186:537–542.

29. Brauer, R. W., Prescott, R. L., and Pizzolato, P. (1951): Isolated rat liver preparation. Bile production and other basic properties. *Proc. Soc. Exp. Biol. Med.,* 78:174–181.
30. Breimer, D. D., and van Rossum, J. M. (1974): Pharmacokinetics of the enantiomers of hexobarbital studied in the same intact rat and in the same isolated perfused rat liver. *Eur. J. Pharmacol.,* 30:349–354.
31. Brigelius, R., Hashem, A., and Lengfelder, E. (1981): Paraquat-induced alterations of phospholipids and GSSG-release in the isolated perfused rat liver; and the effect of SOD-active copper complexes. *Biochem. Pharmacol.,* 30:349–354.
32. Brock, W. J., and Vore, M. (1982): Hepatic morphine and estrone glucuronyl transferase activity and morphine biliary excretion in the isolated perfused rat liver. *Drug Metab. Dispos.,* 10:336–343.
33. Brown, H., and Hardison, W. G. M. (1972): Fluorocarbon sonicated as a substitute for erythrocyte in rat liver perfusion. *Surgery,* 71:388–394.
34. Burk, R. F., Nishiki, K., Lawrence, R. A., and Chance, B. (1978): Peroxide removal by selenium-dependent and selenium-independent glutathione peroxidases in hemoglobin-free perfused rat liver. *J. Biol. Chem.,* 253:43–46.
35. Cohen, G. M., Blake, O. M., and Davis, D. S. (1974): "First-pass" metabolism of paracetamol in rat liver. *J. Pharm. Pharmacol.,* 26:348–351.
36. Collins, F. G., and Skibba, J. L. Improved in situ rat liver perfusion technique. *J. Surg. Res.,* 28:65–70.
37. Condon, R. E., Nyhus, L. M., and Harkins, H. N. (1964): Isolated perfused bovine liver responses to common vasoactive drugs. *Arch. Surg.,* 89:602–608.
38. Conway, J. G., Kauffman, F. C., Ji, S., Lemasters, J. L., and Thurman, R. G. (1982): Rates of sulfation and glucuronidation of 7-hydroxycoumarin in periportal and pericentral of the liver lobule. *Mol. Pharmacol.,* 22:509–516.
39. Craig, A., (1959): Effects of epinephrine on lactic and keto-acid production phosphate balance and pH changes in the isolated perfused frog liver. *Am. J. Physiol.,* 196:959–964.
40. Cummings, J. F., and Mannering, G. F. (1970): Effect of phenobarbital administration on the oxygen requirement of hexobarbital metabolism in the isolated perfused rat liver and in the intact rat. *Biochem. Pharmacol.,* 19:973–978.
41. Elbers, R., Soboll, S., and Kampffmeyer, H. G. (1980): Alterations in cellular intermediary metabolism by 4-dimethylaminophenol metabolism in the isolated perfused rat liver and the implications of 4-dimethylaminophenol toxicity. *Biochem. Pharmacol.,* 29:1747–1753.
42. Erlandersen, E. J., and Gram, L. F. (1982): Imipramine kinetics in the single pass rat liver perfusion model. *Acta Pharmacol. Toxicol.,* 50:137–147.
43. Evans, G. H., Wilkinson, G. R., and Shand, D. G. (1973): The disposition of propranolol IV. A dominant role for tissue uptake in the dose-dependent extraction of propanolol by the perfused rat liver. *J. Pharmacol. Exp. Ther.,* 186:447–454.
44. Exton, J. H., Crobin, J. G., and Harper, S. C. (1972): Control of gluconeogenesis in liver. Effects of fasting, diabetes and glucagon on lactate and endogenous metabolism in the perfused rat liver. *J. Biol. Chem.,* 247:4996–5003.
45. Eyer, P., and Kampffmeyer, H. G. (1978): Biotransformation of 4-dimethylaminophenol in the isolated perfused rat liver and in the rat. *Biochem. Pharmacol.,* 28:2223–2228.
46. Forker, E. L. (1977): Mechanisms of hepatic bile formation. *Annu. Rev. Physiol.,* 39:323–347.
47. Forker, E. L., Luxon, B. A., Snell, M., and Shurmantine, W. O. (1982): Effect of albumin binding on the hepatic transport of rose bengal: Surface-mediated dissociation of limited capacity. *J. Pharmacol. Exp. Ther.,* 223:342–347.
48. Gerber, N., Leger, R. M., Gordon, P., Smith, R. G., Bauer, J., and Lynn, R. K. (1975): The metabolism of *d*-, *l*-, and *dl*-methadone in the isolated perfused rat liver. *J. Pharmacol. Exp. Ther.,* 200:487–495.
49. Gerber, N., Weller, W. L., Lyn, R., Rangno, R. E., Sweetman, B. J., and Bush, M. T. (1971): Study of dose-dependent metabolism of 5,5-diphenylhydantoin in the rat using new methodology for isolation and quantitation of metabolites in vivo and in vitro. *J. Pharmacol. Exp. Ther.,* 178:567–579.
50. Gerstenecker, C., and Sies, H. (1980): Restriction of hexobarbital metabolism by t-butyl hydroperoxide in perfused rat liver. *Biochem. Pharmacol.,* 29:3112–3113.
51. Gibaldi, M., Boyes, R. N., and Feldman, S. (1971): Influence of first-pass effect on availability of drugs on oral administration. *J. Pharm. Sci.,* 60:1338–1340.
52. Gollan, J., Hammaker, L., Licko, V., and Schmid, R. (1981): Bilirubin kinetics in intact rats and isolated perfused liver. Evidence for hepatic deconjugation of bilirubin glucuronides. *J. Clin. Invest.,* 67:1003–1015.
53. Gonzalez, M. C., Sutherland, F., and Simon, F. R. (1979): Regulation of hepatic transport of bile salts. Effect of protein synthesis inhibition on excretion of bile salts and their binding to liver surface membrane fractions. *J. Clin. Invest.,* 63:694–699.
54. Goodman, M., Parrilla, R., and Toews, C. J. (1973): Influence of fluorocarbon emulsions on hepatic metabolism in perfused rat liver. *Am. J. Physiol.,* 225:1384–1388.
55. Gordon, E. R. (1968): The utilization of ethanol by the isolated perfused rat liver. *Can. J. Physiol. Pharmacol.,* 46:609–616.
56. Goresky, C. A., Back, G. G., and Nadeau, B. E. (1973): On the uptake of materials by the intact liver. The transport and net removal of galactose. *J. Clin. Invest.,* 52:991–998.
57. Gräfstrom, R., Ormstad, K., Moldéus, P., and Orrenius, S. (1979): Paracetamol metabolism in the isolated perfused rat liver with further metabolism of a biliary paracetamol conjugate by the small intestine. *Biochem. Pharmacol.,* 28:3573–3579.
58. Groszmann, R. J., Dubin, M., and Royer, M.

(1975): Study of indirect methods for measuring blood flow in the isolated perfused dog liver. *Digestion,* 13:220–231.
59. Hamada, N., and Gessner, T. (1973): A rapid method for the mass spectrometric identification of glucuronides and other polar drug metabolites in permethylated rat bite. *Drug Metab. Dispos.,* 1:489–505.
60. Hems, R., Ross, B. D., Berry, M. N., and Krebs, H. A. (1966): Gluconeogenesis in the perfused rat liver. *Biochem. J.,* 101:284–292.
61. Herz, R., Cueni, B., Bircher, J., and Paumgartner, G. (1973): The excretory capacity of the isolated rat liver. *Naunyn Schmiedebergs Arch. Pharmacol.,* 277:297–304.
62. Hirom, P. C., Millburn, P., Smith, R. L., and Williams, R. T. (1972): The effect of testosterone on the biliary excretion of tartrazine in female rats. *Biochem. J.,* 127:1071–1077.
63. Imamura, T., and Fujimoto, J. M. (1980): Transit patterns of marker compounds given by segmented retrograde intrabiliary injection (SRII) in the isolated in situ perfused rat liver. *J. Pharmacol. Exp. Ther.,* 215:110–115.
64. Inaba, T., Umeda, T., Endrenyi, L., Mahon, W. A., and Kalow, W. (1978): Uptake and metabolism of diphenylhydantoin in the isolated perfused rat liver. *Biochem. Pharmacol.,* 27:1151–1158.
65. Ji, S., Lemasters, J. L., and Thurman, R. G. (1981): A fluorometric method to measure sublobular rates of mixed function oxidation in the hemoglobin-free perfused rat liver. *Mol. Pharmacol.,* 19:513–516.
66. Kahl, G. F., Klaus, E., Legraverend, C., Nebert, D. W., and Pelkonen, O. (1979): Formation of benzo(a)pyrene metabolite-nucleoside adducts in isolated perfused rat and mouse liver and in mouse lung slices. *Biochem. Pharmacol.,* 28:1051–1056.
67. Kashiwagi, T., Ji, S., Lemasters, J. L., and Thurman, R. G. (1981): Rates of alcohol dehydrogenase-dependent ethanol metabolism in periportal and pericentral regions of the perfused rat liver. *Mol. Pharmacol.,* 21:438–443.
68. Kauffman, F. C., Evans, R. K., and Thurman, R. G. (1977): Alterations in nicotinamide and adenine nucleotide systems during mixed-function oxidation of p-nitroanisole in perfused livers from normal and phenobarbital-treated rats. *Biochem. J.,* 166:583–592.
69. Keiding, S., and Chiarantini, E. (1978): Effect of sinusoidal perfusion on galactose elimination kinetics in perfused rat liver. *J. Pharmacol. Exp. Ther.,* 205:465–470.
70. Keiding, S., Johansen, S., Winkler, K., Tonnesesn, K., and Tygstrup, N. (1976): Michaelis-Menten kinetics of galactose elimination by the isolated perfused pig liver. *Am. J. Physiol.,* 230:1302–1313.
71. Koster, H., Halsema, I. C. M., Pang, K. S., Scholtens, E., and Mulder, G. J. (1982): Effect of the inhibition of sulfation on glucuronidation kinetics of harmol in the perfused rat liver preparation. *Biochem. Pharmacol.,* 31:2023–2028.
72. Koster, H., Halsema, I. C. M., Scholtens, E., Meerman, J. H. N., Pang, K. S., and Mulder, G. J. (1982): Pharmacokinetics and characterization of the inhibitory effect of 2,6-dichloro-4-nitrophenol. *Biochem. Pharmacol.,* 31:1919–1924.
73. Krone, W., Huttner, W. B., Kampf, S. C., Rittich, B., Seitz, H. S., and Tarnowski, W. (1974): Long-term perfusion of the isolated rat liver maintenance of its functional state by use of a fluorocarbon emulsion. *Biochem. Biophys. Acta,* 372:55–67.
74. Květina, J., and Guaitani, A. (1969): A versatile method for the in vitro perfusion of isolated organs of rats and mice with particular reference to liver. *Pharmacology,* 2:65–67.
75. Lavy, U. I., Hespe, W., and Meijer, D. K. F. (1972): Uptake of excretion of the quaternary ammonium compound deptropinemethiodide in the isolated perfused rat liver. *Naunyn Schmiedebergs Arch. Pharmacol.,* 275:183–192.
76. Lee, E., Ross, B. D., and Haines, J. R. (1972): The effect of experimental bile-duct obstruction on critical biosynthetic functions of the liver. *Br. J. Surg.,* 59:564–568.
77. Lindros, K. O. (1974): The once-through perfusion technique advantages and limitations. In: *Alfred Benzoin Symposium VI. Regulation of Hepatic Metabolism,* edited by F. Lundqvist and N. Tygstrup, pp. 778–789. Academic Press, Munksgaard, Copenhagen.
78. Lloyd, M. H., Iles, R. A., Walton, B., Hamilton, C. A., and Cohen, R. A. (1975): Effect of phenytoin on gluconeogenesis from lactate and intracellular pH in the isolated perfused guinea pig liver. *Diabetes,* 24:618–620.
79. Long, D. E., and Rickert, D. E. (1982): Metabolism and excretion of 2,6-dinitro [^{14}C]toluene in vivo and in isolated perfused rat livers. *Drug Metab. Dispos.,* 10:455–458.
80. Lynn, R. K., Leger, R. M., and Gerber, N. (1976): Identification of glucuronide metabolites of d- and l-methadone in bile from the isolated perfused rat liver. *Res. Commun. Chem. Pathol. Pharmacol.,* 15:1–10.
81. Lynn, R. K., Smith, R. G., Leger, R. N., Deinzer, M. L., Griffith, D., and Gerber, N. (1977): Identification of glucuronide metabolites of benzomorphan narcotic analgesic drugs in bile from the isolated perfused rat liver by gas chromatography and mass spectrometry. *Drug Metab. Dispos.,* 5:47–55.
82. Mayes, P. A., and Felts, J. M. (1966): Liver function studied by liver perfusion. *Proc. Eur. Soc. Drug Tox.,* 7:47–55.
83. Meerman, J. H. N., Keulemans, K., and Mulder, G. J. (1980): Inhibition of sulfate conjugation of N-hydroxy-2-acetylaminofluorene in isolated perfused rat liver and in the rat in vivo by pentachlorophenol and low sulfate. *Cancer Res.,* 40:3772–3779.
84. Meijer, D. K. F., Keulemans, K., and Mulder, G. J. (1981): Isolated perfused rat liver technique. In: *Methods in Enzymology,* Vol. 77, edited by W. B. Jakoby, pp. 81–94. Academic Press, New York.
85. Meijer, D. K. F., Vonks, R. L., Keulemans, K., and Weitering, J. (1977): Hepatic uptake and biliary excretion of dibromosulfophthalein. Albumin dependence, influence of phenobarbital and nafenopin pretreatment and the role of Y and Z protein. *J. Pharmacol. Exp. Ther.,* 202:8–21.

86. Meijer, D. K. F., Weitering, J., and Vonk, R. J. (1976): Hepatic uptake and biliary excretion of d-tubocurarine and trimethyltubocurarine in the rat in vivo and in isolated perfused rat livers. *J. Pharmacol. Exp. Ther.*, 198:229–239.
87. Miller, L. L. (1973): History of isolated liver perfusion and some still unsolved problems. In: *Isolated Liver Perfusion and Its Applications*, edited by I. Bartošek, A. Guaitani, and L. L. Miller, pp. 1–9. Raven Press, New York.
88. Miller, L. L., Bly, C. G., Watson, M. L., and Bale, W. F. (1951): The dominant role of the liver in plasma protein synthesis. A direct study of the isolated perfused rat liver with the aid of lysine-C^{14}. *J. Exp. Med.*, 94:431–453.
89. Minck, K., Schupp, R. R., Illing, H. P. A., Kahl, G. F., and Netter, K. J. (1973): Inter-relationship between demethylation of p-nitroanisole and conjugation of p-nitrophenol rat liver. *Naunyn Schmiedebergs Arch. Pharmacol.*, 279:347–360.
90. Moldowan, M., and Bellward, D. (1974): Studies on ^{14}C-imipramine metabolism in the isolated perfused rat liver. *Can. J. Physiol. Pharmacol.*, 52:441–450.
91. Montgomery, C., and Vore, M. (1979): The effect of diethylstilbestrol treatment on the metabolism and biliary excretion of [^{14}C]phenytoin in the isolated perfused rat liver. *Biochem. Pharmacol.*, 28:510–519.
92. Mortimore, G. (1961): Effect of insulin on potassium transfer in isolated rat liver. *Am. J. Physiol.*, 200:1315–1319.
93. Mulder, G. J., and Keulemans, K. (1978): Metabolism of inorganic sulphate in the isolated perfused rat liver. Effect of sulphate concentration on the rate of sulphation by phenol sulphotransferase. *Biochem. J.*, 176:959–965.
94. Nastainczyk, W., and Ullrich, V. (1978): Effect of oxygen concentration on the reaction of halothane with cytochrome P450 in liver microsomes and isolated perfused rat liver. *Biochem. Pharmacol.*, 27:387–396.
95. Olson, J. R., and Fujimoto, J. M. (1980): Evaluation of hepatobiliary function in the rat by the segmented retrograde intrabiliary injection technique. *Biochem. Pharmacol.*, 29:205–211.
96. Oomen, H. A. P. C., and Charamalun, R. A. F. M. (1971): Correlation between histological and biochemical parameters of isolated perfused rat liver. *Virchows Arch.* [*Cell Pathol.*], 8:243–251.
97. Otani, G., About-ET-Nakaren, M. M., and Bock, K. W. (1976): UDP-glucuronyl transferase in perfused rat liver and in microsomes III. Effects of galactosamine and carbon-tetrachloride on the glucuronidation of l-naphthol and bilirubin. *Biochem. Pharmacol.*, 25:1293–1297.
98. Pang, K. S. (1979): Dose dependent hepatic elimination of allopurinol in the perfused rat liver *in situ* preparation. *Res. Commun. Chem. Pathol. Pharmacol.*, 26:317–328.
99. Pang, K. S., and Gillette, J. R. (1978): Kinetics of metabolite formation and elimination in the perfused rat liver preparation: Differences between the elimination of preformed acetaminophen and acetaminophen formed from phenacetin. *J. Pharmacol. Exp. Ther.*, 207:178–194.
100. Pang, K. S., and Gillette, J. R. (1979): Sequential first-pass elimination of a metabolite derived from its precursor. *J. Pharmacokinet. Biopharm.*, 7:275–290.
101. Pang, K. S., Glazebrook, P. A., and Lam, D. M.-K. (1983): Characterization of retrograde perfusion of the liver by physical measurements. An electron microscopic and enzyme monitoring study. (*submitted for publication*)
102. Pang, K. S., Koster, H., Halsema, I. C. M., Scholtens, E., and Mulder, G. J. (1981): Aberrant pharmacokinetics of harmol in the perfused rat liver preparation: Sulfate and glucuronide conjugations. *J. Pharmacol. Exp. Ther.*, 219:134–140.
103. Pang, K. S., Koster, H., Halsema, I. C. M., Scholtens, E., Mulder, G. J., and Stillwell, R. N. (1983): Normal and retrograde perfusion to probe the zonal distribution of sulfation and glucuronidation activities of harmol in the perfused rat liver preparation. *J. Pharmacol. Exp. Ther.*, 224:647–653.
104. Pang, K. S., and Rowland, M. (1977): Hepatic clearance of drugs I. Theoretical consideration of a "well-stirred" model and a "parallel tube" model. Influence of hepatic blood flow plasma and blood cells binding and the hepatocellular enzymatic activity on hepatic drug clearance. *J. Pharmacokinet. Biopharm.*, 5:625–654.
105. Pang, K. S., and Rowland, M. (1977): Hepatic clearance of drugs II. Experimental evidence for the acceptance of the "well-stirred" model over the "parallel tube" model using lidocaine in the perfused rat liver *in situ* preparation. *J. Pharmacokinet. Biopharm.*, 5:655–680.
106. Pang, K. S., and Rowland, M. (1977): Hepatic clearance of drugs III. Additional experimental evidence for the acceptance of the "well-stirred" model using metabolite (MEGX) data generated from lidocaine under varying hepatic blood flows in the rat liver perfused *in situ* preparation. *J. Pharmacokinet. Biopharm.*, 5:681–699.
107. Pang, K. S., and Terrell, J. A. (1981): Retrograde perfusion to probe the heterogeneous distribution of hepatic drug metabolizing enzymes in rats. *J. Pharmacol. Exp. Ther.*, 216:339–346.
108. Pang, K. S., and Terrell, J. A. (1981): Sulfate conjugation kinetics of acetaminophen by the perfused rat liver preparation. *Biochem. Pharmacol.*, 30:1959–1965.
109. Pang, K. S., Cherry, W. F., and Terrell, J. A. (1983): Disposition of enalaprilat and its diacid metabolite in the perfused rat liver preparation. Presence of a diffusional barrier into hepatocytes. (*submitted for publication*)
110. Pang, K. S., Waller, L., Horning, M. G., and Chan, K. K. (1982): Metabolite kinetics: Formation of acetaminophen from deuterated and non-deuterated phenacetin and acetanilide on acetaminophen sulfation kinetics in the perfused rat liver preparation. *J. Pharmacol. Exp. Ther.*, 222:14–19.
111. Patel, J. M., Wood, J. C., and Leibman, K. C. (1980): The biotransformation of allyl alcohol and acrolein in rat liver and lung preparations. *Drug Metab. Dispos.*, 8:305–308.

112. Perez, G. O., Reitberg, B., Owens, B., Parker, T., Obaya, H., and Schiff, E. R. (1979): Urea synthesis by perfused rat liver—studies of CCl_4-induced cirrhosis. *Biochem. Pharmacol.,* 28:485–488.
113. Rane, A., Shand, D. G., and Wilkinson, G. R. (1977): Disposition of carbamazepine and its 10,11-epoxide metabolite in the isolated perfused rat liver. *Drug Metab. Dispos.,* 5:179–184.
114. Reichens, J., and Paumgartner, G. (1976): Uptake of bile acids by perfused rat liver. *Am. J. Physiol.,* 231:734–742.
115. Reichert, D., Werner, H. W., and Hensler, D. (1978): Role of liver glutathione in 1,1-dichloroethylene metabolism and hepatotoxicity in intact rats and isolated perfused rat liver. *Arch. Toxicol.,* 41:167–178.
116. Reinke, L. A., Belinsky, S. A., Kauffman, F. C., Evans, R. A., and Thurman, R. G. (1982): Regulation of NADPH-dependent mixed-function oxidation in perfused livers. *Biochem. Pharmacol.,* 31:1621–1628.
117. Reinke, L. A., Belinsky, S. A., Evans, R. K., Kauffman, F. C., and Thurman, R. G. (1981): Conjugation of p-nitrophenol in the perfused rat liver: The effect of substrate concentration and carbohydrate reserves. *J. Pharmacol. Exp. Ther.,* 217:863–870.
118. Reinke, L. A., Kauffman, F. C., Belinsky, S. A., and Thurman, R. G. (1979): Interactions between ethanol metabolism and mixed-function oxidation in perfused rat liver: Inhibition of p-nitroanisole O-demethylation. *J. Pharmacol. Exp. Ther.,* 213:70–78.
119. Reinke, L. A., Kauffman, F. C., and Thurman, R. G. (1979): Stimulation of p-nitroanisole O-demethylation by ethanol in perfused livers from fasted rats. *J. Pharmacol. Exp. Ther.,* 211:133–139.
120. Reinke, L. A., Kauffman, F. C., and Thurman, R. G. (1980): Stimulation of p-nitroanisole O-demethylation in perfused livers by xylitol and sorbitol. *Biochem. Pharmacol.,* 29:813–890.
121. Renaud, G., Foliot, A., and Infante, E. (1978): Inhibitory effect of cholephilic anions on fatty acid uptake by the perfused rat liver. *Biochem. Pharmacol.,* 27:897–902.
122. Ritchie, H. D., and Hardcastle, J. D. (1973): Isolated organ perfusion for physiologic studies. In: *Isolated Organ Perfusion.* Crosby Lockwood Stapes, London.
123. Rogers, R. M., Taylor, S. M., Dickinson, G. R., Ilias, A. M., Lynn, R. K., and Gerber, N. (1980): Mechanism and chloretic effect of naltrexone in the isolated perfused rat liver. *Drug Metab. Dispos.,* 8:390–396.
124. Ross, B. D., (1972): In: *Perfusion Techniques in Biochemistry. A Laboratory Manual,* pp. 135–220. Clarendon Press, London.
125. Roth, R. A. (1979): Use of the isolated perfused lung in biochemical toxicology. *Rev. Biochem. Toxicol.,* 1:287–309.
126. Rowland, M., Benet, L. Z., and Graham, G. G. (1973): Clearance concepts in pharmacokinetics. *J. Pharmacokinet. Biopharm.,* 1:123–136.
127. Schimassek, H. (1962): Perfusion of isolated rat liver with a semi-synthetic medium and control of liver function. *Life Sci.,* 11:629–634.
128. Schimassek, H. (1962): Regulation of lactate and pyruvate levels in perfusion medium by the isolated rat liver. *Life Sci.,* 11:635–638.
129. Schmucker, D. L., and Curtis, J. C. (1974): A correlated study of the fine structure and physiology of the perfused rat liver. *Lab. Invest.,* 30:201–212.
130. Scholz, R., Hansen, W., and Thurman, R. G. (1973): Interaction of mixed-function oxidation with biosynthetic processes. *Eur. J. Pharmacol.,* 38:64–72.
131. Scholz, R., Thurman, R. G., Williamson, J. R., Chance, B., and Bucher, T. (1969): Flavin and pyridine nucleotide oxidation-reduction changes in perfused rat liver. *J. Biol. Chem.,* 244:2317–2324.
132. Shand, D. G., Branch, R. A., Nies, A. S., and Wilkinson, G. R. (1973): The disposition of propranolol VII. The effects of saturable hepatic tissue uptake on drug clearance by the perfused rat liver. *Drug Metab. Dispos.,* 1:679–686.
133. Shand, D. G., Cotham, R. H., and Wilkinson, G. R. (1978): Perfusion-limited effects of plasma drug binding on hepatic drug extraction. *Life Sci.,* 19:125–130.
134. Shand, D. G., Kornhauser, D. M., and Wilkinson, G. R. (1975): Effects of route of administration and blood flow on hepatic drug elimination. *J. Pharmacol. Exp. Ther.,* 195:424–432.
135. Siddik, Z. H., Barnes, B. D., Dring, L. G., Smith, R. L., and Williams, R. T. (1979): The metabolism of lysergic acid di[^{14}C]ethylamide ((^{14}C)LSD) in the isolated perfused rat liver. *Biochem. Pharmacol.,* 28:3081–3091.
136. Sies, H., and Chance, B. (1970): The steady-state level of catalase compound I in isolated hemoglobin-free perfused rat liver. *FEBS Lett.,* 11:172–176.
137. Sies, H., Bartoli, G. M., Burk, R. F., and Wayhas, C. (1978): Glutathione efflux from perfused rat liver after phenobarbital treatment, during drug oxidations, and in selenium deficiency. *Eur. J. Biochem.,* 89:113–118.
138. Skibba, J. L., Jones, F. E., and Condon, R. E. (1982): Altered hepatic disposition of doxorubicin in the perfused rat liver at hyperthermic temperatures. *Cancer Treat. Res.,* 66:1357–1363.
139. Smith, B. R., and Bend, J. R. (1979): Metabolism and toxicity of benzo(a)pyrene-4,5-oxide in the isolated perfused rat liver. *Toxicol. Appl. Pharmacol.,* 43:313–321.
140. Smith, R. L. (1973): In: *The Excretory Function of Bile. The Elimination of Drugs and Toxic Substances in Bile,* pp. 12. Chapman and Hall, London.
141. Soboll, S., Heldt, H.-W., Scholz, R., Muller, M., and Noell, C. (1981): Changes in the subcellular development of metabolites due to ethanol oxidation in the perfused rat liver. *Hoppe-Seyers Z. Physiol. Chem.,* 362:247–260.
142. Sonawane, B. R., Yaffe, S. J., Reinke, L. A., and Thurman, R. G. (1981): Postnatal development of mixed function oxidation and conjugation in he-

moglobin-free perfused rat liver. *J. Pharmacol. Exp. Ther.*, 216:473–478.
143. Steele, J. W., Yagen, B., Hernandez, O., Cox, R. H., Smith, B. R., and Bend, J. R. (1981): The metabolism and excretion of styrene oxide-glutathione conjugates in the rat and by isolated perfused liver, lung and kidney preparations. *J. Pharmacol. Exp. Ther.*, 219:35–41.
144. Stitzel, R. E., Tephly, T. R., and Mannering, G. J. (1968): Inhibition of drug metabolism VI. Inhibition of hexobarbital metabolism in the isolated perfused liver of the rat. *Mol. Pharmacol.*, 4:15–19.
145. Subbiah, M. T., Kuksis, A., and Mookerjea, S. (1969): Secretion of bile salts by intact and isolated rat livers. *Can. J. Biochem.*, 47:847–854.
146. Tavaloni, N., Reed, J. S., Hruben, Z., and Boyer, J. L. (1979): Effect of chlorpromazine in hepatic perfusion and bile secretory functions in the isolated perfused rat liver. *J. Lab. Clin. Med.*, 94:726–741.
147. Terrell, J. A., Pang, K. S., and Nelson, S. D. (1982): *Fed. Proc.*, 41:1731.
148. Thompson, R. M., Gerber, N., Seibert, R. A., and Desidero, D. M. (1973): A rapid method for the mass spectrometric identification of glucuronides and other polar drug metabolites in permethylated rat bile. *Drug Metab. Dispos.*, 1:489–505.
149. Thomson, O., and Larsen, J. A. (1982): Comparison of vanadate and ouabain effects on liver hemodynamics and bile production in the perfused rat liver. *J. Pharmacol. Exp. Ther.*, 221:197–205.
150. Thurman, R. G., Marazzo, D. J., Jones, L. S., and Kauffman, F. C. (1977): The continuous kinetic determination of p-nitroanisole O-demethylation in hemoglobin-free perfused rat liver. *J. Pharmacol. Exp. Ther.*, 201:498–506.
151. Thurman, R. G., and Reinke, L. A. (1979): The isolated perfused liver: A model biochemical mechanism of chemical toxicity. *Rev. Biochem. Toxicol.*, 1:249–285.
152. Thurman, R. G., and Scholz, R. (1969): The effect of aminopyrine on oxygen uptake mixed function oxidation in perfused rat liver. *Eur. J. Biochem.*, 10:459–467.
153. Thurman, R. G., and Scholz, R. (1973): Interaction of mixed-function oxidation with biosynthetic process. *Eur. J. Biochem.*, 38:73–78.
154. Triner, L., Verosky, M., Hanig, D. B., and Nahas, G. G. (1970): Perfusion of isolated liver with fluorocarbon emulsions. *Fed. Proc.*, 29:1778–1781.
155. Trowell, O. A. (1942): Urea formation in the isolated perfused liver of the rat. *J. Physiol. (London)*, 100:432–458.
156. Tygstrup, N., Funding, J., Juul-Nielsen, J., Keiding, S., Koudahl, G., and Ramsoe, K. (1971): The function of the isolated perfused and the in vivo pig liver. *Scand. J. Gastroenterol.* [*Suppl*], 9:131–138.
157. Uetrecht, J. P., Wooseley, R. L., Freeman, R. W., Sweetman, B. J., and Oates, J. A. (1981): Metabolism of procainamide in the perfused rat liver. *Drug Metab. Dispos.*, 9:183–187.
158. Ullrich, V., and Diehl, D. (1971): Uncoupling of monooxygenation and electron transport by fluorocarbons in liver microsomes. *Eur. J. Biochem.*, 20:509–512.
159. van Anda, J., Smith, B. R., and Bend, J. R. (1979): Concentration-dependent metabolism and toxicity of [^{14}C]styrene oxide in the isolated perfused rat liver. *J. Pharmacol. Exp. Ther.*, 211:207–212.
160. von Bahr, C., Borga, O., Fellenius, E., and Rowland, M. (1973): Kinetics of nortriptyline (NT) in rats in vivo and in the isolated perfused liver: Demonstration of a "first pass disappearance on NT in the liver. *Pharmacology*, 9:177–186.
161. Vonk, R. J., Danhoff, M., Coenraads, T., van Doorn, A. B. D., Keulemans, K., Scaf, A. H. J., and Meijer, D. K. F. (1979): Influence of bile salts on hepatic transport of dibromosulfophthalein. *Am. J. Physiol.*, 237:E524–E534.
162. Vonk, R. J., Scholtens, E., Keulemans, G. T. P., and Meijer, D. K. F. (1978): Choleresis and hepatic transport mechanisms IV. Influence of bile salt choleresis on the hepatic transport of the organic cations, D-tubocurarine and N^4-acetylprocainamide ethobromide. *Naunyn Schmiedebergs Arch. Pharmacol.*, 302:1–9.
163. Vonk, R. J., van Doorn, A. B. D., Scaf, A. H. J., and Meijer, D. K. F. (1977): Choleresis and hepatic transport mechanisms III. *Naunyn Schmiedebergs Arch. Pharmacol.*, 300:173–177.
164. Vore, M., Bauer, J., and Pascussi, V. (1978): The effect of pregnancy on the metabolism of [^{14}C] phenytoin in the isolated perfused rat liver. *J. Pharmacol. Exp. Ther.*, 206:439–447.
165. Vu, V. T., and Chen, C.-P. (1982): Effects of *dl*-propanolol on lidocaine disposition in the perfused rat liver. *Drug Metab. Dispos.*, 10:350–355.
166. Williams, R. T. (1959): In: *Detoxification Mechanisms*, 2nd edition, pp. 1–17. Chapman and Hall, London.
167. Williamson, J. R., Browning, E. T., Thurman, R. G., and Scholz, R. (1969): Inhibition of glucagon effects in perfused rat liver by (+)decanoyl-carnitine. *J. Biol. Chem.*, 244:5055–5064.
168. Winkler, K., Bass, L., Keiding, S., and Tygstrup, N. (1974): The effect of hepatic perfusion on assessment of kinetic constants. In: *Alfred Benzoin Symposium VI. The Regulation of Hepatic Metabolism*, edited by F. Lundqvist and N. Tygstrup, pp. 797–807. Munksgaard, Copenhagen.
169. Winkler, K., Juul-Nielsen, J., Iversen Hansen, R., Schmidt, A., and Tygstrup, N. (1971): The Relation between function and perfusion of the isolated pig liver. *Scand. J. Gastroenterol.* [*Suppl.*], 9:139–147.
170. Winkler, K., Keiding, S., and Tygstrup, N. (1973): Clearance as a quantitative measure of liver function. In: *The Liver: Quantitative Aspects of Structure and Function*, edited by P. Paumgartner and R. Presig, pp. 144–155. S. Karger, Basel.
171. Woods, H. F., Stubbs, W. A., Johnson, G., and Sibert, K. G. M. M. (1974): Inhibition by salicylate of gluconeogenesis in the isolated perfused rat liver. *Clin. Exp. Pharmacol. Physiol.*, 1:535–540.
172. Yu, V. C., de Lamirande, E., Horning, M. G., and Pang, K. S. (1982): Dose-dependent kinetics of quinidine in the perfused rat liver preparation: Kinetics of formation of active metabolites. *Drug Metab. Dispos.*, 10:568–572.

Drug Metabolism and Drug Toxicity,
edited by J. R. Mitchell and M. G. Horning.
Raven Press, New York © 1984.

Analytical Methodology for the Study of Metabolites

Marjorie G. Horning,[1] Long-Sheng Sheng, and Khingkan Lertratanangkoon

Institute for Lipid Research, Baylor College of Medicine, Houston, Texas 77030

In the 12 years since the publication of *Fundamentals of Drug Metabolism and Drug Disposition* by La Du, Mandel, and Way (19), new methods and new instrumentation have been developed for the separation and identification of drugs and their metabolites. Because of the sensitivity and selectivity of detection inherent in the new analytical systems, both the size of the biological sample and the time required for isolation and identification has been reduced substantially. Microgram, rather than milligram, quantities of metabolites are required, and often analyses can be carried out with submicrogram quantities without difficulty.

Before initiating studies of drug metabolism, it is necessary to decide on an analytical approach because the analytical procedures selected determine the type of information that will be obtained. For example, in pharmacokinetic studies, only the disappearance of a parent drug and/or the formation of the major metabolites may be of interest. Spectrophotometric methods, paper chromatography, or thin layer chromatography may provide the most effective analytical procedures. In studies of drug toxicity, however, until the toxic metabolite has been identified or the mechanism of toxicity has been established, all of the metabolites are of interest. Inasmuch as it is not possible to predict *a priori* the number or relative amounts of metabolites that may be formed, procedures that provide multicomponent analyses are preferred. At present, multicomponent analyses are carried out most conveniently by high performance liquid chromatography (HPLC) and gas chromatography (GC). Both methods provide profiles of metabolites (or classes of metabolites) that can be used for quantification and identification of the minor as well as the major metabolites. Minor metabolites are of interest because they frequently indicate new pathways or potentially toxic pathways of metabolism. Further, minor metabolites may be important if a very small amount of a metabolite elicits a very toxic response.

In carrying out multicomponent analyses, general procedures that can be used to study the metabolism of a variety of drugs and environmental chemicals, rather than specific procedures designed for the study of individual drugs, are preferred. The analytical methods described in this chapter include procedures for the isolation, separation, quantification, and tentative identification of metabolites. All of the methods involved in these four phases of a metabolic study have been used to investigate the metabolism of a wide variety of drugs and environmental chemicals. It is important, however, to recognize the limitations of a method; therefore, the disadvantages as well as the advantages are discussed in the section entitled Methods. For convenience, the experimental details for several of the methods

[1] *Present address:* Department of Pharmaceutical Analysis, Nanjing College of Pharmacy, Nanjing, China.

are included in the appendix at the end of the chapter.

Although profile analyses have been used primarily for the separation and identification of metabolites, it should be noted that profiles also provide permanent visual records of the metabolism of a drug under a defined set of experimental conditions, and these records frequently contain valuable additional information. The various kinds of information that can be obtained by comparison and reexamination of metabolic profiles are discussed in the section entitled Applications.

METHODS

Isolation of Metabolites from a Biological Matrix (Urine, Plasma, Bile, or Homogenate)

To carry out profile analyses, procedures that ensure the isolation of most of the metabolites are essential. Two procedures, (a) extraction with ammonium carbonate–ethyl acetate (salt-solvent pair extraction) and (b) DEAE-Sephadex chromatography, have been used extensively in our laboratory for the isolation of nonacidic (neutral plus basic) and acidic metabolites. Both procedures can be used with enzymatically hydrolyzed as well as unhydrolyzed samples of urine, bile, plasma, or tissue homogenates. The advantages and disadvantages of the two procedures are discussed below and summarized in Table 1. The neutral and acidic fractions must, of course, be analyzed by either high-pressure liquid chromatography (HPLC) or gas chromatography (GC) in order to evaluate the usefulness of isolation procedures for profiling.

Ammonium Carbonate–Ethyl Acetate Procedure (14)

This extraction procedure is used to separate the metabolites into three fractions: (a) non-

TABLE 1. *Comparison of ammonium carbonate–ethyl acetate and DEAE-Sephadex isolation procedures*

Procedure	Advantages	Disadvantages
Ammonium carbonate–ethyl acetate extraction	Recovery of neutral + basic metabolites is 85 to 100%	Recovery of acidic metabolites from aqueous phase varies from 50 to 100% depending on the structure of acidic metabolites
	Endogenous neutral metabolites (sugars and sugar alcohols) remain in the aqueous and do not interfere with HPLC or GC analyses	Endogenous urinary acids may interfere with subsequent HPLC and GC analyses of ethyl-acetate–soluble acids
	Recovery of ethyl acetate–soluble acids (mercapturic, mercaptolactic and mercaptoacetic acids) is 85 to 100%	Significant quantities of ethyl acetate–insoluble acids may remain in the aqueous phase
DEAE-Sephadex	Recovery of neutral + basic metabolites is 95 to 100%	Endogenous neutral metabolites (i.e., sugars and sugar alcohols) may interfere with HPLC or GC analysis
	Recovery of acidic metabolites is 95 to 100%	Endogenous acidic metabolites (i.e., urinary acids) may interfere with HPLC or GC analysis
	Many columns (10–20) can be run simultaneously	Fractions must be lyophilized before analyses by HPLC or GC
	Profiles of endogenous as well as drug metabolites are obtained	

acidic (ethyl acetate–soluble neutral and basic) metabolites, (b) ethyl acetate–soluble acidic metabolites, and (c) water soluble (ethyl acetate–insoluble) metabolites. (See Appendix for experimental details.)

Nonacidic (Neutral Plus Basic) Fraction

If the neutral and basic metabolites are soluble in ethyl acetate, the ammonium carbonate–ethyl acetate extraction procedure is preferred to the DEAE-Sephadex procedure because it requires less time. The recovery of neutral and basic (nonacidic) metabolites including phenols and catechols is excellent (85–100%). Most of the endogenous neutral metabolites (sugars and sugar alcohols) that might interfere with either the separation or identification of drug metabolites remain in the ammonium carbonate–saturated aqueous phase. Thus, when ethyl acetate extracts are analyzed by either GC or HPLC, metabolites of the administered drug dominate the profiles. This is illustrated in Fig. 1B, which shows a capillary GC analysis of the neutral metabolites of phenanthrene extracted from hydrolyzed rat urine by this procedure. Four major metabolites are labeled on the chart, but approximately 20 of the smaller peaks have been identified as phenanthrene metabolites by GC-MS (23). Additional GC profiles of neutral (nonacidic) metabolites isolated from urine by this procedure are shown in Figs. 11 to 14.

Neutral metabolites isolated by this procedure can also be profiled by HPLC. Figure 2 shows HPLC analyses of the neutral metabolites of carbamazepine (CBZ) extracted from rat and human urine; HPLC analyses of the neutral metabolites of carbamazepine extracted from hydrolyzed rat bile and liver perfusate are compared in Fig. 3A and 3B. Neutral metabolites isolated from microsomes, hepatocytes, and S_9 fractions are also suitable for analyses by GC or HPLC. A GC analysis of the neutral metabolites of biphenyl synthesized by a liver S_9 fraction is shown in Fig. 4. From these illustrations, it is clear that this simple, rapid procedure can be used to isolate neutral metabolites of numerous drugs and environmental chemicals from a variety of biological fluids.

Ethyl Acetate–Soluble Acids

Recovery of acidic drug metabolites by ethyl acetate extraction after acidification of the ammonium carbonate–saturated aqueous phase varies from 50 to 100%, depending on the structure of the acidic metabolites. Many endogenous acids are present in this extract, and glucosiduronic acids may also be present if the sample has not been hydrolyzed. The endogenous acids may complicate both the separation and identification of metabolites when this fraction is analyzed by GC or HPLC. In Fig. 5A and 5B, GC analyses of the ethyl acetate–soluble acids isolated from the urine of a rat and a guinea pig after i.p. injection of styrene oxide are compared. The endogenous acids (hippuric, phenylaceturic, etc.) do not interfere with either the separation or the identification of the isomeric mercapturic acids or mercaptolactic acid derivatives because of the relatively large quantities and long retention times of these bivalent sulfur acids. It was difficult, however, to obtain definitive mass spectra of the two mercaptoacetic acids present in guinea pig urine because an endogenous acid coeluted with the isomeric mercaptoacetic acids. The endogenous acids may interfere with subsequent analyses by GC and HPLC if the ethyl acetate–soluble acidic drug metabolites are excreted in quantities comparable to those of the endogenous acids. Figure 6 illustrates this problem. The mercapturic acid(s) derivative of naphthalene is excreted in large quantities in mouse urine, but four of the acidic bivalent sulfur metabolites are present in quantities similar to those of the endogenous acids. In spite of the large number of endogenous acids present in the extract, it was possible to identify the naphthalene metabolites because they were eluted after most of the endogenous acids.

Many of the endogenous acids, which are soluble in ethyl acetate, absorb in the UV region (hippuric, phenylaceturic, and *p*-hydroxyphenylacetic acids, etc.). These acids

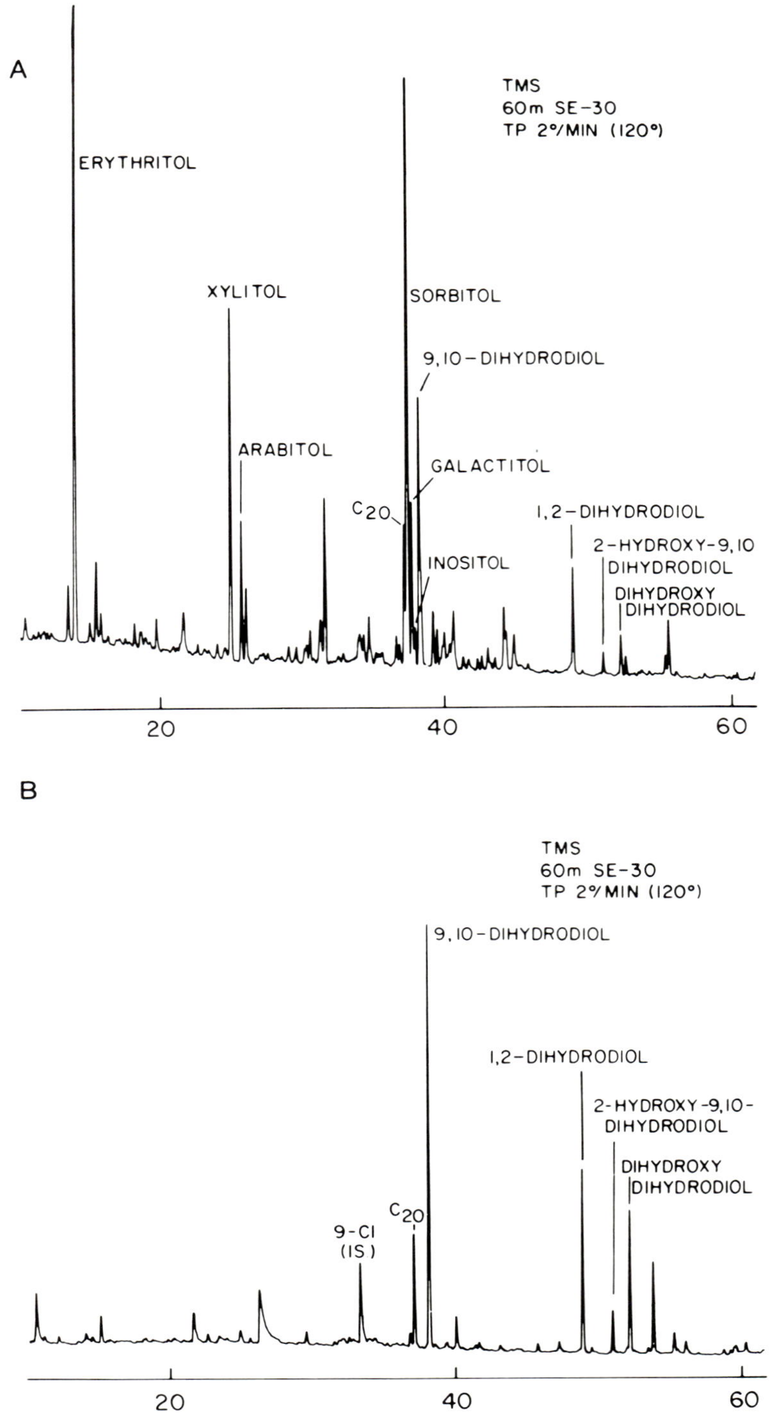

FIG. 1. Comparison of GC separations of the TMS derivatives of neutral phenanthrene metabolites isolated from hydrolyzed rat urine by the DEAE-Sephadex procedure (**A**) and by the ammonium carbonate–ethyl acetate procedure (**B**). The dose of phenanthrene was 50 mg/kg, i.p. The separations were carried out on a 60 meter glass capillary column coated with SE-30. The column was temperature programmed at 2°/min from 120°C. 9-Chlorophenanthrene (9-Cl) was the internal standard and the hydrocarbon eiscosane (C_{20}) was added as an external standard. In addition to the 9,10-dihydrodiol and the 1,2-dihydrodiol, 2,9,10-trihydroxy-9,10-dihydrophenanthrene and a dihydroxy-dihydrodiol metabolite were identified.

may interfere with the HPLC analyses of acidic drug metabolites when UV detection is used. For example, in the HPLC separation shown in Fig. 7, phenylaceturic acid coelutes with the mercaptopyruvic acid metabolite of styrene oxide. From the examples shown in Figs. 5 to 7, it is clear that the acidic bivalent sulfur metabolites can be extracted from acidified urine by ethyl acetate. The recovery of mercapturic, mercaptoacetic, mercaptolactic, and mercaptopyruvic acid metabolites of several environmental chemicals in the ethyl acetate extract is essentially quantitative (23).

Water Soluble Acids

If radioactivity data indicate that a significant percentage of the metabolites remains in the aqueous phase after extraction of ethyl acetate–soluble acids, an alternative procedure which does not involve saturation with ammonium carbonate is used (see Appendix). The ethyl acetate–insoluble metabolites excreted in urine and bile are polar and usually are difficult to convert into volatile derivatives for analysis by GC. These metabolites can frequently be separated by HPLC. An HPLC analysis of the ethyl acetate–insoluble acidic metabolites of phenanthrene excreted in bile is shown in Fig. 8. The structures of the cysteine and glutathione adducts were confirmed by fast-atom–bombardment mass spectrometry (FAB-MS) and by synthesis from phenanthrene 9,10-oxide (23).

DEAE-Sephadex Procedure (18)

A second isolation procedure used extensively in our laboratory involves chromatography on DEAE-Sephadex columns. This procedure separates the metabolites present in urine, bile, plasma, or homogenates into two fractions: (a) nonacidic (neutral plus basic) metabolites that are eluted from the DEAE-Sephadex column with water and (b) acidic metabolites which are eluted from the column with 1.5 M pyridine–acetic acid. (See Appendix for experimental details.) This procedure is very useful for the separation of neutral and acidic metabolites that are not readily extracted by ethyl acetate. Studies with a large number of radioactive reference compounds have shown that most neutral and basic compounds can be completely separated from acidic compounds by this procedure; further, the recovery of metabolites from the column is essentially quantitative (11). After lyophilization, both fractions can be analyzed by either HPLC or GC. Endogenous metabolites will be present in both fractions and may interfere with the separation and identification of metabolites by HPLC or GC unless the metabolites are present in larger quantities than the endogenous metabolites.

Nonacidic (Neutral Plus Basic) Metabolites

A GC analysis of a neutral fraction eluted from a DEAE-Sephadex column is shown in Fig. 1A. The endogenous neutral metabolites (sugar alcohols) do not interfere with the separation and identification of the major metabolites but do interfere with the identification of the minor metabolites of phenanthrene. This profile can be compared with the profile of neutral phenanthrene metabolites obtained by the ammonium carbonate–ethyl acetate procedure (Fig. 1B) because comparable aliquots of the same hydrolyzed rat urine were used for the analyses. It is interesting that the profiles of phenanthrene metabolites obtained by the two procedures are not identical. When compared with the external standard, C_{20}, the dihydroxydihydrodiol peak is much smaller in Fig. 1A than in Fig. 1B, suggesting that some loss of the dihydroxydihydrodiol occurred when phenanthrene metabolites were isolated by the DEAE-Sephadex procedure.

Acidic Metabolites

A GC analysis of an acidic fraction eluted from a DEAE-Sephadex column is shown in Fig. 9. The urine sample that had not been hydrolyzed was obtained from a rat treated with salicylic acid. In this example, the endogenous acids did not interfere with either the identification or quantification of salicylic acid or glucuronic acid. Salicyluric acid, how-

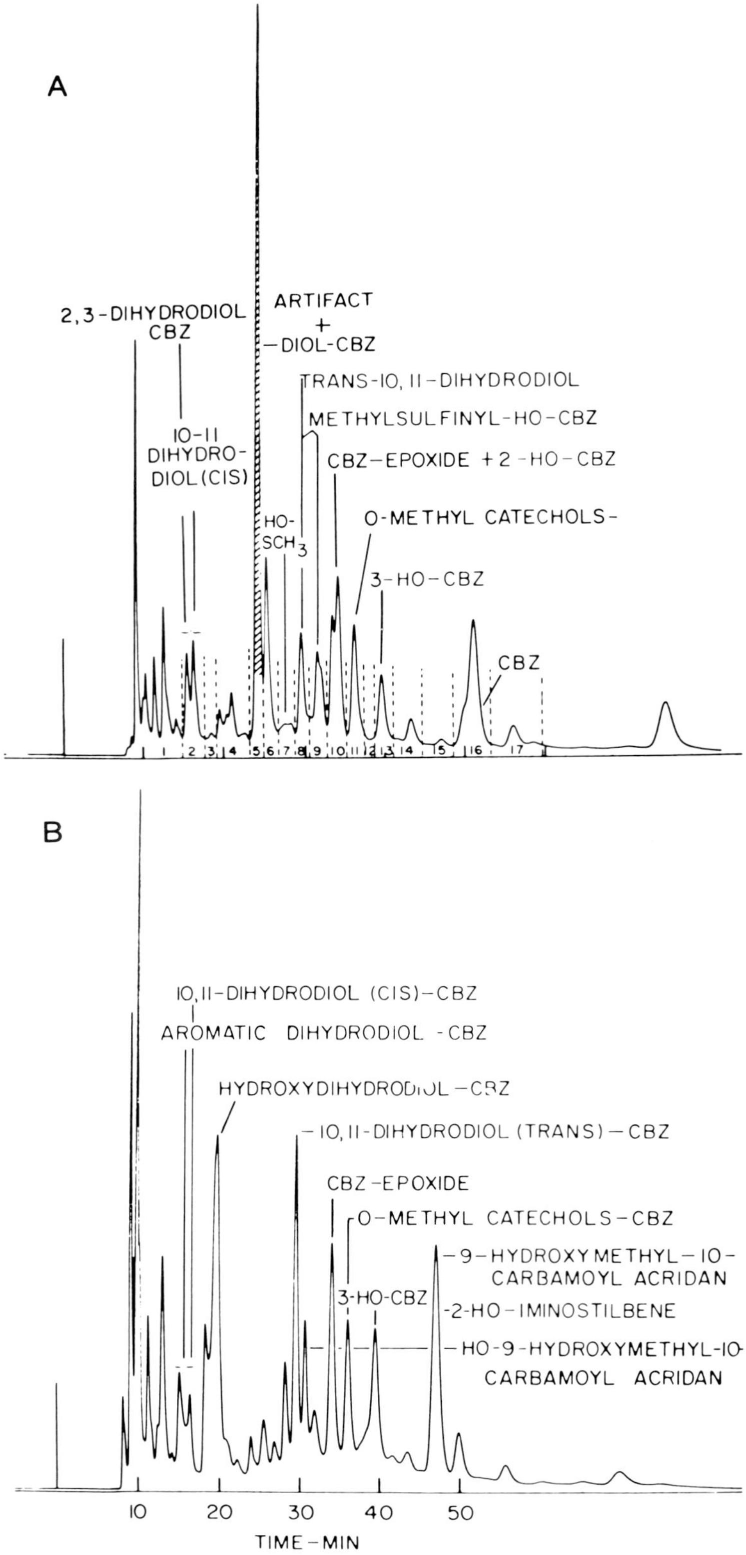

A
2,3-DIHYDRODIOL
CBZ
10-11
DIHYDRO-
DIOL(CIS)
ARTIFACT
+
-DIOL-CBZ
HO-
SCH$_3$
TRANS-10,11-DIHYDRODIOL
METHYLSULFINYL-HO-CBZ
CBZ-EPOXIDE +2-HO-CBZ
O-METHYL CATECHOLS-
3-HO-CBZ
CBZ
1 2 3 4 5 6 7 8 9 10 11 12 13 14 15 16 17
B
10,11-DIHYDRODIOL (CIS)-CBZ
AROMATIC DIHYDRODIOL -CBZ
HYDROXYDIHYDRODIOL-CBZ
-10,11-DIHYDRODIOL (TRANS)-CBZ
CBZ-EPOXIDE
O-METHYL CATECHOLS-CBZ
-9-HYDROXYMETHYL-10-
CARBAMOYL ACRIDAN
3-HO-CBZ
-2-HO-IMINOSTILBENE
-HO-9-HYDROXYMETHYL-10-
CARBAMOYL ACRIDAN
10
20
30
40
50
TIME-MIN

ever, was present in trace quantities and could only be tentatively identified because it coeluted with an endogenous metabolite. If the acidic metabolites are present in much smaller quantities than those shown in Fig. 9, separation (and identification) of metabolites is more difficult because of the large number of endogenous urinary acids. Although Fig. 1A and Fig. 9 illustrate some of the limitations of the DEAE-Sephadex procedure for profiling drug metabolites, the procedure does provide fractions that can be used to obtain excellent profiles of both neutral and acidic drug and endogenous metabolites (11). Profiles of endogenous metabolites can be used to study the effects of toxic doses of drugs and environmental chemicals on endogenous metabolism.

Recovery of Metabolites

Evaluation of the isolation and recovery of metabolites by either procedure is greatly facilitated by the use of radioactive tracers, and whenever possible in animal studies, the administered drug should be labeled with trace quantities of the radioactive drug. Usually 1 to 10 μCi of radioactive drug are adequate in studies with mice, rats, and guinea pigs. The distribution of radioactivity in the various isolated fractions defines the analytical problem. This is illustrated in Table 2, which shows the recovery of radioactivity from rat and guinea pig urine following i.p. administration of phenanthrene (50 mg/kg) labeled with 5 μCi of 9-^{14}C-phenanthrene. When the quantities of metabolites (mg) are calculated from the radioactivity measurements it is clear that a single rat urine will provide sufficient neutral (nonacidic) and ethyl acetate–soluble acidic metabolites for GC and/or HPLC analyses. Further, the data show that milligram quantities of nonacidic metabolites can be isolated by HPLC from two or three guinea pig urine samples for pharmacological or toxicological studies of the metabolites. If, in contrast, calculations based on recovery of radioactivity indicate that the quantities of metabolites are very small (<0.1 mg), several urine samples can be pooled before carrying out subsequent profile analyses. In this example, the data in Table 2 indicate that a significant amount (21%) of the radioactivity excreted in rat urine remained in the aqueous phase whereas only a small amount (5% or less) of the radioactivity in guinea pig urine was not extracted. It probably would be interesting and informative to pool several urines from rats rather than guinea pigs for the identification of water soluble metabolites since the accuracy of the 5% figure is questionable. This type of information, which can be acquired in a few hours when radioactive drugs are used, is very difficult to obtain without radioactivity measurements.

Inasmuch as the recovery of radioactive metabolites by the DEAE-Sephadex procedure is essentially quantitative, this procedure can be used to validate recovery of radioactive metabolites by the ammonium carbonate–ethyl acetate procedure. When duplicate aliquots of the same biological sample are analyzed by the two procedures, the radioactivity in the neutral plus basic fraction obtained by the ammonium carbonate–ethyl acetate extraction should be the same as the radioactivity in the neutral plus basic fraction eluted from a DEAE-Sephadex column, if recovery by extraction is essentially quantitative. This applies to hydrolyzed as well as unhydrolyzed samples.

FIG. 2. Comparison of HPLC separations of the neutral carbamazepine (CBZ) metabolites isolated from hydrolyzed rat (**A**) and human (**B**) urine by the ammonium carbonate–ethyl acetate procedure. The dotted lines indicate the seventeen fractions that were collected for subsequent analyses by GC and MS. Semipreparative μBondapak-C_{18} columns were used for both separations. The solvent system consisted of a mixture of solvent A, methanol-water-acetic acid (33:67:0.1 V/V), and solvent B, methanol-water-acetic acid (50:50:0.1), in which the proportion of B varied from 10 to 90%. A 20-min gradient (gradient 6) was used with a column pressure 800 psi and a flow rate of 1.2 ml/min. The structures of the metabolites are discussed in ref. 20.

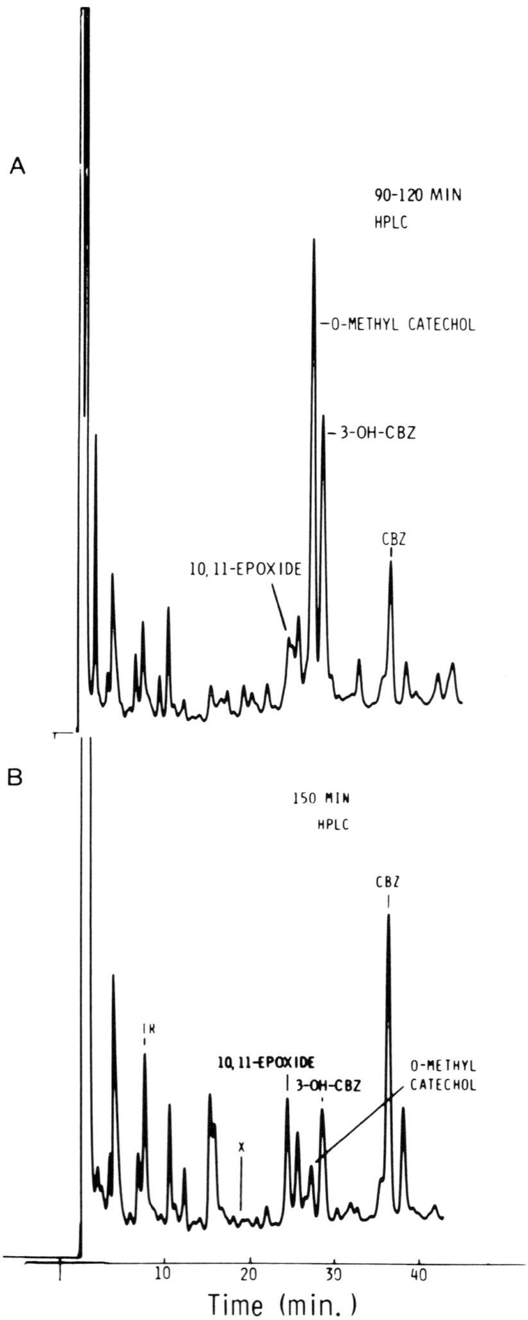

FIG. 3. Comparison of HPLC separations of the neutral carbamazepine metabolites isolated from hydrolyzed rat bile (**A**) and perfusate (**B**) by the ammonium carbonate–ethyl acetate procedure. Analytical μBondapak-C_{18} columns were used for both separations. The solvent system consisted of solvent A, methanol-water-acetic acid (20:80:0.1), and solvent B, methanol-water-acetic acid (50:50:0.1); the percentage of B varied from 10 to 90%. A 40-min gradient system (gradient 6) was used with a column pressure of 1,100 to 1,200 psi and a flow rate of 1.2 ml/min.

Further, when aliquots of hydrolyzed samples are analyzed by the two procedures, a comparison of the radioactivity in the acidic fraction extracted by ethyl acetate (ammonium carbonate procedure) with the radioactivity in the acidic fraction eluted from a DEAE-Sephadex column will help to validate recovery of acidic metabolites by the extraction procedure. If the recovery of radioactive metabolites in the ethyl acetate–soluble acidic fraction is considerably less than the radioactivity recovered in the acid fraction eluted from the DEAE-Sephadex column, significant quantities of ethyl acetate–insoluble acidic (polar) metabolites are present in the aqueous phase. It is, of course, possible to measure the radioactivity in the aqueous phase directly, but the measurements may not be too accurate if the aqueous phase has a high salt content.

If the radioactive drug is not available, it is still possible to quantify the recovery of metabolites by a reisolation procedure, providing the metabolites are easily detected by GC or HPLC. Fortunately, the recovery of a large number of metabolites can be evaluated in a single analysis. (See Appendix.)

Separation of Metabolites

Profiles of metabolites can be obtained most conveniently by HPLC or GC procedures. If the metabolites can be converted quantitatively into stable, volatile derivatives, profile analyses are carried out by capillary GC because the samples used for profiling by GC can also be used for identification of metabolites by mass spectrometry (MS). HPLC is especially useful for profiling polar, nonvolatile, or thermally unstable metabolites that can be detected spectrophotometrically. Fortunately, many metabolites that are not amenable to analysis by GC can be separated by

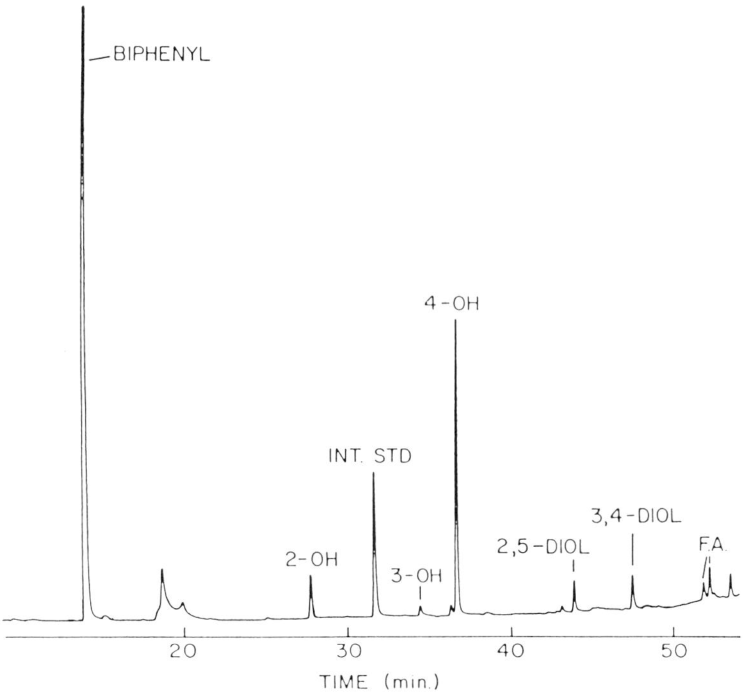

FIG. 4. GC separation of TMS derivatives of the neutral metabolites of biphenyl formed in an incubation of a noninduced mouse 9,000 g supernatant liver fraction with biphenyl. The separation was carried out with a 49 meter SE-30 glass capillary column by temperature programming at 2°/min from 130°C. The metabolites are 2-hydroxybiphenyl (2-OH), 3-hydroxybiphenyl (3-OH), 4-hydroxybiphenyl (4-OH), 2,5-dihydroxybiphenyl (2,5-DIOL), 3,4-dihydroxybiphenyl (3,4-DIOL); fatty acids (FA) were also present. 4-Bromobiphenyl was used as an internal standard (INT. STD.) for quantification.

HPLC. The techniques are complementary, and in most studies of drug metabolism it is advantageous to use both separation procedures.

Both analytical techniques are used so extensively that it is not necessary to present a detailed description of the methods. Some comments, however, pertaining to GC and HPLC analyses may be helpful, and are presented below.

Gas Chromatography

At present, glass capillary columns are preferred to packed columns for profiling metabolites because of the greatly increased resolution obtained with capillary columns. Glass open tubular capillary columns (1% SE-30; 60–75 meters) prepared in our laboratory by the method of German et al. (6) were used for all of the GC separations illustrated in this chapter. Excellent open tubular capillary columns (glass or fused silica) can now be purchased from several sources.

It is usually advisable to convert metabolites into suitable derivatives before carrying out profile analysis by GC because the separation, stability, and quantitation of metabolites are improved by derivatization. Some drug metabolites can be analyzed satisfactorily without derivatization. In most biological samples, however, there are many compounds that may either interfere with the separation and identification of metabolites or decrease the life of the capillary column if the sample is not derivatized. Only a few types of derivatives are employed for most metabolic studies. Trimethylsilylation is used for the derivatization

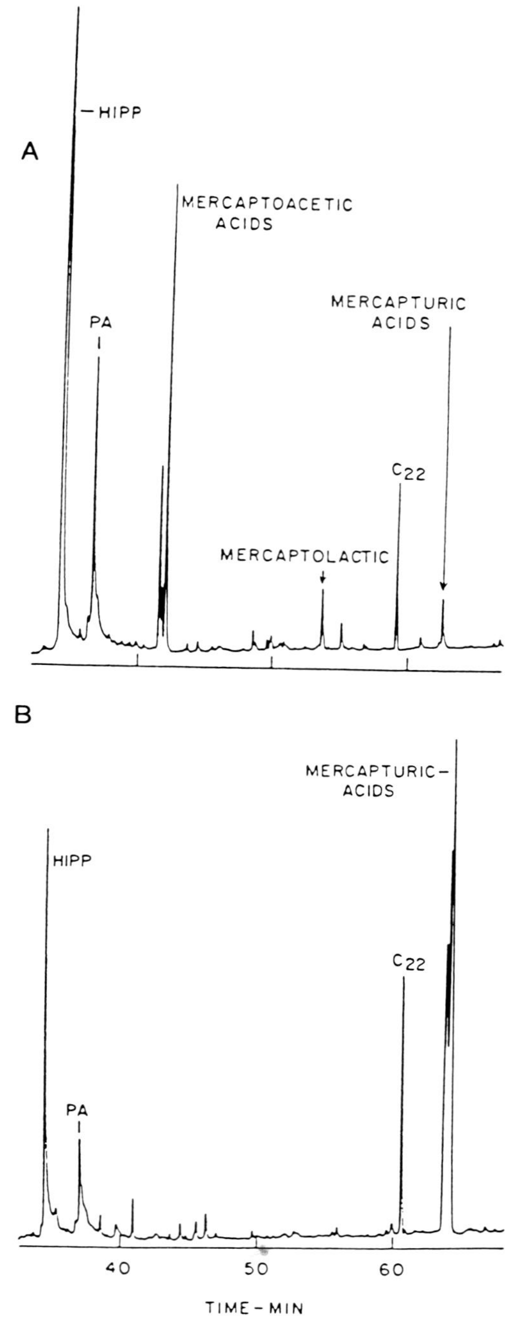

FIG. 5. GC separation of the ME-TMS derivatives of acidic metabolites (ethyl acetate–soluble acids) of styrene oxide isolated from hydrolyzed guinea pig (**A**) and rat (**B**) urine by the ammonium carbonate–ethyl acetate procedure. The separations were carried out on a 60 meter SE-30 glass capillary column by temperature programming at 2°/min from 100°C. Metabolites identified in guinea pig urine included mercaptoacetic acids, positional isomers *S*-(2-hydroxy-2-phenylethyl)mercaptoacetic acid and *S*-(2-hydroxy-1-phenylethyl)mercaptoacetic acid; mercaptolactic acid, *S*-(2-hydroxy-1-phenylethyl)mercaptolactic acid; mercapturic acid, *N*-acetyl-*S*-(2-hydroxy-2-phenylethyl)-L-cysteine; HIPP, hippuric acid; PA, phenaceturic acid; C_{22}, docosane (internal reference compound). Metabolites identified in rat urine included: mercapturic acids, four isomers with structures *N*-acetyl-*S*-(2-hydroxy-1-phenylethyl)-L-cysteine (diastereoisomers) and *N*-acetyl-*S*-(2-hydroxy-2-phenylethyl)-L-cysteine (diastereoisomers not separated); other compounds as indicated on the upper chart.

of most neutral and basic compounds. In Figs. 1A and 1B, the neutral fractions were silylated with *bis*-trimethylsilylacetamide (BSA) in pyridine; all of the hydroxyl groups were converted into trimethylsilyl ethers. Methylation followed by silylation is used for the derivatization of acidic compounds. In Figs. 5A and 5B, the acidic fractions were methylated and then silylated; all of the carboxyl groups were converted into methyl esters and all hydroxyl groups into trimethylsilyl ethers. The formation of these derivatives is rapid and quantitative. Methylation of biological samples is complete in 3 to 15 min and trimethylsilylation is usually complete in 30 to 60 min. (See Appendix for experimental procedures.)

Aliquots of the samples used for the GC analyses shown in Figs. 1A, 1B, 5A, and 5B were analyzed by electron-impact mass spectrometry for identification of metabolites. The identification of all of the labeled peaks was confirmed by MS.

HPLC

Reversed phase columns (μBondapak C_{18}) are used extensively for the separation of neutral, basic, and acidic drug metabolites (Figs. 2, 3, and 8). Frequently, metabolites that cannot be separated satisfactorily on a reversed phase column can be separated on a normal phase column such as Porasil. For example, the four isomeric mercapturic acid metabolites

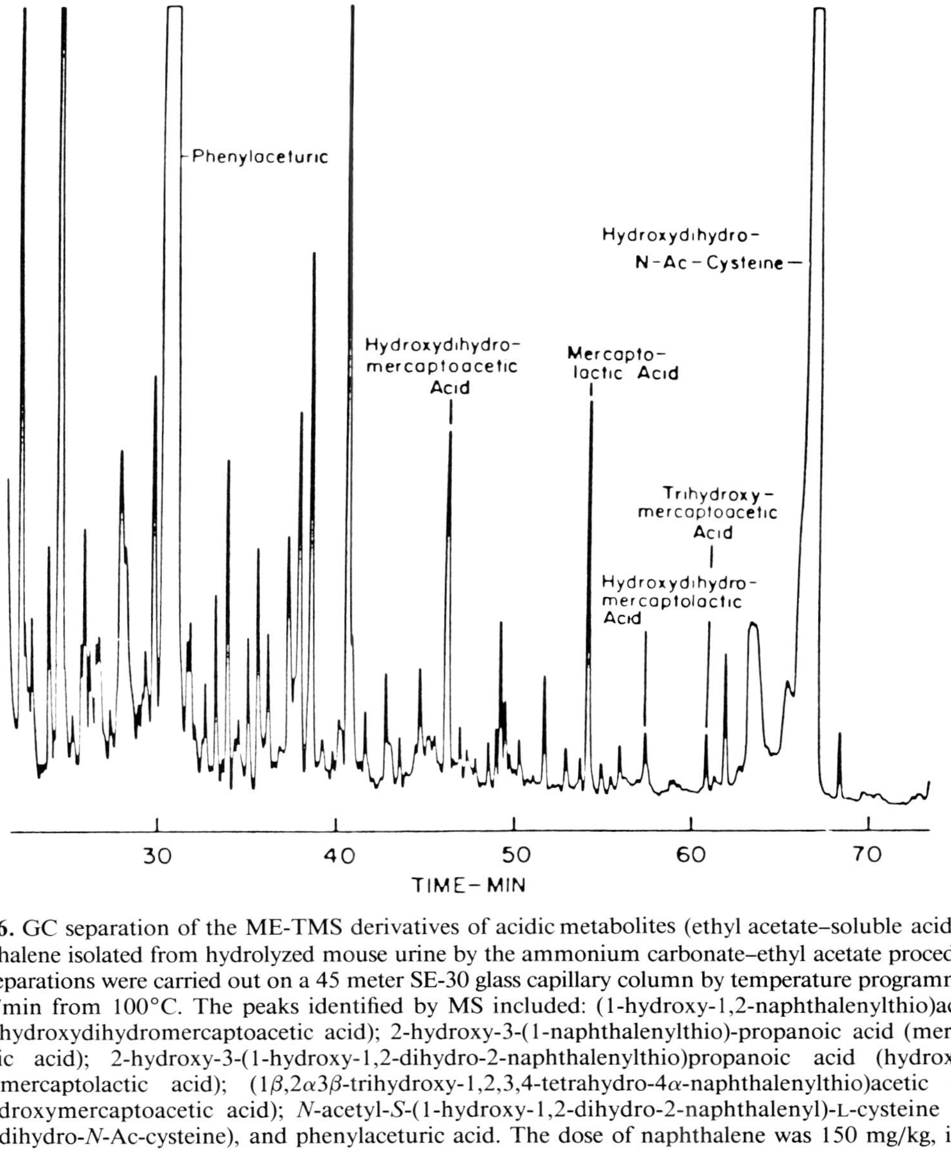

FIG. 6. GC separation of the ME-TMS derivatives of acidic metabolites (ethyl acetate-soluble acids) of naphthalene isolated from hydrolyzed mouse urine by the ammonium carbonate-ethyl acetate procedure. The separations were carried out on a 45 meter SE-30 glass capillary column by temperature programming at 2°/min from 100°C. The peaks identified by MS included: (1-hydroxy-1,2-naphthalenylthio)acetic acid (hydroxydihydromercaptoacetic acid); 2-hydroxy-3-(1-naphthalenylthio)-propanoic acid (mercaptolactic acid); 2-hydroxy-3-(1-hydroxy-1,2-dihydro-2-naphthalenylthio)propanoic acid (hydroxydihydromercaptolactic acid); ($1\beta,2\alpha3\beta$-trihydroxy-1,2,3,4-tetrahydro-4α-naphthalenylthio)acetic acid (trihydroxymercaptoacetic acid); *N*-acetyl-*S*-(1-hydroxy-1,2-dihydro-2-naphthalenyl)-L-cysteine (hydroxydihydro-*N*-Ac-cysteine), and phenylaceturic acid. The dose of naphthalene was 150 mg/kg, i.p.

that separated on a Porasil column (Fig. 10, peaks 1–4) did not separate on a reversed phase HPLC column. Semipreparative columns (7.8 mm × 30 cm) are used to isolate larger quantities (μg to mg) of individual metabolites when they are needed for identification by MS or for pharmacological or chemical studies. Fig. 2A shows the separation of carbamazepine metabolites on a semipreparative μBondapak C_{18} column. Seventeen fractions were collected as indicated by the dotted lines in Fig. 2A. In this example pooled individual fractions from four HPLC runs provided sufficient material for identification of most of the metabolites by GC-MS. Precolumns are used on analytical as well as semipreparative columns to protect and prolong the life of the columns.

Many solvent systems are described in the literature for the separation of drug metabolites. We have found methanol-water-acetic

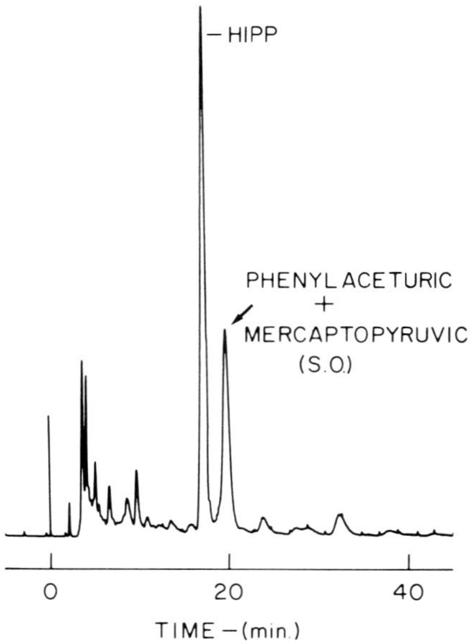

FIG. 7. HPLC separation of ME derivatives of acidic metabolites (ethyl acetate soluble acids) of styrene oxide isolated from hydrolyzed guinea pig urine by the ammonium carbonate–ethyl acetate procedure. The metabolites were separated on an analytical Porasil column by isocratic elution with hexane/ethanol (95:5). The column pressure was 1,100–1,200 psi with a flow rate of 1.2 ml/min. The dose of styrene oxide was 100 mg/kg, i.p.

acid and acetonitrile-water-acetic acid to be the most useful. By varying the proportions of these three solvents in a gradient system, neutral, basic, and acidic metabolites of a large number of drugs have been separated (20,23,32) (K. Lertratanangkoon et al., *unpublished observations*) (Figs. 2, 3, and 8). The inclusion of acetic acid in the solvent system (0.1–2%) rather than salt buffers is preferred because eluted metabolites collected for subsequent use (chemical, pharmacological, or MS studies) will not be contaminated with relatively large quantities of salts.

Because of the wide variation in the polarity of metabolites present in most biological samples, gradient rather than isocratic elution is employed for profiling metabolites. If a gradient is not used, the analysis time may be greatly prolonged, and the peak shape and resolution can deteriorate.

In contrast to GC analysis, derivatization of the biological sample is usually not required for HPLC analysis. Sometimes, however, derivatization improves the separation of metabolites by HPLC just as it does for GC analysis. For example, the four isomeric mercapturic acids, in Fig. 10, were separated as their methyl esters; the free acids were not resolved by gradient or isocratic elution on either normal or reversed phase columns.

Some of the advantages and disadvantages

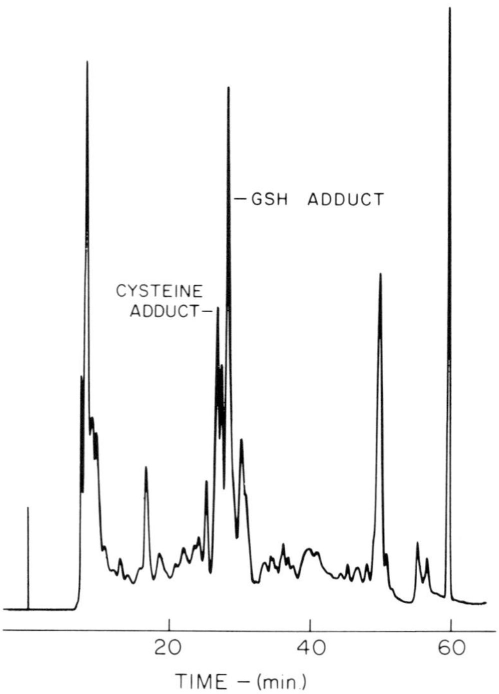

FIG. 8. HPLC separation of the water soluble (ethyl acetate–insoluble) acidic metabolites of phenanthrene isolated from hydrolyzed rat bile by a modified extraction procedure (see Appendix). The metabolites were separated on a semipreparative μBondapak C_{18} column by gradient elution. The solvent system consisted of solvent A, methanol-water-acetic acid (20:80:0.1), and solvent B, methanol-water-acetic acid (80:20:0.1); the percentage of B varied from 10 to 90. The cysteine and glutathione metabolites were identified by MS as *S*-(9-hydroxy-9,10-dihydrophenanthryl)-L-cysteine and *S*-(9-hydroxy-9,10-dihydrophenanthryl)-glutathione. The dose of phenanthrene was 50 mg/kg, i.p.

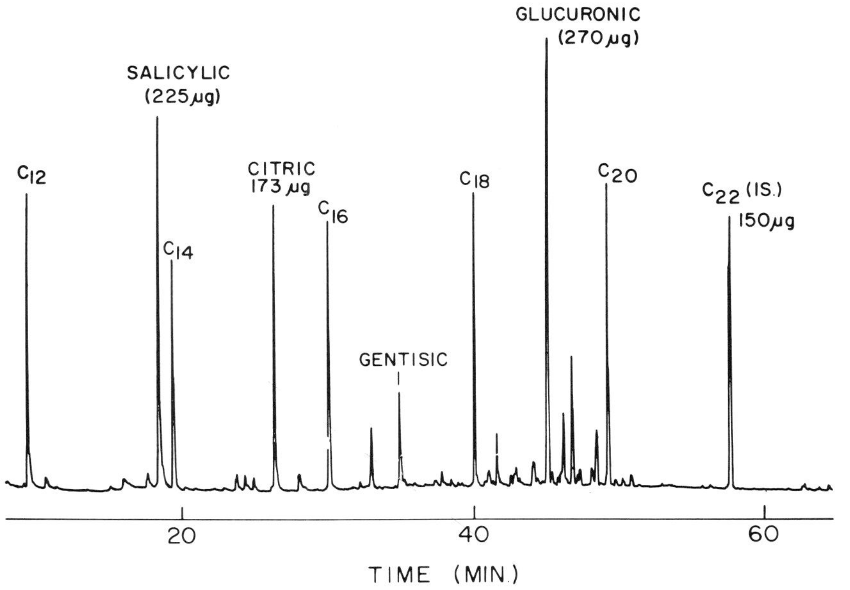

FIG. 9. GC separation of the ME-TMS derivatives of the acidic metabolites of salicylic acid and endogenous acids isolated from unhydrolyzed rat urine by the DEAE-Sephadex procedure. The separation was carried out on a 60 meter SE-30 glass capillary column by temperature programming at 2°/min from 110°C. The dose of salicylic acid was 260 mg/kg, i.p.

of the two separation techniques listed in Table 3 are illustrated in several of the figures. For example, the neutral and ethyl acetate–soluble acidic metabolites of phenanthrene isolated from hydrolyzed urine were analyzed by GC (Fig. 1B and 17) because the derivatized samples used for GC analyses could also be used for identification of metabolites by GC-MS. The time required for GC-MS analysis and interpretation of the mass spectra was approximately 2 hr for each sample. Both fractions can be profiled by HPLC, but the time required for the separation and subsequent identification of the metabolites by GC-MS

TABLE 2. *Recovery of radioactive metabolites from urine*[a]

Sample	Species	0–24 hr
Total urine		
% of administered dose	Rat[b]	35 (3.5 mg)
	Guinea pig[c]	67 (20.0 mg)
Hydrolyzed urine		
% Recovered as nonacidic metabolites[a]	Rat	46 (1.61 mg)
	Guinea pig	81 (16.2 mg)
% Recovered as ethyl acetate soluble acids	Rat	33 (1.15 mg)
	Guinea pig	14 (2.8 mg)
% Acidic metabolites remaining in aqueous phase	Rat	21 (0.74 mg)
	Guinea pig	<5 (1.0 mg)

[a] Recovery by the ammonium carbonate–ethyl acetate procedure.
[b] 10 mg (50 mg/kg) phenanthrene administered i.p.
[c] 30 mg (50 mg/kg) phenanthrene administered i.p.

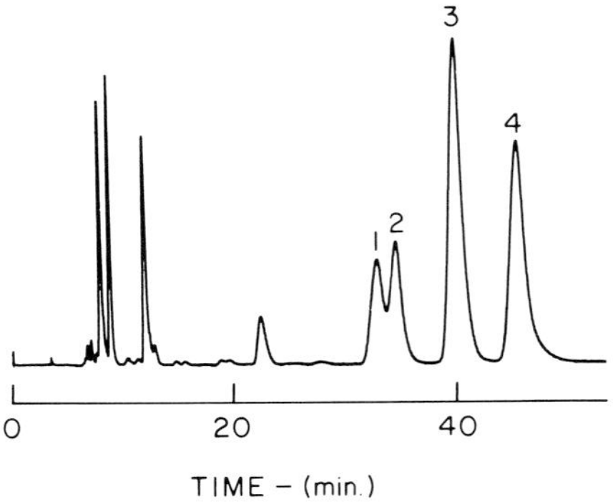

FIG. 10. HPLC separation of the methyl esters of the four isomeric mercapturic acid derivatives of styrene oxide. The separation was carried out on an analytical Porasil column by isocratic elution with hexane/ethanol (95:5). Peaks 1 and 2 are the diastereoisomers of *N*-acetyl-*S*-(2-hydroxy-2-phenylethyl)-L-cysteine and peaks 3 and 4 are the diastereoisomers of *N*-acetyl-*S*-(2-hydroxy-1-phenylethyl)-L-cysteine.

makes the analytical approach impractical. HPLC was used, however, to separate the nonvolatile cysteine and glutathione adducts (ethyl acetate–insoluble acids) excreted in bile after administration of phenanthrene (Fig. 8). Approximately 2 to 3 days were required for the separation and identification of the two adducts. In order to obtain sufficient quantities of metabolites, four to six HPLC separations were carried out on a semipreparative column. After pooling the individual fractions, removing the organic solvents (Rotovap) and lyophilizing the individual fractions, the residues were identified by FAB-MS. The GC analyses of this fraction provided no useful information and consequently the time spent on the HPLC separation and subsequent identification was not excessive.

Although the separation and subsequent identification of metabolites eluted from an HPLC column can be a very time consuming process, it is frequently necessary to carry out profile analyses by HPLC because of thermal instability of metabolites under GC conditions. The metabolites of carbamazepine that rearrange to iminostilbene and acridine derivatives during GC analysis exemplify this problem. When profile analyses were carried out by HPLC, it was clear that a large number of carbamazepine metabolites were present in hydrolyzed urine (Fig. 2A and 2B). It was also clear that the metabolites were not completely separated on the HPLC column and that individual fractions eluted from the HPLC column would have to be separated on another HPLC column or analyzed by GC or GC-MS. Seventeen fractions, indicated by the dotted lines in Fig. 2A, were collected, pooled, and

TABLE 3. *Comparison of GC and HPLC separation procedures*

Procedure	Advantages	Disadvantages
GC (packed or capillary columns)	Derivatized sample can be used directly for identification by MS	Samples usually require derivatization before GC analysis
	Can be used with any metabolite (or derivative) that can be volatilized	Not suitable for thermally unstable and nonvolatile compounds
HPLC	Derivatization of sample is usually not required	Most useful for metabolites that can be detected spectrophotometrically
	Can be used for separation of thermally unstable compounds	Samples eluted from HPLC column require considerable work-up for identification by MS
	Can be used for separation of very polar and nonvolatile compounds	

lyophilized. After derivatization the fractions were analyzed by GC and GC-MS. In spite of their thermal instability, most of the metabolites could be identified by GC-MS because each of the 17 fractions contained only one to three metabolites. It was necessary, however, to use desorption chemical-ionization mass spectrometry (DCI-MS) to identify the methylsulfinyl-hydroxy metabolites of CBS (20).

A total of 30 metabolites of carbamazepine, including 18 that had not been reported previously, were identified by MS as a result of profiling by HPLC. Both DCI and FAB mass spectrometry are extremely useful for the identification of metabolites eluted from the HPLC. Although the isolation requires a considerable amount of time, the mass spectrometric analyses of the individual fractions by DCI or FAB can be carried out very rapidly; only 5 to 10 min are required for each analysis. Clearly, a combined HPLC-MS analytical system would be useful for identification of metabolic eluting from an HPLC column. Analytical systems in which the effluent from an HPLC column is introduced directly into a mass spectrometer are under development.

Identification of Metabolites

Identification of metabolites present in either GC or HPLC profiles generally is based on mass spectrometric analysis. GC-MS systems operated in the electron impact (EI) or chemical ionization (CI) mode have been used extensively for this purpose during the past decade. More recently, desorption chemical-ionization (DCI) and fast-atom–bombardment (FAB) mass spectrometry have made possible the identification of nonvolatile and very polar metabolites. Identification by these analytical techniques is discussed in the following chapter.

Tentative identification of metabolites is established by comparing the retention times of HPLC peaks or the methylene unit (MU) values of GC peaks in the metabolite profiles with (a) the retention times or MU values of reference standards or (b) the retention times or MU values of metabolites previously identified by MS. Retention times and MU values obtained from the literature are helpful if comparable analytical conditions are employed. If good HPLC columns are used, retention times (measured in minutes from the time of injection of the sample) are very reproducible. MU values determined by GC with *n*-alkanes as reference compounds are also very reproducible (±0.03 MU). Methylene unit (MU) values obtained with a packed GC column (1% SE-30, 3 meters) may, however, differ slightly from values obtained with a glass capillary column (1% SE-30, 60 meters). (See Appendix, for the method of calculating MU values.) Figure 9 shows an analysis of a sample to which the alkanes C_{12}-C_{22} had been added in order to calculate MU values for the ME-TMS derivatives of salicylic acid (MU = 13.80), citric acid (MU = 15.28), gentisic acid (MU = 17.08), and glucuronic acid (MU = 19.08).

It should be emphasized that it is not unusual for two metabolites to have very similar retention times and/or MU values. For this reason it is advisable to check the homogeneity and identity of the peaks of interest by mass spectrometry, particularly when changes in experimental parameters (induction, inhibition) are involved. For example, in the HPLC analysis in Fig. 2B, two metabolites, 9-hydroxymethyl-10-carbamoylacridan and 2-hydroxyiminostilbene, eluted as a single symmetrical peak. MS and GC analyses, however, indicated that two metabolites were present. In the GC analysis in Fig. 5, an endogenous urinary acid, p-hydroxyphenyllactic acid (ME-TMS derivative) coeluted with one of the isomeric mercaptoacetic acids (ME-TMS derivative); GC-MS analysis proved that two compounds were present. The homogeneity and identity of the peaks must be established if the profiles are to be used for quantitative analysis.

Quantitation of Metabolites

Both HPLC and GC profiles can be used for quantitative analyses. Ideally, an internal standard (IS) should be added to the biological sample before isolation of the metabolites is initiated. If suitable internal standards are not available, external standards (ES) can be used; the external standard is added to the extract or to the sample before or after derivatization. In Fig. 1, the internal standard, 9-chlorophenanthrene, was added to the urine before extraction by the ammonium carbonate–ethyl acetate procedure; the C_{20} hydrocarbon was added as an external standard before derivatization.

In quantitative analysis by GC and HPLC, response factors (RF) should be determined for the metabolites with respect to the internal or external standard. When packed GC or HPLC columns are used, calculations are usually based on peak area rather than peak height. When capillary columns are employed in GC analyses, calculations of response factors are based on peak height:

$$\mathrm{RF} = \frac{\text{peak height of metabolite/mg metabolite}}{\text{peak height IS (or ES)/mg IS (or ES)}}$$

If the metabolites to be quantified are not available as reference compounds, a response factor of 1 with respect to the internal or external standard is assumed. In these circumstances valid ratio measurements can be made; that is, the percentage increase or decrease in the amount of a metabolite can be determined precisely, but the amount of metabolite expressed in mg (or μg) is a relative number (mg $\times$ RF). In reporting quantitative results, it should be clearly stated whether response factors were determined for metabolites or a response factor of 1 was assumed.

In Fig. 1B, a response factor of 1 was assumed because most of the metabolites were not available as pure reference compounds. In the study of biphenyl metabolism, however, most of the metabolites could be obtained from commercial sources, and response factors were determined for the metabolites with respect to the internal standard, bromobiphenyl (Fig. 4). Similarly, in the study with salicylic acid (Fig. 9) the response factors for salicylic, gentisic, citric, and glucuronic acids (ME-TMS derivatives) were determined with respect to the hydrocarbon docosane (C_{22}). In this example docosane was added as an external standard. Because of the diverse structures of the urinary acids, it is simpler to use a hydrocarbon as an external standard than to add suitable internal standards for each of the acids of interest.

In HPLC studies with radioactive drugs, quantitation of metabolites can also be based on the radioactivity present in the eluted metabolite peaks, if the specific activity of the administered drug is known, and if each of the HPLC peaks to be quantified contains only one radioactive metabolite.

The precision of quantitative profile analysis by either HPLC or GC is excellent if the peaks are symmetrical, well resolved, and homogeneous. For example when quadruplicate GC analyses were carried out with the same derivatized samples of biphenyl, bromobenzene, and phenanthrene metabolites (Figs. 1B, 4, 9, 12, 14 to 16) the standard error of the instrumental analyses was $<3\%$ for the major metabolites. Similar results were obtained when quadruplicate samples were analyzed by HPLC.

It should be emphasized that for quantitative analysis, peaks must be symmetrical in shape, well resolved, and homogeneous. In the GC analysis shown in Fig. 5A and 5B, the peaks labeled HIPP (hippuric acid) and PA (phenylaceturic acid) are not suitable for quantitation because of poor peak shape (trailing). In Fig. 5B, the mercapturic acids cannot be quantified because of inadequate resolution. In Figs. 1B, 4, 9, 12, and 14 to 16, however, the homogeneity of the symmetrical peaks was established by MS analysis and the labeled peaks were quantified. The HPLC analyses in Fig. 2A and 2B which were used for tentative identification of carbamazepine metabolites, were not considered useful for quantitation because of inadequate resolution of the peaks (for example, fractions 2, 9, 10, and 16 in Fig. 2A). The inhomogeneity of these peaks was confirmed by GC and MS analyses. The carbamazepine metabolites separated in the HPLC analyses shown in Fig. 3A and 3B were quantified by measuring the radioactivity in the individual peaks eluted from the HPLC column.

In order to quantify minor metabolites, it is necessary to inject larger samples or to increase the sensitivity of detection, so that the peak height or peak area can be measured with reasonable precision. In Fig. 4, the peak labeled 3-OH (3-hydroxybiphenyl) is too small to be measured reliably; in order to quantify this metabolite, a larger sample was injected on the GC.

The advantage of multicomponent analysis in quantitative studies is that a large number of metabolites of diverse structure can be quantified in a single GC or HPLC analysis that requires no more than 80 min and frequently only 20 to 30 min.

APPLICATIONS

Profiling procedures have been used primarily for the separation and identification of metabolites. Even a superficial inspection of the profiles, however, yields information about the number and relative quantities of metabolites. This is apparent from a comparison of the neutral metabolites in Figs. 2 and 11. Considerable additional information can be obtained about the metabolism and toxicity of drugs and environmental chemicals if the metabolic profiles are studied carefully after the metabolites have been identified and quantified. Metabolic profiles can be used (a) to detect new metabolites and metabolites present in trace quantities, (b) to study species differences in metabolism, (c) to study the effect of inducers and inhibitors on metabolism, (d) to define the differences between *in vivo* and *in vitro* metabolism, (e) to study the effect of drug administration on the metabolism of endogenous compounds, and (f) to define new pathways of metabolism. Examples of the applications are described below.

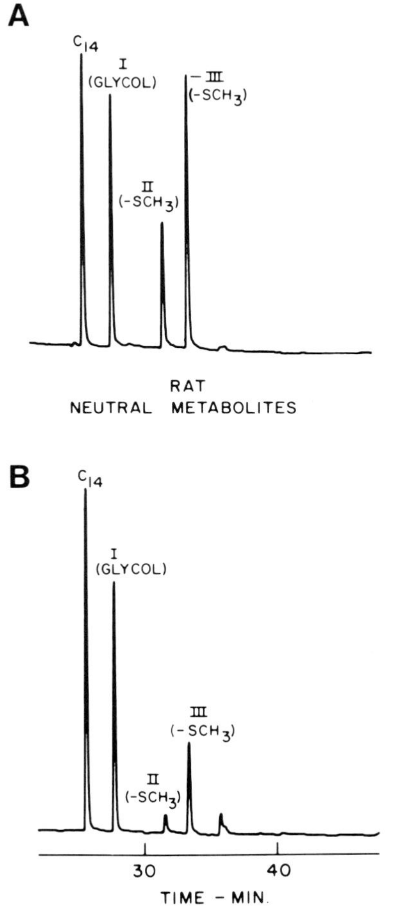

FIG. 11. Comparison of the GC separations of the TMS derivatives of the neutral styrene oxide metabolites isolated from hydrolyzed guinea pig (**A**) and rat (**B**) urine by the ammonium carbonate–ethyl acetate procedure. The separations were carried out on a 60 meter SE-30 glass capillary column by temperature programming at 2°/min from 110°C. The dose of styrene oxide was 100 mg/kg, i.p.

Separation and Identification of New Metabolites, Including Trace Metabolites

When the metabolites of drugs or environmental chemicals are profiled by HPLC or capillary GC, new metabolites are usually detected. This is due in part to the selectivity and sensitivity of detection by GC and HPLC and in part to the isolation procedures which were developed for profiling by GC and HPLC. The new metabolites are not necessarily trace metabolites. For example, in Fig. 11 two of the three major neutral metabolites of styrene oxide, 1-hydroxy-2-methylthio-1-phenylethane (II) and 2-hydroxy-1-methylthio-1-phenylethane (III), had not been identified previously (25). The HPLC profiles of carbamazepine metabolites provide another example; the 2,3-dihydrodiol and the methylsulfinylhydroxycarbamazepine metabolites present in urine in significant quantities (Fig. 2A) were only identified recently (20).

The identification of trace metabolites is illustrated in Figs. 12A and 13 which show profiles of neutral metabolites of bromobenzene isolated from hydrolyzed guinea pig urine. Two of the peaks labeled (OH, SCH_3) in Fig. 12A qualify as trace metabolites if trace is defined as <2% of the total metabolites in a profile. Figure 13 shows an analysis of the same sample on the same GC column when both the size of the injected sample and the sensitivity of detection were increased; under these conditions three methylthiohydroxydihydrobromobenzene and four aromatic methylthiohydroxybromobenzene metabolites were identified by GC and GC-MS. Bromobenzene is not an isolated example. Very small peaks in the GC and/or HPLC profiles have been identified as trace metabolites of phenanthrene (23), naphthalene (16), biphenyl (7), styrene oxide (25), carbamazepine (20), safrole (29), methaqualone (30), and the barbiturates (10). In all of these examples, the tentative identification of metabolites by MU values or retention times was confirmed by GC-MS.

Both the isolation and identification of new metabolites are important because they frequently demonstrate that (a) alternate pathways of metabolism are operative or (b) that reactive or potentially toxic intermediates have been formed. In the references cited above, dihydrodiols or diols were identified as urinary metabolites demonstrating that these environmental chemicals and drugs are metabolized via the epoxide-diol pathway.

Species Differences in Metabolism

Profiles of drug metabolites are ideally suited for studies of species differences in metabolism because both qualitative and quantitative differences in metabolism are recorded. In studies of the metabolism of styrene oxide, significant qualitative differences were observed when profiles of the bivalent sulfur acids excreted by the rat and guinea pig were compared. The two isomeric mercaptoacetic acid derivatives, *S*-(2-hydroxy-2-phenylethyl)mercaptoacetic acid and *S*-(2-hydroxy-1-phenylethyl)mercaptoacetic acid, are the major bivalent sulfur acids in guinea pig urine, whereas only the four isomeric mercapturic acids are present in rat urine (Fig. 5A and 5B). Quantitative rather than qualitative differences were observed in the profiles of neutral metabolites of styrene oxide (Fig. 11A and 11B). In hydrolyzed guinea pig urine the excretion of the isomeric methylthio ethers II and III exceeded the excretion of the glycol I. The ratio was reversed in hydrolyzed rat urine; the excretion of glycol was considerably larger than the excretion of methylthio ethers.

Both qualitative and quantitative differences were observed when the rat and guinea pig profiles of neutral metabolites of bromobenzene were compared (Figs. 12A, 12B, 13). The 3,4-dihydrodiol of bromobenzene, a major metabolite in hydrolyzed rat urine, was not detected in guinea pig urine. It is interesting that the 2,3-dihydrodiol was also missing from the guinea pig profile. Seven methylthio ethers (OH, SCH_3) excreted in the guinea pig urine, however, were not detected in rat urine. In addition to these qualitative differences, quantitative differences in the ratio of 3-hydroxy to 4-hydroxybromobenzene were observed in the profiles of the two species. These results suggest that different metabolic pathways are operative in the rat and guinea pig (22).

Quantitative differences in metabolite profiles can demonstrate that different pathways of metabolism are dominant in the various species. In comparing the profiles of neutral

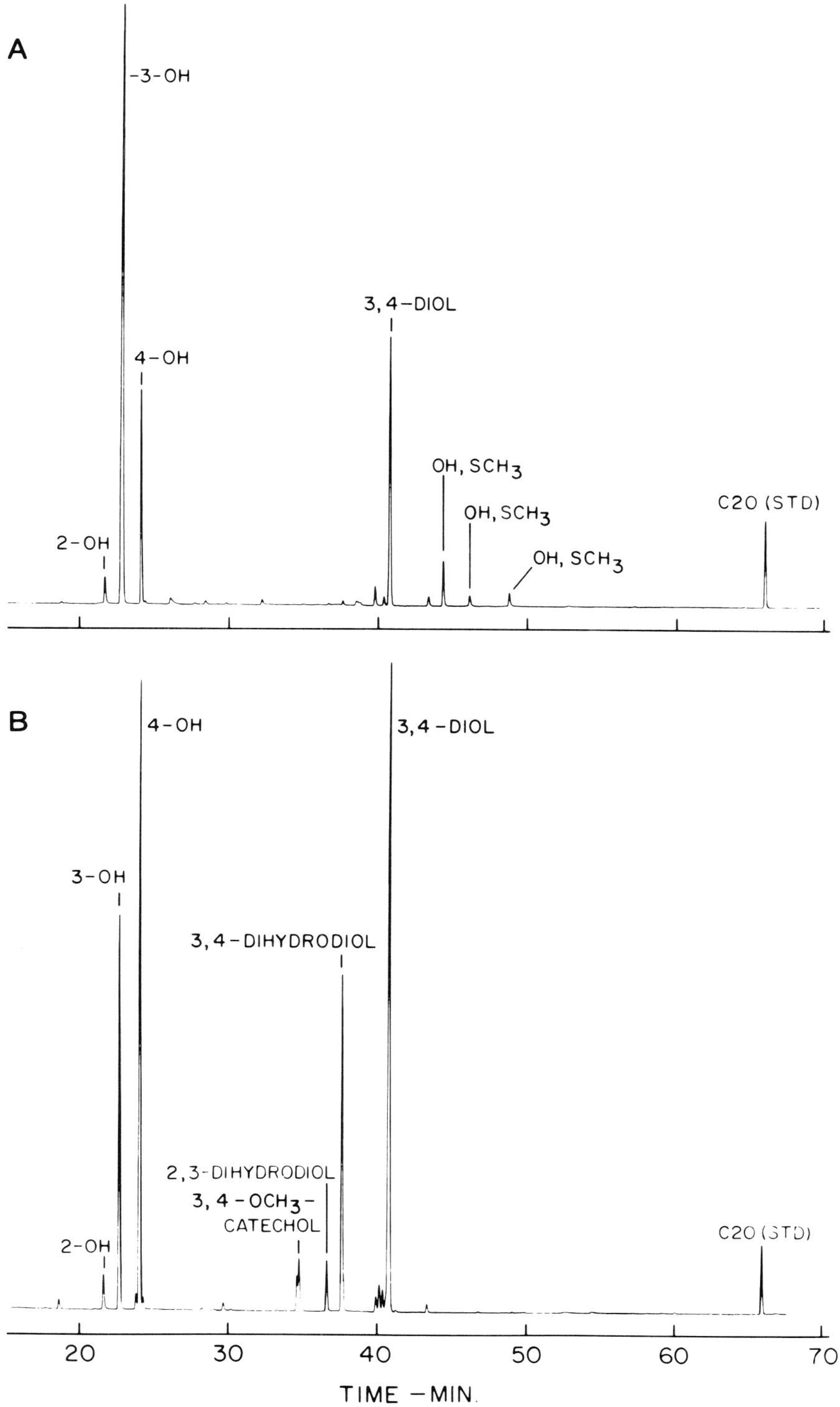

FIG. 12. Comparison of the GC separations of the TMS derivatives of the neutral bromobenzene metabolites isolated from hydrolyzed guinea pig (**A**) and rat (**B**) urine by the ammonium carbonate–ethyl acetate procedure. The separations were carried out on a 70 meter SE-30 glass capillary column by temperature programming at 2°/min from 100°C. The dose of bromobenzene was 0.8 ml/kg, i.p. The peaks identified included: 2-hydroxybromobenzene (2-OH); 3-hydroxybromobenzene (3-OH); 4-hydroxybromobenzene (4-OH); 2,3-dihydroxy-2,3-dihydrobromobenzene (2,3-dihydrodiol); 3,4-dihydroxy-3,4-dihydrobromobenzene (3,4-dihydrodiol); 3,4-dihydroxybromobenzene (3,4-diol); 3-methoxy-4-hydroxybromobenzene (3,4-OCH_3catechol) and three methylthio-hydroxybromobenzenes (OH, SCH_3). The hydrocarbon C_{20} was added as an external standard.

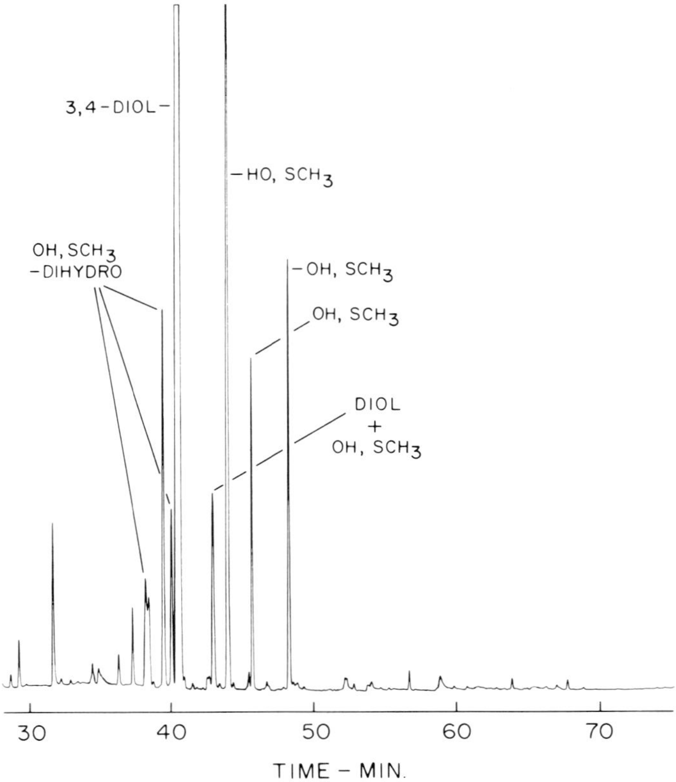

FIG. 13. GC analysis of the sample shown in Fig. 12**A**. The separation conditions were the same as those described in Fig. 12**A**; a larger aliquot, however, was injected on the column.

metabolites of biphenyl it was found that the major diol excreted by the rat was 4,4′-dihydroxybiphenyl, whereas the major diol excreted by the mouse was the catechol, 3,4-dihydroxybiphenyl (Fig. 14A and 14B). Both species metabolize biphenyl to the 4-hydroxybiphenyl, but in the mouse the second hydroxylation occurs predominantly on the ring already hydroxylated, and in the rat the second hydroxylation occurs preferentially on the unoxidized ring (8).

Qualitative differences in metabolic profiles can also indicate that different pathways are operative in two species. When profiles of carbamazepine metabolites were compared (Fig. 2A and 2B), it was found that 9-hydroxymethylacridan was present in significant amounts in human urine; this metabolite was present in trace quantities in rat urine. Thus, ring contraction of the 10,11-epoxide or the corresponding *trans*-10,11-dihydrodiol of carbamazepine to an acridan derivative occurs

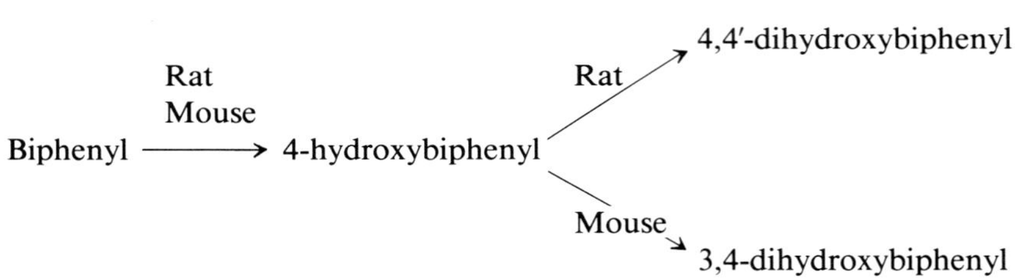

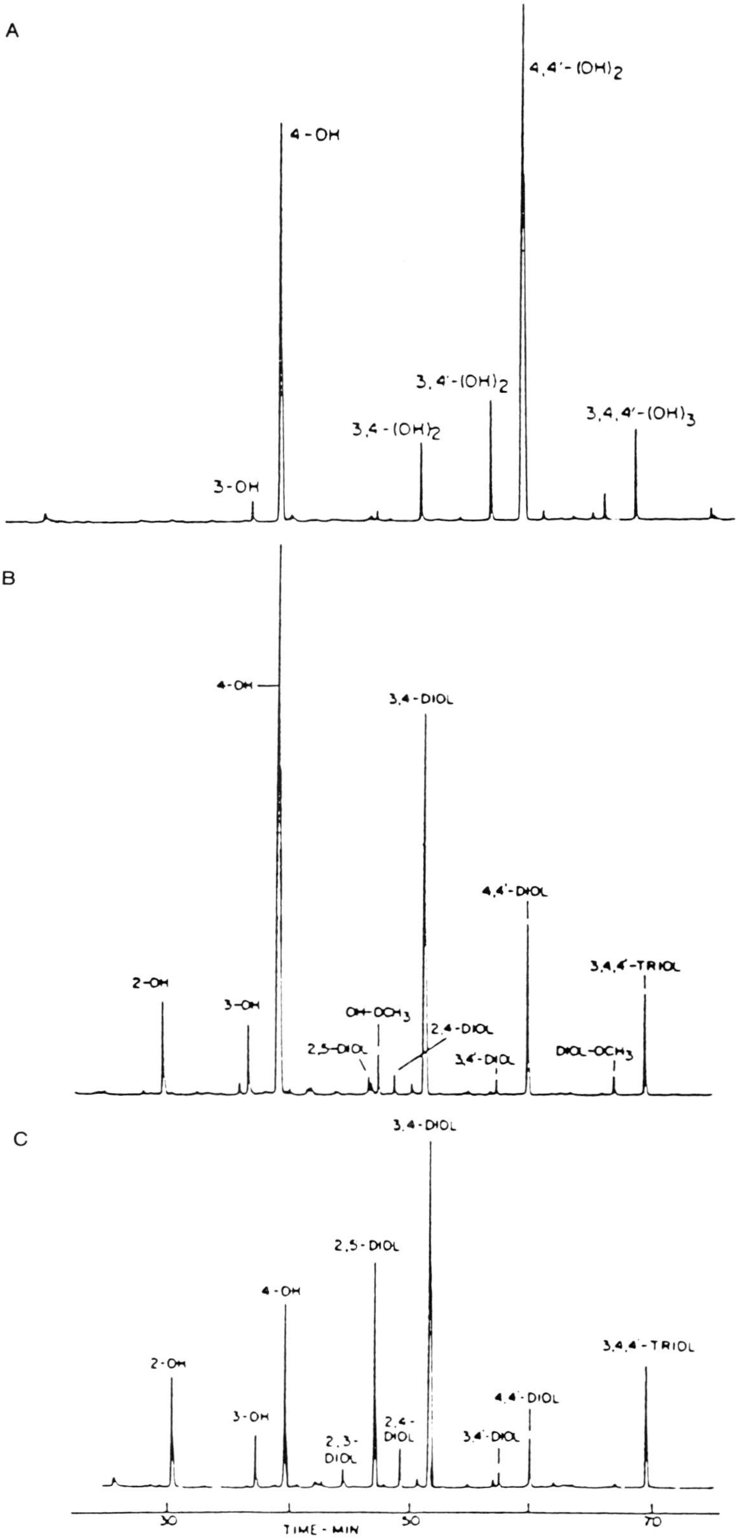

FIG. 14. Comparison of the GC separations of the TMS derivatives of the neutral biphenyl metabolites isolated from hydrolyzed control rat (**A**) control C57Bl/6Tex mouse (**B**) and β-naphthoflavone induced C57Bl/6Tex mouse (**C**) urine by the ammonium carbonate–ethyl acetate procedure. The separations were carried out on a 75 meter SE-30 glass capillary column by temperature programming at 2°/min from 140°C. Mice received 60 mg/kg, i.p. and rats 30 mg/kg, i.p. of biphenyl. In addition to the metabolites identified in Fig. 4, 2,3-dihydroxy-(2,3-diol), 2,4-dihydroxy-(2,4-diol), 3,4′-dihydroxy-(3,4′-diol), 4,4′-dihydroxy-(4,4′-diol), and 3,4,4′-trihydroxybiphenyl (3,4,4′-triol) were identified.

readily in man, but this ring contraction is a very minor pathway in the rat (20).

Effect of Inducing Agents

Inducing agents affect the activity of a number of enzymes involved in the metabolism of drugs and environmental chemicals, and these alterations in enzyme activity could lead to changes in profiles of metabolites. Studies carried out in the C57Bl/6Tex mouse provided an interesting example of the effects of the inducing agent β-naphthoflavone on the profile of biphenyl metabolites (Fig. 14B and 14C). Following induction, the excretion of 4-hydroxybiphenyl decreased markedly and the excretion of 2,5-dihydroxy biphenyl increased approximately fourfold. The 2,5-diol, present in trace quantities in the noninduced C57Bl/6Tex mouse, is formed by hydroxylation of either 2-hydroxy- or 3-hydroxybiphenyl. Thus, a pathway involving sequential oxidation that was barely operative in the noninduced mouse became a major pathway in the β-naphthoflavone induced mouse (8).

Comparison of *In Vivo* and *In Vitro* Metabolism

The profiles of metabolites formed *in vitro* by S_9 fractions or microsomes may be quite different from the profiles obtained when studies are carried out *in vivo*. In whole animal studies, extensive recycling (sequential oxidation) of metabolites frequently occurs, whereas very little sequential oxidation normally occurs with *in vitro* preparations. The metabolism of biphenyl illustrates this point. The profile of biphenyl metabolites formed by an S_9 fraction (Fig. 4) is very different from the profile of metabolites formed *in vivo* (Fig. 14A). The major metabolite excreted in rat urine is the diol, 4,4′-dihydroxybiphenyl, whereas the major metabolite formed *in vitro* is 4-hydroxybiphenyl; the 4,4′-diol was not detected *in vitro*. The profiles did not change significantly when the incubations were carried out with S_9 fractions prepared from rats induced with phenobarbital, 3-methylcholanthrene, or Arochlor 1254 (9). In this example, the *in vitro* system is not a good model for *in vivo* metabolism. If mutagenic or toxic metabolites are formed by sequential oxidation in the whole animal, *in vitro* systems will not

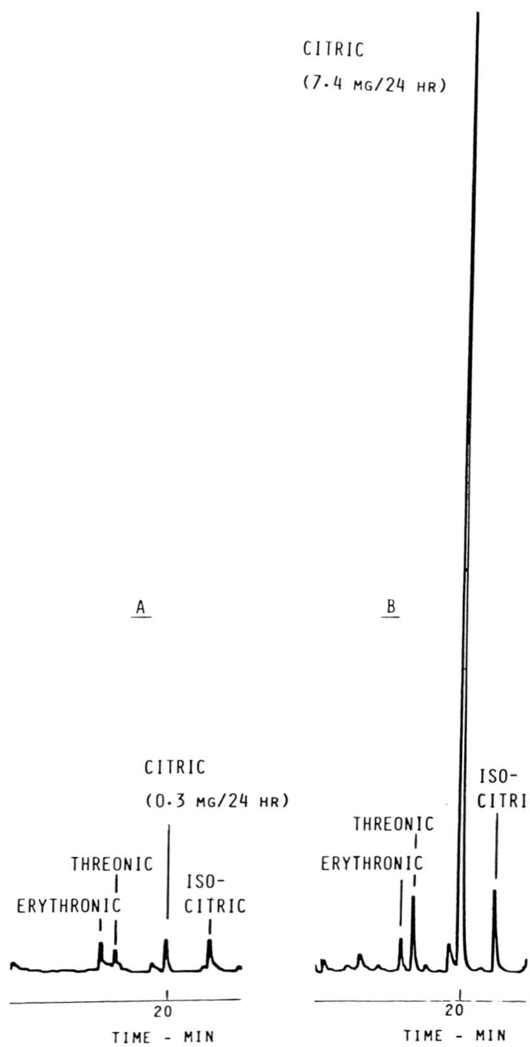

FIG. 15. Comparison of the GC separations of the ME-TMS derivatives of urinary acids isolated from control rat (**A**) and galactosamine-treated rat (**B**) urine by the DEAE-Sephadex procedure. The separations were carried out on a 60 meter SE-30 glass capillary column by temperature programming at 2°/min from 100°C. The dose of galactosamine was 375 mg/kg, i.p.

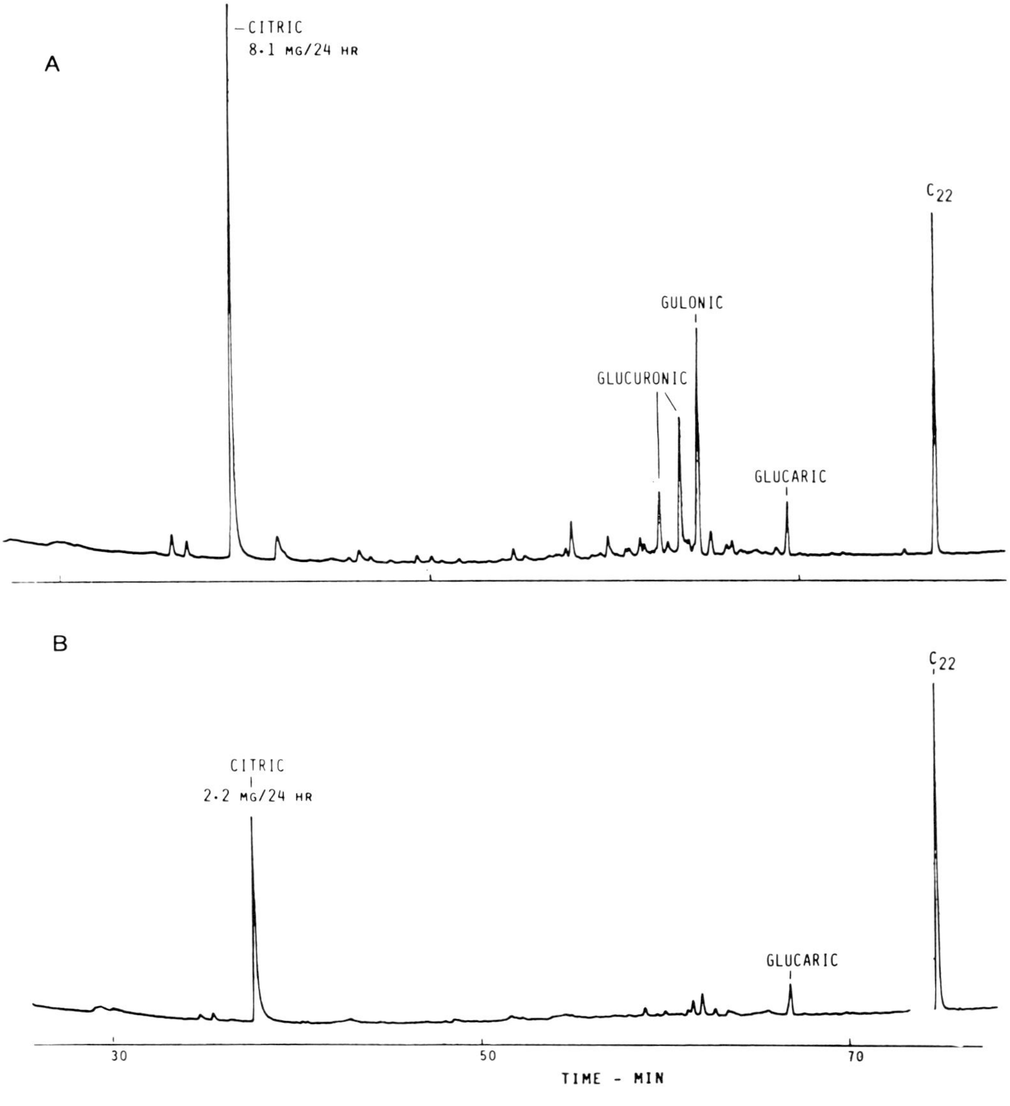

FIG. 16. Comparison of the GC separations of the ME-TMS derivatives of the acids isolated by the DEAE-Sephadex procedure from urine of rats treated with 1.5 ml/kg, i.p. (**A**) and 0.45 ml/kg, i.p. (**B**) of carbon tetrachloride in 0.5 ml of corn oil. The separations were carried out as described in Fig. 15.

accurately reflect the mutagenic or toxic potential of the parent compound.

Effect of Drugs on Endogenous Metabolism

If an administered drug or environmental chemical affects endogenous metabolism, changes may occur in the profiles of endogenous metabolites. Any variations in the excretion of neutral or acidic endogenous metabolites are readily observed when the DEAE-Sephadex procedure is used to isolate these fractions. For example, Fig. 15A and 15B show the effect of administration of an hepatotoxic dose of galactosamine on the profile of urinary acids. The only acid which changed significantly was citric acid. The normal excretion of citric acid by the rat is 0.2 to 1.0 mg/24

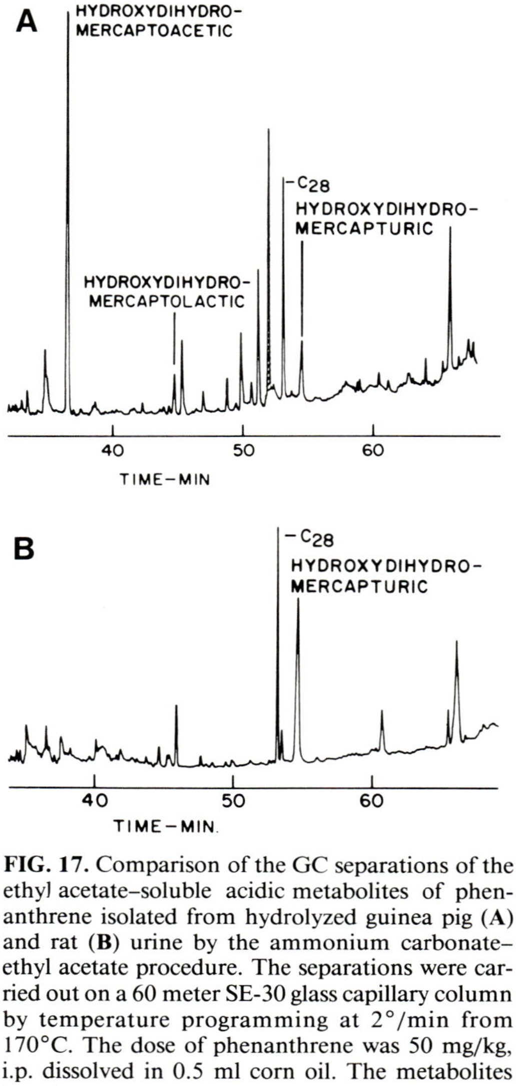

FIG. 17. Comparison of the GC separations of the ethyl acetate–soluble acidic metabolites of phenanthrene isolated from hydrolyzed guinea pig (**A**) and rat (**B**) urine by the ammonium carbonate–ethyl acetate procedure. The separations were carried out on a 60 meter SE-30 glass capillary column by temperature programming at 2°/min from 170°C. The dose of phenanthrene was 50 mg/kg, i.p. dissolved in 0.5 ml corn oil. The metabolites identified in guinea pig and rat urine were: *S*-(9-hydroxy-9,10-dihydro-10-phenanthryl) mercaptoacetic acid (hydroxydihydromercaptoacetic), 2-hydroxy-*S*-(9′-hydroxy-9′,10′-phenanthryl)-3-mercaptopropanoic acid (hydroxydihydromercaptolactic), and *N*-acetyl-*S*-(9-hydroxy-9,10-dihydro-10-phenanthryl)-L-cysteine (premercapturic).

hr. After administration of galactosamine, the excretion was 7.4 mg/24 hr, approximately a 10- to 20-fold increase. This increased excretion of citric acid was dose dependent.

Dose-dependent changes in several endogenous urinary acids were observed after administration of carbon tetrachloride, another hepatoxin (Fig. 16A and 16B). Following a dose of 0.45 ml/kg of carbon tetrachloride, the citric acid excretion increased from control levels to 2.2 mg/24 hr, and after a dose of 1.5 ml/kg the excretion rose to 8.1 mg/24 hr. The excretion of gulonic acid and glucuronic acid also increased significantly after administration of carbon tetrachloride. Changes in profiles of endogenous metabolites may help in defining the chemical basis of drug toxicity. It is possible that binding of a reactive metabolite of carbon tetrachloride to the "iron-sulfur center" of aconitase had occurred, and that inhibition of aconitase resulted in increased excretion of citric acid.

New Pathways of Metabolism

Metabolites present in trace quantities sometimes provide evidence for a new pathway of metabolism. In a recent study we identified *cis*-1,4-dihydroxy-1,4-dihydronaphthalene (1,4-dihydrodiol) as a minor urinary metabolite of naphthalene (16). Although Sims (28) had reported that 1,4-epoxy-1,4-dihydronaphthalene was metabolized by rats to the 1,4-dihydrodiol, he concluded that the 1,4-epoxide was not formed *in vivo* because the 1,4-dihydrodiol was not detected in urine following naphthalene administration. Inasmuch as the 1,4-dihydrodiol has now been isolated from rat urine, the *in vivo* formation of a 1,4-epoxide must be considered as a very likely possibility.

Another 1,4-dihydrodiol, a 1,4-dihydroxy-1,4-dihydro metabolite of carbamazepine (Fig. 2A, fraction 3) has been isolated from both human and rat urine (20). Presumably this metabolite is also formed from an intermediate 1,4-epoxide. These two examples suggest that aromatic compounds can be metabolized by a new pathway involving a 1,4-epoxide or possibly a 1,4-peroxide.

Sometimes major rather than minor metabolites prove that a new pathway is operative. When profile analysis was used to study the acidic bivalent sulfur metabolites of phenanthrene (23), styrene oxide (25), and bro-

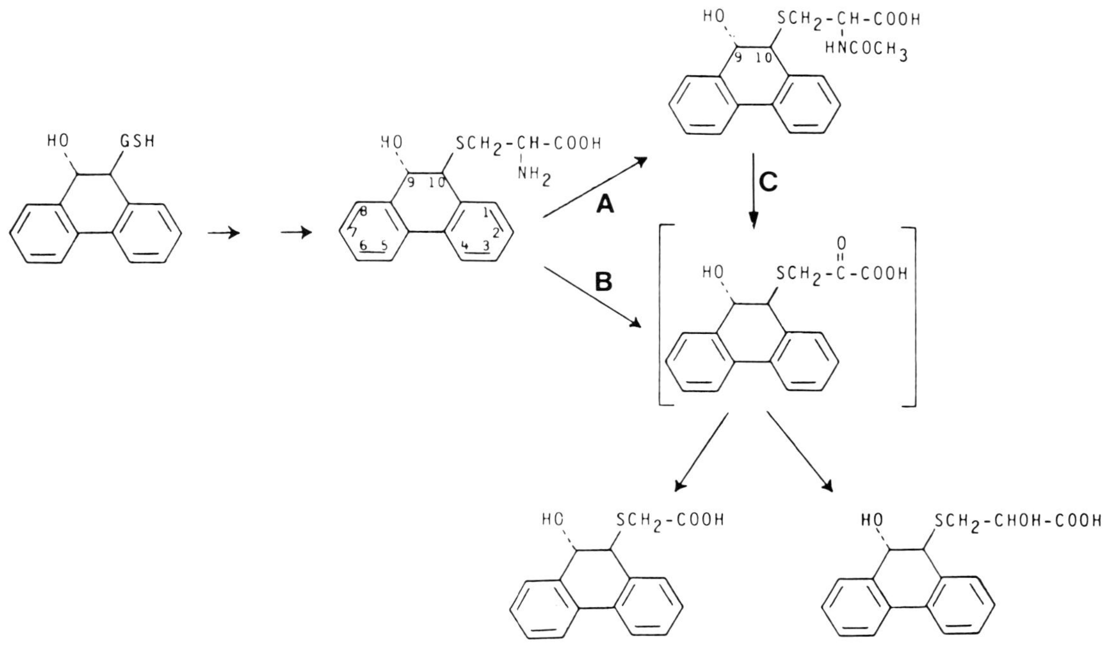

SCHEME 1. Proposed pathways for the formation of bivalent sulfur acids.

mobenzene (21), it was found that the guinea pig metabolized glutathione and/or cysteine adducts quite differently from the rat. The guinea pig excretes primarily mercaptoacetic acid derivatives instead of the mercapturic acids excreted by the rat (Figs. 5 and 17). The excretion of mercaptoacetic and mercaptolactic acids by the guinea pig may be due to a failure to acetylate the cysteine adducts or to deacylation of the mercapturic acids. The two possible pathways are shown for phenanthrene in Scheme 1. If acetylation does not occur, metabolism follows pathway B. If the excretion of mercaptoacetic and mercaptolactic acids is the result of deacylation, then metabolism follows pathway A → C. When synthetic mercapturic acids prepared from styrene oxide and phenanthrene were administered to guinea pigs, extensive deacylation of mercapturic acids occurred and mercaptoacetic and mercaptolactic acid as well as the mercapturic acids were excreted in urine. When the same mercapturic acids were administered to rats, the only bivalent sulfur acids recovered from urine were the unchanged mercapturic acids (17). Regardless of the sequence of reactions, the guinea pig metabolizes cysteine adducts by a new pathway. Although it has been established that humans excrete mercapturic acids, it is not known whether the human profile of bivalent sulfur acids is closer to that of the rat or the guinea pig because no one has looked for these new bivalent sulfur acids in human urine.

APPENDIX

Isolation of Drug and Metabolites from Urine or Bile by DEAE-Sephadex Chromatography (18)

The anion exchanger DEAE-Sephadex (A-25, Sigma) was cycled with 0.5 N hydrochloric acid, distilled water, 0.5 N sodium hydroxide solution and distilled water as recommended by the supplier. An aqueous suspension of the exchanger is poured into a chromatographic column (0.9 cm i.d.) to give a column 6 cm in height. After washing the exchanger with 10 ml of water and with 40 ml of 0.5 M aqueous pyridine-acetate solution (39.5 ml of pyridine and 30 ml of glacial acetic acid diluted with distilled water to 1 liter), 1 to 2 ml of urine (pH 4.5 to 5.0) is transferred to the column. Basic and neutral compounds are eluted by washing with

25 ml of glass distilled water. An acidic fraction is eluted with 35 ml of 1.5 M pyridine acetate solution (119 ml of pyridine and 90 ml of glacial acetic acid diluted with glass-distilled water to 1 liter). After lyophilization, the two fractions are transferred with methanol to calibrated screw-capped centrifuge tubes and stored at −20°C until analyzed. The separation including washing the exchanger on the column requires about 90 to 120 min; however, several columns can be run simultaneously. Lyophilization takes 2 to 3 hr. When larger urine samples are chromatographed, a larger column (1.3 cm i.d.) filled to a height of 9 cm is used and the solvent volumes are increased fourfold.

Isolation of Drug and Drug Metabolites by the Ammonium Carbonate-ethyl Acetate Procedure (14)

a. *Isolation of nonacidic metabolites from urine or bile.* One to 5 ml of urine or bile is transferred to a 12 ml calibrated centrifuge tube fitted with a Teflon-lined screw cap, and powdered anhydrous ammonium carbonate is added to saturation (approximately 1 g/ml of urine or bile). After adding 5 to 7 ml of ethyl acetate, the contents of the tube are mixed thoroughly by inversion and then agitated with a vortex-type mixer for 20 sec. The phases are separated by centrifugation (10 min) and the organic phase is transferred with a Pasteur pipet to a screw-capped centrifuge (12 ml) tube. The extraction is repeated with 2 × 5 ml of solvent. The combined solvent extracts are taken to dryness under a nitrogen stream. The residue containing drugs and their metabolites is dissolved in 0.5 ml of methanol either for storage (−20°C) or for conversion to derivatives and subsequent analysis by HPLC, GC, or GC-MS.

Emulsion formation has not been observed with urine or bile samples and only rarely with plasma or homogenate samples. If an emulsion is present after centrifugation, careful inversion of the tube and mixing followed by centrifugation is usually sufficient to break the emulsion.

Although other salt-solvent pairs have been employed (1,13), we prefer to use ammonium carbonate–ethyl acetate because recovery of metabolites has always been better with this salt-solvent pair.

b. *Isolation of nonacidic metabolites from plasma or tissue homogenates.* An aliquot of plasma (1 to 2 ml) or tissue homogenate (0.2 to 2.0 ml) is transferred to a 15 ml calibrated screw-capped centrifuge tube, diluted with three volumes of glass-distilled water and saturated with powdered anhydrous ammonium carbonate. Drugs and their metabolites are extracted with 3 × 5 ml of ethyl acetate. Although the mixture may appear unmanageable, the aqueous and organic phase separate cleanly after centrifugation. The combined ethyl acetate extracts are taken to dryness and the residue dissolved in 0.5 ml methanol for storage (−20°C) or conversion to derivatives.

c. *Isolation of ethyl acetate–soluble acidic metabolites from urine, bile, plasma or homogenate (23).* After extraction of the neutral metabolites, the chilled aqueous layer is carefully acidified (pH 2) with 6 N sulfuric acid, and the acids are extracted with 3 × 5 ml of ethyl acetate. The aqueous and organic phases are separated by centrifugation. The solvent is removed (nitrogen stream) from the pooled extracts and the residue of acidic drug metabolites and ethylacetate–soluble endogenous acids are redissolved in methanol and stored at −20°C for subsequent analysis by HPLC or GC. If acidification is not carried out carefully, the carbon dioxide liberated by acidification of the ammonium-carbonate–saturated aqueous phase may cause the solution to foam out of the tube.

d. *Isolation of acidic metabolites insoluble in ethyl acetate.* If the recovery of radioactive metabolites indicates that a significant percentage of metabolites remains in the aqueous phase, the following modified procedure is used to isolate these polar metabolites. One to 5 ml of hydrolyzed urine or bile is transferred to a 12 ml calibrated centrifuge tube fitted with a Teflon-lined screw cap and acidified with 3 N sulfuric acid to pH 2.0. Saturation with salts is omitted because a high salt content may interfere with subsequent analyses. The neutral and ethyl acetate–soluble acidic metabolites are extracted with 4 × 5 ml of ethyl acetate; the aqueous and organic phases are separated by centrifugation. After removal of the small amount of solvent remaining with the aqueous phase (nitrogen stream), the aqueous phase containing the ethyl acetate–insoluble metabolites is lyophilized. The residue is suspended in methanol and centrifuged to remove any insoluble material. The methanolic solution can be used for HPLC analysis of metabolites exhibiting UV absorption (Fig. 8).

Reisolation Procedure for Evaluating Recovery of Metabolites

If radioactive drugs are not available as tracers in recovery experiments, it is possible to use a reisolation procedure to quantitate recovery of metabolites. In this procedure an aliquot (1/3) of the neutral metabolites (ethyl acetate extract) or ethyl acetate–soluble acids isolated from urine is analyzed by either GC or HPLC. A second aliquot (1/3) is dissolved in a reasonable volume of control urine, and the isolation of the same fraction (neutral or acidic) is repeated. The analysis of the reisolated metabolites by GC or HPLC is compared with the analysis of the first isolate. From the number and height of the peaks in the GC or HPLC charts it is possible to evaluate the recovery of the metabolites. When a suitable internal or external standard is added to both aliquots, quantitative comparisons can be made. The same reisolation procedure can be applied to bile, plasma, or tissue fractions.

Derivatization

Silylation

Trimethylsilyl (TMS) derivatives are prepared by evaporating the solvent (used for extraction or storage of the sample) and redissolving the residue of drug and metabolites in a small volume of pyridine. For the urinary aliquots described in the isolation procedures, usually 20 to 50 μl of pyridine is sufficient. The pyridine solution of metabolites is silylated with 30 to 60 μl of BSA and then heated at 60°C for 30 to 60 min. If the metabolites have hindered (tertiary) hydroxyl groups, TSIM (trimethylsilylimidazole) or BSA plus TMCS (trimethylchlorosilane) is used instead of BSA, and the silylation is carried out at 90°C for 1 hr. TSIM does not form *N*-silyl derivatives readily and can be used when the formation of *N*-silyl derivatives is undesirable. This procedure converts hydroxyl groups into trimethylsilyl ethers and carboxyl groups into trimethylsilyl esters. Trimethylsilyl esters are less stable than methyl esters, and for this reason the use of methyl esters is preferred.

Deuterated trimethylsilyl derivatives are prepared by substituting d_{18}-BSA or d_9-TSIM for the protonated analogs. Deuterated derivatives may have different retention times (HPLC) and MU values (GC) from the protonated analogs if the number of deuterium atoms introduced is large compared with the number of hydrogen atoms in the molecule (15,24,26).

Methylation

After evaporation of the solvent used for extraction, a suitable aliquot (1/3) of drug and metabolites is dissolved in 0.5 ml of methanol and an excess of ethereal diazomethane (prepared from Diazald) is added. After standing at room temperature for 2 to 15 min, the excess ether, diazomethane, and methanol are removed with a nitrogen stream. The residue is dissolved in a suitable solvent for subsequent analysis by HPLC or in pyridine (20 to 50 μl) for silylation by BSA (20 to 50 μl) and subsequent analyses by GC.

Methylation converts aromatic hydroxyl groups into methyl ethers, and carboxyl groups into methyl esters (ME). In addition acidic -NH groups (barbiturates, hydantoins) are converted into *N*-methyl derivatives. If a short methylation of 1 to 2 min is employed, usually only the carboxyl groups are methylated.

A short methylation followed by silylation converts methyl esters into methyl ester–trimethylsilyl ethers (ME-TMS). Both aromatic and nonaromatic hydroxyl groups are converted into trimethylsilyl ethers.

Ethylation

Ethylated derivatives are prepared by treating an ethanolic solution (0.5 ml) of drugs and drug metabolites with an excess of ethereal solution of diazoethane for 15 min. The diazoethane is prepared from *N*-ethyl-*N*′-nitro-*N*-nitrosoguanidine according to the directions supplied by Aldrich Chemical Co. After removal of the excess reagents (N_2 stream), the residue is dissolved in a suitable solvent for analysis or in pyridine for silylation. When ethylation is used, it is possible to distinguish catechols (as diethoxy derivatives) from *O*-methylcatechols (ethoxy, methoxy derivatives) by GC and GC-MS.

The preparation, use and storage of diazoalkanes is hazardous, and for this reason other alkylating procedures are frequently employed. For example, barbiturates can be alkylated with methyl or ethyl iodide in acetone-solid potassium carbonate (3,4). 5,5-Disubstituted hydantoins can be quantitatively alkylated with methyl or ethyl iodide in the presence of potassium hydroxide (27). Diazomethane is, however, the most convenient reagent for esterifying acidic fractions isolated from biological samples. Apparatus for the preparation of small quantities (<1 mmol) of diazomethane is available from Aldrich Chemical Co.

Oximation

Neutral metabolites (2,25). The solvent is removed from a suitable aliquot of the extract containing drug and metabolites and the residue dissolved in 50 μl of a pyridine solution of *O*-benzylhydroxylamine (or a suitable alkyl hydroxylamine) hydrochloride (50 mg/ml pyridine). After heating the solution for 1 hr at 80°C, the pyridine is evaporated (nitrogen stream) to approximately 20 μl, and 30 μl of BSA is added and the solution heated at 60°C for 1 hr.

The neutral metabolites containing a ketone group are converted into benzyloxime (BO) derivatives or into benzyloxime-trimethylsilyl ether (BO-TMS) derivatives if hydroxyl groups are present in the molecule.

Acidic metabolites (12,31). The methyl esters, prepared as described, are dissolved in a pyridine solution of *O*-benzylhydroxylamine hydrochloride or another suitable alkyl hydroxylamine hydrochloride. After heating for 1 hr at 80°C, the pyridine is evaporated and the sample is silylated as described above.

The acidic metabolites containing a ketone group are converted into benzyloxime-methyl ester (BO-ME) derivatives or into benzyloxime-methyl ester-trimethylsilyl ether (BO-ME-TMS) derivatives if hydroxyl groups are also present in the molecule.

The use of benzyloxime derivatives is preferred because the retention time is increased by approximately 7 methylene units, which facilitates identification by GC.

Enzymatic Hydrolysis of Conjugates (Glucuronides and Sulfates)

Usually 1 to 5 ml of urine or 1 ml of bile is hydrolyzed with an appropriate quantity of Glusulase. After the addition of 0.5 g of sodium acetate, the pH of the sample is adjusted to 4.5 to 4.8 with glacial acetic acid and 0.4 ml of Glusulase is added. After incubation for 15 hr (overnight) at 37°C, the metabolites are isolated by either the DEAE-Sephadex procedure or the ammonium carbonate–ethyl acetate procedure.

Although acid hydrolysis can be used, enzymatic hydrolysis is preferred because acid hydrolysis may decompose or destroy reactive intermediates.

Gas Chromatography

Glass open tubular capillary columns 40 to 75 meters in length prepared by the method of German et al. (6) are used. The best procedure for preparing SE-30 columns is to use a two-step coating process of a silanized glass capillary 0.3 mm I.D. and 1.0 mm O.D. The initial coating containing Silanox, (Grade 101; Cabot, Boston, MA, USA) is applied by using a dynamic coating process in which a suspension of Silanox (2 g/100 ml) in carbon tetrachloride containing SE-30 (0.5 g/100 ml) is propelled through the column. After drying, a second coat of SE-30 is applied by forcing a 2% solution of SE-30 in isooctane through the column. Columns prepared in this way show approximately 100,000 theoretical plates for tetracosane at 250°C (HETP 0.60 mm); the highest value observed for a 60 meter column was 150,000 theoretical plates (HETP 0.40 mm).

The injection system includes a precolumn packed with about 1 cm of 10% SE-30 on Gas Chrom Q and a gas phase splitter (5). The precolumn provides complete sample evaporation before the splitter zone, traps contaminating nonvolatiles, and prevents decomposition of components. Frequent changes of the precolumn, especially after injection of acid samples, prolong the life of capillary columns considerably. Capillaries prepared by this procedure are stable up to 325°C and will last 12 to 18 months.

The separations are usually carried out by temperature programming at 2°/min from 100 to 300°C. However, an appropriate temperature range and rate of programming can be selected after the methylene unit values have been determined for the metabolites.

Calculation of Methylene Unit Values

In temperature-programmed GC analyses, methylene unit (MU) values are determined with a series of even-numbered *n*-alkanes as reference compounds. The *n*-alkane tetradecane (C_{14}) has an MU value of 14 and hexadecane (C_{16}) has an MU value of 16, etc. (Fig. 9). The retention values for the metabolites are obtained by interpolating between values for the nearest neighboring hydrocarbons. For example, in Fig. 9, the ME-TMS derivative of citric acid is eluted between C_{14} and C_{16}. The MU value for this derivative is 15.28, indicating that the derivative is eluted 0.64× the interval (2 MU) between C_{14} and C_{16}. If x is the distance between C_{14} and the citric acid peak and y is the distance between C_{14} and C_{16}, the methylene unit is described by the equation:

$$MU_{\text{citric acid}} = MU_{C_{14}} + (x/y \times 2)$$

$$= 14 + (0.64 \times 2) = 15.28$$

REFERENCES

1. Bastos, M. L., Kananen, G. E., Young, R. M., Montforte, J. R., and Sunshine, I. (1970): Detection of basic organic drugs and their metabolites in urine. *Clin. Chem.*, 16:931–940.
2. Devaux, P. G., Horning, M. G., Hill, R. M., and Horning, E. C. (1971): O-Benzyloximes: Derivatives for the study of ketosteroids by gas chromatography. Applications to urinary steroids of the newborn human. *Anal. Biochem.*, 41:70–82.
3. Dünges, W. (1973): Alkylation of acidic organic compounds for gas chromatographic analysis. *Chromatographia*, 6:196–197.
4. Dünges, W., and Bergheim-Irps, E. (1973): A new methylation method for the gas chromatography of barbituric acids. *Anal. Letters*, 6:185–195.
5. German, A. L., and Horning, E. C. (1972): Capillary column inlet system for the gas chromatography of biological samples. *Anal. Letters*, 5:619–628.
6. German, A. L., Pfaffenberger, C. D., Thenot, J.-P., Horning, M. G., and Horning, E. C. (1973): High resolution gas chromatography with thermostable glass capillary columns. *Anal. Chem.*, 45:930–935.
7. Halpaap, K., Horning, M. G., and Horning, E. C.

(1978): Metabolism of biphenyl in the rat. *J. Chromatogr.,* 166:479–490.
8. Halpaap-Wood, K., Horning, E. C., and Horning, M. G. (1981): The effect of phenobarbital and β-naphtho-flavone induction in the metabolism of biphenyl in the rat and mouse. *Drug Metab. Dispos.,* 9:97–102.
9. Halpaap-Wood, K., Horning, E. C., and Horning, M. G. (1981): The effect of 3-methylcholanthrene, Aroclor 1254 and phenobarbital induction on the metabolism of biphenyl by rat and mouse 9000 g supernatant liver fractions. *Drug Metab. Dispos.,* 9:103–107.
10. Harvey, D. J., Glazener, L., Johnson, D. B., Butler, C. M., and Horning, M. G. (1977): Comparative metabolism of four allylic barbiturates and hexobarbital by the rat and guinea pig. *Drug Metab. Dispos.,* 5:527–546.
11. Horning, E. C., and Horning, M. G. (1971): In: *Methods in Medical Research, Vol. 12,* edited by R. E. Olson, pp. 369–411. Yearbook Med. Pub., Chicago.
12. Horning, M. G., Boucher, E. A., Moss, A. M., and Horning, E. C. (1968): Gas chromatographic study of derivatives of acids of the Krebs cycle and related compounds. *Anal. Letters,* 1:713–723.
13. Horning, M. G., Boucher, E. A., Stafford, M., and Horning, E. C. (1972): A rapid procedure for the isolation of drugs and drug metabolites from plasma. *Clin. Chem. Acta,* 37:381–386.
14. Horning, M. G., Gregory, P., Nowlin, J., Stafford, M., Letratanangkoon, K., Butler, C., Stillwell, W. G., and Hill, R. M. (1974): Isolation of drugs and drug metabolites from biological fluids by use of salt-solvent pairs. *Clin. Chem.,* 20:282–287.
15. Horning, M. G., Thenot, J.-P., Bouwsma, O., Nowlin, J. G., and Lertratanangkoon, K. (1978): In: *Advances in Pharmacology and Therapeutics,* edited by J. P. Tillement, pp. 245–256. Pergamon Press, Oxford.
16. Horning, M. G., Stillwell, W. G., Griffin, G. W., and Tsang, W.-S. (1980): Epoxide intermediates in the metabolism of naphthalene by the rat. *Drug Metab. Dispos.,* 8:404–414.
17. Horning, M. G., Lertratanangkoon, K., Hugenroth, S., Middleditch, B. S., Tsang, W.-S., and Griffin, G. W. (1982): Metabolism of exogenous mercapturic acids by rat and guinea pig. *The Pharmacologist,* 24:128.
18. Jaakonmaki, P. I., Knox, K. L., Horning, E. C., and Horning, M. G. (1967): The characterization by gas-liquid chromatography of ethyl β-D-glucosiduronic acid as a metabolite of ethanol in rat and man. *Eur. J. Pharmacol.,* 1:63–70.
19. LaDu, B. N., Mandel, H. G., and Way, E. L. (1971): *Fundamentals of Drug Metabolism and Drug Disposition.* Williams and Wilkins, Baltimore.
20. Lertratanangkoon, K., and Horning, M. G. (1981): Metabolism of carbamazepine. *Drug Metab. Dispos.,* 10:1–10.
21. Lertratanangkoon, K., and Horning, M. G. (1982): Bivalent sulfur metabolites of bromobenzene. *Fed. Proc.,* 41:1572.
22. Lertratanangkoon, K., Horning, M. G., and Middleditch, B. S. (1982): Comparison of the hydroxylated metabolites of bromobenzene excreted by the rat and guinea pig. *The Pharmacologist,* 24:94.
23. Lertratanangkoon, K., Horning, M. G., Middleditch, B. S., Tsang, W.-S., and Griffin, G. W. (1982): Urinary bivalent sulfur metabolites of phenanthrene excreted by the rat and guinea pig. *Drug Metab. Dispos.,* 10:614–623.
24. McCloskey, J. A., Lawson, A. M., and Leemans, F. A. J. M. (1967): Gas chromatographic and mass spectrometric properties of perdeuterated fatty acid methyl esters. *Chem. Comm.,* 1967:285–287.
25. Nakatsu, K., Hugenroth, S., Sheng, L.-S., Horning, E. C., and Horning, M. G. (1983): Metabolism of styrene oxide in the rat and guinea pig. *Drug Metab. Dispos.,* 11:463–470.
26. Oates, J. A., Seyberth, H. W., Frolich, J. C., Sweetman, B. J., and Watson, J. T. (1978): In: *Stable Isotopes: Applications in Pharmacology, Toxicology and Clinical Research,* edited by T. A. Baillie, pp. 281–287. The Macmillan Press Ltd., London.
27. deSagher, R., Pocius, J., and Thenot, J.-P. (1978): Alkylation studies of 5,5-disubstituted hydantoins. *J. Chromatogr.,* 156:43–53.
28. Sims, P. (1965): Metabolism of polycyclic compounds. *Biochem. J.,* 95:608–611.
29. Stillwell, W. G., Carman, M. J., Bell, L., and Horning, M. G. (1974): Metabolism of safrole and 2′,3′-epoxysafrole in the rat and guinea pig. *Drug Metab. Dispos.,* 2:489–498.
30. Stillwell, W. G., Gregory, P. A., and Horning, M. G. (1975): Metabolism of methaqualone by the epoxide-diol pathway in man and the rat. *Drug Metab. Dispos.,* 3:287–296.
31. Vane, F., and Horning, M. G. (1969): Separation and characterization of the prostaglandins by gas chromatography and mass spectrometry. *Anal. Lett.,* 2:357–371.
32. Yu, V. C., de Lamirande, E., Horning, M. G., and Pang, K. S. (1982): Dose-dependent kinetics of quinidine in the perfused rat liver preparation. *Drug Metab. Dispos.,* 10:568–572.

Drug Metabolism and Drug Toxicity,
edited by J. R. Mitchell and M. G. Horning.
Raven Press, New York © 1984.

Bioanalytical Systems Based on Mass Spectrometry

E. C. Horning, D. I. Carroll, R. N. Stillwell, M. G. Horning, J. G. Nowlin, H. Hughes, and J. R. Mitchell

Institute for Lipid Research, Baylor College of Medicine, Houston, Texas 77030

Many years ago Claude Bernard wrote (16) in *An Introduction to the Study of Experimental Medicine* that ". . . In the experimental sciences all progress is measured by improvement in the means of investigation. . . . Every time that a new and reliable means of experimental analysis makes its appearance, we invariably see science make progress in the questions to which this means of analysis can be applied. . . ." The use in pharmacological and toxicological sciences of bioanalytical systems based on mass spectrometry illustrates the validity of these statements.

Mass spectrometry (MS) is a relatively old field of science. Its development has been marked by intermittent surges of high activity in the design of new types of instruments, and these periods of activity have led in turn to new uses of MS and to much new knowledge in each area of application. The development of the combined gas chromatograph–mass spectrometer (GC-MS), which started about 25 years ago, is summarized very briefly in this chapter. The current period is again one of high activity in the design of new types of instruments, and in the development of new analytical uses of mass spectrometry.

Two highly important changes in instrument design and use occurred a few years ago. For many years it was believed that the conversion of a nonvolatile organic compound to gas phase ions was very difficult to accomplish. This was because of the absence of both a theoretical background and easily repeatable experimental methods. It is, in fact, very easy to obtain gas phase ions from nonvolatile organic compounds under a variety of circumstances, and several new types of sources and instruments are now used for this purpose. At the same time, new methods for the study of ion structures, based on what is usually called MS/MS, or tandem MS, were developed. Triple quadrupole mass spectrometers (a form of tandem MS) are likely to be widely used in the future in many applications. Much new knowledge is certain to result from the use of these new instruments and new methods. It is also likely that the development of new instruments will continue at an accelerated rate.

DEVELOPMENT OF GC-MS INSTRUMENTS

Until very recently, the most powerful methods of analysis of complex mixtures of biologic origin, for compounds other than macromolecules, were based upon the use of GC-MS–computer bioanalytical systems of early design. The MS in these systems is usually a quadrupole or magnetic sector instrument with a single mass analyzer. In some instances, a double-focusing MS, with an electrical sector and a magnetic sector (usually of Nier–Johnston geometry for quantitative analysis or Mattauch–Herzog geometry for structural studies), is employed. The GC may use a packed column or an open tubular capillary column; fused silica open tubular capillary columns with suitable injection devices are available for use in most instruments. The computer and peripherals are used for operating these systems and for acquiring, processing, analyzing, and recording data that were previously recorded as intensity measurements on light-sensitive paper or on photographic plates. These systems for chemical analysis are in wide use in structural studies of organic compounds, in identification work and in many kinds of multicomponent quantitative analytical applications including trace organic analysis.

The first commercially available combined GC-MS instrument was the LKB 9000. This was the result of work started before 1960 by several Swedish scientists, with the leadership of Sune Bergström, at the Karolinska Institute in Stockholm. The major problem in design and operation was that of concentrating volatile organic compounds in a flowing gas stream, so that the pressure in the MS source could be kept sufficiently low to permit electron impact mass spectra to be taken. This problem was solved by the development of the jet-orifice separator by Ragnar Ryhage (119). A prototype GC-MS instrument was constructed in the laboratories of the Karolinska Institute. An additional prototype instrument was based on a MAT CH4 MS which was modified to include a GC, a "molecule separator," and faster scan capabilities; this instrument was assembled in Stockholm for use at Baylor College of Medicine in Houston through support from the Robert A. Welch Foundation and an NIH grant.

GC was in a primitive state when this work was started, but rapid progress was made in biologic applications after it was demonstrated in 1959–1960 that steroids and other compounds of interest in biology and medicine could be separated through use of GC column packings prepared with thin films of highly thermostable polysiloxanes on deactivated supports (68,130,140–143,145,146). Techniques for the derivatization of steroids (95,96,139,144) and many other polyfunctional compounds, primarily through the formation of trimethylsilyl (TMS) ethers, were found and applied rapidly. These methods came into universal use. Many variations in methods of derivative formation, and in the preparation of column packings, were published over the next 10 to 15 years. The chief advance in GC methodology in recent years was the introduction of improved techniques for open tubular capillary chromatography. Quantitative analyses by GC for components of biologic interest should always be carried out by open tubular capillary methods, with satisfactory sample injection devices, because of the greater efficiency of capillary columns with respect to packed columns (64,65).

The original purpose of developing a combined GC-MS instrument was to identify compounds present in highly complex mixtures of biologic origin. It was assumed that quantitative analyses would be carried out by GC methods, but in 1967–1968 Bo Holmstedt (also at the Karolinska Institute) showed that GC-MS instruments could be used in quantitative analysis with high sensitivity and selectivity in detection (71). The method was based on an earlier study by Sweeley et al. (129) of selective detection of a stable isotope labeled compound. The technique was called "mass fragmentography" at that time, but it is now usually called "selected ion detection." It is in universal use.

For many years, the only type of mass spectrum of interest in bioanalytical studies was that obtained by electron impact ionization (EI). Organic compounds lose an electron (called a Rydberg electron in inorganic chemistry) rather easily when internal energy is supplied, and in all GC-MS instruments of early design the ion source was an EI source. Parent positive radical ions are formed under these conditions with a range of internal energies, and many (sometimes all) parent ions are converted in a very short time (these are often picosecond reactions) into fragment ions. If the process is relatively slow, metastable ions are observed. The fragmentation process involves bond-breaking, and may also involve extensive rearrangement. Most of the mass spectra of organic compounds that have been published in journal articles, or that are available in compendia or computer-readable files, are EI mass spectra. Mass spectra of individual compounds may be obtained with a GC-MS instrument by manual operation of the MS whenever a peak of interest is observed in the total ion current chart. With computer-based instrumental systems, a continuous record of MS scans may be obtained for an entire run. "Reconstructed" GC separation charts are obtained in this way; single MS scans can also be recalled for study.

At the start of this period, GC-MS instrument combinations were almost always based on magnetic sector mass spectrometers. Electrical field instruments of the multipole type (and monopole instruments) were believed to be unsuitable in GC-MS combinations because of their limited mass range. When it was realized that derivative formation greatly extended the scope of GC, and that many polyfunctional compounds of biologic interest could be separated by GC methods after conversion to derivatives (often with a considerable increase in molecular mass), this point of view was widely accepted. Improvements in design soon occurred, however, and electrical field instruments are now in wide use. The early Finnigan MS, used in GC-MS combination as Model 1015, was the first commercially available quadrupole MS designed with a range to m/z 750. These instruments are highly compatible with computer systems, and the development of GC-MS–computer bioanalytical systems based on quadrupole and related designs is continuing.

The chief limitation of these combined instruments is that samples must be volatilized for the GC separation. During the past few years, numerous methods have been developed for obtaining mass spectra of nonvolatile compounds, and much work will be done in the future with nonvolatile samples of biologic origin. Mass spectra obtained by these new methods are not EI mass spectra; they resemble chemical ionization (CI) mass spectra. Typical CI spectra involve protonation to form MH^+ ions, followed by a limited degree of fragmentation with loss of neutral molecules. Many strong gas phase bases show only MH^+ ions; weaker gas phase bases with hydroxyl groups may show only fragment ions corresponding to $(MH\text{-}18)^+$, $(MH\text{-}36)^+$ and so forth. The terminology implies that ionization occurs by ion molecule reactions, rather than by electron molecule reactions. Gas phase reagents that have been used in CI studies include CH_5^+, $C_4H_7^+$, NH_4^+, H_3O^+, $(CH_3)_3Si^+$, and $NO^{+\bullet}$. The first four reagents act primarily by proton transfer. Reaction with the TMS ion leads to TMS adduct ions, and reaction with $NO^{+\bullet}$ leads primarily to electron transfer and to the formation of radical ions. If helium or nitrogen is employed as a reagent gas at an appropriate pressure, the sample is ionized by electron transfer, and the resulting mass spectra are indistinguishable from EI mass spectra. Bioanalytical systems of current design have capabilities for obtaining both EI and CI mass spectra.

Most organic compounds give uncomplicated CI mass spectra containing relatively few ions, and the interpretation of CI mass spectra is often not difficult. Fragment ions are almost always formed by loss of neutral molecules, and it is widely believed that CI mass spectra contain relatively little structural information. With increasing use of collision-induced fragmentation methods, however, CI procedures will be much more widely used in structural studies of both volatile and nonvolatile compounds. Examples of CI mass spectra of nonvolatile compounds are in the next section.

Bioanalytical systems with a single mass analyzer are widely used in quantitative analytical applications because the limit of detection and the selectivity in detection is much beyond that available with less specific detection methods. They often show, however, relatively high chemical noise and less than adequate specificity in detection for organic trace analysis when operated in positive ion mode, and this makes it difficult to use these systems in applications that require subpicogram detection. Double focusing instrumental systems show very low chemical noise, and relatively high specificity in detection, and for this reason GC-MS–computer systems with double focusing mass spectrometers are used in trace organic analysis. Subpicogram detection was achieved some time ago with atmospheric pressure ionization mass spectrometers (34,73), and subpicogram detection limits should be available with triple quadrupole bioanalytical systems. Problems of quantitative trace organic analysis are discussed in a later section.

Instrumental systems which include a GC, an MS with a single mass analyzer, and a computer or microprocessor with its peripherals, will probably continue in use for a long time because of their effectiveness in providing both qualitative and quantitative multicomponent analytical data for highly complex mixtures and for relatively small samples of biologic origin. Their use in research applications frequently requires a considerable degree of experimental skill in preparing samples for analysis, and considerable expertise in interpreting EI mass spectral data. Methods for the study of metabolites are discussed in the preceeding chapter of this volume. Numerous monographs dealing with the interpretation of EI mass spectral data and with special topics in MS, have been published.

MASS SPECTRA OF NONVOLATILE COMPOUNDS

Obtaining a mass spectrum of a nonvolatile compound was believed for many years to be extremely difficult. There were few guidelines in chemical theory, and very few avenues of investigation seemed open. It is now known that there are numerous ways, rather than only a few, of obtaining gas phase ions of nonvolatile compounds. The spectra that are obtained are similar to CI mass spectra; the processes that are most widely used do not lead to positive radical molecular ions. The methods listed in Table 1 are of greatest interest at the present time. Additional methods have been described in the literature.

TABLE 1. *Ionization of nonvolatile compounds*

Fast atom bombardment (glycerol; Ar or Xe)
Secondary ion MS (glycerol; Cs^+ or Ar^+)
Desorption chemical ionization (with or without molecular adduct formation)
^{252}Cf or ^{127}I particle bombardment
Laser ionization
Field desorption ionization
Spray/aerosol evaporation (with or without electron beam)

Pioneering studies with nonvolatile compounds were carried out in several laboratories. Field desorption ionization, based on applying a high field to an emitter surface coated with a thin film of a nonvolatile organic compound, was developed over a period of years, and for some time this provided the only useful method of obtaining mass spectra of compounds that could not thermally be volatilized. The experimental procedures were difficult to reproduce, however, and this method is not widely used. The work of Macfarlane and Torgerson (98), with a time of flight MS, and with bombardment of a thin film of compound (from the rear side) by nuclear fission particles from ^{252}Cf, demonstrated that gas phase ions (typically MH^+ and MHM^+) could be obtained from nonvolatile compounds by highly localized and rapid energy transfer. Although this is a relatively high energy process, the physical entities that are ejected from the film into the gas phase are packets made up of neutral molecules and ions, and the dispersed MH^+ and MHM^+ ions are relatively stable (indicative of low internal energy). For this reason, this and related processes are often called "soft ionization" methods, in contrast to methods that result in much fragmentation of parent ions.

Later, it was found that other methods of bombardment could be used to obtain gas phase ions of nonvolatile organic compounds (13,14,46,47). Bombardment of a metal surface with high energy ion beams or neutral atom beams results in the ejection of metal ions (sputtering) (12) from the surface of the target. This procedure yields ions when applied to organic compounds. When dissolved in a liquid matrix (6–9) and placed in film form on a support, however, most organic compounds will give gas phase ions very readily under sputtering conditions. The physical process, as in the case of nuclear particle bombardment, is believed to involve the ejection (or sputtering) of multiunit packets from the surface of the liquid film (13,27,46,47). The size and charge state of these packets has not been fully defined, but dissociation of the packets is believed to occur very rapidly to yield a mixture of gas phase ions (usually M^+, MHM^+, and $(M\text{-}H)^-$, and possibly fragment ions) and neutral molecules from both the liquid matrix (which may include more than one component) and the sample (which may have one or many components). Ions from matrix molecules are always generated along with ions from the sample, and the spectra usually show much chemical noise when organic solvents are used. Glycerol is the most widely used liquid matrix; samples should be in solution, and they can be added to glycerol in polar solvents including methanol or pyridine. Nonpolar solvents can be used in place of glycerol, but most nonvolatile organic compounds are polyfunctional and require polar solvents for solution. Ammonium chloride has also been recommended as a matrix (27).

A different experimental procedure, without a matrix, can also be used. Samples are heated in a CI source with the electron beam in operation, so that the source contains energized neutral molecules or atoms as well as ions. The support should be inert; we use a gold wire for this purpose, and the sample should not be exposed directly to the electron beam (36,76,113,114,127). It was thought initially that CI proton donor ions were required for sample ion formation, but this is now known to be incorrect (127). Mass spectra can be obtained by this desorption chemical ionization (DCI) process with nitrogen or argon as the source gas, and the resulting spectra resemble those obtained by methods based upon bombardment. An advantage of these procedures is that a reagent may be added to the source gases. For example, stable isotope labeled molecular adduct ions may be obtained readily under these conditions (36,127), but not under the lower pressure conditions that involve ion or atom beams. Particle bombardment methods and time of flight instruments may be required for compounds of very high molecular mass.

The lowest internal energy for MH^+ ions should be associated with processes that involve the least amount of energy transfer, and this condition may be achieved by aerosol evaporation without an electron beam. Ions that are present in solution can be desolvated under mild conditions to yield MH^+ ions with minimal fragmentation. This method (136) is not in wide use, and it is not yet known if the late stage of the desolvation process is much the same as the disintegration of charged packets generated by particle, ion beam, or atom beam bombardment methods.

Much experimental work has been carried out with the aim of developing high-performance liquid chromatography (HPLC)-MS–computer bioanalytical systems analogous to GC-MS–computer systems, but this may not be the critical issue in obtaining mass spectra of nonvolatile compounds. The great significance of these advances in ionization techniques lies in the possibility of extending gas phase chemical methodology to organic compounds generally, rather than only to thermally volatile compounds. When these methods are joined to new capabilities for working with gas phase ions provided by the development of triple quadrupole MS, the entire field of gas phase organic ion chemistry will advance rapidly.

The following sections contain brief summaries of several current experimental methods for obtaining mass spectra of nonvolatile compounds. Recent summaries include those by Fenselau (56) and McNeal (108).

Fast Atom Bombardment Ionization with a Liquid Matrix and Secondary Ion MS with a Liquid Matrix

The fast atom bombardment (FAB) ionization technique, as described in the initial studies of Barber and his colleagues (6,7), involved the bombardment of a liquid film containing the sample with a beam of energized atoms. Argon or xenon is usually used; the source is open and the gases are removed as rapidly as possible. The most widely used liquid is glycerol, and the sample should be in solution. The sample may be added to glycerol in water, methanol, or pyridine. Although the energy of the atomic beam is high (for example, if the liquid film is not present, metal ions from the probe tip will be observed), the internal energy of organic ions from the sample is relatively low, so that only a small degree of fragmentation is usually observed. Ions from the liquid matrix are also always present in the mass spectrum.

Ionization in secondary ion MS (SIMS) is not greatly different for organic compounds. An energetic ion beam is used, and the sample is present in a liquid or solid matrix, or as a solid film. Variations in the technique include the use of a liquid metal ion primary source (10). Cesium (1,37,105,118) and argon (27,54) sources have been described in recent papers. FAB and SIMS techniques are quite similar, and the mass spectra obtained in each case are essentially the same (1,10). The mechanism of ion formation is presumably the same in both instances, and the key to an effective and generally useful ionization process is the use of a matrix.

Many variations may be made in details of these ionization techniques. The composition of the liquid film can be varied, and additives can be used (acids and metal ions have been employed to aid the ionization process). In some instances biologic fluids (for example, urine) or plant tissue can be analyzed without a separation step. Negative ions corresponding to $(M\text{-}H)^-$, or in some instances $M^{-\bullet}$, are generated along with positive ions. In general, polar compounds give good results, while hydrocarbons do not. Operating conditions for FAB MS have been defined (103).

Figure 1 shows a FAB mass spectrum of ecdysterone in glycerol, with the sample added in pyridine solution. This is a typical high noise positive ion spectrum, but the major ions corresponding to MH^+, $(MH\text{-}18)^+$, $(MH\text{-}36)^+$, and $(MH\text{-}54)^+$ are clearly evident. Ecdysterone contains a ketone group and six hydroxyl groups (three are tertiary), and the fragmentation is due to loss of water (four elimination reactions are evident in the mass spectrum). Figure 2 shows a FAB mass spectrum of adenosine 5′-triphosphate (ATP) as the disodium salt. Oxalic acid was added; a water solution was added to glycerol. The major ions include MH^+ ions for ATP, monosodium ATP, and disodium ATP. Fragment ions include MH^+ ions for the monophosphate

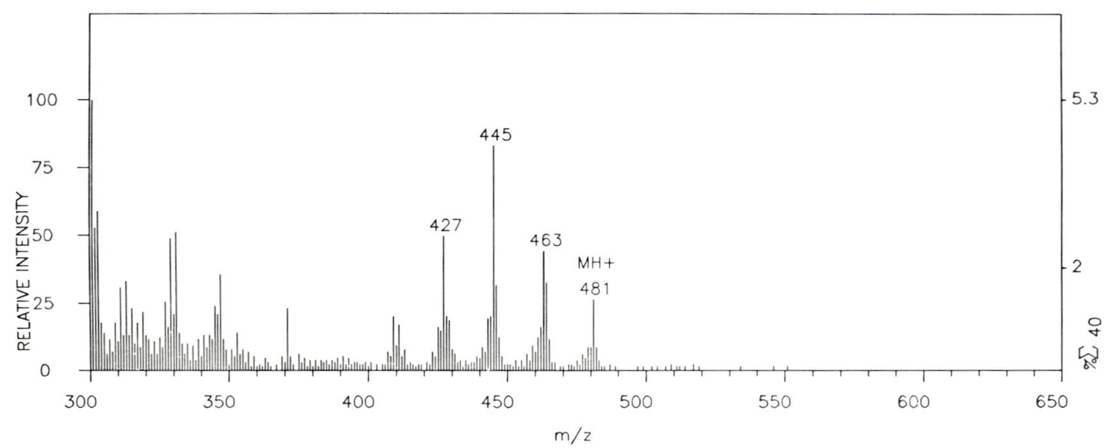

FIG. 1. FAB mass spectrum of ecdysterone in a pyridine–glycerol matrix. The major ions are MH^+, $(MH\text{-}18)^+$, $(MH\text{-}36)^+$, and $(MH\text{-}54)^+$. This mass spectrum should be compared with the DCI mass spectrum in Fig. 9.

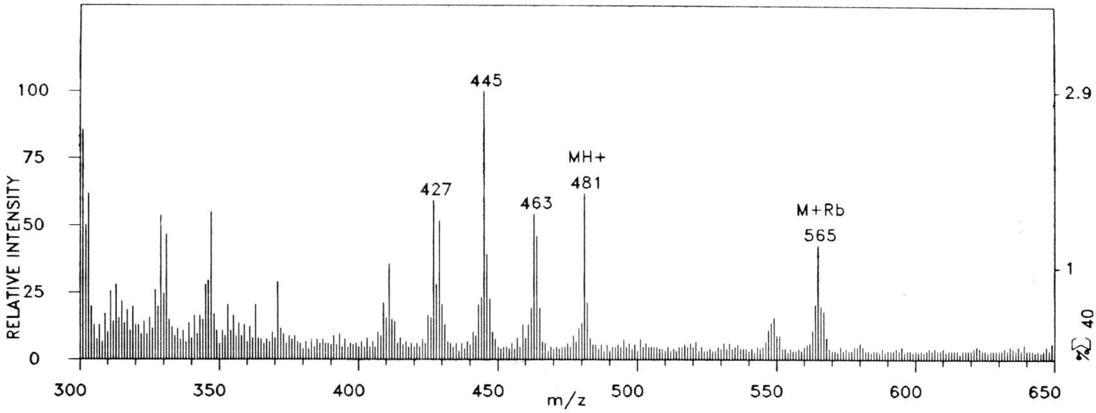

FIG. 6. FAB mass spectrum of ecdysterone in a pyridine–water–glycerol matrix containing Rb^+ ions. The Rb^+ adduct ion is present, in addition to ions corresponding to MH^+, $(MH\text{-}18)^+$, $(MH\text{-}36)^+$, and $(MH\text{-}54)^+$.

DCI

Chemical ionization sources are usually operated at 0.5 to 1 torr pressure, and the residence time of reagent ions is adjusted to allow sufficient time for their reaction with sample molecules (although thermal and chemical equilibration is not established within the source). The usual purpose is to obtain protonated sample ions. Special conditions can be used to obtain $M^{-\bullet}$ or $(M\text{-}H)^-$ ions, and positive ion mass spectra equivalent to EI spectra can be obtained by charge or energy transfer with appropriate gases.

DCI techniques (36,76,113,114,127) require very little modification of sources, probes, and circuits. We use a gold wire probe extension (heated by the probe) with an unheated source. The support extends into the source, but is not in a direct line with the electron beam. Samples of nonvolatile compounds are placed on the tip by evaporation of solutions, and in instances where adsorption is a problem, a thin film of polymethylsiloxane (SE-30) is

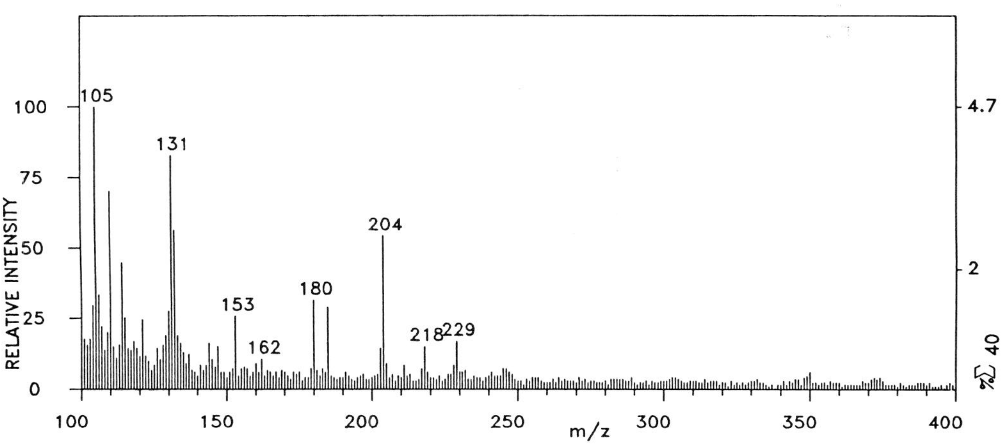

FIG. 7. FAB mass spectrum of a urine sample, in glycerol, of a patient with Reyes' syndrome. The sample was untreated. Ions at *m/z* 204 and 218 are from acetylcarnitine and propionylcarnitine, respectively. The compound responsible for the ion at *m/z* 229 has not been identified.

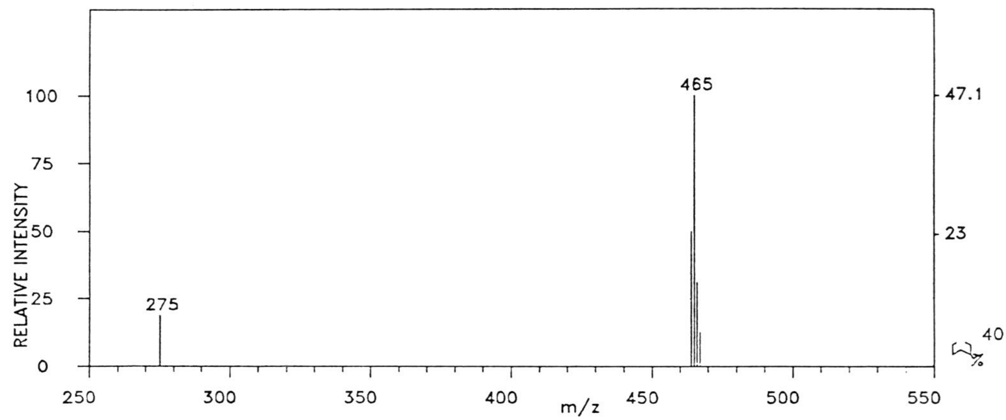

FIG. 8. FAB negative ion mass spectrum for androsterone glucuronide. The matrix was glycerol. The major ion corresponds to $(M\text{-}H)^-$.

placed on the gold surface before the sample is added. As the sample is heated, gas phase ions are formed in a sequence that resembles a GC peak. If thermal decomposition of the sample occurs at the same time as gas phase ion formation, the total ion current chart usually shows a late shoulder or extensive trailing.

This technique provides mass spectra of the CI type which closely resemble those obtained by FAB/SIMS techniques, and it is probable that the mechanism of ion formation is essentially the same under DCI conditions as in ion beam, atom beam, and particle bombardment methods (127). For example, Fig. 9 shows a DCI mass spectrum of ecdysterone, with nitrogen as the source gas. The spectrum is similar to that shown in Fig. 1. If the current hypothesis of gas phase ion formation for nonvolatile compounds is correct, the physical entities entering the gas phase under DCI conditions are multiunit charged packets which disintegrate very rapidly after leaving the surface. The products are neutral molecules, MH^+, MHM^+, and $(M\text{-}H)^-$ or $M^{-\bullet}$. Fragment ions resulting from energized MH^+ ions, and possibly some neutral fragments, are most likely formed from collisions occurring during the disintegration process.

DCI procedures have two advantages with respect to FAB/SIMS ionization methods.

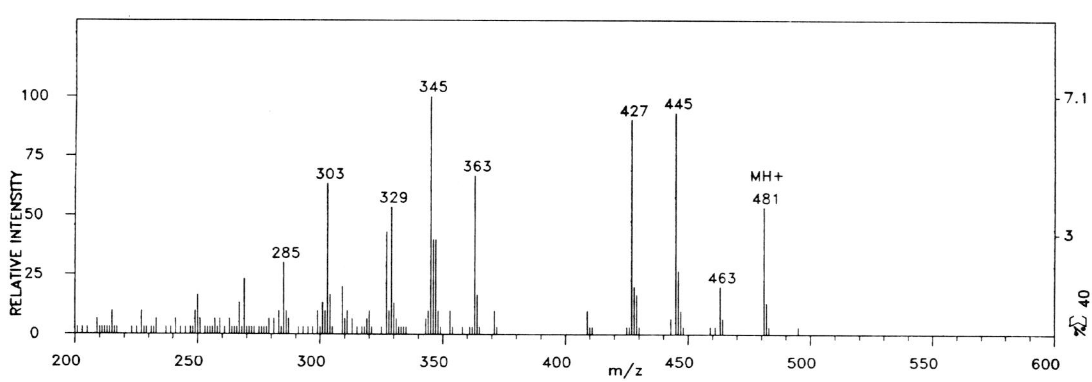

FIG. 9. DCI mass spectrum of ecdysterone, with nitrogen as the source gas. The major ions correspond to MH^+, $(MH\text{-}18)^+$, $(MH\text{-}36)^+$, $(MH\text{-}54)^+$, and a second series of fragment ions. This should be compared with the mass spectrum in Fig. 1.

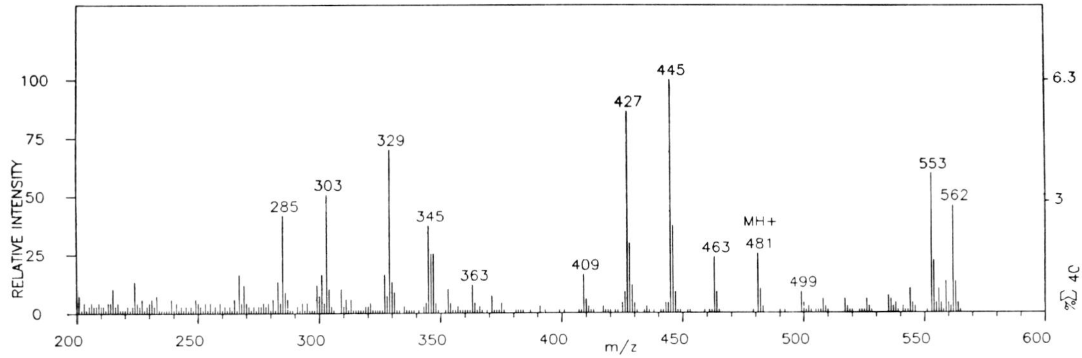

FIG. 10. DCI mass spectrum of ecdysterone, with nitrogen as the source gas and tetramethylsilane-tetramethylsilane-d_{12} as reagents. The molecular adduct ions are at m/z 553 and 562 for the unlabeled and labeled ions, respectively.

Very little instrument or source modification is required, and it is possible to add gas phase reagents to the source in order to characterize ions containing intact molecules. The technique of molecular adduct ion formation, with a labeled reagent, is illustrated in Fig. 10 for ecdysterone. The TMS ion (73 amu), and its deuterium-labeled form (82 amu), can be generated easily in a CI source from tetramethylsilane and tetramethylsilane-d_{12}. These ions add to most neutral organic compounds that contain a functional group to form $(M + TMS)^+$ ions, and the adducts are immediately recognizable because of the isotope distribution (twin-ion technique). The molecular adduct ions serve to define the m/z value of MH^- (which may or may not be present) and it is then possible to recognize ion sequences derived from MH^+ by elimination reactions. Figure 11 shows another example of molecular adduct ion formation for prostaglandin $F_{2\alpha}$; this is based on adduct formation with pyridine.

If the structure of a compound is known, it is usually not difficult to assign structures to ions in a CI or DCI mass spectrum. In the upper chart of Fig. 11, for example, it is clear that an MH^+ ion is not present, and that the major ions correspond to protonated structures in a series corresponding to $(MH\text{-}18)^+$, $(MH\text{-}36)^+$. . . . If an unlabeled reagent is added, the $(MH + pyr)^+$ ion is present, but if unknowns are under study, or if samples are impure, there would be no way of immediately recognizing the identity of the adduct ion. When the twin-ion technique is used, as shown in the lower chart in Fig. 11, the molecular adduct ions are clearly indicated. In this instance, MH^+ ions are still missing, but the m/z value for MH^+ can be deduced from the molecular adduct ion, and the major ion products can in turn be identified as corresponding to the series $(MH\text{-}18)^+$, $(MH\text{-}36)^+$, and $(MH\text{-}54)^+$. Other examples of DCI mass spectra are shown in Figs. 12–14. Conjugated compounds usually give very good DCI spectra, with ions corresponding both to MH^+ and to protonated molecules formed by cleavage reactions at the site of conjugation. This effect is illustrated in Fig. 12 for two related glycosides. Nucleosides give good DCI mass spectra. The bases show MH^+ and adduct ions, alone and as fragments from nucleosides, as shown in Fig. 13. Negative radical ions may also be obtained; this is illustrated in Fig. 14. In this instance, $M^{-\cdot}$ ions are probably formed by electron capture by gas phase neutral molecules released from charged packets ejected from the surface. Spectra can be obtained for anthracycline antibiotics with 1 ng samples (126).

A disadvantage of DCI methods with respect to FAB/SIMS procedures is that the upper mass limit may be relatively low, and some

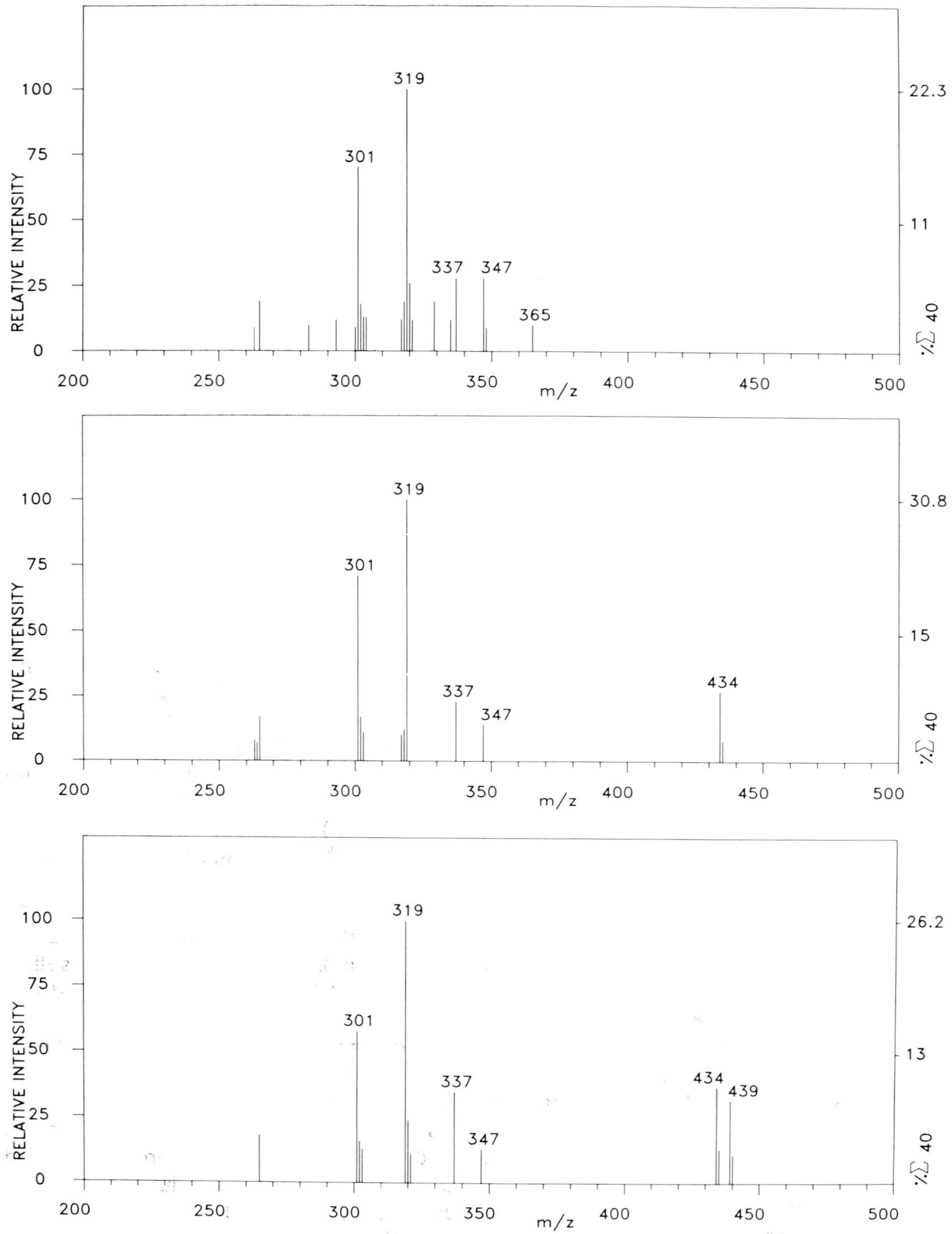

FIG. 11. DCI mass spectra of prostaglandin $F_{2\alpha}$. **Upper chart:** Mass spectrum with methane as the source gas; the MH^+ ion is missing. **Middle chart:** Mass spectrum with methane as the source gas, and pyridine as a reagent; the MH^+ ion is missing, but a molecular adduct ion is present. **Lower chart:** Mass spectrum with methane as the source gas, and pyridine-pyridine-d_5 as reagents; the MH^+ ion is missing, but molecular adduct ions at m/z 434 and 439 are present. The twin ion technique permits immediate recognition of the adducts in this chart and in Fig. 10.

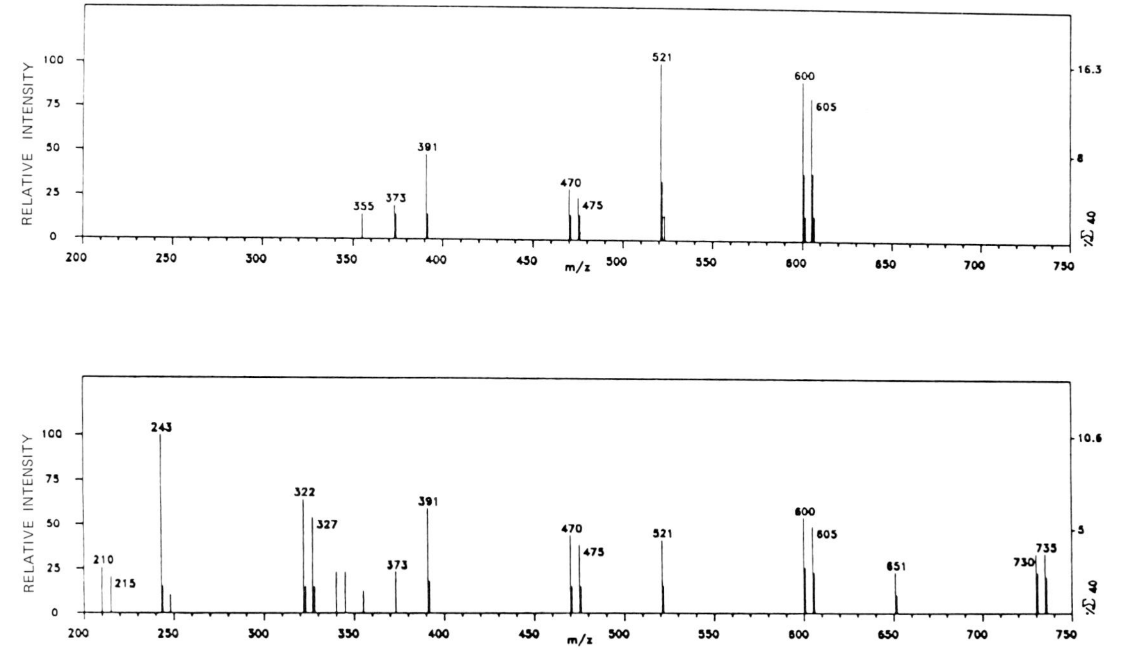

FIG. 12. DCI mass spectra for digoxigenin monodigitoxoside (**upper chart**) and digoxigenin didigitoxoside (**lower chart**) with isobutane as the source gas and pyridine-pyridine-d_5 as reagents. The molecular adduct ions can be recognized by the twin ion effect. They are present for the aglycone, the monodigitoxoside, and the didigitoxoside. Cleavage of conjugates as a consequence of protonation is a frequent occurrence.

ionic compounds may not give good spectra. The use of a liquid matrix under DCI conditions has not been fully explored; it may be possible to extend the process to higher mass samples by using liquid films. Limits of detection for positive ions are discussed in a later section.

^{252}Cf Desorption Ionization and Related Ionization Methods

These ionization processes depend on the bombardment of a thin film of a nonvolatile organic compound (usually supported on aluminized Mylar film) with energetic particles. The positive ion products are typically MH^+ and MHM^+, and the mechanism is related to that discussed earlier (the bombarding particles pass through the Mylar film and the film of organic compound; localized energy transfer leads to localized ionization and the ejection of charged packets which dissociate into ions and neutral molecules). A time of flight MS is employed; the measurement of time (or its inverse, frequency) can now be carried out with great precision, and the flight path need not be inordinately long (35–40 cm is adequate). In the Macfarlane design (98,99,108) ^{252}Cf was used as a nuclear particle source, and mass spectra were obtained for many high mass polar organic compounds. This work was very important in showing that high mass gas phase organic ions could be generated and detected.

A related instrument employing a beam of 90-MeV ^{127}I ions (+20 charge state) was employed in a study of mass spectra of bovine insulin (70). The positive ion mass spectrum contained MH^+ ions at m/z 5730 ± 10 and two fragment ions at m/z 3415 ± 3 and 2350 ± 1. An MHM^+ ion was present in the vicinity of m/z 12,000 (not examined in de-

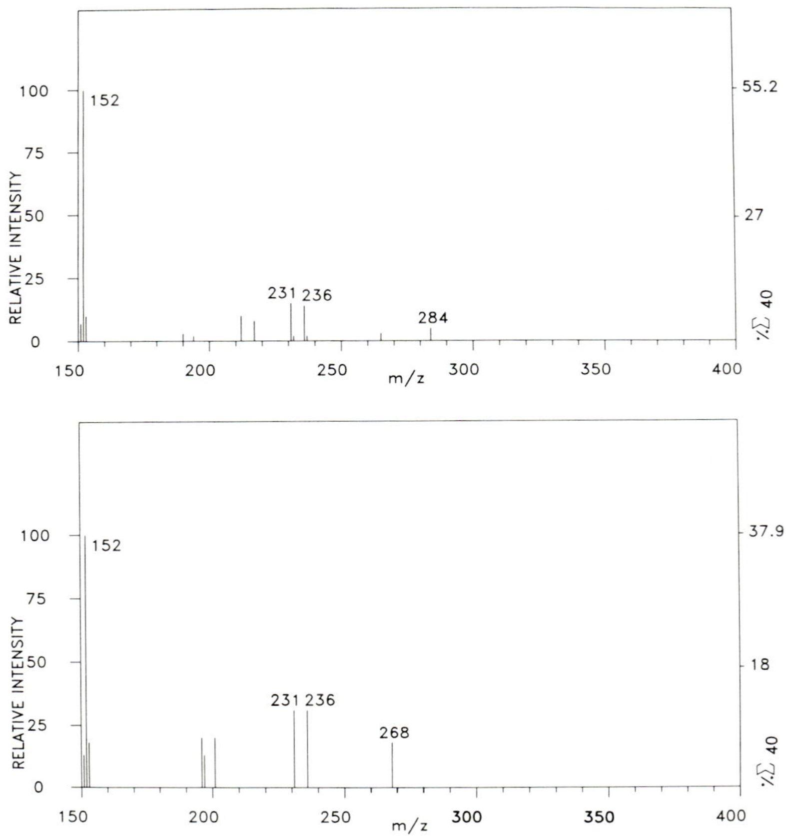

FIG. 13. DCI mass spectrum of guanosine (**upper chart**) and of 2-deoxyguanosine (**lower chart**). The source gas was isobutane, with pyridine-pyridine-d_5 as reagents. The nucleosides do not form molecular adducts with pyridine, but adducts are formed with the bases.

tail). The fragment ions were derived from the α- and β-chains. The negative ion mass spectrum showed ions at m/z 5785 ± 10, 3407 ± 3, and 2356 ± 1. The isotopically averaged molecular mass of bovine insulin is 5733 (the negative ion may be hydrated).

In the future, it may be possible to determine the molecular mass of many relatively high mass polar organic compounds and biopolymers, both by these methods and by FAB/SIMS procedures. An advantage of a time of flight MS of the Macfarlane design is that ions of high mass may be studied; for example, an ion at 12,637 amu was observed. A disadvantage of time of flight instruments is that the ions are not available for further study by MS/MS techniques.

HPLC-MS Combined Instruments: The Introduction of MS Samples in Solution

A variety of approaches has been taken to the design of HPLC-MS–computer analytical systems which are analogs of existing systems with GC separation. Moving belt devices for sample introduction, with arrangements for the removal of HPLC solvents under reduced pressure, were developed some time ago, and these devices have given good results with some types of samples (32,58). Compounds that are not highly volatile (which would be lost in the solvent removal step), but which can be volatilized thermally, often give good mass spectra. Nonvolatile compounds are less likely to be ionized in satisfactory fashion, de-

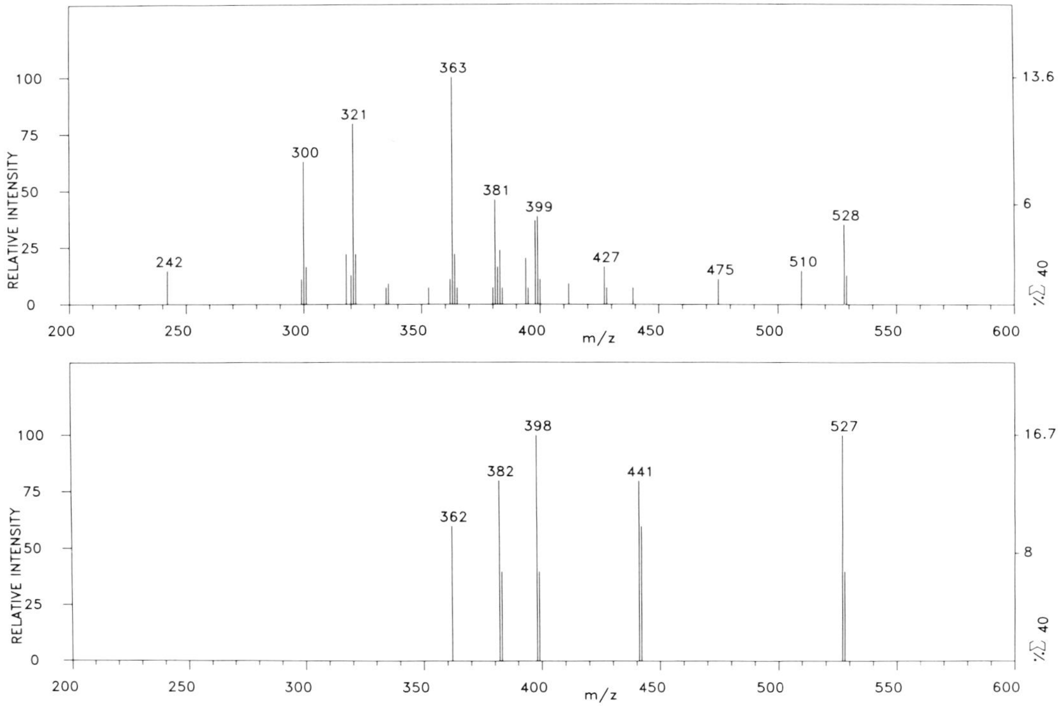

FIG. 14. DCI positive ion mass spectrum (**upper chart**) and DCI negative ion mass spectrum (**lower chart**) of daunorubicin. The source gas was methane. Ions corresponding to MH^+ and to $M^{-\bullet}$ are present.

pending on the design, in contrast to results observed when samples are ionized by FAB/SIMS, DCI, or ^{252}Cf desorption ionization, and for this reason moving belt devices are not in wide use.

Most current studies of combined instruments are based on the view that nonvolatile samples which are in solution in HPLC solvents should be introduced into the MS source in solution, leading to the formation of an aerosol. Numerous different types of source design and desolvation techniques have been used, but in all instances the HPLC solvents accompany the sample through the ionization process, and in most or all instances the desolvation sequence goes through an aerosol phase. One of the first HPLC-MS combinations involved the injection of samples in organic solvents (or water-organic solutions) into an atmospheric pressure ionization (API) source (35,74). Desolvation was carried out thermally (the solutes were volatile and thermally stable) and most sample ions were solvated. It was recently found that an aerosol spray technique could be used with a large volume API source, and that ions could be desolvated by a collision technique prior to entry into the mass analyzer (136). Chemical and thermal equilibration of product ions and neutral molecules occurs in API sources, but most reversed phase HPLC solvents (for example, methanol–water mixtures containing a little acetic acid, and acetonitrile–water mixtures) are weak gas phase bases, and would not deionize MH^+ sample ions from strongly basic solutes. Strong gas phase bases, and acids which are ionized in solution, do not require an energetic ionization condition in an API source; the only processes that are involved are spray/aerosol desolvation and ion desolvation. Further studies of spray/aerosol injection into API sources may lead to HPLC-

MS(API) combined instruments which will generally be useful with reversed phase HPLC separation procedures.

Spray injection of solutions into heated CI sources involves numerous technical difficulties, but this method has been successfully used. The early studies of Baldwin and McLafferty (5) indicated that difficulties were associated with the conversion of an HPLC effluent into a suitable spray, and with solvent vapor removal from the source and from the region before the mass analyzer (in order to maintain suitable pressure relationships). Several commercial GC-MS–computer bioanalytical systems have been modified in design to permit their operation as HPLC-MS-computer systems with spray introduction of the column effluent stream. Current studies (2,24,148,150) are concerned with design of the interface and with the operating parameters of temperature, pressure, and solvent composition. The usual assumption is that reversed phase HPLC will be used with either a split effluent stream from an analytical column or the entire stream from a micro liquid chromatograph. Satisfactory results have been reported, particularly in the negative ion mode, but the technique is not yet in wide use.

A different approach described as "thermospray" is under study (17). An HPLC effluent stream is vaporized, under conditions of relatively high temperature and pressure, in a narrow bore entry to a source chamber that need not have an electron beam or other initiator of ionization. Most of the solvent vapor/aerosol mixture is removed under reduced pressure; the chamber is sampled in much the same way as in most API sources. The details of the ionization process have not been established, and further evaluation work is needed.

All techniques for the introduction into an MS of samples in solution, whether the samples have been purified separately or are in an HPLC effluent stream, require the removal from the system of relatively large volumes of vaporized solvent(s). The inclusion in the solution of substances which aid the HPLC separation may or may not lead to additional complications. The initially formed ions from polar nonvolatile compounds (many applications will involve compounds of this type) are often solvated, and these ions should be desolvated before mass analysis.

Sample ions from nonvolatile compounds, whether obtained from an HPLC effluent stream with an HPLC-MS combined instrument or through the use of a FAB, SIMS, or other source, are of the CI type. The major problems to be studied in the future are the use of CI ion products in structural and identification work, and the establishment of quantitative analytical methods (particularly those involving trace organic analysis) (43) for nonvolatile organic compounds. The question of whether samples should be introduced sequentially (for example, in DCI, FAB, SIMS, or ^{252}Cf sources) or continuously in an HPLC effluent stream may not have a simple answer. Most likely, both approaches will be used. A bibliography of HPLC-MS work has been published (52).

MS/MS INSTRUMENTS: GAS PHASE ORGANIC ION CHEMISTRY

For many years, studies of gas phase organic ion chemistry were concerned with unimolecular fragmentation reactions of positive radical ions, and with positive radical ion structures. This was because $M^{+\bullet}$ ions with relatively high internal energies are formed in EI sources, and reactions leading to fragment ions from $M^{+\bullet}$ ions with high internal energy are usually fast, extensive, and complicated. These studies were extremely valuable both in establishing much new knowledge in an essentially new field of organic chemistry (gas phase organic radical ion chemistry) and in providing an approach to the determination of the chemical structure of novel types of new compounds (often of biologic origin) by methods which were quite different from earlier classical procedures.

In the course of these studies it was found that relatively stable positive radical ions, formed in ordinary EI sources, could be made to undergo fragmentation reactions as a consequence of collisions or near-collisions with neutral atoms or molecules (for example, with helium, argon, or nitrogen as collision gases). This led to the development of new types of mass spectrometers, and new analytical systems, which are based on what is now usually termed MS/MS or tandem MS (106,107). In the simplest types of MS/MS instruments, mass-analyzed ions are directed through a reaction region (usually leading to fragmentation) and product ions are mass analyzed. The descriptive terminology refers to the mode of mass analysis (B, magnetic sector; E, electrical sector; Q, quadrupole); instrumental combinations include BE, BEB, EBE, EBEB, and QQQ. Much of the work that has been published, aside from matters of instrument design, involves two approaches: the study of ion structures and fragmentation reactions, and mixture analysis. Fragmentation reactions, based on collision-induced dissociation or collisionally activated dissociation, are of critical importance in both theory and applications. Mixture analysis largely involves analytical applications, and at present is based on fragmentation reactions. The literature is too extensive to permit a detailed discussion, with individual references, of MS/MS work. The following sections summarize current knowledge; work with QQQ instruments is emphasized.

Reaction Conditions

Analytical systems based on a QQQ combination, or a QQ combination with an enclosed collision region, have a reaction chamber which may be used in several different ways. When fragmentation reactions are under study, the pressure is usually 1 to 4 millitorr, and the collision gas is usually helium, argon, or nitrogen. If the pressure in the reaction chamber is raised, thermal and chemical equilibration occurs without major loss in ion transmission. It is also possible, under conditions of increased pressure, to carry out functional group reactions through the introduction of reagents into the collision chamber.

Fragmentation reactions can be studied with all types of MS/MS instrumental combinations, but the QQQ combination is best suited for studies of ion molecule reactions with added gas phase reagents. The basic design of a QQQ instrument is relatively simple; Yost et al. (157) and Yost and Enke (156) showed that low energy collisions are highly effective in leading to ion fragmentation, and their work started the development of commercially available QQQ instruments.

Fragmentation Reactions of Positive Ions

The fragmentation of a positive radical ion in an EI source leads to the same ion products as those resulting from fragmentation or dissociation of the ion in a collision region. A unit resolution EI mass spectrum cannot serve to distinguish ions of the same mass but different structure, and it is usually not possible to determine unequivocally all pathways of fragment ion formation from parent $M^{+\bullet}$ ions by study of the mass spectrum. When positive radical ions from an EI source are introduced serially into a collision chamber (QQQ), or into the corresponding collision region of other types of instrumental systems (for example, BE or EBE), the mass spectrum of each ion shows the charged fragments derived from the ion. It is possible, with this information, to construct a chart of relationships or pathways of formation, for ions in the original EI mass spectrum. It is also possible to reverse the procedure; the precursor(s) of an ion can be found by scanning with the first mass analyzer while the second mass analyzer is acting to select only the product ion.

Studies of positive radical ion fragmentation reactions by MS/MS techniques lead to extensions of basic knowledge relating to gas phase organic ion chemistry, and this is important for future structural studies. Many future structural problems will involve nonvolatile compounds, however, and the ions produced in DCI, FAB/SIMS and direct liquid introduction sources are typical CI ions and not radical ions. The statement is frequently made that CI mass spectra contain no structural information, and that the only use of CI data is to define the molecular mass. Current studies suggest that this conclusion is premature, and that most future structural studies will probably also involve fragmentation studies of CI ions. The problem is illustrated by the mass spectrum in Fig. 15. A number of different steroids give relatively simple CI mass spectra under DCI and FAB/SIMS conditions (35,37). Neutral molecules are eliminated from different parent MH^+ ions, and the ion of lowest molecular mass in several spectra is at *m/z* 255. This is clearly a hydrocarbon ion corresponding to protonated $C_{19}H_{26}$, but it is not possible, by comparisons of ordinary CI spectra, to determine if the same +255 ion is formed from different steroids. Figure 15 shows the mass spectrum of this hydrocarbon ion. The same spectrum was obtained when the +255 ion from several steroids was examined (QQQ data). The ions in Fig. 15 are not present as ion products in the original CI mass spectra; they may be observed only through collision studies. When a hydrocarbon ion is present in a CI mass spectrum (this is the case when CHO compounds are under study), additional CI mass spectra of this kind should be obtained.

A related circumstance is illustrated in Fig. 16. A positive ion CI mass spectrum of benzene shows an MH^+ ion at *m/z* 79, indicating the nominal molecular mass. The mass spectrum of this ion is shown in Fig. 16 (QQQ data). The elimination of hydrogen and acetylene from a CI ion is unusual, when compared with typical losses of water, ethylene, and other neutral molecules, and this spectrum serves to characterize the MH^+ ion from benzene. These ions are not present in an ordinary CI mass spectrum of benzene.

Secondary mass spectra of peptides, obtained by MS/MS techniques, provide amino acid sequence data (78,106), and similar methods are being used in other applications.

Additional studies are needed to evaluate the information content of QQQ mass spectral data for CI ions; the CI spectral data which can now be obtained are far more extensive than was realized earlier.

Fragmentation Reactions of Negative Ions

Comparatively few studies have been made of negative ion fragmentation reactions. In some instances, the effect of a collision on an

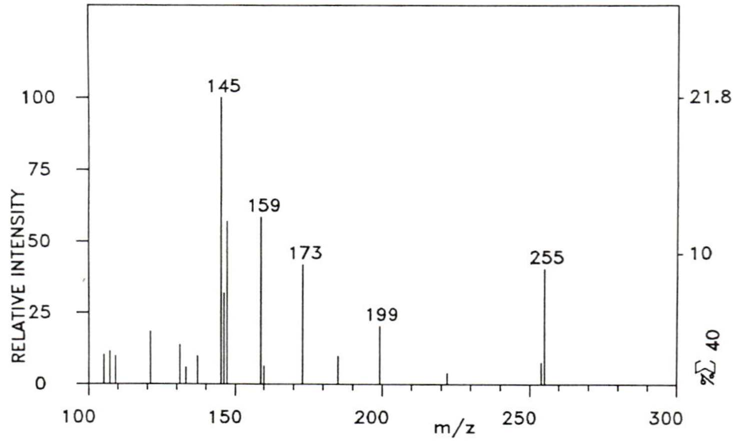

FIG. 15. Collision-induced dissociation mass spectrum of the *m/z* 255 hydrocarbon ion from a steroid DCI mass spectrum. These are hydrocarbon ions generated in the collision chamber of a QQQ instrument with argon as the collision gas at 2 millitorr pressure.

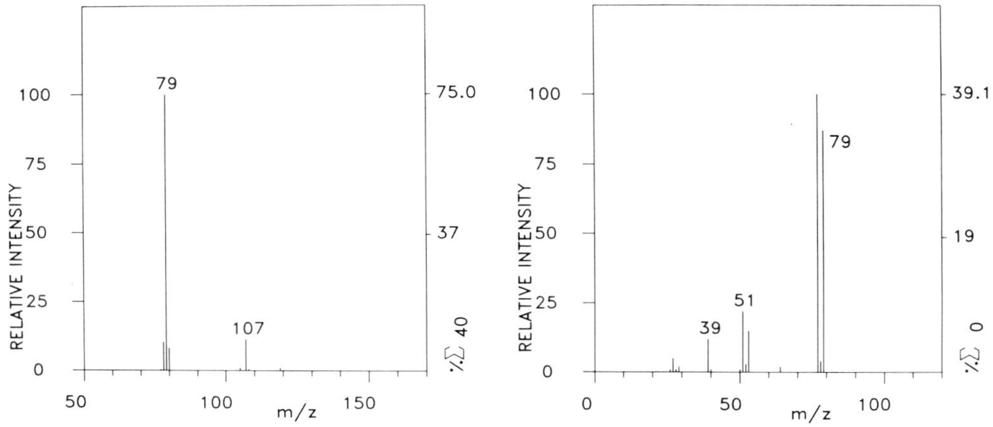

FIG. 16. Left chart: CI mass spectrum of benzene, with methane as the reagent gas. The principal ion at *m/z* 79 is MH^+. **Right chart:** Collision-induced dissociation mass spectrum of the *m/z* 79 ion from the left chart. These ions were generated in the same way as in Fig. 15.

$M^{-\bullet}$ ion is loss of the electron, but fragment ion formation occurs for some negative ions, and studies have been made of the possibility of charge reversal. The chief use of negative ion MS at present is in mixture analysis, and this is discussed in a later section.

Functional Group Reactions of Protonated Ions

Few studies of functional group reactions of protonated ions have been carried out with QQQ systems. The usual gas phase reaction of compounds with protonated functional groups is loss of a neutral molecule related to the functional group, but in some instances specific gas phase synthetic reactions can be carried out with appropriate reagents. The liquid phase analogs of these reactions are acid-catalyzed syntheses; some of these have been studied in the gas phase. For example, protonated carboxylic acids react with methanol in the gas phase to form protonated methyl esters. It may be possible to recognize or characterize functional groups in this way; the necessary QQQ studies have not yet been made. The general problem of functional group recognition by gas phase ion molecule reactions has been discussed by Keogh (88); dimethyl ether was recommended as a reagent.

Ion Exchange Reactions

The collision chamber of QQQ systems can be used for ion exchange reactions. Under conditions of chemical equilibration, the protonated ions leaving the chamber will be those of the strongest gas phase base(s). If a reagent is introduced into the chamber under these conditions, the only ions leaving the chamber will be from compounds that are stronger gas phase bases than the reagent. In practice, this may provide a rapid way of determining proton affinities.

Mixture Analysis Based on Fragmentation of Positive Ions

Current aspects of qualitative and quantitative mixture analysis are discussed later, but fragmentation reactions are important in this context, and QQQ systems may be used widely in the future in quantitative analytical applications. The current use of GC-MS systems in analytical work of many kinds is based on the much greater specificity of detection provided by MS, when compared with other instrumental methods (for example, ultraviolet absorption spectrometry), and upon the relatively low limit of detection that can be achieved. Analytical systems with a single mass analyzer are suitable in many bioanalytical applications, but they are generally not satisfactory for trace organic analysis except under special conditions; the specificity of detection and the limits of detection may not be adequate. Systems of the QQQ type have greatly increased specificity of detection, and a lower limit of detection, in most applications. The increased specificity of detection is due to the use of two related ions (a fragment ion and a parent ion), in the instrumental procedure. Ions of the same nominal mass, but with different structure, will give different ions in a collision-induced or collisionally activated fragmentation reaction. This leads to very high specificity in detection in mixture analysis. The detection process in a QQQ system is not different from that in a Q system, but the limit of detection and the limit of quantitation is determined by the signal-to-noise ratio, and the chemical noise is very low in QQQ systems. Losses in ion transmission are also low.

Specificity in detection can also be achieved by scanning in the linked scan technique. In a profile separation of the type now carried out with GC-MS systems, for example, both mass analyzers may be used in a scanning mode with a selected mass difference. All compounds showing this mass difference in their spectra will be detected; other compounds will not be observed. Linked mass analysis, with selection of two ion masses, can also be carried out in analogy to the selected ion detection technique used in GC-MS analyses.

Mixture analysis can be carried out both with QQQ instruments (low energy) and magnetic sector instruments (high energy) (44). Little or no processing of samples is needed in some applications (79); the lettuce leaf example cited by McLafferty (106) illustrates this point.

A novel design of a magnetic sector instrument (single mass analyzer) for MS/MS studies has been described (128); the collision chamber is placed between the source and the mass analyzer.

NEGATIVE ION MS

Most bioanalytical systems based on MS are now designed for operation in a negative ion mode as well as in a positive ion mode, or concurrently in both modes by rapid switching. Early bioanalytical systems were always designed for operation in the positive ion mode alone. This was because most organic compounds, when ionized under EI conditions, give only a few negative ions of low molecular mass which are not highly useful in either structural studies or mixture analysis.

Most current studies of negative ion formation involve conditions of ionization that were not used in earlier investigations. The relatively high energy (low pressure) CI condition developed by Brandenberger (20,21,59,120) is useful in forensic studies, and it is based on the formation of structurally significant negative fragment ions from parent negative ions. The initiating step may be either an electron molecule reaction or an ion molecule reaction with O^-. When ordinary CI conditions (0.5–1.0 torr pressure) are used for negative ion formation, the initiating step (unless special reagents are added) is an electron molecule reaction (electron capture) or reaction with $O_2^{-\bullet}$ which is unavoidably present in CI sources unless special precautions are taken. Reagents leading to HO^- can be employed; the usual reaction under these circumstances is $(M\text{-}H)^-$ formation. Negative ions observed under API conditions are formed in the same way as in a CI source, but the chemical equilibration occurring in an API source may lead to ion products different from those observed under CI conditions when mixtures are present.

The principal applications of negative ion MS are in forensic chemistry and in trace organic analysis. The reason for the great value of negative ion mass spectra in forensic work is that organic compounds with an electron affinity greater than that of oxygen are toxic to aerobic life forms, and most of the toxic organic agents likely to be encountered in forensic analytical circumstances are in this group. It is not certain why this is true, but in most instances the reaction of these compounds with electrons leads to a neutral radical and a stable even-electron negative ion, and the toxicity of these compounds may be due to the formation of neutral radicals during oxidative metabolism in the body (73). In some instances, stable $M^{-\bullet}$ ions are formed by electron molecule reactions (for example, from quinones and α,β-diketones), and examples are known of fragmentation reactions leading to stable negative radical ions. When oxygen is present, complex reactions with $O_2^{-\bullet}$ may occur. These reactions usually lead to neutral radicals and to stable even-electron negative ions through *ipso* substitution (for aromatic compounds) or displacement through a mechanism similar to S_N2 substitution reactions (for aliphatic and alicyclic compounds) (73).

Negative ions resulting from reaction with electrons or $O_2^{-\bullet}$ may be formed under API conditions, ordinary CI conditions, or the low pressure CI conditions developed by Brandenberger. The latter conditions are preferred for analytical studies that involve compound identification, and all forensic laboratories should have capabilities for negative ion MS.

There is a very close relationship between reactions that occur in an electron-capture detector and those that occur in a CI or API source with electrons or $O_2^{-\bullet}$ ions as reagents (73). Most pesticides, herbicides, and related toxic compounds used for other purposes show an electron capture response. This response is relatively nonspecific, however, and for this reason identification studies should not be based on electron capture response data.

Most organic compounds do not react in the gas phase with thermal or near-thermal electrons. Consequently, when mass spectrometers are operated in the negative ion mode with CI or API sources, the chemical noise is extremely low (the chemical noise in an electron-capture detector is also normally very low for the same reason). This circumstance suggests that negative ion MS involving electron molecule reactions, or reactions with $O_2^{-\bullet}$, should be particularly useful in quantitative analytical applications. This is true (examples are cited in a later section), except that for chlorinated compounds the product ion is often Cl^- (a ubiquitous ion whose formation is not usually the basis of a mass spectrometric analytical method).

It is possible to define and study gas phase acidity, involving the formation of $(M\text{-}H)^-$ ions by proton transfer, in much the same way that gas phase basicity can be defined and studied. Comparatively few uses have been published, however, of $(M\text{-}H)^-$ ions in structural studies or in mixture analysis. In instances where $(M\text{-}H)^-$ ions are formed readily, or where negative molecular adduct ions are formed, the parent ions are useful in indicating molecular mass.

IDENTIFICATION AND STRUCTURAL STUDIES BY MS

Classical methods for determining the structure of newly isolated organic compounds (often from a natural source) always assumed that the initial requirement was that of obtaining samples of high purity, and the most widely used method for defining chemical reaction products obtained in structural studies was through elemental analysis by combustion. Much time and effort was expended in obtaining highly purified samples which were burned in order to determine empirical formulas.

The development of instrumental methods of structural analysis started slowly but progressed rapidly, and structural information can now be obtained in many ways. Mass spectrometric methods are usually employed at as early a stage as possible, in part because small samples are used, and in part because elemental composition data and much structural information can often be obtained very rapidly through the use of high resolution instruments and bioanalytical systems.

Structural problems in drug metabolism, and drug toxicity studies, are generally greatly simplified because the precursors have known structures, and because many of the major pathways of drug metabolism have been defined. In many instances the chief problem is to find a suitable isolation procedure and suitable methods of derivative formation so that GC-MS or GC-MS/MS analytical methods may be used. It is not necessary to isolate individual samples of high purity unless other instrumental methods are to be used. Samples obtained by metabolic profile procedures are generally highly complex mixtures, but these mixtures can usually be analyzed by MS with bioanalytical systems as effectively (or more effectively) as individual samples of high purity. The most useful derivatives in identification studies are those which are stable in the analytical system, which reduce hydrogen bonding by converting polar functional groups into nonpolar groups, and which can be prepared with stable isotope labels.

Until very recently, identification and structural studies based on MS were almost entirely limited to applications where EI mass spectra could be obtained. CI mass spectral data were used largely to confirm the molecular mass. The reason for this circumstance is evident in a comparison of Figs. 17 and 18. Figure 17 shows the EI mass spectrum of the N,N′-dimethyl derivative of phenobarbital. This mass spectrum was obtained in a conventional fashion with a GC-MS bioanalytical system, and it shows ions that are dissociation products of parent $M^{+\bullet}$ ions. Some structural information can be deduced from the *m/z* values of the major ions, and the spectrum is characteristic of this phenobarbital derivative. A CI (methane) positive ion mass spectrum of the same compound is shown in Fig. 18. This mass spectrum contains many fewer data than the spectrum in Fig. 17. It may be inferred that the molecular mass is 260, from the *m/z* values for MH^+, $(M + 29)^+$, and $(M + 41)^+$, but this information is not sufficient for identification purposes. The great power of GC-MS and GC-MS/MS methods is due to the specificity of detection (along with high sensitivity of detection) that is attainable even when highly complex mixtures are under study. This is because both physical properties and chemical reaction properties are involved in the analysis. The retention behavior is dependent on a physical property (the free energy of solution of the solute in the liquid phase), while an EI mass spectrum is based upon a chemical reaction property (the unimolecular decomposition of an energized $M^{+\bullet}$ ion). Other types of reactions (for example, reaction with

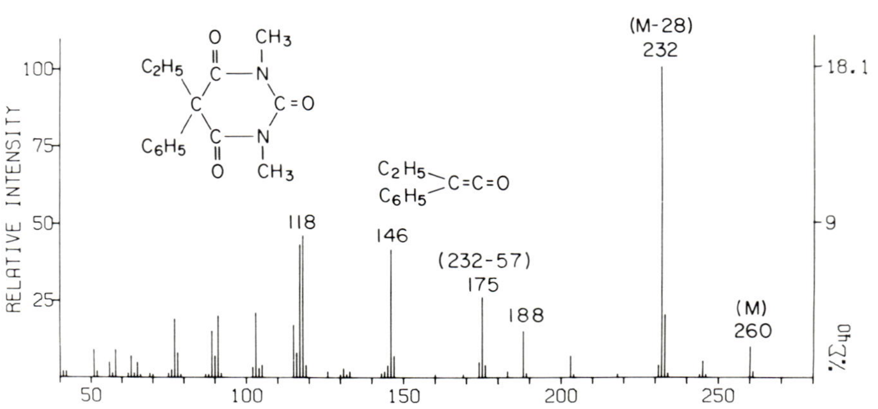

FIG. 17. EI ionization mass spectrum of the N,N′-dimethyl derivative of phenobarbital. The fragment ions provide structural information. The information content of an EI mass spectrum is generally greater than that of a CI mass spectrum.

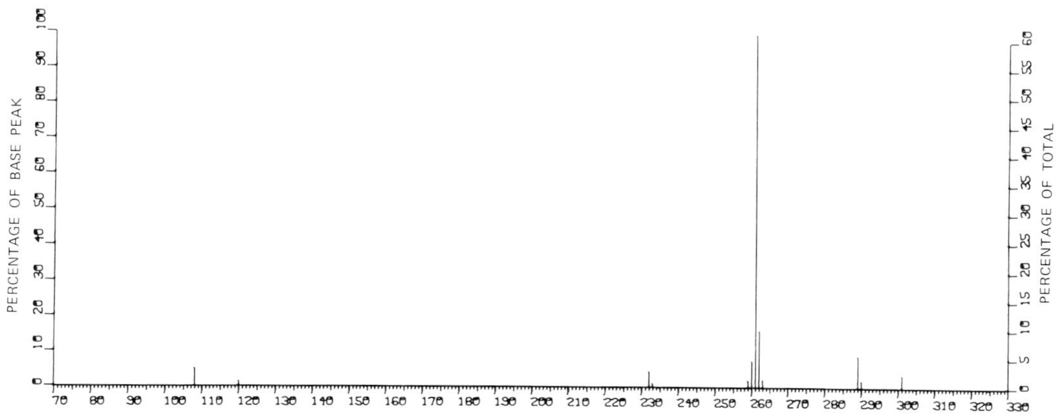

FIG. 18. Chemical ionization (CI) mass spectrum of the N,N′-dimethyl derivative of phenobarbital. The major ion corresponds to MH^+, and very little fragmentation is observed. Ions at $(M + 29)^+$ and $(M + 41)^+$ are usually also present when methane is used as the reagent.

$O_2^{-\bullet}$) may be used in quantitative work, but EI conditions are employed in structural studies.

Figure 19 shows an early example of a structural problem in drug metabolism. One of the metabolites of 5,5-diphenylhydantoin was found to contain two hydroxyl groups, and the EI mass spectrum of the N-methyl-O-TMS ether (Me-TMS) derivative contained an ion at *m/z* 191 which is characteristic of a TMS derivative of a vicinal glycol. This ion was at *m/z* 209 for the deuterium-labeled compound. This metabolite was assigned a dihydrodiol structure on the basis of its molecular mass and EI mass spectrum, and many metabolites of this type are now known. This was one of the first examples of a dihydrodiol metabolite of a drug to be studied by GC-MS analytical methods (77), and at that time other methods of instrumental study were also employed (41). In current studies of aromatic compounds, with TMS derivatives, an EI mass spectrum with an ion at *m/z* 191, moved to *m/z* 209 for the deuterium analog, is a virtually certain indication of a dihydrodiol structure.

Figure 20 shows the mass spectrum of the methyl ester-TMS ether (Me-TMS) derivative of the glucuronide of 9-phenanthrol. Ions at *m/z* 406/407 are characteristic of glucuronides derivatized in this way, and the *m/z* values for $M^{+\bullet}$ and $(M\text{-}15)^{+\bullet}$ correspond to a phenanthrol structure. After hydrolysis, the phen-

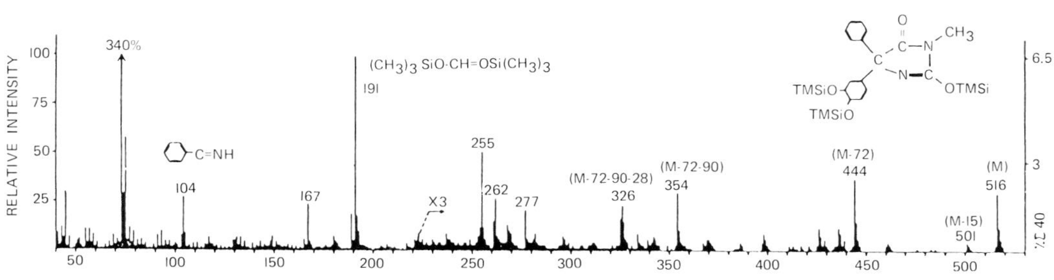

FIG. 19. EI ionization mass spectrum of the methyl-TMS ether (Me-TMS) derivative of a 5,5-diphenylhydantoin metabolite from human urine. This compound is a dihydrodiol which was formed from an intermediate epoxide. A prominent ion at *m/z* 191 is present in the mass spectrum of most metabolites of this kind (as TMS derivatives).

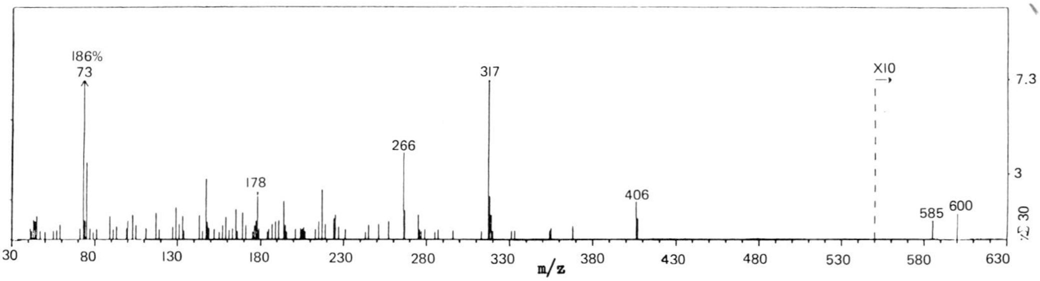

FIG. 20. EI ionization mass spectrum of the methyl ester-TMS ether (Me-TMS) derivative of the glucuronide of 9-phenanthrol. Ions at 406/407 are characteristic of TMS derivatives of glucuronides.

anthrol was identified as 9-phenanthrol. This urinary metabolite of phenanthrene was found during a study of phenanthrene metabolism in the guinea pig (89). A recent study by Cairns and Siegmund (31) describes a way of recognizing glucuronides by their CI (ammonia) mass spectra, and this procedure should be useful in studies of glucuronides separated by HPLC and analyzed without derivative formation.

Figure 21 shows the EI mass spectrum of the methylthio analog of the 9,10-dihydro-9,10-diol of phenanthrene, as the TMS ether. Methylthio compounds of this kind show $(M-47)^{+}$ and $(M-48)^{+\cdot}$ ions. In this instance, a reference sample of the compounds was prepared from the 9,10-oxide of phenanthrene in order to confirm the identity of the metabolite (89).

Chemical ionization MS is useful in sequence determination studies, and in general, in studies of conjugates of many kinds. A recent example is the study by Suzuki, Tatematsu and their colleagues of permethylated oligosaccharides (72). Another example is the study of the 22-phosphates of ecdysone and related compounds by FAB MS (81). Similar methods were used in identifying carboxylic acids related to ecdysone (80).

Negative ion mass spectra are highly useful

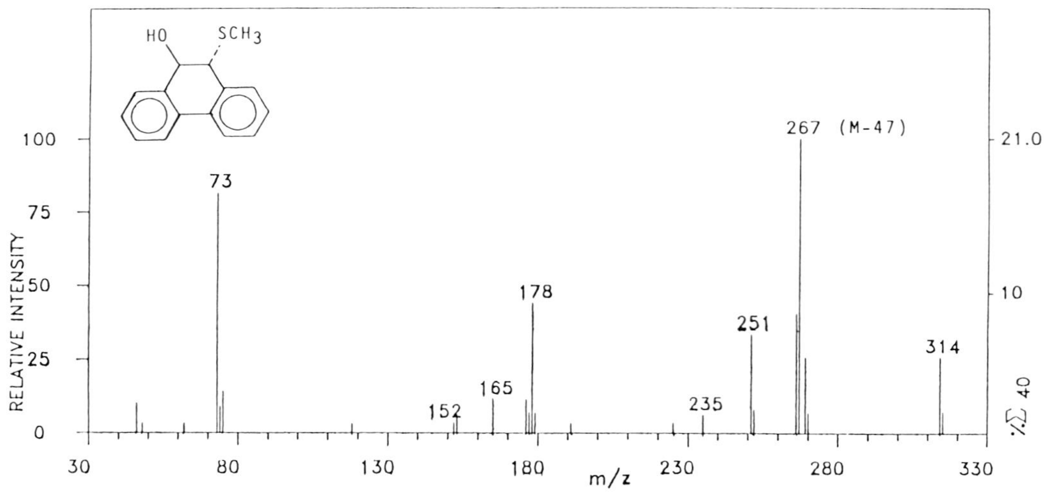

FIG. 21. EI ionization mass spectrum of the TMS derivative of the methylthio analog of the 9,10-dihydrodiol of phenanthrene. The precursor of this metabolite of phenanthrene is the 9,10-oxide.

for identification purposes in forensic work. They have also been employed recently in studies of pyrrolizidine alkaloids (51), in the classification of crude oils (26) by reaction with HO^-, and in the detection of chlorinated alkanes in fish (67).

Severe problems in identification with GC-MS systems are usually due to the presence of multiple isomers or great complexity of the sample. The approaches that have been used in these instances include increasing the separation capabilities through the use of open tubular capillary columns with special phases (104) and with two columns with different phases when necessary (104,116), and using selective ionizing reagents. An example of the latter is the use of chlorobenzene as a reagent gas for ionizing aromatic components in petroleum products (124).

Structural and identification studies by MS/MS techniques are likely to increase greatly as these analytical systems come into wider use. Recent investigations include those by McLafferty of fentanyl derivatives (42), studies of peptides (a recent example is the work of Hunt and his associates (78) on peptide sequencing); and a recent study by Gross of ornithine-containing lipids which employed both positive and negative ion modes (137).

The detection and identification of specific compounds in mixtures can often be carried out very effectively by MS/MS methods; this approach has been used by McLafferty and by Cooks in several investigations for example, in a study of quaternary alkaloids in cacti (45), and it is likely to become one of the major uses of MS/MS analytical systems. Other recent examples include the identification of sulfonamide drugs in swine liver (25); the identification of drugs in equine serum (23); and the identification of sulfur compounds in petroleum distillates (79).

The determination of absolute configuration and the identification and separate determination of enantiomers cannot be accomplished by MS alone. Chromatographic methods, however, can be used to separate enantiomers either directly (use of a chiral phase) or after appropriate derivatization (to form diastereoisomers). Recent examples include a study of ant 3-octanol (3) and of the enantiomers of γ-vinyl-γ-aminobutyric acid in the human (69).

QUANTITATIVE ANALYSIS OF COMPLEX MIXTURES

For compounds that are volatile, or that can be converted to volatile derivatives for separation by gas chromatography, the most useful form of quantitative analysis is by GC-MS bioanalytical systems with an EI or CI source. Analytical methods that are particularly useful for drug metabolism studies are generally called metabolic profile analyses; these methods were developed soon after GC-MS combined instruments came into use, and they are described in the preceding chapter. The very high degree of specificity in detection which is inherent in these methods is due to the use of both GC data and MS(EI) data; a combination of GC and MS(CI) data is less specific. Mass spectra (EI) are sometimes said to have the specificity of fingerprints, but this is not so; stereoisomers of some types give virtually identical EI spectra, and there is no difference in the mass spectrum of R- and S-forms. Positional isomers usually show different EI mass spectra. The GC retention behavior of positional isomers and diastereoisomers is usually not the same, and by combining a GC separation with EI mass spectral data it is possible to identify and quantify many compounds in complex mixtures. It is not unusual to find a large number of drug metabolites in an analysis of urine, for example, and detailed studies of the constituents of tobacco smoke and plant-derived odors have resulted in the identification of hundreds of compounds in mixtures. These separations can usually be quantified.

In most current quantitative work it is desirable to combine qualitative analytical methods with the capability of acquiring quantitative data at the same time. The increasing need for quantitative data in many applications has also led to the development of many different types of analytical methods that are rapid and that can be automated or easily reduced to routine operation. In most of these instances, analytical methods of higher specificity are needed to serve as definitive procedures, and very often the highest degree of specificity is provided by systems based upon MS.

One of the great advantages of mass spectrometric quantitative analysis is that small amounts of sample may be used. Many methods based on samples varying in amount from low picograms (or less) to low micrograms have been described. There was a tendency in early work to use relatively large samples because many GC columns were of low quality and component loss by adsorption was a common occurrence. With improvements in GC technology, and improved adsorption test procedures, sample sizes have decreased.

The chief disadvantage of mass spectrometric analytical methods, until recently, was the requirement for volatility of the organic compounds under study. Most organic compounds, with the exception of macromolecules, can now be converted into gas phase ions of the CI type, and both qualitative and quantitative analytical methods are now under development for use with DCI and FAB/SIMS sources. Current studies indicate that the most useful type of bioanalytical system for work of this kind will be a QQQ system (or a QQ equivalent) with a DCI or FAB/SIMS source. Analyses have been carried out with sample components as low as 10 to 15 ng.

Quantitative Analysis by Selected Ion Detection with GC-MS Bioanalytical Systems

These instrumental systems, in their current design, usually have capabilities for operation in either positive or negative ion mode (or concurrently by switching), and in either EI or CI mode, with the option of using either a packed or open tubular capillary GC column, and with a variety of options in computer and/or microprocessor-based operations related to obtaining, analyzing, and recording data. Other options usually include capabilities for obtaining mass spectra of nonvolatile compounds with DCI or FAB/SIMS techniques. Older systems may be limited to use in an EI positive ion mode, and early GC-MS combined instruments were manually operated.

The basic design of these bioanalytical systems includes, for the MS, an ion source, a mass analyzer, and a detector. Critical issues in quantitative analysis include the linearity of the instrumental response with respect to the amount of sample, the upper limit of the linear range, and the limit of detection. The characteristics of the GC column are also important; these include the polarity, efficiency, adsorption behavior, and bleed rate. Overall, the specificity of detection and the limit of detection, and the precision and accuracy of the analyses, will also be determined by the degree of skill and experience in preparing samples and in operating these systems that is available in the laboratory.

Figure 22 shows a comparison of positive ion and negative ion detection for ions generated in an API source by ion molecule and by electron molecule reactions, respectively (34). Samples were introduced by GC (packed column; SE-30 liquid phase). The linearity of response with respect to the amount of sample is evident, and similar data can be obtained with both CI and EI sources. The limit of detection is not the same for positive and negative ions. With most systems that have a single mass analyzer, the chemical noise is much higher in the positive ion mode than in the negative ion mode. The limit of detection is determined by the signal-to-noise ratio, and the difference in chemical noise in the two modes of operation is sufficiently high to have a marked effect on the detection limit. There may also be a difference in the rates of electron

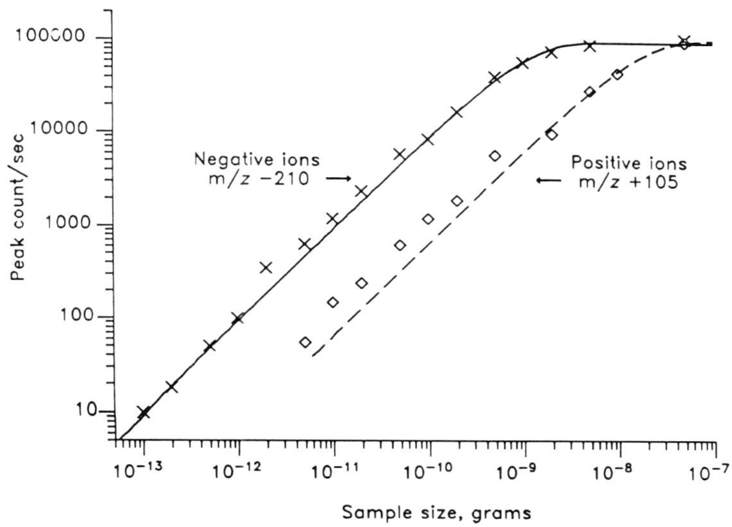

FIG. 22. Responses observed for positive and negative ions with benzil as the test compound and with an API source.

molecule reactions and ion molecule reactions, which leads to a lower limit of detection in the negative ion mode when this is based on electron capture reactions.

In many applications, adequate amounts of samples are available and quantitative data are required for only a few components of the sample. In these instances, the operating conditions involve stable, low noise baselines, and adsorption/decomposition of sample components is not usually encountered in the GC column or GC-MS interface. Internal standards are added as early as possible in the analytical scheme. The most useful internal standards are stable isotope-labeled compounds, but it should be realized that deuterium substitution may lead to small but easily observable alterations in GC behavior. This effect does not occur for ^{13}C, ^{15}N, or ^{18}O labeling. Homologs and analogs of compounds under study are also often used as internal standards.

Selected ion detection is carried out by rapid switching, on a continuing basis, between *m/z* values for the compounds under study and the internal standards. The data, when converted to strip chart records, resemble GC separation data (in effect, the MS is acting as a selective detector) and analytical results may be calculated on the basis of peak areas (peak heights can often be used in temperature programmed separations). Most computer-based systems provide programs that carry out the required calculations, but experience is required in establishing the conditions of analysis (both GC and MS). The ions that are monitored are usually relatively high intensity ions in the EI or CI mass spectrum. There are a number of technological problems associated with the use of stable isotope-labeled internal standards, with the design and execution of analytical schemes and with estimating the precision and accuracy of a specific analytical method. These are mentioned in a later section.

Analyses of this kind, where only one or a few components of the sample are of interest, and where the determinations are not carried out near the limit of detection, are used in a variety of ways. One use is to establish the validity of other methods of analysis ("definitive methods"). They are also used in environmental analyses, in therapeutic drug monitoring, in pharmacokinetic studies, and in drug metabolism studies.

Multicomponent Quantitative Analyses by Programmed Data Analysis with GC-MS Bioanalytical Systems

Most systems now include computer-based or microprocessor-based capabilities for carrying out analyses that are based on repetitive scanning. When this technique is used, together with a temperature programmed GC separation, it is possible to carry out multicomponent quantitative analyses by programmed analysis of the GC-MS data. External standards (usually long chain alkanes) are added in order to monitor the separation process; internal standards are added as usual. It is generally not possible to add as many internal standards as might be desirable, and when this is the case response factors are needed to complete the calculations. When expressed in strip chart form, these data are usually called "reconstructed gas chromatograms" or "reconstructed GC data." The reconstruction may be on the basis of total ion current (to show all components of the sample) or on the basis of selected ions which are specific for the compounds under study.

It is usually best to use EI conditions and packed columns when this method of analysis is employed. The specificity of the method in each application depends upon the ions chosen as the basis for the analysis, and the relatively long cycle time of many systems may not be compatible with the narrow peak width characteristic of open tubular capillary columns.

Variations of this method include selected ion detection during "windows" based on timed intervals or intervals between alkane peaks. In all instances programmed analyses are designed for repetitive use under uniform conditions, but the precision and accuracy of the results are not the same for all components and may vary with variations in individual samples. They are particularly useful in metabolic profile studies of all kinds where many components are quantified. The only comparable method of analysis of complex mixtures is by GC separation with open tubular capillary columns with 100,000 or higher theoretical plate efficiency, and when GC alone is used (with nonspecific detection by a hydrogen flame detector) it is necessary to carry out detailed identification studies by GC-MS methods in order to validate the GC procedure.

Quantitative Analyses with HPLC-MS Systems

The technological problems associated with HPLC-MS analyses are quite different from those encountered with GC-MS systems, and a generally useful HPLC-MS instrumental system which can be used for multicomponent quantitative analyses of nonvolatile samples has not yet been developed. Most current work with HPLC-MS systems is directed to the development of appropriate interfaces and sources, and to obtaining qualitative analytical data. There is no reason, however, why quantitative methods should prove to be unattainable. Some studies of quantitative methods have been carried out, and a few comparisons have been made of GC-MS and HPLC-MS data (58).

Quantitative Analyses with MS/MS Systems Without Chromatography

There is a general belief that quantitative single component or multicomponent analyses may be carried out with MS/MS systems, without chromatography, and with direct introduction of samples by probe or with use of DCI or FAB/SIMS sources. Our experience confirms this view, but in fact there are very few published data derived from quantitative methods. In almost all instances an internal standard was not used, and the results are treated on the basis of pattern recognition (presence or absence of specific compounds) or comparisons of selected ion intensities in different samples ("high" or "low" values). These studies were essentially concerned with detection and identification problems, rather than with problems of quantitative analysis, but it is usually assumed that the methods could be converted in the future to quantitative procedures by adding an internal standard(s) to the sample. Very high specificity in detection, and very low chemical noise, are characteristics of MS/MS systems, and these are valuable in quantitative work. The chief technological problems, as yet unresolved, are those involved in introducing internal standards into solid samples containing insoluble components, and generally of unwanted matrix effects in the ion source.

Recent Examples of Applications

The major quantitative uses of MS, since the development of GC-MS combined instruments, have been in biologic applications and in environmental analyses. Mass spectrometric quantitative analytical methods were introduced many years ago in the petroleum/petrochemical industry, and these uses are continuing, along with related applications in the chemical industry. It is not possible, because of the volume of literature describing both specific methods and general problems in biologic applications, to do more than provide a brief statement with a few examples of current work.

In recent years the symposia organized by De Leenheer and his colleagues, under the title "International Symposia on Quantitative Mass Spectrometry in Life Sciences," and held at the University of Ghent, have been a forum for the presentation and discussion of this subject, and the resulting journal articles (*Biomed. Mass Spectrom.*, 10(3), 1983, for example) reflect the state of the art. Numerous symposia and conferences continue to be concerned with environmental analyses and problems of environmental toxicology, and the regulatory aspects have led to detailed studies of mass spectrometric analytical methodology. The review by Cairns and his colleagues (33) contains a discussion of current approaches to a major problem—toxic agents in food and feed commodities. An earlier review (97) described the general problem of analytical methodology involving low concentrations of organic compounds.

It should be emphasized that the general principles of quantitative analysis apply to mass spectrometric analyses, and these are not new or unrecognized. The relatively great difference in results that still exists between many laboratories is due to the fact that personal experience and experimental skills are involved in many new applications. Fully automated systems may eliminate this factor in routine analyses, but it will always be present when new instruments and new methods are under development.

Methods that have the greatest degree of accuracy within a group of instrumental analytical methods, but which are not suitable for routine applications (because of time or cost considerations), are usually called "definitive methods," and they are used to validate other (usually routine) procedures. This is an important matter in studies of new therapeutic agents and in the work of clinical chemistry laboratories. Almost always, definitive procedures are based upon mass spectrometric analytical systems. At present, this usually means use of a GC-MS bioanalytical system; in the future, GC-MS/MS (QQQ) systems may be used more often. A recent example is the work of Jonckheere and De Leenheer (84) on the determination of cortisol in human serum.

The determination of endogenous compounds in blood, urine, and other tissues (human, animal, or plant), and of foreign compounds and their metabolites, is very often carried out with GC-MS systems. Recent examples include the work of Setchell et al. (122) on lignans excreted by humans; the studies of Liebich (91) on 4-heptanone; the determination of estrogens in serum (125,138); and the determination of mandelic acid (94), ketobemidone (19), melperone (40), and harringtonine and homoharringtonine (117) in plasma or serum.

Sweeley developed several GC-MS human metabolic profile analytical methods which involve programmed analysis. These include metabolic profiles for organic acids in urine (61,62,131), organic acids in plasma (82), and steroids in urine (151). Shackleton developed a metabolic profile method for human urinary steroids (123); Fennessey also used steroid profiles (55). Jellum (83) developed and described a group of metabolic profile screening procedures. These methods for multicomponent analyses require computer programs, and these can also be used with the metabolic profile procedures described in the previous chapter. It is not always realized that GC separations with an open tubular capillary column and hydrogen flame detection may have greater precision than computer-based programmed analyses of GC-MS repetitive scan data (because of ion statistics), but when GC separations are used for quantitative analysis the identities of the components should be established by GC-MS identification procedures.

Quantitative studies of steroid sulfates with a FAB source were carried out by Gaskell et al. (60). The magnitude of matrix effects in quantitative work with FAB/SIMS sources is not yet fully known.

PRECISION, ACCURACY, LIMIT OF DETECTION, LIMIT OF QUANTITATION, QUALITY CONTROL; TECHNOLOGICAL PROBLEMS; AND COMPARISONS OF METHODS

Evaluation of Data

The development and use of a new quantitative analytical method should include estimates of the precision and accuracy, and of the limit of detection. The limit of quantitation, a more recently defined term (97), is a larger value than the limit of detection; it is not possible to carry out quantitative analyses in an effective fashion at the limit of detection of an analytical system. Quality control measures should be instituted whenever analyses (new or old) are carried out.

In practice, it may be less easy to establish these values, and to establish adequate quality control guidelines, than to agree that this should always be done. In part, this is due to the fact that opinions differ with respect to the statistical approaches that should be used. This problem is illustrated in a recent discussion of ways of defining the limit of detection (92). The urgency of arriving at a more uniform approach to these matters, and to problems of quality control, increased greatly when environmental analyses became involved in regulatory decisions. Recommendations for quantitative analytical work, particularly where trace analysis methods are used, have been published (97).

A greater difficulty lies in the fact that accuracy is often more difficult to estimate than precision. Precision is defined in statistical terms (standard deviation expressions include standard deviation of the mean, pooled standard deviation, and relative standard deviation) and it is estimated without an estimate of accuracy. The accuracy of a procedure will not be better than the precision, but it may be considerably worse, and it may be subject to unexpected variation. The accuracy of a routine method may be estimated by comparisons with data from a definitive method. In many instances, however, accuracy is estimated by comparing data from blank samples with data from spiked or reference samples. In general, the validation of a quantitative method should follow current considerations (97).

The limit of quantitation (97) is currently defined as being 100 above the signal due to the blank; the limit of detection (92) is 30 above the blank signal. When larger samples are used in mass spectrometric methods, blank values are generally low and the often troublesome problems arising in trace analysis are greatly decreased or not present.

Quality control is a necessity in all quantitative work, but it is difficult to reduce this view to specific recommendations that cover all situations. Interlaboratory comparisons of data are usually the best way of demonstrating inadequate quality control or defects in methods. When reliable reference samples are available, however, it is possible to institute satisfactory quality control measures. The most difficult circumstance occurs when new methods are subject to error by apparently minor changes in procedure or reagents.

The precision attainable with mass spectrometric systems is very high, and the accuracy is usually only slightly poorer. It should not be concluded, however, that this means that all procedures based on mass spectrometry uniformly show high precision and accuracy. It was shown in a detailed study of the determination of cholesterol in serum by a bioanalytical system based on MS [the study was mentioned by Markey (101)] that the precision of the mass spectrometric measurements was better than that of the volumetric measurements of serum samples. The overall precision, with the use of pipetted samples, was determined by the mode of sample measurement and not by the bioanalytical system. Precision in analysis can be lost in many ways; the use of an MS does not lead instantly to high precision.

Technological Problems

Recurring technological problems are a frequent source of difficulty in quantitative work. It is not possible, in a brief review, to discuss these problems in detail, but several should be mentioned because of their general occurrence.

Stable isotope-labeled compounds are widely used as internal standards. Unlabeled material is always present in these compounds, and this may or may not lead to a noticeable effect on accuracy. This is a significant problem in trace analysis, and it has been discussed recently in terms of proposed programmed data analysis procedures (85,111,155).

Multicomponent analyses which include compounds present in low concentration, and trace analyses, are subject to losses arising from adsorption/decomposition on GC columns and in GC-MS interfaces. The usual cause of column loss is either an unsatisfactory column packing, or the presence of column adsorption sites in open tubular capillary columns that have not been bonded. Good columns, however, may be damaged by the use of samples which destroy the bonding used to deactivate surfaces. The usual remedy in these instances is to replace a few centimeters of column packing at the head of a packed column, or to remove a turn or two of an open tubular capillary column. Active adsorption sites are also the origin of loss in the heated connecting lines in GC-MS interfaces. These effects are minimized by allowing column bleed to coat the lines, and by frequent use of nonacidic silylating reagents.

The preparation of derivatives by appropriate methods is a critical matter in much GC-MS work. Many detailed studies have been reported; the early work of Brooks et al. (4,22), Chambaz and Horning (38,39), Devaux et al. (49,50), Horning and Maume (75), and Thenot and Horning (132–135) on steroid derivatives is an example. Good instrumental practices cannot compensate for unsatisfactory sample preparation. Matrix effects in MS and MS/MS procedures are known to occur (27,87,149), but they have not yet received adequate study for FAB/SIMS sources.

Comparison of Methods

In the field of environmental analysis, a number of comparisons have been made of analytical methods based on MS. A study that compared GC-MS (high resolution), GC-MS/MS and MS/MS with probe introduction of samples was recently carried out for polychlorinated biphenyls and 2,3,7,8-tetrachlorodibenzofuran (149). The paper should be consulted for details of the work. It was concluded that GC-MS (high resolution) and GC-MS/MS gave more reliable results than the

MS/MS procedure without chromatography because of matrix effects. The use of fused silica capillary columns was compared with the use of packed columns in a GC-MS system for the determination of organic contaminants in water (53). The sweep time was 4.3 sec for the packed column procedure and 1 sec for the open tubular capillary method. The relative standard deviations were about the same for both procedures. A comparison was made of response factors for 53 priority pollutants determined with a GC/MS and a GC-MS/MS (triple quadrupole) system (121). The values were not greatly different ($\pm15\%$) and the precision was about the same for the two instrumental systems. The chief differences that would be expected in comparing GC-MS and GC-MS/MS methods are a lower detection limit in the positive ion mode, and better accuracy in the analysis of complex samples, for GC-MS/MS systems. Precision and accuracy of sediment analyses were studied (93).

TRACE ORGANIC ANALYSIS IN BIOLOGIC STUDIES

Trace organic analyses usually require the use of instrumental systems with subpicogram limits of detection. In the positive ion mode, this detection limit can be attained with GC-MS (high resolution) and GC-MS/MS (QQQ) systems, but generally not with GC-MS systems. In the negative ion mode, this limit is attainable with all systems, and there may be no advantages gained by using a GC-MS/MS or GC/MS (high resolution) system. There are also a number of important trace analyses that can be carried out when the detection limit is about 10 to 100 pg in the positive ion mode, and this is usually attainable with GC/MS systems. The limit of quantitation is 3.3-fold above the detection limit; the precision normally improves as the sample size increases above this limit.

Trace analyses require much attention to all steps in the analytical procedure. These usually include isolation of a chemical sample of the analyte(s) from the biologic sample, derivative formation, and instrumental analysis. In some instances, near-trace analyses can be carried out with a minimum amount of sample processing. Almost always, the instrumental analysis is carried out near or beyond the manufacturer's specification of quantitation limits, and good instrumental practices must be followed.

Mass spectrometric methods have been used for many years in prostaglandin studies, both for structural determinations and for tissue analyses. Two recent methods illustrate different approaches to quantitative analytical procedures. In each instance, new derivatization sequences were developed. Early work on GC derivatives (147) indicated that TMS ester-TMS ether and methoxime-TMS ester-TMS ether (MO-TMS) derivatives could be used in GC and GC-MS studies of most prostaglandins. Continued experience, however, indicated that it would be desirable in this and other applications to use derivatives showing greater stability toward hydrolysis than TMS esters. In extended studies by Miyazaki and his colleagues, it was found that isopropyldimethylsilyl derivatives (ethers and esters) were much more stable than the corresponding TMS derivatives, and that the rate of their formation was not too slow for general use. An analytical method for prostaglandins was developed, based on the formation of methyl ester-isopropyldimethylsilyl ether and methoxime-methyl ester-isopropyldimethylsilyl ether derivatives, and on the use of a GC-MS system in the positive ion mode (110). The limit of detection was about 5 pg.

tert-Butyldimethylsilyl ether derivatives, introduced by Corey in synthetic studies, were used as prostaglandin derivatives by Mai et al. (100). These derivatives are much more resistant to hydrolysis than TMS ethers.

A different approach to the instrumental analysis of prostaglandins was taken by Blair, Barrow, and their associates (11,152). In order to use the negative ion mode of analysis, a new sequence was established for derivative formation. This was based upon the formation of methoxime-pentafluorobenzyl ester-TMS ether derivatives. A new isolation procedure was also developed. The instrumental analyses were carried out with a GC-MS system in the negative ion mode (loss of the pentafluorobenzyl radical) and with an open tubular capillary column. The method was developed for the determination of 6-oxoprostaglandin $F_{1\alpha}$, it was also suitable for thromboxane B_2. The limit of detection was 2 pg in the negative ion mode (CI-methane), and about 500 pg in the positive ion mode (EI).

The negative ion mode of operation with a GC-MS system was used by Markey in studies of biologic amines. An analytical method for melatonin was developed (90,101); this was based upon a rearrangement product (formed in a hot injection zone or in a hot source) of the pentafluoropropionyl derivative. A similar method was later used for the determination of serotonin (102). The limit of quantitation was estimated to be about 10 pg for serotonin.

A negative ion mass spectrometric method was developed by Foltz et al. (57) for the determination of Δ^9-tetrahydrocannabinol (and two metabolites). An open tubular capillary column was used in the GC-MS system.

The detection and determination of highly toxic substances in human or animal tissues (and in air, water, plants and plant products, or soil) often requires trace analyses by mass spectrometric methods. Many of these compounds do not require derivatization before the instrumental analysis step, but very high specificity in detection is needed. In these instances, the most suitable systems are GC-MS (high resolution), GC-MS/MS (QQQ), GC-MS (API), or GC-MS (API)/MS (QQQ). An example of the use of a GC-MS (high resolution) system is the determination of N-nitrosodimethylamine by Webb et al. (153). The limit of detection was 300 fg.

The problem of nicotine analysis in plasma was studied by Enzell and his colleagues (86). A GC/MS (high resolution) system was used. In our experience, based upon MS (API) analyses for nicotine, all individuals in an urban environment, and working in air-conditioned buildings, show low plasma concentrations of nicotine. This is because of the prevalence of cigarette smoking and the transfer of nicotine by air. The nicotine in laboratory or office air (vaporized or on aerosol particulates) may be sufficiently high to require the use of glove boxes in sample handling. Plasma samples that do not contain nicotine can only be obtained from individuals who have no direct or indirect contact with cigarette smoking. Relatively high plasma concentrations can be determined in a variety of ways; the plasma half-life is short, however, and low concentrations should be determined by mass spectrometric methods.

Environmental studies of 2,3,7,8-tetrachlorodibenzodioxin (2,3,7,8-TCDD) require reliable methods of analysis. The chief difficulties, aside from the fact that low concentrations must be detected and quantified, arise from the fact that isomers and analogs of 2,3,7,8-TCDD are also usually present (there are 22 positional TCDD isomers, and 75 chlorinated dibenzodioxins), and from the ubiquitous presence of polychlorobiphenyls in concentrations that may be many times greater than that of 2,3,7,8-TCDD. Chlorinated methoxybiphenyls may also be present (115). The Seveso incident (28) led to increased concern about the biologic effects of 2,3,7,8-TCDD, and this has continued because of the exposure of many individuals to Agent Orange. Several analytical methods based on high resolution MS have been described. The analytical problem was reviewed by Cairns et al. (30). Mitchum and his colleagues developed a method based upon API MS (109). The gas phase reaction of 2,3,7,8-TCDD with $O_2^{-\bullet}$ leads to a negative semiquinone ion, and this is a highly specific method. The chromatographic separation is also critical because of the possible presence of other chlorinated compounds. A study by Buser and Rappe (29) indicated that an unequivocal identification of 2,3,7,8-TCDD can be made by using a system with appropriate open tubular capillary columns.

Analyses of urine for 2,3-dibromopropanol, a metabolite of "tris" (the phosphate ester of

2,3-dibromopropranol), were carried out by GC-MS (API) with detection of Br^- ions (18). The specificity of detection was increased by the fact that bromine has two stable isotopes.

Environmental analyses based upon GC-MS/MS systems are now being reported. In all trace analyses, it would be helpful if analytical data could be obtained in several different types of mass spectrometric systems. This may become possible in the future.

Numerous additional trace analysis methods have been published. These examples were chosen to illustrate current or recent problems and a range of methods.

EXACT MASS DETERMINATION

Exact mass determinations are valuable in structural studies. The most precise and accurate measurements of mass are those made by ion cyclotron resonance/Fourier transform MS, but at present it is difficult to use these instruments in analytical studies of moderately large molecules that are not highly volatile. The method has been described for use with and without a calibrant (154). The most widely used methods in the past were based upon the use of photographic plates in EB instruments with Mattauch–Herzog geometry, or upon peak matching devices. The increasing use of FAB/SIMS sources for studies of nonvolatile compounds, and of MS/MS instruments as well as high resolution instruments to obtain unmixed ion species, has led to renewed interest in peak matching devices. When a rotatable probe was used with a FAB source (in order to generate strong signals from both "unknown" and calibrant), the error in exact mass measurement, made to mass values above 1500, was 1 to 2 ppm (66). Peak matching in the negative ion mode, with a high resolution instrument, was also recently reported (51). If some structural information is available, exact mass measurements are helpful in confirming ion identities.

ISOTOPE RATIO MEASUREMENTS

Measurements of isotope ratios, with mass spectrometers designed for that purpose, are carried out in specialized laboratories. The methods are not within the scope of this summary.

CONCLUSION

The most effective methods now known for the analysis of complex mixtures of biologic origin are based upon MS. Earlier methods were essentially restricted to volatile compounds or to compounds that could be converted to volatile derivatives. Although further work on quantitative methodology is needed, the methods can now be extended to nonvolatile compounds, except for macromolecules. The scope of gas phase organic ion chemistry has also widened to provide new methods for structural and identification studies. Very high specificity, and a very low limit of detection, can be attained in quantitative work in single or multicomponent analyses.

REFERENCES

1. Aberth, W., Straub, K. M., and Burlingame, A. L. (1982): Secondary ion mass spectrometry with cesium ion primary beam and liquid target matrix for analysis of bioorganic components. *Anal. Chem.*, 54:2029–2034.
2. Arpino, P. J., Bounine, J. P., Dedieu, M., and Guiochon, G. (1983): Optimization of the instrumental parameters of a combined liquid chromatograph-mass spectrometer, coupled by an interface for direct liquid introduction. IV. A new desolvation chamber for droplet focusing or Townsend discharge ionization. *J. Chromatogr.*, 271:43–50.
3. Attygalle, A. B., Morgan, E. D., Evershed, R. P., and Rowland, S. J. (1983): Comparison of three derivatives for the enantiomeric separation of chiral alcohols and the absolute configuration of *Myrmica* ant 3-octanol. *J. Chromatogr.*, 260:411–417.
4. Baillie, T. A., Brooks, C. J. W., and Horning, E. C. (1972): O-Butyloximes and O-pentyloximes as derivatives for the study of ketosteroids by gas chromatography. *Anal. Lett.*, 5:351–361.
5. Baldwin, M. A., and McLafferty, F. W. (1973): Direct chemical ionization of relatively involatile samples. Application to underivatized oligopeptides. *Org. Mass Spectrom.*, 7:1353–1356.
6. Barber, M., Bardoli, R. S., Elliott, G. J., Sedgwick, R. D., and Tyler, A. N. (1982): Fast atom bombardment mass spectrometry. *Anal. Chem.*, 54:645A–657A.
7. Barber, M., Bardoli, R. S., Sedgwick, R. D., and Tyler, A. N. (1981): Fast atom bombardment of

solids (F.A.B.): A new ion source for mass spectrometry. *J. Chem. Soc. Chem. Commun.*, 325–327.
8. Barber, M., Bordoli, R. S., Sedgwick, R. D., and Tyler, A. N. (1981): Fast atom bombardment of solids as an ion source in mass spectrometry. *Nature*, 293:270–275.
9. Barber, M., Bardoli, R. S., Sedgwick, R. D., and Tyler, A. N. (1981): Fast atom bombardment mass spectrometry of cobalamines. *Biomed. Mass Spectrom.*, 8:492–495.
10. Barofsky, D. F., Giessman, U., Bell, A. E., and Swanson, L. W. (1983): Molecular secondary ion mass spectrometry with a liquid metal ion primary source. *Anal. Chem.*, 55:1318–1323.
11. Barrow, S. E., Waddell, K. A., Ennis, M., Dollery, C. T., and Blair, I. A. (1982): Analysis of picomolar concentrations of 6-oxoprostaglandin $F_{1\alpha}$ in biological fluids. *J. Chromatogr.*, 239:71–80.
12. Behrisch, R., Editor (1980): *Sputtering by Ion Bombardment*. Springer, Heidelberg.
13. Benninghoven, A. (1982): Secondary ion mass spectrometry of organic compounds. *Trends Anal. Chem.*, 1:311–314.
14. Benninghoven, A., and Sichterman, W. (1977): Secondary ion mass spectrometry: A new analytical technique for biologically important compounds. *Org. Mass Spectrom.*, 12:595–597.
15. Benninghoven, A., and Sichtermann, W. (1978): Detection, identification and structural investigation of biologically important compounds by secondary ion mass spectrometry. *Anal. Chem.*, 50:1180–1184.
16. Bernard, C. (1865): *Introduction a l'Étude de la Médecin Experimentale*, Chapter 1. Bailliere, Paris.
17. Blakley, C. R., and Vestal, M. L. (1983): Thermospray interface for liquid chromatography/mass spectrometry. *Anal. Chem.*, 55:750–754.
18. Blum, A., Gold, M. D., Ames, B. N., Kenyon, C., Jones, F. R., Hett, E. A., Dougherty, R. C., Horning, E. C., Dzidic, I., Carroll, D. I., Stillwell, R. N., and Thenot, J.-P. (1978): Children absorb *tris*-BP flame retardant from sleepwear: Urine contains the mutagenic metabolite, 2,3-dibromopropanol. *Science*, 201:1020–1023.
19. Boudesson, U., Hartvig, P., Abrahamsson, L., and Ahnfelt, N.-O. (1983): Simultaneous determination of ketobemidone and its N-demethylated metabolite in patient plasma samples by gas chromatography mass spectrometry with selected ion monitoring. *Biomed. Mass Spectrom.*, 10:283–286.
20. Brandenberger, H. (1979): Negative ion mass spectrometry—A new tool for the forensic toxicologist. In: *Instrumental Applications in Forensic Drug Chemistry*, edited by M. Klein, A. V. Kruegel, and S. P. Sobol, pp. 48–59. U.S. Government Printing Office, Washington, D.C.
21. Brandenberger, H., and Ryhage, R. (1978): In: *Recent Developments in Mass Spectrometry in Biochemistry and Medicine*, edited by A. Frigerio, pp. 327–341. Plenum, New York.
22. Brooks, C. J. W., and Middleditch, B. J. (1972): Uses of chloromethyldimethylsilyl ethers as derivatives for combined gas chromatography-mass spectrometry of steroids. *Anal. Lett.*, 5:611–618.
23. Brotherton, H. O., and Yost, R. A. (1983): Determination of drugs in blood serum by mass spectrometry/mass spectrometry. *Anal. Chem.*, 55:549–553.
24. Bruins, A. P., and Dreuth, B. F. H. (1983): Experiments with the combination of a micro liquid chromatograph and a chemical ionization mass spectrometer, using a capillary interface for direct liquid introduction. Some theoretical considerations concerning the evaporation of liquids from capillaries into vacuum. *J. Chromatogr.*, 271:61–71.
25. Brumley, W. C., Min, Z., Matusik, J. E., Roach, J. A. G., Barnes, C. J., Sphon, J. A., and Fazio, T. (1983): Identification of sulfonamide drugs in swine liver by collision-induced dissociation/mass spectrometry. *Anal. Chem.*, 55:1405–1409.
26. Burke, P., Jenninger, K. R., Morgan, R. P., and Gilchrist (1982): Identification of crude oils by selective chemical ionization mass spectrometry. *Anal. Chem.*, 54:1304–1308.
27. Busch, K. L., Hsu, B. H., Xie, Y.-X., and Cooks, R. G. (1983): Matrix effects in secondary ion mass spectrometry. *Anal. Chem.*, 55:1157–1160.
28. Buser, H. R. (1982): The Seveso accident—An environmental application of mass spectrometry. *Trands Anal. Chem.*, 1:318–321.
29. Buser, H. R., and Rappe, C. (1980): High-resolution gas chromatography of the 22 tetrachlorodibenzo-*p*-dioxin isomers. *Anal. Chem.*, 52:2257–2262.
30. Cairns, T., Fishbein, L., and Mitchum, R. K. (1980): Review of the dioxin problem. Mass spectrometric analyses of tetrachlorodioxins in environmental samples. *Biomed. Mass Spectrom.*, 7:484–492.
31. Cairns, T., and Siegmund, E. G. (1982): Characterization of glucuronides by chemical ionization mass spectrometry with ammonia as reagent gas. *Anal. Chem.*, 54:2456–2461.
32. Cairns, T., Siegmund, E. G., and Dovse, G. M. (1983): Liquid chromatography mass spectrometry of thermally labile pesticides. *Biomed. Mass Spectrom.*, 10:24–29.
33. Cairns, T., Siegmund, E. G., Jacobson, R. A., Barry, T., Petzurger, G., Morris, W., and Heikes, A. A. (1983): Application of mass spectrometry in the regulatory analysis of pesticides and industrial chemicals in food and feed commodities. *Biomed. Mass Spectrom.*, 10:301–315.
34. Carroll, D. I., Dzidic, I., Horning, E. C., and Stillwell, R. N. (1981): Atmospheric pressure ionization mass spectrometry. *Appl. Spectrom. Rev.*, 17:337–406.
35. Carroll, D. I., Dzidic, I., Stillwell, R. N., Horning, M. G., and Horning, E. C. (1974): A subpicogram detection system for gas phase analysis based upon atmospheric pressure ionization (API) mass spectrometry. *Anal. Chem.*, 46:706–710.
36. Carroll, D. I., Nowlin, J. G., Stillwell, R. N., and Horning, E. C. (1981): Adduct ion formation in chemical ionization mass spectrometry of nonvolatile organic compounds. *Anal. Chem.*, 53:2007–2013.
37. Chait, B. T., and Standing, K. G. (1981): A time-of-flight mass spectrometer for measurement of secondary ion mass spectra. *Int. J. Mass Spectrom. Ion Phys.*, 40:185–193.
38. Chambaz, E. M., and Horning, E. C. (1967): Steroid trimethylsilyl ethers. *Anal. Lett.*, 1:201–211.

39. Chambaz, E. M., and Horning, E. C. (1969): The conversion of steroids to trimethylsilyl derivatives for gas phase analytical studies. Reactions of silylating reagents. *Anal. Biochem.*, 30:7–24.
40. Chan, K. Y., and Okerholm, R. A. (1983): Quantitative analysis of melperone in human plasma by gas chromatography-mass spectrometry-selected ion monitoring. *J. Chromatogr. Biomed. Appl.*, 274:121–127.
41. Chang, T., Savory, A., and Glazko, A. J. (1970): A new metabolite of 5,5-diphenylhydantoin (Dilantin). *Biochem. Biophys. Res. Commun.*, 38:444–449.
42. Cheng, M. T., Kruppa, G. H., McLafferty, F. W., and Cooper, D. A. (1982): Structural information from tandem mass spectrometry for China White and related fentanyl derivatives. *Anal. Chem.*, 54:2204–2207.
43. Christensen, R. G., White, E., Meiselman, S., and Hertz, H. S. (1983): Quantitative trace analysis by reversed-phase liquid chromatography mass spectrometry. *J. Chromatogr.*, 271:61–70.
44. Clupek, J. D., Zakett, D., and Cooks, R. G. (1982): High and low energy collision mass spectrometry/mass spectrometry of aza and amino polynuclear aromatic compounds in coal-derived liquids. *Anal. Chem.*, 54:2215–2219.
45. Davis, D. V., Cooks, R. G., Meyer, B. N., and McLaughlin, J. L. (1983): Identification of naturally occurring quaternary compounds by combined laser desorption and tandem mass spectrometry. *Anal. Chem.* 55:1302–1305.
46. Day, R. J., Unger, S. E., and Cooks, R. G. (1980): Molecular secondary ion mass spectrometry. *Anal. Chem.*, 52:557A–572A.
47. Day, R. J., Unger, S. E., and Cooks, R. G. (1980): Phenanthroline cationization by various methods in secondary ion mass spectrometry. *Anal. Chem.*, 52:353–354.
48. Dell, A., and Morris, H. R. (1982): Fast atom bombardment-high field magnet mass spectrometry of 6000 dalton polypeptides. *Biochem. Biophys. Res. Commun.*, 106:1456–1462.
49. Devaux, P. G., and Horning, E. C. (1969): Testosterone heptafluorobutyrates: Derivatives for gas chromatography. *Anal. Lett.*, 2:637–648.
50. Devaux, P. G., Horning, M. G., and Horning, E. C. (1971): Benzyloxime derivatives of steroids. A new metabolic profile procedure for human urinary steroids. *Anal. Lett.*, 4:151–160.
51. Drelfuss, P. A., Brumley, W. C., Sphon, J. A., and Caress, E. A. (1983): Negative ion chemical ionization mass spectrometry of pyrrolizidine alkaloids with hydroxide reactant ion. *Anal. Chem.*, 55:1036–1040.
52. Edmonds, C. G., McCloskey, J. A., and Edwards, V. A. (1983): A bibliography of combined liquid chromatography mass spectrometry. *Biomed. Mass Spectrom.*, 10:237–238.
53. Eichelberger, J. W., Kerns, E. H., Olynyk, P., and Budde, W. L (1983): Precision and accuracy in the determination of organics in water by fused silica capillary column gas chromatography/mass spectrometry and packed column gas chromatography/mass spectrometry. *Anal. Chem.*, 55:1471–1479.
54. Eicke, A., Anders, V., Junack, M., Sichtermann, W., and Benninghoven, A. (1983): Secondary ion mass spectrometry of folic acid analogues. *Anal. Chem.*, 55:178–182.
55. Fennessey, P. V., Marsh, P. G., Orr, E. R., Burnstein, P., and Betz, G. (1983): Determination of steroid profiles in healthy and diseased states: Identification and quantification of a block of 17α-hydroxylase. *Clin. Chim. Acta,* 129:3–11.
56. Fenselau, C. C. (1982): Mass spectrometry of middle molecules. *Anal. Chem.*, 54:105A–116A.
57. Foltz, R. L., McGinnis, K. M., and Chinn, D. M. (1983): Quantitative measurement of Δ^9-tetrahydrocannabinol and two major metabolites in physiological specimens using capillary column gas chromatography negative ion chemical ionization mass spectrometry. *Biomed. Mass Spectrom.*, 10:316–323.
58. Foster, M. G., Meresz, O., Graves, D. E., Lant, M. S., and Westwood, S. A. (1983): Capillary gas chromatographic mass spectrometric and microbore liquid chromatographic mass spectrometric studies of a test well sample from a landfill site. *Biomed. Mass Spectrom.*, 10:338–342.
59. Frangi-Schnyder, D., and Brandenberger, H. (1978): Anion-CI-mass spectrometry of the main classes of hypnotics. *Z. Anal. Chem.*, 290:153–154.
60. Gaskell, S. J., Brownsey, B. G., Brooks, P. W., and Green, B. N. (1983): Fast atom bombardment mass spectrometry of steroid sulfates: Qualitative and quantitative analyses. *Biomed. Mass Spectrom.*, 10:215–219.
61. Gates, S. C., Dendramis, N., and Sweeley, C. C. (1978): Automated metabolic profiling of organic acids in human urine. I. Description of methods. *Clin. Chem. (Winston-Salem, N.C.),* 24:1674–1679.
62. Gates, S. C., and Sweeley, C. C. (1978): Quantitative metabolic profiling based on gas chromatography. *Clin. Chem. (Winston-Salem, N.C.),* 24:1663–1673.
64. German, A. L., and Horning, E. C. (1973): Thermostable open tube capillary columns for the high resolution gas chromatography of human urinary steroids. *J. Chromatogr. Sci.*, 11:76–82.
65. German, A. L., Pfaffenberger, C. D., Thenot, J.-P., Horning, M. G., and Horning, E. C. (1973): High resolution gas chromatography with thermostable glass capillary columns. *Anal. Chem.*, 45:930–935.
66. Gilliam, J. M., Landis, P. W., and Occolowitz, J. L. (1983): Accurate mass measurement in fast atom bombardment mass spectrometry. *Anal. Chem.*, 55:1531–1533.
67. Gjos, N., and Gustavsen, K. O. (1982): Determination of chlorinated paraffins by negative ion chemical ionization mass spectrometry. *Anal. Chem.*, 54:1316–1318.
68. Haahti, E. O. A., VandenHeuvel, W. J. A., and Horning, E. C. (1961): Separation of urinary 17-ketosteroids by gas chromatography. *Anal. Biochem.*, 2:182–187.
69. Haegele, K. D., Schoun, J., Alken, R. G., and Huebert, N. D. (1983): Determination of the R(−) and S(+)-enantiomers of γ-vinyl-γ-aminobutyric acid in human body fluids by gas chromatography-mass spectrometry. *J. Chromatogr. Biomed. Appl.*, 274:103–110.

70. Hakansson, P., Kamensky, I., Sundqvist, B., Fohlman, J., Peterson, P., McNeal, C. J., and Macfarlane, R. D. (1982): ^{127}I-Plasma desorption mass spectrometry of insulin. *J. Am. Chem. Soc.*, 104:2948–2949.
71. Hammar, C. G., Holmstedt, B., and Ryhage, R. (1968): Mass fragmentography: Identification of chlorpromazine and its metabolites in human blood by a new method. *Anal. Biochem.*, 25:532–548.
72. Harada, K., Ito, S., Takeda, N., Suzuki, M., and Tatematsu, A. (1983): Sequence determination of permethylated oligosaccharides by chemical ionization mass spectrometry. *Biomed. Mass Spectrom.*, 10:5–12.
73. Horning, E. C., Carroll, D. I., Dzidic, I., and Stillwell, R. N. (1981): In: *Electron Capture: Theory and Practice in Chromatography,* edited by A. Zlatkis and C. F. Poole, pp. 359–375. Elsevier, Amsterdam.
74. Horning, E. C., Horning, M. G., Carroll, D. I., Dzidic, I., and Stillwell, R. N. (1973): A new picogram detection system based on a mass spectrometer with an external ionization source at atmospheric pressure. *Anal. Chem.*, 45:936–943.
75. Horning, E. C., and Maume, B. F. (1969): Derivatives of aldosterone for gas phase analysis. *J. Chromatogr. Sci.*, 7:411–418.
76. Horning E. C., Mitchell, J. R., Horning, M. G., Stillwell, W. G., Stillwell, R. N., Nowlin, J. G., and Caroll, D. I. (1979): Plasma desorption mass spectrometry. *Trends Pharmacol. Sci.*, 3:76–80.
77. Horning, M. G., Stratton, C., Wilson, A., Horning, E. C., and Hill, R. M. (1971): Detection of 5-(3,4-dihydroxy-1,5-cyclohexadien-1-yl)-5-phenyl hydantoin as a major metabolite of 5,5-diphenylhydantoin (Dilantin) in the newborn human. *Anal. Lett.*, 4:537–545.
78. Hunt, D. F., Buko, A. M., Ballard, J. M., Shabanowitz, J., and Giordani, A. B. (1981): Sequence analysis of polypeptides by collision activated dissociation on a triple quadrupole mass spectrometer. *Biomed. Mass Spectrom.*, 8:397–408.
79. Hunt, D. F., and Shabanowitz, J. (1982): Determination of organosulfur compounds in hydrocarbon matrices by collision-activated dissociation mass spectrometry. *Anal. Chem.*, 54:574–578.
80. Isaac, R. E., Milner, N. P., and Rees, H. H. (1983): Identification of ecdysonoic acid and 20-hydroxyecdysonoic acid isolated from developing eggs of *Schistocerca gregaria* and pupae of *Spodoptera littoralis. Biochem. J.*, 213:261–265.
81. Isaac, R. E., Rose, M. E., Rees, H. H., and Goodwin, T. W. (1983): Identification of the 22-phosphate esters of ecdysone, 2-deoxyecdysone, 20-hydroxyecdysone and 2-deoxy-20-hydroxyecdysone from newly laid eggs of the desert locust, *Schistocerca gregaria. Biochem. J.*, 213:533–541.
82. Issachar, D., Holland, J. F., and Sweeley, C. C. (1982): Metabolic profiles of organic acids from human plasma. *Anal. Chem.*, 54:29–32.
83. Jellum, E. (1979): Profiling of human body fluids in healthy and diseased states using gas chromatography and mass spectrometry, with special reference to organic acids. *J. Chromatogr. Biomed. Appl.*, 143:427–462.
84. Jonckheere, J. A., and De Leenheer, A. P. (1983): Candidate definitive method for the determination of cortisol in human serum. *Biomed. Mass Spectrom.*, 10:197–202.
85. Jonckheere, J. A., De Leenheer, A. P., and Steyaert, H. L. (1983): Statistical evaluation of calibration curve nonlinearity in isotope dilution gas chromatography/mass spectrometry. *Anal. Chem.*, 55:153–155.
86. Jones, D., Curvall, M., Abrahamsson, L., Kazemi-Vala, E., and Enzell, C. (1982): Quantitative analysis of plasma nicotine using selected ion monitoring at high resolution. *Biomed. Mass Spectrom.*, 9:539–545.
87. Kallos, G. J., Caldecourt, V., and Tou, J. C. (1982): Matrix effects in quantitation and identification by chemical ionization mass spectrometry. *Anal. Chem.*, 54:1313–1316.
88. Keogh, T. (1982): Dimethyl ether as a reagent gas for organic functional group determination by chemical ionization mass spectrometry. *Anal. Chem.*, 54:2540–2547.
89. Lertratanangkoon, K., Horning, M. G., Middleditch, B. S., Tsang, W.-S., and Griffin, G. W. (1982): Urinary bivalent sulfur metabolites of phenanthrene excreted by the rat and guinea pig. *Drug Metab. Dispos.*, 10:614–623.
90. Lewy, A. J., and Markey, S. P. (1978): Analysis of melatonin in human plasma by gas chromatography negative chemical ionization mass spectrometry. *Science,* 201:741–743.
91. Liebich, H. M. (1983): Gas chromatographic-mass spectrometric determination of total 4-heptanone, a new marker in diabetes mellitus. *J. Chromatogr. Biomed. Appl.*, 273:67–75.
92. Long, G. L., and Winefordner, J. R. (1983): Limit of detection. *Anal. Chem.*, 55:713A–724A.
93. Lopez-Avila, V., Northcutt, R., Onstot, J., and Wickham, M. (1983): Determination of 51 priority organic compounds after extraction from standard reference materials. *Anal. Chem.*, 55:881–889.
94. Luthe, H., Ludwig-Kohn, H., and Langenbeck, U. (1983): Quantitative gas chromatographic mass spectrometric determination of mandelic acid in blood plasma: Comparison of deuterated and homologous internal standards. *Biomed. Mass Spectrom.*, 10:183–186.
95. Luukkainen, T., VandenHeuvel, W. J. A., Haati, E. V. A., and Horning, E. C. (1961): Gas chromatographic behavior of trimethylsilyl ethers of steroids. *Biochem. Biophys. Acta,* 52:599–601.
96. Luukkainen, T., VandenHeuvel, W. J. A., and Horning, E. C. (1962): An estrogen determination method using gas chromatography. *Biochem. Biophys. Acta,* 62:153–159.
97. MacDougall, D., et al. (1980): Guidelines for data acquisition and data quality evaluation in environmental chemistry. *Anal. Chem.*, 52:2242–2249.
98. Macfarlane, R. D., and Torgerson, D. F. (1976): Californium-252 plasma desorption mass spectrometry. *Science,* 191:920–925.
99. Macfarlane, R. D. (1982): Particle-induced mass spectrometry of large involatile biomolecules: Surface

chemistry in the high energy-short time domain. *Acc. Chem. Res.*, 15:268–275.

100. Mai, J., German, B., and Kinsella, J. E. (1983): Prostaglandins and thromboxane; *tert*-butyldimethylsilyl ethers as derivatives for their analyses by gas chromatography-mass spectrometry-selection ion monitoring. *J. Chromatogr.*, 254:91–108.
101. Markey, S. P. (1981): Quantitative mass spectrometry. *Biomed. Mass Spectrom.*, 8:426–430.
102. Markey, S. P., Colburn, R. W., and Johannessen, J. N. (1981): Efficient extraction and mass spectrometric assay of serotonin in biological fluids. *Biomed. Mass Spectrom.*, 8:301–304.
103. Martin, S. A., Costello, C. E., and Biemann, K. (1983): Optimization of experimental procedures for fast atom bombardment mass spectrometry. *Anal. Chem.*, 54:2362–2368.
104. Mazer, T., Hileman, F. D., Noble, R. W., and Brooks, J. J. (1983): Synthesis of the 38 tetrachlorodibenzofuran isomers and identification by capillary column gas chromatography/mass spectrometry. *Anal. Chem.*, 55:104–110.
105. McEwen, C. N. (1983): Source-mounted cesium ion gun for obtaining liquid matrix secondary ion mass spectra of organics. *Anal. Chem.*, 55:967–968.
106. McLafferty, F. W. (1982): MS/MS: Cloned mass spectrometers. *Trends Anal. Chem.*, 1:298–300.
107. McLafferty, F. W., Editor (1982): *Tandem Mass Spectrometry*. Wiley, New York.
108. McNeal, C. J. (1982): Symposium on fast atom and ion induced mass spectrometry of nonvolatile organic solids. *Anal. Chem.*, 54:43A–50A.
109. Mitchum, R. K., Moler, G. F., and Korfmacher, W. A. (1980): Combined capillary gas chromatography/atmospheric pressure negative chemical ionization/mass spectrometry for the determination of 2,3,7,8-tetrachlorodibenzo-*p*-dioxin in tissue. *Anal. Chem.*, 52:2278–2282.
110. Miyazaki, H., Ishibashi, M., Yamashita, K., and Nishikana, Y. (1981): Dimethylisopropylsilyl ether derivatives in gas chromatography mass spectrometry of prostaglandins and thromboxane B_2. *Biomed. Mass Spectrom.*, 8:521–526.
111. Moler, G. F., Delongchamp, R. R., Korfmacher, W. A., Pearce, B. A., and Mitchum, R. K. (1983): Confidence limits in isotope dilution gas chromatography/mass spectrometry. *Anal. Chem.*, 55:835–841.
112. Morris, H. R., Panico, M., and Haskins, N. J. (1983): Comparison of ionization basis in FAB mass spectra. *Int. J. Mass Spectrom. Ion Phys.*, 46:363–366.
113. Nowlin, J. G., Carroll, D. I., Dzidic, I., Horning, M. G., Montgomery, F. E., Stillwell, R. N., and Horning, E. C. (1979): Chemical ionization mass spectrometry of nonvolatile organic compounds. *Anal. Chem.*, 51:1858–1860.
114. Nowlin, J. G., Carroll, D. I., Dzidic, I., Horning, M. G., Stillwell, R. N., and Horning, E. C. (1979): Plasma desorption ionization mass spectra of unconjugated human steroids. *Anal. Lett.*, 12:573–580.
115. Phillipson, D. W., and Puma, B. J. (1980): Identification of chlorinated methoxybiphenyls as contaminants in fish and as potential interference in the determination of chlorinated dibenzo-*p*-dioxins. *Anal. Chem.*, 52:2328–2332.
116. Rasmussen, P. (1983): Identification of volatile components of jackfruit by gas chromatography/mass spectrometry with two different columns. *Anal. Chem.*, 55:1331–1335.
117. Roboz, J., Greaves, J., Jui, H., and Holland, J. F. (1982): Quantification of homoharringtonine and harringtonine in serum by chemical ionization mass spectrometry. *Biomed. Mass Spectrom.*, 9:510–514.
118. Rudat, M. A., and McEwen, C. N. (1983): New on-source miniature atomic FAB and alkali ion SIMS sources. *Int. J. Mass Spectrom. Ion Phys.*, 46:351–354.
119. Ryhage, R. (1964): Use of a mass spectrometer as a detector and analyzer for effluents emerging from high temperature gas liquid chromatography columns. *Anal. Chem.*, 36:759–764.
120. Ryhage, R., and Brandenberger, H. (1978): Negative ion mass spectrometry of phenothiazines. *Biomed. Mass Spectrom.*, 5:615–620.
121. Sauter, A. D., Betowski, L. D., and Ballard, J. M. (1983): Comparison of priority pollutant response factors for triple and single quadrupole mass spectrometers. *Anal. Chem.*, 55:116–119.
122. Setchell, K. D. R., Lawson, A. M., McLaughlin, L. M., Patel, S., Kirk, D. N., and Axelson, M. (1983): Measurement of enterolactone and enterodiol, the first mammalian lignans, using stable isotope dilution and gas chromatography mass spectrometry. *Biomed. Mass Spectrom.*, 10:277–235.
123. Shackleton, C. H. L. (1983): Inborn errors of steroid biosynthesis: Detection by a new mass spectrometric method. *Clin. Chem. (Winston-Salem, N.C.)*, 29:246–249.
124. Sieck, L. W. (1983): Determination of molecular weight distribution of aromatic components in petroleum products by chemical ionization mass spectrometry with chlorobenzene as reagent gas. *Anal. Chem.*, 55:38–41.
125. Siekmann, L., Siekmann, A., Breuer, H., and Dehennin, L. (1983): Measurement by isotope dilution mass spectrometry of equiline and oestrone in serum of women taking tablets of equine oestrogens. *Biomed. Mass Spectrom.*, 10:168–174.
126. Smith, R. G. (1982): Characterization of anthracycline antibiotics by desorption chemical ionization mass spectrometry. *Anal. Chem.*, 54:2006–2008.
127. Stillwell, R. N., Carroll, D. I., Nowlin, J. G., and Horning, E. C. (1983): Formation of trimethylsilyl molecular adduct ions in desorption chemical ionization mass spectrometry of nonvolatile organic compounds. *Anal. Chem.*, 55:1313–1318.
128. Stults, J. T., Enke, C. G., and Holland, J. F. (1983): Mass spectrometry/mass spectrometry by time-resolved magnetic dispersion. *Anal. Chem.*, 55:1323–1330.
129. Sweeley, C. C., Elliott, W. A., Fries, I., and Ryhage, R. (1966): Mass spectrometric determination of unresolved components in gas chromatographic effluents. *Anal. Chem.*, 38:1549–1553.
130. Sweeley, C. C., and Horning, E. C. (1960): Micro-

analytical separation of steroids by gas chromatography. *Nature,* 187:144–145.

131. Sweeley, C. C., Vrbanac, J., Pinkston, D., and Issachar, D. (1981): Quantitative profiling of organic acids in complex mixtures. *Biomed. Mass Spectrom.,* 8:436–439.
132. Thenot, J.-P., and Horning, E. C. (1971): Gas chromatography of 17-ketosteroid oximes. Formation of nitriles by Beckmann fission. *Anal. Lett.,* 4:683–694.
133. Thenot, J.-P., and Horning, E. C. (1972): MO-TMS derivatives of human urinary steroids for GC and GC-MS studies. *Anal. Lett.,* 5:21–33.
134. Thenot, J.-P., and Horning, E. C. (1972): GC behavior of 3-ketosteroid methoximes. Application to GC studies of adrenocortical steroid hormone MO-TMS derivatives. *Anal. Lett.,* 5:801–814.
135. Thenot, J.-P., and Horning, E. C. (1972): GC-MS derivatization studies: The formation of dexamethasone MO-TMS. *Anal. Lett.,* 5:905–913.
136. Thomson, B. A., Iribarne, J. V., and Dziedzic, P. J. (1982): Liquid ion evaporation/mass spectrometry/mass spectrometry for the detection of polar labile molecules. *Anal. Chem.,* 54:2219–2224.
137. Tomer, K. B., Crow, F. W., Knoche, H. W., and Gross, M. L. (1983): Fast atom bombardment and mass spectrometry/mass spectrometry for analysis of a mixture of ornithine containing lipids from *Thiobacillus thioxidans. Anal. Chem.,* 55:1033–1036.
138. Tserng, K.-Y., Danish, R. K., and Bendt, J. S. (1983): Rapid simultaneous assay of serum estrone, estradiol and estriol in pregnant women using methyl ether acetate derivatives by capillary gas chromatography and electron-impact mass spectrometry. *J. Chromatogr. Biomed. Appl.,* 272:223–241.
139. VandenHeuvel, W. J. A., Creech, B. G., and Horning, E. C. (1962): Separation and estimation of the principal human urinary 17-ketosteroids as trimethylsilyl ethers. *Anal. Biochem.,* 4:191–197.
140. VandenHeuvel, W. J. A., Haahti, E. O. A., and Horning, E. C. (1961): A new liquid phase for gas chromatographic separations of steroids. *J. Am. Chem. Soc.,* 83:1513–1514.
141. VandenHeuvel, W. J. A., and Horning, E. C. (1960): Gas chromatography of adrenal cortical steroid hormones. *Biochem. Biophys. Res. Commun.,* 3:356–360.
142. VandenHeuvel, W. J. A., and Horning, E. C. (1961): Gas chromatographic separation of sapogenins. *J. Org. Chem.,* 26:634–635.
143. VandenHeuvel, W. J. A., Horning, E. C., Sato, Y., and Ikekawa, N. (1961): Gas chromatographic separation of steroidal amines. *J. Org. Chem.,* 26:628–629.
144. VandenHeuvel, W. J. A., Sjovall, J., and Horning, E. C. (1961): Gas chromatographic behavior of trifluoroacetoxy steroids. *Biochem. Biophys. Acta,* 48:596–599.
145. VandenHeuvel, W. J. A., Sweeley, C. C., and Horning, E. C. (1960): Separation of steroids by gas chromatography. *J. Am. Chem. Soc.,* 82:3481–3482.
146. VandenHeuvel, W. J. A., Sweeley, C. C., and Horning, E. C. (1960): Microanalytical separations by gas chromatography in the sex hormone and bile acid series. *Biochem. Biophys. Res. Commun.,* 3:33–36.
147. Vane, F., and Horning, M. G. (1969): Separation and characterization of the prostaglandins by gas chromatography and mass spectrometry. *Anal. Lett.,* 2:357–371.
148. Voyksner, R. D., Hass, J. R., and Bursey, M. M. (1982): Analysis of the chemical ionization reagent plasma produced in liquid chromatography/mass spectrometry by direct liquid introduction mass spectrometry/mass spectrometry. *Anal. Chem.,* 54:2465–2470.
149. Voyksner, R. D., Hass, J. R., Sovocool, G. W., and Bursey, M. M. (1983): Comparison of gas chromatography/high resolution mass spectrometry and mass spectrometry/mass spectrometry for detection of polychlorinated biphenyls and tetrachlorodibenzofuran. *Anal. Chem.,* 55:744–749.
150. Voyksner, R. D., Parker, C. E., Hass, J. R., and Bursey, M. M. (1982): Effects of pressure, temperature and solvent composition in analysis by direct liquid introduction liquid chromatography/mass spectrometry. *Anal Chem.,* 54:2583–2586.
151. Vrbanac, J. J., Sweeley, C. C., and Pinkston, J. D. (1983): Automated metabolic profiling analysis of urinary steroids by a gas chromatography-mass spectrometry data system. *Biomed. Mass Spectrom.,* 10:155–161.
152. Waddell, K. A., Blair, I. A., and Wellby, J. (1983): Combined capillary column gas chromatography negative ion chemical ionization mass spectrometry of prostanoids. *Biomed. Mass Spectrom.,* 10:83–88.
153. Webb, K. S., Gough, T. A., Carrick, A., and Hazelby, D. (1979): Mass spectrometric and chemiluminescent detection of picogram amounts of N-nitrosodimethylamine. *Anal. Chem.,* 51:989–992.
154. White, R. L., Onyiriuka, C., and Wilkins, C. L. (1983): Exact mass measurement in the absence of calibrant by Fourier transform mass spectrometry. *Anal. Chem.,* 55:339–343.
155. Yap, W. T., Schaffer, R., Hertz, H. S., White, E., and Welch, M. J. (1983): On the difference between using linear and non-linear models in bracketing procedures in isotope dilution mass spectrometry. *Biomed. Mass Spectrom.,* 10:262–264.
156. Yost, R. A., and Enke, C. G. (1978): Selection ion fragmentation with a tandem quadrupole mass spectrometer. *J. Am. Chem. Soc.,* 100:2274–2275.
157. Yost, R. A., Enke, C. G., McGilvery, D. C., Smith, D., and Morrison, J. D. (1979): High efficiency collision-induced dissociation in an rf-only quadrupole. *Int. J. Mass Spectrom. Ion Phys.,* 30:127–136.

Subject Index